# Basic Clinical Radiobiology

FIFTH EDITION

# Basic Clinical Radiobiology

Edited by

## Michael C. Joiner PhD
Professor of Radiobiology
Wayne State University School of Medicine
Detroit, Michigan, USA

## Albert J. van der Kogel PhD
Professor of Radiobiology
University of Wisconsin School of Medicine and Public Health
Madison, Wisconsin, USA

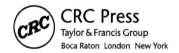

**CRC Press**
Taylor & Francis Group
Boca Raton  London  New York

CRC Press is an imprint of the
Taylor & Francis Group, an **informa** business

CRC Press
Taylor & Francis Group
6000 Broken Sound Parkway NW, Suite 300
Boca Raton, FL 33487-2742

© 2019 by Taylor & Francis Group, LLC
CRC Press is an imprint of Taylor & Francis Group, an Informa business

No claim to original U.S. Government works

Printed in Canada on acid-free paper

International Standard Book Number-13: 978-1-4441-7963-7 (Hardback)

**Library of Congress Cataloging-in-Publication Data**

Names: Joiner, Michael, editor. | Kogel, Albert van der, editor.
Title: Basic clinical radiobiology / edited by Michael C. Joiner and Albert J. Van der Kogel.
Description: Fifth edition. | Boca Raton, FL : CRC Press/Taylor & Francis Group, [2018] | Includes bibliographical references and index.
Identifiers: LCCN 2018002257| ISBN 9781444179637 (hardback : alk. paper) |
ISBN 9780429490606 (ebook : alk. paper)
Subjects: | MESH: Neoplasms--radiotherapy | Cell Survival--radiation effects | Dose-Response Relationship, Radiation
Classification: LCC RM847 | NLM QZ 269 | DDC 615.8/42--dc23
LC record available at https://lccn.loc.gov/2018002257

**Visit the Taylor & Francis Web site at**
**http://www.taylorandfrancis.com**

**and the CRC Press Web site at**
**http://www.crcpress.com**

# Contents

# Preface

Welcome to *Basic Clinical Radiobiology*, which was first published 25 years ago under the editorship of Gordon Steel, who was also successful in taking the book to its second and third editions. This is now the fifth edition and second under the current editorship and we hope that within this latest dark-blue cover, we have maintained and even improved the high standard of content, presentation and accessibility that has always been an integral part of this trans-generational project.

This book has always been directed at an international audience and arose originally to support the teaching courses organized by the European Society for Radiotherapy and Oncology (ESTRO) for students of radiotherapy, radiation physics and radiobiology. These courses still take place once or twice a year and now occur worldwide, which is reflected in the reach of *Basic Clinical Radiobiology* into every important place that is teaching radiation oncology. In this new edition, as previously, the truly multi-national authorship includes some of the top radiation oncologists, biologists and physicists from North America and Europe who regularly teach this material both nationally and internationally, focusing on core principles of radiobiology which are useful anywhere on the planet.

Our successful previous fourth edition has well stood the test of time yet clearly now must give way to this new edition to take account of all the very positive advances in radiation oncology that have occurred over the past 10 years. All chapters have therefore been revised and updated and three additional new chapters have been added on 'Stem cells in radiotherapy', 'Tissue response models', and 'Physics of radiation therapy for the radiobiologist' which assists us all in seeing how radiobiology and physics are closely connected, for example in the increasing use of proton and light-ion beams and image guidance. Thus, these topics have become important in teaching radiation biology.

We continue to provide in-depth coverage of the more established subjects of dose responses and fractionation including the linear-quadratic framework, time factors and dose rate effects, volume effects and retreatment tolerance, tumour radiobiology, combined modality therapy, LET and RBE, the oxygen effect, the pathogenesis of normal tissue side effects and radiotherapy-induced second cancers. And, the more topical subjects of image-guided radiotherapy, biological response modifiers, the tumour microenvironment, the molecular description of the DNA damage response, cell death and molecular targeting and individualization.

Above all, we have taken much care to retain the emphasis on solid science which is not 'current fashion', here today and gone tomorrow, but is well understood, well proven in clinical practice and here to stay. Yet, we believe we have achieved the same high levels of accessibility and assimilation that have always been associated with *Basic Clinical Radiobiology* and which we hope will again make this fifth edition an essential companion to everyone involved in radiation oncology, whatever their contribution and level of expertise.

**Michael C. Joiner**
**Albert J. van der Kogel**

# Contributors

**Michael Baumann**
Division of RadioOncology/RadioBiology
German Cancer Research Center (DKFZ)
Heidelberg, Germany

**Adrian C. Begg**
Division of Experimental Therapy
Netherlands Cancer Institute
Amsterdam, The Netherlands

**Søren M. Bentzen**
Department of Epidemiology and Public Health
Division of Biostatistics and Bioinformatics
University of Maryland School of Medicine
Baltimore, Maryland

**Robert G. Bristow**
Manchester Cancer Research Centre
University of Manchester
Manchester, United Kingdom

**J. Martin Brown**
Department of Neurology
Stanford University
Stanford, California

**Jay W. Burmeister**
Wayne State University School of Medicine
Karmanos Cancer Institute
Gershenson ROC
Detroit, Michigan

**Robert P. Coppes**
Department of Cell Biology
and
Department of Radiation Oncology
University Medical Center Groningen
University of Groningen
Groningen, The Netherlands

**Wolfgang Dörr**
Department of Radiation Oncology
Medical University of Vienna
Vienna, Austria

**Dorota Gabryś**
Radiotherapy Department
Maria Sklodowska – Curie Memorial Cancer Center and
Institute of Oncology
Gliwice, Poland

**Vincent Grégoire**
Department of Radiation Oncology
Léon Bérard Cancer Center
Lyon, France

**Karin Haustermans**
Department of Radiation Oncology
Leuven Cancer Institute
University Hospital Gasthuisberg
Leuven, Belgium

**Richard P. Hill**
Departments of Medical Biophysics and Radiation Oncology
University of Toronto
Toronto, Canada

**Michael R. Horsman**
Department of Experimental Clinical Oncology
Aarhus University Hospital
Aarhus, Denmark

**Michael C. Joiner**
Department of Oncology
Wayne State University School of Medicine
Detroit, Michigan

**Marianne Koritzinsky**
Department of Radiation Oncology
Institute of Medical Sciences
Princess Margaret Cancer Center
University of Toronto
Toronto, Canada

**Mechthild Krause**
Department of Radiotherapy and Radiation Oncology
and OncoRay
National Center for Radiation Research in Oncology
Faculty of Medicine and University Hospital Carl Gustav Carus
Technische Universität Dresden
Dresden, Germany

**John Lee**
Center for Molecular Imaging and Experimental
Radiotherapy
Université Catholique de Louvain
St-Luc University Hospital
Brussels, Belgium

**Jean-Pascal Machiels**
Department of Medical Oncology
St-Luc University Hospital
Brussels, Belgium

**Jens Overgaard**
Department of Experimental Clinical Oncology
Aarhus University Hospital
Aarhus, Denmark

**G. Gordon Steel**
Institute of Cancer Research
Royal Marsden Hospital
Surrey, United Kingdom

**Fiona A. Stewart**
Division of Experimental Therapy
Netherlands Cancer Institute
Amsterdam, The Netherlands

**Klaus Rüdiger Trott**
Department of Radiation Oncology
Technical University Munich
Munich, Germany

**Albert J. van der Kogel**
Department of Human Oncology
University of Wisconsin
School of Medicine and Public Health
Madison, Wisconsin

**Peter van Luijk**
Department of Radiation Oncology
University Medical Center Groningen
Groningen, The Netherlands

**Conchita Vens**
Division of Experimental Therapy
Netherlands Cancer Institute
Amsterdam, The Netherlands

**Catharine M.L. West**
Translational Radiobiology Group
Division of Cancer Sciences
University of Manchester
Christie Hospital Withington
Manchester, United Kingdom

**Bradly G. Wouters**
University Health Network
Princess Margaret Cancer Centre
Toronto, Canada

**Daniel Zips**
University Department of Radiation Oncology
CCC Tübingen-Stuttgart
University Hospital Tübingen
Tübingen, Germany

# Introduction: The significance of radiobiology and radiotherapy for cancer treatment

MICHAEL C. JOINER, ALBERT J. VAN DER KOGEL AND G. GORDON STEEL

## 1.1 THE ROLE OF RADIOTHERAPY IN THE MANAGEMENT OF CANCER

Radiotherapy has consistently remained one of the most effective treatments for cancer, with around half of all patients receiving radiotherapy at some point during their management (1,3,4,13). Therefore, particularly due to aging populations in North America, Europe and China, and increased diagnosis and treatment of cancers in low- to middle-income countries, worldwide use of radiotherapy is increasing, which requires a corresponding increase in support, education and training (6,8,9,10,11,15).

Surgery, with a longer history than radiotherapy, is also in many tumour types the primary form of treatment and it leads to good therapeutic results in a range of early non-metastatic malignancies. Radiotherapy is a good alternative to surgery for the long-term control of many cancers of the head and neck, lung, cervix, bladder, prostate and skin, in which it often achieves a reasonable probability of tumour control with good cosmetic results. In addition to these examples of the curative role of radiation therapy, many patients gain valuable palliation by radiation.

Chemotherapy is the third most important treatment modality. Many patients receive chemotherapy at some point in their management and useful symptom relief and disease arrest are often obtained. Following the early use of nitrogen mustard during the 1920s, cancer chemotherapy has emerged to the point where a very large choice of drugs is available (7). New targeted agents (also called *small* or *smart molecules*) are being introduced into clinical practice all the time, and many have been associated with radiotherapy and shown good clinical results, as have the more traditional drugs like cisplatin which continue to be used. In all such combination therapies of local solid cancers, it is the radiotherapy (or surgery) that still does the 'heavy lifting'.

Table 1.1, adapted from Barton et al. (1), illustrates the proportions of patients who should optimally receive radiotherapy for cancers in different sites, derived from evidence-based guidelines. The following briefly outlines examples of the role of radiotherapy in different disease sites:

- *Breast*: Early breast cancers, not known to have meta-stasised, are usually treated by surgery (e.g. lumpectomy or tumourectomy), and this has a tumour control rate in the region of 50%–70%. Post-operative radiotherapy given to the breast and regional lymph nodes increases control by up to 20% and improves long-term survival. Hypofractionation is common. Hormonal therapy and chemotherapy also have significant impact on patient survival. In patients who have evidence of metastatic spread at the time of diagnosis the outlook is poor.

- *Lung*: Most locally advanced lung tumours are inoperable and in these, the 5-year survival rate for radiotherapy combined with chemotherapy is in the region of 5%. However, studies have shown high local tumour control in early disease following hypofractionated radiotherapy with high doses per fraction (stereotactic body radiation therapy [SBRT]).

- *Prostate*: Surgery and radiotherapy have a similar level of effectiveness, with excellent long-term outcome. Early stage disease is often treated with radiotherapy alone, either by external beam or by brachytherapy, with 5-year disease-specific control rates more than 95%. Hypofractionation can be used. Locally more advanced tumours may require an association between anti-hormonal treatment and external radiotherapy. Chemotherapy makes a limited contribution to local tumour control.

- *Cervix*: Disease that has developed beyond the *in situ* stage is often treated by a combination of intracavitary and external-beam radiotherapy; in more advanced stages radiotherapy is frequently combined with chemotherapy. The control rate varies widely with the stage of the disease, from around 70% in stage I to perhaps 7% in stage IV.

- *Head and neck*: Early stage disease can be cured with either surgery or radiotherapy (external beam and/or brachytherapy). For more advanced diseases, radiotherapy is typically delivered with alternative fractionation (e.g. accelerated treatment or hyperfractionation), or with concomitant chemo-radiotherapy. Concomitant association of epidermal growth factor receptor (EGFR) inhibitors (e.g. cetuximab) and radiotherapy has also been validated. Post-operative radiotherapy or concomitant chemo-radiotherapy is also often used after primary surgery for locally advanced diseases.

- *Lymphoma*: In early disease Hodgkin lymphoma, radiotherapy alone achieves a control rate of around

Table 1.1 Optimal radiotherapy utilization rate by cancer type

| Tumour type | Proportion of all cancers (%) | Proportion of patients receiving radiotherapy (%) | Patients receiving radiotherapy (% of all cancers) |
|---|---|---|---|
| Bladder | 2.0 | 47 | 0.9 |
| Brain | 1.4 | 80 | 1.1 |
| Breast | 12.2 | 87 | 10.6 |
| Cervix | 1.0 | 71 | 0.7 |
| Colon | 8.4 | 4 | 0.3 |
| Gall bladder | 0.6 | 17 | 0.1 |
| Head and neck | 3.3 | 74 | 2.4 |
| Kidney | 2.3 | 15 | 0.3 |
| Leukaemia | 2.3 | 4 | 0.1 |
| Liver | 1.2 | 0 | 0 |
| Lung | 9.0 | 77 | 6.9 |
| Lymphoma | 4.2 | 73 | 3.1 |
| Melanoma | 9.9 | 21 | 2.1 |
| Myeloma | 1.2 | 45 | 0.5 |
| Oesophagus | 1.2 | 71 | 0.9 |
| Ovary | 1.1 | 4 | 0.04 |
| Pancreas | 2.1 | 49 | 1.0 |
| Prostate | 18.4 | 58 | 10.7 |
| Rectum | 4.2 | 60 | 2.5 |
| Stomach | 1.8 | 27 | 0.5 |
| Testis | 0.8 | 7 | 0.1 |
| Thyroid | 1.8 | 4 | 0.1 |
| Unknown primary | 2.4 | 61 | 1.5 |
| Uterus | 1.8 | 38 | 0.7 |
| Vagina | 0.1 | 94 | 0.1 |
| Vulva | 0.3 | 39 | 0.1 |
| Other | 5.0 | 19 | 1.0 |
| Total (all cancers) | 100.0 | | 48.3 |

From (1) with permission.

80%–90%, but nowadays is more often associated with chemotherapy allowing for smaller irradiated volumes and lower doses of radiation.

- *Bladder*: The success of surgery or radiotherapy varies widely with stage of the disease; both approaches give 5-year survival rates in excess of 50%. For early stage bladder cancer, organ-preserving (partial) bladder irradiation is a good alternative to surgery with comparable local control rates.
- *Other tumour sites*: Radiotherapy alone or combined with chemotherapy is also frequently used as a post-operative modality in brain tumours, pancreatic tumours or sarcoma, or as a pre-operative modality in oesophageal, rectal or gastric tumours.

Substantial numbers of patients with common cancers achieve long-term tumour control largely by the use of radiation therapy. Broad estimates over 30 years ago by DeVita et al. (5) and Souhami and Tobias (12) suggested that local treatments, including surgery and/or radiotherapy, even then could be expected to be successful

in approximately 40% of these cases; in perhaps 15% of all cancers, radiotherapy would be the principal form of treatment. In contrast, many patients receive chemotherapy but their contribution to the overall cure rate of cancer may be as low as 2%, with some prolongation of life in perhaps another 10%. This is because the diseases in which chemotherapy alone does well are rare. Given these figures are correct, it may be that around seven times as many patients are cured by radiotherapy as by chemotherapy. This is not to undervalue the important benefits of chemotherapy in a number of chemosensitive diseases and as an adjuvant treatment, but to stress the greater role of radiotherapy as the curative agent (14).

Considerable efforts are being devoted at the present time to the improvement of radiotherapy and chemotherapy. Wide publicity is given to the newer areas of drug development such as lymphokines, immunologics, growth factors and gene/protein targeting. But if we were to imagine aiming to increase the cure rate of cancer by say, 2%, it would seem on a realistic estimation that this would more likely be achieved by increasing the results of radiotherapy alone from say 15% to 17% than by doubling the results achieved by chemotherapy alone.

There are four main ways in which such an improvement in radiotherapy might be obtained:

1. By raising the standards of radiation dose prescription and delivery to those currently in use in the best radiotherapy centres
2. By improving radiation dose distributions beyond those that have been already achieved, either by using techniques of highly conformal radiotherapy and intensity modulation with photons, or by the use of proton or carbon-ion beams
3. By integrating image guidance more tightly into daily treatment delivery
4. By exploiting radiobiological initiatives

The proportion of radiotherapists worldwide who work in academic centres is probably less than 5%. They are the clinicians who may have access to new treatment technologies, for instance ion-beam therapy and image guidance, or to new radiosensitizers or to new agents for targeted therapy. Chapters of this book allude to these exciting developments which may well have a significant impact on treatment success in the future. But it should not be thought that the improvement of radiation therapy lies exclusively with clinical research in the specialist academic centres. It has widely been recognised that by far the most effective way of improving cure rates on a national or international scale is by quality assurance in the prescription and delivery of radiation treatment. Chapters 9–12 of this book deal with the principles on which fractionation schedules should be optimised, including how to respond to unavoidable gaps in treatment. For many radiotherapists, this will be the most important part of this book, for even in the smallest department it is possible, even without access to greatly increased funding, to move closer to optimum fractionation practices.

## 1.2 THE ROLE OF RADIATION BIOLOGY

Experimental and theoretical studies in radiation biology contribute to the development of radiotherapy at three different levels, moving in turn from the most general to the more specific:

*Ideas*: Providing a conceptual basis for radiotherapy, identifying mechanisms and processes that underlie the response of tumours and normal tissues to irradiation and which help to explain observed phenomena. Examples are knowledge about hypoxia, reoxygenation, tumour cell repopulation or mechanisms of repair of DNA damage.

*Treatment Strategy*: Development of specific new approaches in radiotherapy. Examples are hypoxic cell sensitizers, targeted agents, high-linear energy transfer radiotherapy, accelerated radiotherapy and hyperfractionation.

*Protocols*: Advice on the choice of schedules for clinical radiotherapy, for instance, conversion formulae for changes in fractionation or dose rate, or advice on whether to use chemotherapy concurrently or sequentially with radiation. We may also include under this heading methods for predicting the best treatment for the individual patient (individualised radiotherapy).

There is no doubt that radiobiology has been very fruitful in the generation of new ideas and in the identification of potentially exploitable mechanisms. A variety of new treatment strategies have been produced, but unfortunately few of these have so far led to demonstrable clinical gains. In regard to the third of the levels listed above, the newer conversion formulae based on the linear-quadratic (LQ) equation seem to be successful. But beyond this, the ability of laboratory science to guide the radiotherapist in the choice of specific protocols is limited by the inadequacy of the theoretical and experimental models: it will always be necessary to rely on clinical trials for the final choice of a protocol.

## 1.3 THE TIMESCALE OF EFFECTS IN RADIATION BIOLOGY

Irradiation of any biological system generates a succession of processes that differ enormously in timescale. This is illustrated in Figure 1.1 where these processes are divided into three phases (2).

The *physical phase* consists of interactions between charged particles and the atoms of which the tissue is composed. A high-speed electron takes about $10^{-18}$ seconds to traverse the DNA molecule and about $10^{-14}$ seconds to pass across a mammalian cell. As it does so it interacts mainly with orbital electrons, ejecting some of them from atoms (ionization) and raising others to higher energy levels within an atom or molecule (excitation). If sufficiently energetic, these secondary electrons may excite or ionize other atoms near which they pass, giving rise to a cascade of ionization events. For 1 Gy of absorbed radiation dose, there are in excess of $10^5$ ionizations within the volume of every cell of diameter 10 μm.

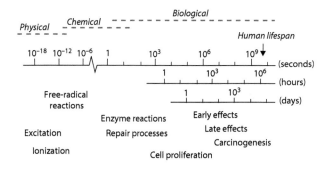

Figure 1.1 Timescale of the effects of radiation exposure on biological systems.

The *chemical phase* describes the period in which these damaged atoms and molecules react with other cellular components in rapid chemical reactions. Ionization and excitation lead to the breakage of chemical bonds and the formation of broken molecules, known as 'free radicals'. These are highly reactive and they engage in a succession of reactions that lead eventually to the restoration of electronic charge equilibrium. Free-radical reactions are complete within approximately 1 ms of radiation exposure. An important characteristic of the chemical phase is the competition between scavenging reactions, for instance with sulphydryl compounds that inactivate the free radicals, and fixation reactions that lead to stable chemical changes in biologically important molecules.

The *biological phase* includes all subsequent processes. These begin with enzymatic reactions that act on the residual chemical damage. The vast majority of lesions, for instance in DNA, are successfully repaired. Some rare lesions fail to repair and it is these that lead eventually to cell death. Cells take time to die; indeed after small doses of radiation, they may undergo a number of mitotic divisions before dying. It is the killing of stem cells and the subsequent loss of the cells that they would have given rise to that causes the early manifestations of normal tissue damage during the first weeks and months after radiation exposure. Examples are breakdown of the skin or mucosa, denudation of the intestine and haemopoietic damage (see Chapter 14). A secondary effect of cell killing is compensatory cell proliferation, which occurs both in normal tissues and in tumours. At later times after the irradiation of normal tissues the 'late reactions' appear. These include fibrosis and telangiectasia of the skin, spinal cord damage and blood vessel damage. An even later manifestation of radiation damage is the appearance of secondary tumours (i.e. radiation carcinogenesis). The timescale of the observable effects of ionizing radiation may thus extend up to many years after exposure.

## 1.4 RESPONSE OF NORMAL AND MALIGNANT TISSUES TO RADIATION EXPOSURE

Much of the text of this book focuses on effects of radiation exposure that become apparent to the clinician or the patient during the weeks, months and years after radiotherapy. These effects are seen both in the tumour and in the normal tissues that are unavoidably included within the treatment plan and exposed to radiation. The primary tasks of radiation biology as applied to radiotherapy are to explain observed phenomena, and to suggest improvements to existing therapies (as outlined in Section 1.2).

The response of a tumour is seen by *regression*, often followed by *regrowth* (or recurrence), but perhaps with failure to regrow during the normal lifespan of the patient (which we term *cure* or more correctly, *local control*). These italicized terms describe the tumour responses that we seek to understand. The cellular basis of tumour response, including tumour control, is dealt with in Chapter 8.

The responses of normal tissues to therapeutic radiation exposure range from those that cause mild discomfort to others that are life threatening. The speed at which a response develops varies widely from one tissue to another and often depends on the dose of radiation which the tissue receives. Generally speaking, the haemopoietic and epithelial tissues manifest radiation damage within weeks of radiation exposure, while damage to connective tissues becomes important at later times. A major development in the radiobiology of normal tissues during the 1980s was the realization that early and late normal tissue responses are differently modified by a change in dose fractionation and this gave rise to the interest in hyperfractionation (see Chapter 11).

The first task of a radiobiologist is to measure a tissue response accurately and reliably. The term *assay* is used to describe such a system of measurement. Assays for tumour response are described in Chapter 8. For normal tissues, the following three general types of assay are available:

*Scoring of Gross Tissue Effects*: It is possible to grade the severity of damage to a tissue using an arbitrary scale as is done for example in Figures 13.7 and 13.9. In superficial tissues this approach has been remarkably successful in allowing isoeffect relationships to be determined.

*Assays of Tissue Function*: For certain tissues, functional assays are available that allow radiation effects to be documented. Examples are the use of breathing rate as a measure of lung function in mice, ethylenediamine tetra-acetic acid clearance as a measure of kidney damage (Figure 9.4) or blood counts as an indicator of bone marrow function.

*Clonogenic Assays*: In some tumours and some normal tissues it has been possible to develop methods by which the colony of cells that derive from a single irradiated cell can be observed. In tumours this is particularly important because of the fact that regrowth of a tumour after subcurative treatment is caused by the proliferation of a small number of tumour cells that retain colony-forming ability. This important area of radiation biology is introduced in Chapter 4.

## 1.5 RESPONSE CURVES, DOSE-RESPONSE CURVES AND ISOEFFECT RELATIONSHIPS

The damage that is observed in an irradiated tissue increases, reaches a peak, and then may decline (Figure 1.2a). How should we quantify the magnitude of this response? We could use the measured response at some chosen time after irradiation, such as the time of maximum response, but the timing of the peak may change with radiation dose and this would lead to some uncertainty in the interpretation of the results. A common method is to calculate the *cumulative* response by integrating this curve from left to right (Figure 1.2b). Some normal tissue responses give a cumulative curve that rises to a plateau, and the height of the plateau is a good

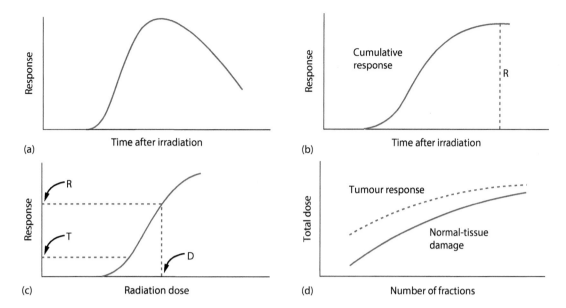

**Figure 1.2** Four types of charts leading to the construction of an isoeffect plot. (a) Time-course of development of radiation damage in normal tissue. (b) The cumulative response. (c) A dose-response relationship, constructed by measuring the response (R) for various radiation doses (D). (d) Isoeffect plot for a fixed level of normal tissue damage (also a similar plot for tumour response).

measure of the total effect of that dose of radiation on the tissue. Other normal tissue responses, in particular the late responses seen in connective and vascular tissues, are progressive and the cumulative response curve will continue to rise (Figures 14.7 and 14.8). The quantification of clinical normal tissue reactions is dealt with in Chapter 14.

The next stage in a study of the radiation response of a tissue will be to vary the radiation dose and thus to investigate the *dose-response relationship* (Figure 1.2c). Many examples of such curves are given throughout this book, for instance Figures 5.6 and 23.8. Cell survival curves (see Chapter 4) are further examples of dose-response curves that are widely used in radiobiology. The position of the curve on the dose scale indicates the sensitivity of the tissue, tumour or cells to radiation; its steepness also gives a direct indication of the change in response that will accompany an increase or decrease in radiation dose. These aspects of dose-response curves are dealt with in detail in Chapter 5.

The foregoing paragraphs have for simplicity referred to 'dose' as though we are concerned only with single radiation exposures. It is a well-established fact in radiation oncology that multiple radiation doses given over a period of a few weeks give a better curative response than can be achieved with a single dose. Diagrams similar to Figures 1.2a–1.2c can also be constructed for fractionated radiation treatment, although the results are easiest to interpret when the fractions are given over a time that is short compared with the timescale of development of the response. If we change the schedule of dose fractionation, for instance by giving a different number of fractions, changing the fraction size or radiation dose rate, we can then investigate the therapeutic effect in terms of an *isoeffect plot* (Figure 1.2d).

Experimentally this is done by performing multiple studies at different doses for each chosen schedule and calculating a dose-response curve. We then select some particular level of effect (R in Figure 1.2c) and read off the total radiation dose that gives this effect. For effects on normal tissues the isoeffect will often be some upper limit of *tolerance* of the tissue, perhaps expressed as a probability of tissue failure (see Chapters 5 and 16) and maybe choosing a lower level of effect (T in Figure 1.2c) will be more appropriate. The isoeffect plot shows how the total radiation dose for the chosen level of effect varies with dose schedule. Examples are Figures 9.2 and 11.3, and recommendations for tolerance calculations are set out in Chapters 9 and 10. The dashed line in Figure 1.2d illustrates how therapeutic conclusions may be drawn from isoeffect curves. If the curve for tumour response is flatter than for normal tissue tolerance, then there is a therapeutic advantage in using a large number of fractions: a tolerance dose given using a small number of fractions will be far short of the tumour-effective dose, whereas for large fraction numbers it may be closer to an effective dose.

## 1.6 THE CONCEPT OF THERAPEUTIC INDEX

Any discussion of the possible benefit of a change in treatment strategy must always consider simultaneously the effects on tumour response and on normal tissue damage. A wide range of factors enter into this assessment. In the clinic, in addition to quantifiable aspects of tumour response and toxicity, there may be a range of poorly quantifiable factors such as new forms of toxicity or risks to the patient, or practicality and convenience to hospital staff, and also cost implications. These must be balanced in the clinical setting.

The role of radiation biology is to address the *quantifiable biological aspects* of a change in treatment.

In the research setting, this can be done by considering dose-response curves. As radiation dose is increased, there will be a tendency for tumour response to increase, and the same is also true of normal-tissue damage. If, for instance, we measure tumour response by determining the proportion of tumours that are controlled, then we expect a sigmoid relationship to dose (for fractionated radiation treatment we could consider the total dose or any other measure of treatment intensity). This is illustrated in the upper part of Figure 1.3. If we quantify normal tissue damage in some way for the same treatment schedule, there will also be a rising curve of toxicity (lower panel). The shape of this curve is unlikely to be the same as that for tumour response and we probably will not wish to determine more than the initial part of this curve since a high frequency of severe damage is unacceptable. By analogy with what must be done in the clinic, we can then fix a notional upper limit of tolerance (see Chapter 16). This fixes, for that treatment schedule, the upper limit of radiation dose that can be tolerated, for which the tumour response is indicated by the point in Figure 1.3 labelled A.

Consider now the effect of adding treatment with a cytotoxic drug. We plan that this will increase the tumour response for any radiation dose and this will be seen as a movement to the left of the curve for tumour control (Figure 1.3). However, there will probably also be an increase in damage to normal tissues which again will consist of a leftward movement of the toxicity curve. The relative displacement of the curves for the tumour and normal tissues will usually be different and this fact makes the amount of benefit from the chemotherapy very difficult to assess. How do we know whether there has been a real therapeutic gain? For studies on laboratory animals, there is a straightforward way of asking whether the combined treatment is better than radiation alone: for the same tolerance level of normal tissue damage (the broken line), the maximum radiation dose (with drug) will be lower and the corresponding level of tumour control is indicated by point B in the figure. If B is higher than A, then the combination is better than radiation alone and represents a therapeutic gain, because it gives a greater level of tumour control for the same level of morbidity.

This example illustrates the radiobiological concept of *therapeutic index*: it is the tumour response for a fixed level of normal tissue damage (see Chapter 5). The term *therapeutic window* describes the (possible) difference between the tumour control dose and the tolerance dose. The concept can in principle be applied to any therapeutic situation or to any appropriate measures of tumour response or toxicity. Its application in the clinic is, however, not a straightforward matter, as indicated in Chapter 19. Therapeutic index carries the notion of 'cost-benefit' analysis. It is impossible to reliably discuss the potential benefit of a new treatment without reference to its effect on therapeutic index.

## 1.7 THE IMPORTANCE OF RADIATION BIOLOGY FOR THE FUTURE DEVELOPMENT OF RADIOTHERAPY

Radiation oncology, more than any of the other modalities for cancer treatment, is to a large extent a technical discipline. Improvements in the treatment of cancer with radiotherapy over the last decades have resulted mainly from improvements in technology, combining new methods of precision in dose delivery with new imaging tools. A major development was the introduction of intensity modulation in combination with various functional imaging modalities such as functional magnetic resonance imaging and positron emission tomography/computed tomography. This has led to new concepts like 'biological target volume', 'dose painting' and 'theragnostic imaging' (see Chapter 22). These developments will undoubtedly lead to further improvements in tumour control rates and reductions in morbidity.

In parallel with these technological advances, new developments have taken place in radiobiology, encompassing the understanding of cancer biology in general, and the radiation response in particular. These fundamental and preclinical research efforts in biology hold great promise, just as the technical innovations, for improving the radiotherapy of cancer. It is even possible that the expected improvements from technical innovations will reach a limit, and the next breakthroughs will come from biological innovations, such as the application of molecularly targeted drugs (see

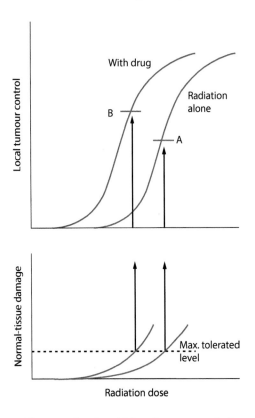

Figure 1.3 The procedure by which an improvement in therapeutic index might be identified, as a result of adding chemotherapy to radiotherapy.

Chapters 20 and 24) in combination with high-precision methods to deliver radiation.

It is interesting to note that the recent rapid progress in knowledge of the biology of cancer is itself also partly due to technological innovations, especially in high-throughput methods to study the genetics of the whole cell. There are now several methods to look at the genes (DNA) and expression of those genes (RNA and protein) in high numbers (tens of thousands) all at once. The trend here is away from the study of single genes or parameters towards genome-wide studies. The many different potential causes of failure, or of severe normal tissue reactions, necessitate such multi-parameter/multi-gene studies. Next to this, methods to selectively manipulate gene expression represent another revolution in biology, allowing one to quickly assess the importance of any given gene by reducing or eliminating its expression (RNA interference and microRNA methods). Radiation biologists are now exploiting these techniques to better understand the molecular pathways which determine how cells respond to damage. This should lead to identification not only of new targets, but targets which are specifically deregulated in tumours, providing the all important tumour specificity of therapy. This should also lead to the development of more robust and accurate predictors of which tumours or normal tissues will respond well to standard radiotherapy and which will not, which could significantly improve individualized radiotherapy (see Chapter 21).

Over the last decade we have seen a change from 'classic radiobiology' which has often focused on fractionation, the LQ model and the phenomenology of repair in terms of 'sublethal' and 'potentially lethal' damage. However, fractionation remains an important core understanding for the application of radiation therapy, particularly in the day-to-day treatment of patients, and the development of the LQ model, together with elucidation of the importance of repopulation, has been central in understanding fractionation, leading to new and better clinical fractionation schemes and the ability to predict the response of normal tissue and tumours to non-standard schedules (see Chapters 9–13). It is of great interest to see a change developing in the established concept of high $\alpha/\beta$ values for head-and-neck and lung tumours and early responding tissues, and low $\alpha/\beta$ values for late responding tissues. This 'dogma' has now evolved into a more differentiated view, indicating that some tumours have a *lower* $\alpha/\beta$ value than surrounding normal tissues, requiring a very different approach to the design of treatment schedules. This new knowledge is now being applied to the design of hypofractionated schedules, such as for the treatment of breast and prostate tumours, which is a dramatic deviation from clinical practice in the last decades.

In a similar manner, simple descriptions of repair and recovery have been supplemented by increasing knowledge and understanding of the molecular pathways involved in various types of repair including those for base damage, single-strand DNA breaks and double-strand breaks. This is leading to new ways to target deregulated repair pathways, with the promise of improving radiotherapy

(see Chapter 21). An example is the link between the EGFR pathway and DNA double-strand break repair, relevant to radiotherapy as blocking EGFR has been shown to improve the effect of radiotherapy in some head and neck cancers (see Chapter 20).

Hypoxia has always been a focus in radiation research, given its large influence on radiosensitivity (see Chapter 17). However, here again, phenomenology has now been replaced by a huge plethora of molecular studies illuminating how cells respond to hypoxia of different degrees and fluctuating over time. Hypoxia is also an important issue for other disciplines apart from cancer, and so an enormous amount of fundamental information has been contributed by these different areas, which radiation biologists can also exploit. This has led to several novel ways to either attack or exploit tumour hypoxia clinically (see Chapters 17 and 18).

Indirectly related to hypoxia is the tumour vasculature and blood supply, and this component of the tumour microenvironment has been a target for therapy for many years now. One approach is to block one of the most important growth factors involved in new vessel formation and the maintenance of blood vessels, vascular endothelial growth factor. Another approach is to modify the function of mature blood vessels. Since radiation therapy is a balancing act between damage to tumours and normal tissues, sparing the latter has always attracted the attention of radiation scientists. The trends in radiation studies of normal tissues, as above, are to elucidate the molecular pathways determining response, and by an increased understanding, to both predict and ameliorate severe side effects (see Chapter 24).

Radiation oncology has always been at the interface of physics, biology and medicine, and with new developments in the technology of high-precision beam delivery with functional and molecular imaging, these are exciting times. Clearly, today's new radiation oncologists and clinical physicists need to obtain a solid understanding of both radiation biology as well as the new developments in molecular radiation oncology. That is the purpose of this book.

---

## Key points

1. Radiotherapy is a very important curative and palliative modality in the treatment of cancer, with around half of all patients estimated to receive radiotherapy at some point during their management.
2. The effects of radiation on mammalian tissues should be viewed as a succession of processes extending from microseconds to months and years after exposure. In choosing one endpoint of effect, it is important not to overlook the rest of this process.
3. Therapeutic index is always 'the name of the game' in curative cancer therapy.
4. Significant gains are still to be made by the optimization of biological and physical factors, particularly in the domain of 'biologically based

treatment planning', use of high doses per fraction, and image-guided therapy.

5. Further gains will also accrue from the increasing knowledge of the molecular mechanisms underlying all radiation responses, enabling more tumour-specific targeting of radiosensitization.

## ■ BIBLIOGRAPHY

1. Barton MB, Jacob S, Shafiq J et al. Estimating the demand for radiotherapy from the evidence: A review of changes from 2003 to 2012. *Radiother Oncol* 2014;112:140–144.

2. Boag JW. The time scale in radiobiology. 12th Failla memorial lecture. In: Nygaard OF, Adler HI and Sinclair WK, editors. *Radiation Research. Proceedings of the 5th International Congress of Radiation Research.* New York, NY: Academic Press; 1975. pp. 9–29.

3. Delaney G, Jacob S, Featherstone C, Barton M. The role of radiotherapy in cancer treatment: Estimating optimal utilization from a review of evidence-based clinical guidelines. *Cancer* 2005;104:1129–1137.

4. Delaney GP, Barton MB. Evidence-based estimates of the demand for radiotherapy. *Clin Oncol (R Coll Radiol)* 2015;27:70–76.

5. DeVita VT, Oliverio VT, Muggia FM et al. The drug development and clinical trials programs of the division of cancer treatment, National Cancer Institute. *Cancer Clin Trials* 1979;2:195–216.

6. Joiner MC, Tracey MW, Kacin SE, Burmeister JW. IBPRO – A novel short-duration teaching course in advanced physics and biology underlying cancer radiotherapy. *Radiat Res* 2017;187:637–640.

7. National Cancer Institute. A to Z list of cancer drugs. 2017; https://www.cancer.gov/about-cancer/treatment/drugs

8. Pan HY, Haffty BG, Falit BP et al. Supply and demand for radiation oncology in the United States: Updated projections for 2015 to 2025. *Int J Radiat Oncol Biol Phys* 2016;96:493–500.

9. Salminen E, Izewska J, Andreo P. IAEA's role in the global management of cancer – Focus on upgrading radiotherapy services. *Acta Oncol* 2005;44:816–824.

10. Smith BD, Haffty BG, Wilson LD, Smith GL, Patel AN, Buchholz TA. The future of radiation oncology in the United States from 2010 to 2020: Will supply keep pace with demand? *J Clin Oncol* 2010;28:5160–5165.

11. Smith BD, Smith GL, Hurria A, Hortobagyi GN, Buchholz TA. Future of cancer incidence in the United States: Burdens upon an aging, changing nation. *J Clin Oncol* 2009;27:2758–2765.

12. Souhami RL, Tobias JS. *Cancer and Its Management.* Oxford: Blackwell Scientific; 1986.

13. Tobias JS. The role of radiotherapy in the management of cancer – An overview. *Ann Acad Med Singapore* 1996; 25:371–379.

14. Tubiana M. The role of local treatment in the cure of cancer. *Eur J Cancer* 1992;28A:2061–2069.

15. Wong K, Delaney GP, Barton MB. Evidence-based optimal number of radiotherapy fractions for cancer: A useful tool to estimate radiotherapy demand. *Radiother Oncol* 2016;119:145–149.

## ■ FURTHER READING

16. Bentzen SM, Thames HD. A 100-year Nordic perspective on the dose-time problem in radiobiology. *Acta Oncol* 1995; 34:1031–1040.

17. Feinendegen L, Hahnfeldt P, Schadt EE, Stumpf M, Voit EO. Systems biology and its potential role in radiobiology. *Radiat Environ Biophys* 2008;47:5–23.

18. Willers H, Beck-Bornholdt HP. Origins of radiotherapy and radiobiology: Separation of the influence of dose per fraction and overall treatment time on normal tissue damage by Reisner and Miescher in the 1930s. *Radiother Oncol* 1996; 38:171–173.

# Irradiation-induced damage and the DNA damage response

## CONCHITA VENS, MARIANNE KORITZINSKY AND BRADLY G. WOUTERS

## 2.1 DNA DAMAGE BY IONIZING RADIATION

Ionizing radiation (IR) consisting of electromagnetic radiation, or photons, is the type of radiation most commonly used for the treatment of patients with radiotherapy. Typical photon energies produced by 4–25 MV linear accelerators found in radiotherapy departments range from less than 100 keV to several MeV (the maximum energy of the machine being used). The principal damaging effects of this type of radiation arise from its ability to eject electrons from (ionize) molecules within cells. Almost all the photons produced by linear accelerators have sufficient energy to cause such ionizations. Most biological damage, however, is done by the ejected electrons themselves, which go on to cause further ionizations in molecules they collide with, progressively slowing down as they go. At the end of electron tracks, interactions become more frequent, giving rise to clusters of ionizations (12). The pattern and density of ionizations and their relationship with the size of the DNA double helix are shown in Figure 2.1. DNA, present in the cell nucleus, comprises two opposing strands linked by hydrogen bonds forming a double-helical structure. Each strand is a linear chain of the four bases adenine (A), cytosine (C), guanine (G) and thymine (T) connected by sugar molecules and a phosphate group, the 'sugar-phosphate backbone' (Figure 2.2). The bases on opposite DNA strands are complementary, forming base pairs where A is paired up with T and C is paired up with G. The order of the bases is the code defining regulatory elements and the protein amino acid sequence. The scales of radiation-induced ionization clusters are such that many ionization events can occur within a few base pairs of the DNA. These clusters are a unique characteristic of IR, in contrast to other forms of radiation such as ultraviolet (UV), or DNA damaging drugs such as topoisomerase inhibitors. Only a small percentage of the radiation damage is clustered, but when these clusters occur in DNA, the cell has particular difficulty coping with the damage.

Ionized molecules are highly reactive and undergo a rapid cascade of chemical changes, which can lead to the breaking of chemical bonds and disruption of macromolecular structure. IR deposits its energy randomly, thus causing damage to all molecules in the cell. However, there are multiple copies of most molecules (e.g. water, mRNA,

proteins and others), and most undergo a continuous rapid turnover, limiting the consequences of damaging just a few molecules of one type. In contrast, DNA is present in only two copies, has very limited turnover, is the largest molecule thus providing the biggest target, and is central to all cellular functions. The consequence of permanent damage to DNA can therefore be serious and often lethal.

There is compelling historical experimental evidence that the DNA is the principal target for radiation-induced cell killing. Elegant experiments were carried out irradiating individual cells with small polonium needles producing short-range alpha particles (23). High doses could be given to plasma membranes and cytoplasm without causing cell death. However, as soon as the needle was placed so that the nucleus received even one or two alpha particles, cell death resulted. Other experiments used radioactively labelled compounds to irradiate principally the plasma membrane ($^{125}$I-concanavalin), or principally the DNA ($^3$H-labeled thymidine), and compared this with homogeneous cell irradiations with X-rays. Cell death closely correlated only with dose to the nucleus, and not to either the plasma membrane or the cytoplasm (Table 2.1).

Due to the importance of DNA, cells and organisms have developed a complex series of processes and pathways for ensuring the DNA remains intact and unaltered in the face of continuous attack from within (e.g. oxidation and alkylation due to metabolism) and outside (e.g. ingested chemicals, UV and IR) (15). These include different forms of DNA repair to cope with the different forms of DNA damage induced by different agents.

Specialized repair systems have evolved to detect and repair damage to bases (base excision repair [BER]), single-strand breaks (single-strand break repair [SSBR], closely related to BER), double-strand breaks (double-strand break repair [DSBR]) and cross links (interstrand cross link [ICL] repair). All of these lesions are produced by IR, and each of these repair pathways is described in more detail in Section 2.7. There are also other DNA repair pathways, such as those for correcting mismatches of base pairs in DNA which can occur during replication (mismatch repair [MMR]) and for repairing bulky lesions or DNA adducts such as those formed by UV light and some drugs like cisplatin (nucleotide excision repair [NER]). However, neither MMR

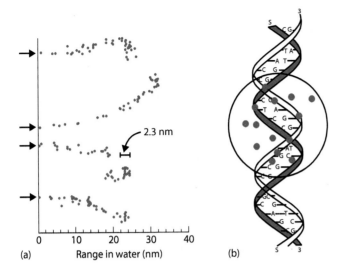

**Figure 2.1** (a) Computer-simulated tracks of 1 keV electrons. Note the scale in relation to the 2.3 nm diameter of the DNA double helix. (b) The concept of a local multiply damaged site produced by a cluster of ionizations impinging on DNA. ([a] Adapted from (4).)

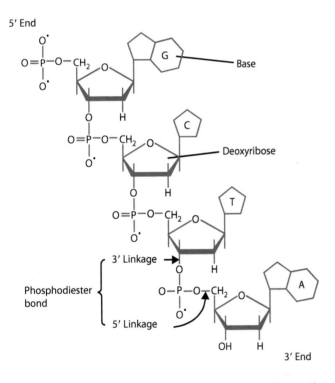

**Figure 2.2** The structure of DNA, in which the four bases (G, C, T, A) are linked through the sugar-phosphate backbone.

nor NER appear to be important for survival after IR, since cells with mutations or deletions in genes governing these pathways are not more sensitive to IR. Such repair processes are still important in order to prevent mutations occurring as a consequence of DNA damage. In contrast, mutations or deletions in BER, SSBR and DSBR genes can all lead to increased radiosensitivity.

To give an idea of the scale and nature of the damage, 1 Gy of irradiation will cause in each cell approximately

**Table 2.1** Toxicity of radioisotopes depends upon their subcellular distribution

| Radiation source/type | Radiation dose to part of the cell[a] Gy | | |
| --- | --- | --- | --- |
| | **Nucleus** | **Cytoplasm** | **Membranes** |
| X-ray | 3.3 | 3.3 | 3.3 |
| $^3$H-thymidine | 3.8 | 0.27 | 0.01 |
| $^{125}$I-concanavalin | 4.1 | 24.7 | 516.7 |

Data from (32).

[a] For each of these three treatments a dose has been chosen that gives 50% cell killing in CHO cells. The absorbed radiation doses to the nucleus, cytoplasm or membranes have then been calculated. $^3$H-thymidine is bound to DNA, $^{125}$I-concanavalin to cell membranes. It is the *nuclear* dose that is constant and thus correlates with cell killing, not the cytoplasmic or membrane doses.

$10^5$ ionizations, more than 1000 damages to DNA bases, around 1000 single-strand DNA breaks (SSBs) and around 20–40 double-strand DNA breaks (DSB). To put this into further perspective, 1 Gy will only kill about 30% of cells from a typical mammalian cell line. This relatively limited cytotoxicity, despite large numbers of induced lesions per cell, is the consequence of efficient DNA repair.

DSBs are considered the most lethal of all lesion types, as they constitute breaks that cause problems during chromosome segregation in mitosis. DSBs can arise from primary radiation lesions or as a consequence of conversion from other types of DNA damage. For example, DSBs can be caused by unresolved replication blocks due to DNA strand cross links, complex base damage or loss of bases. Such replication-induced DSBs after radiation are chemically distinct from those caused by primary lesions, and they can appear hours after radiation. SSBs can also result in secondary DSBs during replication or due to stability issues during the repair process.

The DNA double helix is wound at regular intervals around a complex of proteins called *histones*, forming nucleosomes, resembling beads on a string. Many other proteins are also associated with the DNA, which control DNA metabolism, including transcription, replication and repair. The DNA plus its associated proteins is called *chromatin*. There are further levels of folding and looping, finally making up the compact structure of the chromosomes. This structure poses various challenges to the cell for repairing DNA damage. First, specialized proteins have to be sufficiently abundant and mobile to detect damage within seconds or minutes of it occurring. Second, the chromatin usually needs to be remodelled (e.g. the structure opened up) to allow access of repair proteins (31). This may entail removal of nucleosomes close to the break, among other changes. The correct repair, accessory and signalling proteins then need to be recruited, often mediated by histone modifications, and tightly coordinated. This includes stopping various processes such as transcription and cell-cycle progression to concentrate on repair. Repair progress needs to be continually monitored so that the chromatin will be reset to its original state after completion of repair, and then normal cellular processes resumed. These concerted events are termed the *DNA damage response* (DDR).

## 2.2 THE DNA DAMAGE RESPONSE

The DDR is a highly complex and coordinated system that determines the cellular outcome of DNA damage caused by radiation. The DDR is not a single pathway, but rather a group of highly interrelated signalling pathways, each of which controls different effects on the cell. This system can be divided into several parts, the *sensors* of DNA damage and the *transducers* and *effectors* of damage response (Figure 2.3). The sensors consist of a group of proteins that actively survey the genome for the presence of damage. These proteins then signal the damage through transducers to three main effector pathways that together determine the outcome for the cell. Additional proteins that function as *activators* or *adaptors* can amplify and regulate the signal. The effector pathways include (1) programmed cell death pathways that kill damaged cells, (2) DNA repair pathways that physically repair DNA and (3) pathways that cause temporary or permanent blocks in the progress of cells

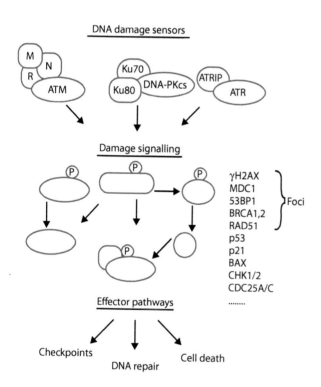

Figure 2.3 The DDR can be divided into sensors and effectors. The sensors consist of protein complexes which recognize DNA damage and include MRN/ATM, Ku/DNAPKcs and ATRIP/ATR. These proteins signal to many other proteins which activate three important effector pathways: cell-cycle checkpoints, DNA repair and cell death. Examples of some of the proteins which signal from the sensors to the effector pathways are listed.

through the cell cycle – the DNA damage checkpoints. Cellular responses after radiation also include adaptive effects on gene transcription, mRNA translation and protein modification and degradation.

## 2.3 DNA DAMAGE SENSORS

DNA damage sensor proteins recognize specific DNA lesions and initiate the DDR. These initial events form the basis for the DDR cascade and the recruitment of repair factors to the site of the lesions. This recruitment of various proteins that cluster at the lesion site can be visualised microscopically as small regions or speckles in the nucleus after DNA damage following staining with antibodies to these proteins (Figure 2.4). Other visualisation methods couple the involved proteins with different fluorescent peptides and tags. These sub-nuclear regions are commonly referred to as IR-induced 'foci' (IRIF). The analysis of such IRIF has helped to identify the factors involved in DNA repair and to monitor their recruitment and interdependencies.

The nature of the lesion dictates the presence of the initial damage-sensing protein. For example, base lesions are recognized by specific glycosylases that are designed to identify and remove the damaged base, while the loss of bases or phosphodiester bonds within DNA quickly activates poly (ADP-ribosylation)-polymerases (PARPs). DSBs are recognized by the MRN complex, consisting of three proteins: MRE11, RAD50 and NBS1. Notably, the NBS1 protein is the product of the gene that is mutated in Nijmegen breakage syndrome (NBS). As its central function in DSB recognition and repair suggests, patients with this syndrome are radiosensitive. The Ku proteins (Ku70 and 80) can also recognize and efficiently bind the ends of DSBs. Single-stranded DNA regions generated during replication or during DSBR are coated by the RPA complex. These initial DNA damage sensing events influence repair pathway choice and dictate DDR signalling through engaging different signal transduction proteins and mechanisms.

## 2.4 DNA DAMAGE SIGNALLING TRANSDUCERS

Upon DNA damage sensing, signals are required to engage repair proteins, cell death mechanisms or cell-cycle checkpoints. Transduction of the signal from the sensors to the effectors is realized through post-translational modification and/or relocalisation of intermediate signalling proteins. These modifications can be phosphorylation (the addition of phosphate groups), ubiquitylation (addition of ubiquitin peptides), sumoylation (addition of sumo peptides), acetylation (addition of acetyl groups) or poly (ADP-ribosylation) performed by various enzymes. Post-translational modifications typically affect the chromatin surrounding the DNA damage to 'mark' and prepare the

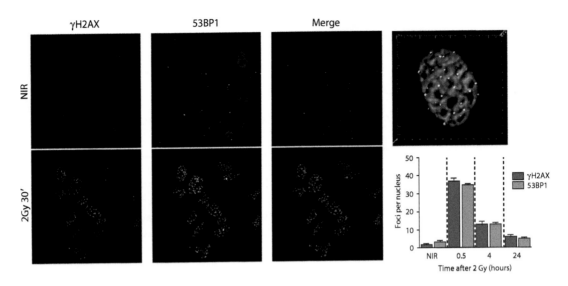

**Figure 2.4** Examples of IRIF. Non-irradiated (NIR) and irradiated (2 Gy) cells have been fixed and stained with antibodies that recognize phosphorylated H2AX protein (γH2AX) and 53BP1. Quantification of IRIF as a function of time reflects repair kinetics. (Courtesy of Jallai and Bristow, Princess Margaret Cancer Centre.)

site, and to help recruitment of crucial repair proteins. Modifications can also alter protein activity or complex formation to initiate downstream signalling to other effector pathways.

## Ataxia-telangiectasia mutated protein

One of the earliest signalling events known to occur in the DDR is the activation of the ataxia-telangiectasia mutated (ATM) protein. ATM protein is mutated in the autosomal recessive syndrome ataxia-telangiectasia (AT), which presents clinically as oculocutaneous telangiectasia and progressive cerebella ataxia (24). These patients are frequently found to be highly radiosensitive and have an increased risk of developing cancer, and cells from these patients are partially defective in many aspects of the DDR. ATM protein is recruited to DSBs with the help of MRN, and is essential to DSB repair and signalling. ATM is a kinase that phosphorylates itself, MRN and numerous other proteins (26). Two important target proteins are CHK2 and p53 which ultimately provide the link to cell-cycle checkpoints and programmed cell death (see Sections 2.5 and 2.6). Another important target of ATM is the histone protein H2AX (27).

## H2AX

H2AX is a variant of histone H2A, a component of the core nucleosome structure around which DNA is packaged. Starting within a few minutes of DSB formation, H2AX becomes phosphorylated at the DSB site. The phosphorylated form of H2AX is termed *γH2AX*. The phosphorylation of H2AX proteins spreads over relatively large chromatin regions (megabases) in both directions of the DSB, an event

that is regulated by an additional protein called MDC1. MDC1 acts as an adaptor by directly binding to both ATM and to γH2AX and in this way is able to amplify ATM-mediated γH2AX in both directions of the break. This amplification significantly alters the chromatin structure around the DSB and is thought to be important for access of other DNA repair proteins to the break. The presence of large areas of γH2AX around a single DSB facilitates the detection of γH2AX foci using microscopy and specific antibodies. In addition to ATM, two other kinases have been shown to phosphorylate H2AX at the sites of DSBs: DNA-dependent protein kinase catalytic subunit (DNA-PKcs) and AT-related (ATR) protein (7).

## DNA-dependent protein kinase catalytic subunit

DNA-PKcs is a kinase that is structurally related to ATM and also responds specifically to DNA damage, in particular to DSBs. Like ATM, DNA-PKcs is unable to act as a sensor of damage itself. This sensor function is carried out by the Ku70/Ku80 complex mentioned previously, which directly binds to the ends of DSBs and recruits DNA-PKcs allowing phosphorylation of H2AX. DNA-PKcs also phosphorylates a number of other target proteins involved in checkpoints and repair.

## ATR-ATRIP

The third kinase that quickly responds to DNA damage and is capable of phosphorylating H2AX is ATR. In contrast to ATM and DNA-PKcs, ATR does not appear to play any substantial role in signalling initiated by radiation-induced DSBs. Instead, it phosphorylates H2AX in response to other types of DNA damage and abnormalities such as single-stranded DNA and stalled or broken replication forks. ATR is thus very important for the types of damage that occur during normal DNA replication. Single-stranded DNA regions coated with RPA recruit the mediator protein ATRIP (ATR interacting protein) and ATR. Although ATR is less important in the initial processing of radiation-induced DSBs, it does play a role in this pathway after ATM is activated. Activation of the ATM-MRN complex leads to processing of the DNA at sites of DSB. This processing can create stretches of single-stranded DNA through extensive DSB end resection, which will then activate ATR. Thus, ATR can be activated 'downstream' of ATM activation. ATR is also activated as a consequence of replication problems following irradiation. DNA strand cross links and oxidized bases caused by radiation interfere with replication and activate ATR (20). ATR shares some of the phosphorylation targets of ATM but also phosphorylates a distinct set of proteins that participate in the DDR. Consequently, components of the DDR effector pathways (DNA repair, checkpoints and cell death) are also dependent on ATR after radiation treatment. For example, the ATR kinase phosphorylates crucial checkpoint proteins such as CHK1, thereby providing a strong link to cell-cycle regulation.

## Poly (ADP-ribosylation)-polymerase

PARPs are enzymes that catalyse the formation of a branched polymer from ADP ribose, termed *poly (ADP-ribose) (PAR)*. As explained previously, those are initial events that occur on chromatin and repair proteins at the site of damage. At least two of the large PARP family members, PARP1 and PARP2, are involved in the recognition and signalling of radiation-induced DNA damage such as abasic sites, SSBs, DNA nicks and DSBs. PARP1 and PARP2 have many protein targets whose activities are altered as a consequence of PARylation. This ultimately results in the regulation of signalling pathways such as those related to inflammation or metabolic responses known to occur after oxidative stress. Thus, PAR-mediated responses may strongly affect radiation-induced inflammatory processes that underline normal tissue toxicities.

Activation of ATM, ATR, DNA-PKcs and PARPs leads to the modification of many other cellular proteins. Studies show that as many as thousands of proteins are substrates for the ATM and ATR kinases or PARP in response to DNA damage (9,22,26). Phosphorylation and PARylation of these other proteins act as the 'signals' to activate the various different downstream effectors of the DDR (most importantly apoptosis, cell-cycle checkpoints and DNA repair).

## 2.5 EFFECTOR PATHWAYS: PROGRAMMED CELL DEATH – APOPTOSIS

Two important proteins which are phosphorylated following activation of ATM are p53 and MDM2. One of

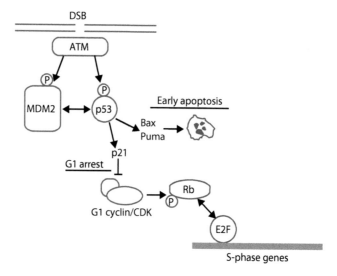

**Figure 2.5** Cells irradiated in the G1 phase are influenced by the action of p53. ATM is activated by DSBs and phosphorylates both mdm2 and p53. This leads to stabilization and activation of p53 which then induces genes that can promote apoptosis (Bax, Puma) and induce cell-cycle checkpoints. Induction of p21 inhibits the action of cyclin/CDK complexes that are necessary for the entry into S phase. Consequently, cells are blocked at the G1/S border after irradiation. In many cancer cells, this checkpoint is abrogated through mutation of p53 or other proteins.

the most commonly mutated tumour suppressors is p53, whose function is to regulate genes that control both cell-cycle checkpoints (see Section 2.6) and programmed cell death through a death mechanism known as apoptosis (see Chapter 3). Consequently, activation of p53 after irradiation can lead either to a block in proliferation or directly to cell death (Figure 2.5).

The p53 protein abundance is regulated by binding to its partner MDM2. This association leads to rapid ubiquitination and destruction of p53 through the proteasome pathway. Thus, in unstressed normal cells, p53 is continuously made but degraded and is thus non-functional. Following DNA damage, ATM phosphorylates both p53 and MDM2. These events destabilize the p53-MDM2 interaction, and as a result the p53 protein is no longer degraded and accumulates in the cell. In addition to this stabilization, direct phosphorylation of p53 by ATM leads to its activation as a transcription factor and thus the upregulation of its many target genes. These target genes include the pro-apoptotic genes BAX and PUMA, which in certain cells can be sufficient to induce cell death. Thus, in some cells, activation of the DDR itself can lead to rapid induction of cell death through apoptosis. The ability to induce apoptosis may contribute to the function of p53 as a tumour suppressor protein. Because DNA damage can lead to dangerous mutations, it may be more beneficial to the organism to eliminate the cell rather than trying to repair the damage (see Chapter 3).

## 2.6 EFFECTOR PATHWAYS: CELL-CYCLE CHECKPOINTS

The second major effector pathway of the DDR is the activation of cell-cycle checkpoints. Treatment of cells with IR causes delays in the movement of cells through the G1, S and G2 phases of the cell cycle (Table 2.2) (16). This occurs through the activation of DNA damage checkpoints, which are specific points in the cell cycle at which progression of the cell into the next phase can be blocked or slowed. The DDR activates four distinct checkpoints in response to irradiation that take place at different points within the cell cycle. These checkpoints can be thought of as delays that would allow cells more time to repair DNA damage and prevent the propagation of damage and associated mutations. By blocking proliferation, cell-cycle checkpoints also reduce the probability of conversion of some lesions into more deleterious lesions through replication or mitotic processes.

All movement through the cell cycle is driven by cyclin-dependent kinases (CDKs). CDKs phosphorylate other proteins to initiate the processes required for progression through the cell cycle. A CDK is active only when associated with a cyclin partner (hence their name), and different cyclin/CDK complexes are active at different points within the cell cycle. For example, cyclinD/CDK4 is active in G1, cyclinB/CDK1 is active in G2 and mitosis and cyclinA with CDK1 and CDK2 during the S phase. Checkpoint activation requires inhibition of the cyclin/CDK complexes, and after radiation this occurs through two main mechanisms. The first is by activation of other proteins that directly inhibit the cyclin/CDK complex, the 'cyclin-dependent kinase inhibitors' (CDKIs). The second is by affecting phosphorylation and activity of the CDK enzyme.

### G1/S checkpoint

Cells contain a checkpoint at the transition between the G1 and S phases that plays an important normal role in the decision of the cell to initiate DNA replication for subsequent cell division. This checkpoint is thus sensitive to growth factors, nutrients and other conditions that favour proliferation. The transition from G1 to the S phase is controlled by the activation of the E2F transcription factor which is important for regulating many of the genes necessary to initiate DNA replication. E2F is kept inactive in G1 by binding to the retinoblastoma (Rb) protein. As cells normally move from G1 into S, the Rb protein becomes phosphorylated by cyclinD/CDK4 and cyclinE/CDK2. This phosphorylation causes release of Rb from E2F, allowing E2F to function as a transcription factor and initiate the S phase. As described previously, irradiation leads to an ATM-dependent stabilization and activation of p53. One of the genes that are upregulated by p53 is the CDKI p21 (CDKN1A). The p21 inhibits the G1 cyclin/CDK complexes, thereby preventing phosphorylation of Rb and entry into the S phase. As a result, cells that are irradiated while in the G1 phase will exhibit a delay prior to entry into the S phase that is dependent on both p53 and p21.

### S-phase checkpoint

Cells that are in S phase at the time of irradiation demonstrate a dose-dependent reduction in the rate of DNA synthesis and as a result, the overall length of time that cells need to replicate their DNA substantially increases. This S-phase checkpoint is controlled by two highly related proteins known as CHK1 and CHK2 (Figure 2.6) (1). CHK1 and CHK2 are direct targets of ATR and ATM, respectively, and are activated by phosphorylation. They in turn phosphorylate the proteins CDC25A and CDC25C, which leads to their destruction or inactivation. CDC25A and CDC25C are phosphatases that keep CDK2 in its active dephosphorylated form. As a result, CHK1 and CHK2 activation by ATR and ATM results in an increase in the amount of phosphorylated CDK2 and thus slows progression through the S phase.

Although ATM-CHK2 and ATR-CHK1 activation and inhibition of CDC25A/C is the main mechanism for initiation of the S-phase checkpoint, several other proteins in the DDR can also influence this response. This includes the BRCA1 and BRCA2 proteins, whose main function is in the homologous recombination branch of DNA repair (see Section 2.7). This suggests a complex relationship between checkpoint activation and DNA repair.

### G2 checkpoints

There are two checkpoints in G2, both of which operate along similar lines to that in the S phase (35). The G2 checkpoint termed 'early' is ATM-CHK2-CDC25A/C dependent and applies to cells that are irradiated while in G2. This checkpoint is activated by relatively low doses of radiation (1 Gy is enough) and results in a block of cell-cycle progression at the end of G2.

Table 2.2 Radiation-induced cell-cycle checkpoints and their characteristics

| Position | Primary signalling proteins | Applies to cells irradiated in | Features |
|---|---|---|---|
| G1 | ATM, p53, p21 | G1 | Prevents entry into S |
| S | ATM, CHK1/2, CDC25A/C, BRCA1,2 | S | Slows progression through S |
| 'Early' G2 | ATM, CHK1/2, CDC25A/C, BRCA1,2 | G2 | Prevents entry into mitosis |
| 'Late' G2 | ATR, CHK1, CDC25A/C | All phases | Prevents entry into mitosis |

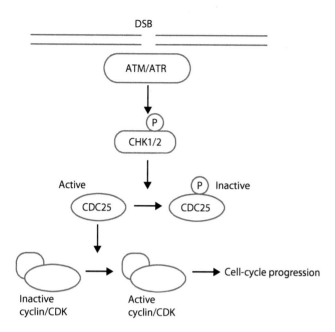

**Figure 2.6** The S, 'early' G2 and 'late' G2 checkpoints are all activated by a similar mechanism. ATM and/or ATR are activated by DSBs and phosphorylate the Chk1/2 kinases. These kinases then phosphorylate and inactivate CDC25A/C. CDC25A/C are required for progression through S phase and into mitosis because they activate the required cyclin/CDK complexes in both parts of the cell cycle. Thus, when CHK1/2 are phosphorylated by ATM, cell-cycle checkpoints in both S and G2 are activated.

The target of ATM-CHK2-CDC25A/C signalling in this case is the mitotic cyclinB/CDK1 complex which, like CDK2 in the S-phase, must be dephosphorylated on specific sites to become active. It is called the early G2 checkpoint because it applies to cells that are irradiated while in the G2 phase and rapidly blocks their movement into mitosis. As a result, there is a drop in the number of cells within mitosis at short times after irradiation.

In contrast, the 'late' G2 checkpoint describes a G2 delay that is observed at longer times after irradiation and is applicable to cells that reach G2 after being previously irradiated while in the G1 or S phases. These cells may experience transient G1- and S-phase checkpoints, but when they arrive in the G2 phase many hours later, they experience a second delay prior to entry into mitosis. Unlike the early G2 checkpoint, this delay is strongly dose dependent, and can last many hours after high doses of radiation. In addition, unlike all the other damage checkpoints, this late G2 checkpoint is independent of ATM. Instead, the principal signalling axis occurs from ATR to CHK1 to CDC25A/C. The late G2 checkpoint is thus mechanistically similar to the S and early G2 checkpoints, and likely arises from a fundamentally different and replication-associated type of DNA damage.

## Checkpoints, cancer and radiosensitivity

In a large proportion of tumour cells, one or more of the G1/S, S, and early G2 checkpoints are disabled due to genetic changes that occur during tumourigenesis. These checkpoint responses have been linked to a tumour suppressor function that must be disrupted to allow oncogene-induced proliferation. This is thought to occur following activation of growth-promoting oncogenes which induce 'inappropriate replication' and DNA damage from replication stress. When functional, the checkpoints block further proliferation of these cells and can thus actively suppress cancer development. This idea is supported by the finding that many early cancer lesions show widespread activation of checkpoint activity.

Mutations in genes that influence checkpoint activation will result in the failure to delay cell-cycle progression in response to irradiation. This may have an important consequence for genetic instability after irradiation and tumour progression but does not necessarily influence overall cellular radiosensitivity. Thus, although the checkpoints are often described as providing extended time for repair, this extra time seems to be more important for maintaining genome integrity than supporting cell survival. For example, most cancer cells have defects in the G1- and S-phase cell-cycle checkpoints due to mutation or loss of tumour suppressor proteins such as p53 or Rb, but are not particularly radiosensitive. Even in isogenic cell models, loss of the protein p21 abrogates the radiation-induced G1/S checkpoint without significantly impacting radiosensitivity (34). In contrast, G2 checkpoints that prevent cells from entering mitosis with DNA damage are important for cell survival after radiation. Cells which fail to activate the 'early' ATM-dependent G2 checkpoint in response to very low radiation doses (<1 Gy) display low-dose hyper-radiosensitivity (6,21) (see Chapter 4), and genetic disruption of the 'late' ATR-dependent G2 checkpoint also leads to radiosensitivity, especially in combination with defects in other checkpoints. It has therefore been proposed that inhibition of ATR signalling may specifically radiosensitize cancer cells that lack other checkpoints due to mutations in proteins such as p53.

Importantly, although the G1 and S checkpoints do not necessarily affect the radiosensitivity of cells to single doses of radiation, they may affect the response to multiple (fractionated) doses. The presence or absence of checkpoints will affect the redistribution of cells in the cell cycle after irradiation. Since DNA repair capacity changes during the course of the cell cycle (see the following section), this may indirectly affect the sensitivity of cells to subsequent doses of radiation. Coordination of tissue architecture and growth kinetics may also render cell-cycle checkpoints more important for radiation response *in vivo* and in some normal tissues (28,33).

## 2.7 EFFECTOR PATHWAYS: DNA REPAIR

As previously discussed, DNA lesions are detected by specialized sensing proteins which signal to the cell that damage has occurred, thereby initiating the DNA damage response. This response effectively focuses the cell's attention on the damage, stopping other processes like transcription and cell-cycle progression, and importantly, initiating DNA repair. Radiation induces a large burden of oxidized base lesions and SSBs, as well as more cytotoxic DSBs. The main repair pathways that tackle these lesions are BER, SSBR and DSBR pathways, of which DSBR is the most important for radiosensitivity (3). Notably, many of the involved repair proteins have been discovered through radiation response analysis, as evident from names such as 'XRCC' (X-ray repair cross complementing) or 'RAD' (radiation).

## Base excision repair and single-strand break repair

Base damages and SSBs far outweigh DSBs in number after radiation, being up to 50 times more frequent. Notably, similar base damages and SSBs also occur without irradiation as a consequence of normal metabolism producing reactive oxygen species. The BER and SSBR pathways have therefore evolved to repair such damage efficiently to maintain genome integrity (8).

As outlined previously, one of the initial lesion sensing events is the activation of PARP and the formation of PAR on chromatin at the lesion sites. SSBs and abasic sites cause a quick PAR response that facilitates repair protein recruitment. PAR polymers are then removed by poly (ADP-ribose)-glycohydrolase (PARG). An outline of the BER and SSBR events that follow is shown in Figure 2.7. Briefly, in

BER, most of the damaged bases in the DNA will be detected and removed by specialized glycosylase proteins which remove the damaged base, resulting in an abasic site. This will be recognized by an AP endonuclease (APE), which will cut the DNA backbone leaving a nick, or SSB. Subsequent repair follows one of two pathways called short patch or long patch. In short patch, the damaged base is replaced by DNA polymerase β (POLβ) in the presence of XRCC1, followed by ligation of the DNA ends by ligase 3 (LIG3). In long patch, up to 10 nucleotides surrounding the damaged site are replaced by DNA polymerase δ or ε in the presence of PCNA, while Flap endonuclease 1 (FEN1) removes the overhanging nucleotides, followed by ligation by ligase 1 (LIG1).

SSBR applies many of the same enzymes as BER. PAR mediates XRCC1 recruitment, which strongly supports BER and SSBR through its close interaction with ligase 3 and other proteins. The radiation-induced SSBs are often more complex than those created endogenously, presenting DNA ends with oxidized nucleotides and lacking the phosphate group linked ends needed for ligation. They are not recognized by ligases or polymerases and therefore require end processing. Such processing can be realized by enzymes such as PNK (polynucleotide kinase), PNKP (polynucleotide kinase 3'-phosphatase) or AP endonucleases. Once a clean end is produced, repair can follow (29). Notably, mutation, deletion or inhibition of either of the main BER/SSBR enzymes can lead to reduced radiation damage repair and relatively mild radiosensitization. The reason why a defective SSBR pathway does not substantially radiosensitize cells is probably because there are efficient backup pathways.

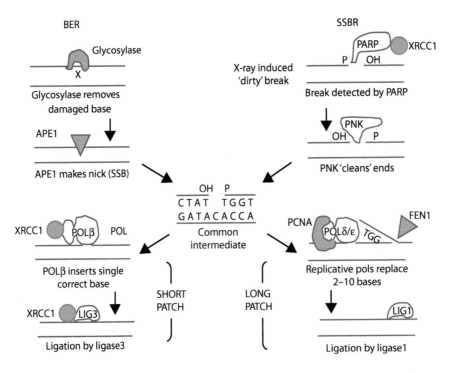

**Figure 2.7** The related pathways of BER and SSBR. The X (top left) represents a damaged base. Different base damages are recognized and removed by different glycosylases as the first step in BER. Both pathways result in a common nicked intermediate, which is processed by short- or long-patch repair.

Unrepaired SSBs can ultimately result in DSBs, which subsequently can be repaired by the DSB repair machinery. However, targeting SSBR in tumours with DSBR defects can represent an attractive therapeutic strategy.

## Double-strand break repair

Radiation can cause direct DSBs that result in chromosome or chromatid damage if misrepaired or not repaired. The two main mechanisms of DSBR are homologous recombination (HR) and non-homologous end joining (NHEJ). As the names imply, HR uses the replicated homologous sister chromatid as a template for repairing DSBs, while NHEJ does not. This renders HR a high-fidelity repair mechanism that restores the original DNA sequence, while NHEJ is error prone and often results in permanent changes to DNA. Whether a DSB is repaired by HR or NHEJ depends on the chromatin structure as well as the cell-cycle phase (11). Typically around 90% of the DNA exists within euchromatin which is lightly packed and can be transcriptionally active. DSBs within euchromatin are mainly repaired by NHEJ with rapid kinetics. For the 10% of DNA that exists within the more densely packed superstructures of the transcriptionally inactive heterochromatin, the choice of repair mechanism depends on cell-cycle stage. In the absence of a replicated sister chromatid, such as in G1 and early S phase, these DSBs must also be repaired by NHEJ. However, if the broken DNA has already been replicated, such as in the G2 phase, these breaks will be repaired by HR. Remodelling of heterochromatin is necessary for DSBR, and this depends on activation of ATM by MRN and subsequent phosphorylation of KAP1 and the endonuclease ARTEMIS. Repair of DSBs within heterochromatin occurs with slower kinetics. The importance of proper repair of DNA within heterochromatin is evidenced by the severe radiosensitivity of cells or patients lacking functional ATM.

A number of proteins help decide whether to engage the NHEJ or HR process in repairing a DSB. CDK1 activity regulates DNA end resection required for HR, thereby preventing cells from attempting HR in G1. Furthermore, phosphorylation of H2AX promotes ubiquitylation of H2A proteins by RNF8 and RNF168 in the surrounding chromatin, which serves as a signalling platform for the attraction of pathway-specific repair factors. Mono-ubiquitylated H2A attracts the protein 53BP1 which directs repair towards NHEJ in G1 by mediating end resection at DNA breaks that directly antagonize HR factors (25). Poly-ubiquitinition chains on the chromatin conversely attract the adaptor protein RAP80 which recruits the HR protein machinery (5).

## Non-homologous end joining

NHEJ simply joins two DNA DSB ends together (19). The general scheme of NHEJ is shown in Figure 2.8. The first event after the binding of the Ku70/80 heterodimer to the DNA ends

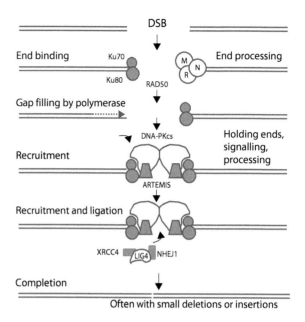

**Figure 2.8** DSB repair by NHEJ. Binding of the Ku70/80 heterodimer mediates recruitment of DNA-PKcs, DNA end processing and ligation. The repair process often results in permanent genetic alterations. For clarity, processes such as end binding have been shown on one side of the break only.

is the recruitment of the DNA-PKcs. It is a large protein and can therefore form a physical bridge between the two ends, helping to keep them in close proximity for subsequent repair events. DNA-PKcs also becomes activated as a kinase when bound to the Ku complex at break sites. DSBs can present 'overhangs' (non-blunt ends) or remnants of sugar groups which make them incompatible for ligation. The PNK, the endonuclease ARTEMIS and polymerases process the damaged DNA ends to facilitate ligation by DNA ligase 4, aided by XRRC4 and NHEJ1. However, this processing can also result in loss or gain of DNA giving rise to permanent deletions, insertions and mutations. Given that NHEJ is the only DSBR mechanism in G1, and responsible for repairing 90% of DSBs in G2, it is not surprising that loss of essential NHEJ proteins such as DNA-PKcs or ligase 4 results in severe radiosensitivity. Another consequence of low repair capacity is the lack of sparing by dividing a single dose into multiple dose fractions. This results in cellular dose-response curves that are relatively straight, i.e. have a high $\alpha/\beta$ value (see Chapter 4). Since the NHEJ machinery also contributes to the V(D)J recombination of antibodies and T-cell receptors, patients with mutations in these genes often present with severe immunodeficiency. Similarly, the commonly used laboratory 'SCID' mouse strain lacks DNA-PKcs activity, underlying both its compromised immune system and radiosensitive phenotype.

## Homologous recombination

As described previously, HR uses replicated homologous undamaged DNA as a template for repair. This restricts

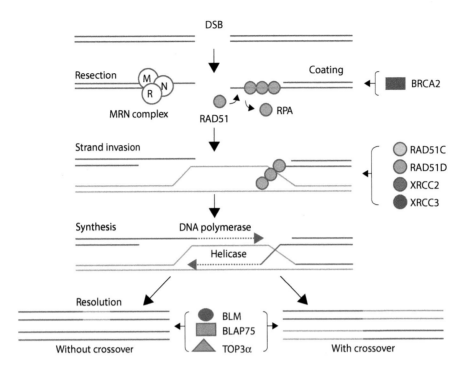

**Figure 2.9** DSB repair by HR. Binding of MRN mediates resection and single-strand invasion of the undamaged sister chromatid (light coloured lines) to use this as a template for high-fidelity repair. The repair process results in error-free DNA, with possible DNA crossover between sister chromatids.

activity to the S and G2 phase of the cell cycle. However, by using DNA with the same sequence as a template, the repair process can be error free, re-establishing the DNA as it was prior to the damage. The general scheme for HR is illustrated in Figure 2.9. Single-stranded regions are created around each side of the break. MRN and other exonucleases such as Exo1 have a crucial role in generating those. As it exposes single-stranded regions, this step is followed by their coating with specialized proteins, such as RPA. These single-stranded nucleoprotein filaments are now capable of invading undamaged double-stranded DNA from the sister chromatid. RAD51 loaded onto these regions guides this process, assisted by BRCA2 (the product of the breast cancer susceptibility gene, type 2). Several RAD51 paralogs help with the search for homologous DNA and sister chromatid invasion processes, including RAD51B, RAD51C, RAD51D, XRCC2 and XRCC3. Deletion or mutation of any of these genes can severely impair homologous recombination.

To enable homology search, invasion and annealing, helicases such as BLM help unwind DNA from its tightly organized structure. When an undamaged DNA template is identified and presented, DNA polymerases can synthesize across the missing regions of the damaged site, thereby accurately repairing the break. The crossover structure that results from this has to be reversed to reset the chromatin to its original configuration. This is done with specialized nucleases which cut or resolve the junctions, followed finally by ligation of adjacent ends. Structure-specific endonucleases such as the human MUS81 complex and SLX4 and SLX1 are also involved in untangling the DNA and assist the resolution

of these complicated structures that are formed during strand invasion and template replication. The RMI complex (BLM, BLAP75, TOP3α) is important to limit DNA crossover. Cells become more radiation resistant in late S and G2 phases of the cell cycle as HR becomes available as a DSBR pathway (30).

The HR machinery is also used in the repair of DNA interstrand cross-link (ICL) damage which causes stalling of replication forks. The Fanconi Anaemia (FA) family of proteins is particularly important for ICL (36), and cells with FA gene mutations show increased sensitivity to DNA cross-linking agents. The core FA complex (involving FANC-A,-B,-C,-E,-F,-G,-L,-M) ubiquitylates FANC-D2 and -I, causing signalling to downstream targets (FANC-D1,-J,-N) that ultimately engages proteins to remove the cross-linked DNA by digestion, synthesize new DNA across the break and assemble the repaired DNA sequence. Many HR proteins bear alternative names that reflect their involvement in this process, such as BRCA2/FANC-D1 and RAD51/FANC-O. As the name implies, patients with FA mutations present with bone marrow failure, but are also prone to developing acute myelogenous leukaemia (AML). Likewise, carriers of germline mutations in HR genes *BRCA1* and *BRCA2* have a much elevated lifetime risk of developing cancer, in particular breast and ovarian cancers. The roles described above of the HR and FA pathways in DSBR and replication-associated stress render cells deficient in HR and FA proteins moderately radiosensitive. This has raised concerns regarding the risk of normal tissue toxicities and second cancers in breast cancer patients carrying *BRCA1/BRCA2* mutations. However, there is currently no evidence for increased adverse effects in this patient population after radiation, likely because the normal cells carry a wild-type (non-mutated) allele that is functionally sufficient (2). There is great interest in therapeutically exploiting defects in HR. One strategy with demonstrated efficacy is to block SSBR using PARP inhibitors in tumours that lack BRCA1 or BRCA2. When PARP is inhibited, stalled replication forks are converted to DSBs which require HR for repair. The specific loss of BRCA in tumour cells thereby provides a therapeutic ratio for this approach.

## Mismatch repair

The MMR pathway corrects mis-paired nucleotides (e.g. other than A-T and C-G). As with all repair pathways it comprises a recognition step, an excision and re-synthesis step, and ligation. Most studies with knockout cells for one or more MMR genes have not found a substantial increase in radiosensitivity. However, this pathway clearly has relevance for cancer treatment, since MMR-deficient cells have altered sensitivity to some chemotherapy agents (e.g. cisplatin and temozolomide). In addition, radiosensitization by thymidine analogues such as IUdR is enhanced in MMR-deficient cells because of their inability to remove the modified base. MMR status of cells can therefore be of importance for outcome after radiotherapy in combination with other agents. Furthermore, tumours with MMR defects have an exceptionally high mutational load which produces antigens that renders them sensitive to immune checkpoint blockade (17). Based on this, the U.S. Food and Drug Administration approved in 2017 for the first time a pan-cancer treatment based on a genetic biomarker, namely, immune checkpoint blockade for tumours carrying MMR defects.

## Nucleotide excision repair

NER copes with bulky lesions at one strand of the DNA that distorts the DNA helix, such as those caused by UV light (thymine dimers) or DNA adducts induced by cross-linkers such as cisplatin. The DNA flanking the damage site is cleaved by the NER proteins ERCC1 and XPF. This generates a large single-stranded gap that is filled in by polymerases to restore the DNA helix. Dysfunctional NER genes have in general little effect on sensitivity to IR.

## 2.8 RADIATION QUALITY, CELL TYPES AND CELLULAR CONTEXT

The clustered damage produced by IR may present the greatest challenge to the cell (20). For example, if base damage occurs on the opposite strand to a radiation-induced SSB, the temporary nick formed during BER can cause a DSB when combined with the radiation break on the opposite strand. These complex lesion sites that require a high degree of DDR coordination result in higher levels of mutagenicity and cytotoxicity. Radiation modalities that create more clustered damage and complex lesions are in consequence relatively more efficient (see Chapter 6).

DNA repair capacity differs between cell types of various origins, between stem cells and differentiated cells, and between cancer cells and normal cells. These differences may affect both normal tissue and tumour response to radiation. Stem cells, which are relevant for both, have been shown to have a higher capacity for HR than differentiated cells, perhaps reflecting the importance of avoiding mutations in these cells. The use of HR is restricted to proliferating cells, rendering most non-proliferative normal tissue cells (resting in G0) to rely on NHEJ for repair of DSBs. Radiotherapy and other exposures to IR can contribute to carcinogenesis through the propagation of normal cells with mis-repaired DNA damage and a higher load of mutations and chromosomal aberrations. The radiation-induced dose-dependent increased relative risk of cancer has been deduced from large cohorts of atomic bomb survivors and radiation-monitored workers (e.g. [13,18]) (see Chapter 27).

A key characteristic of cancer cells is the lack or alteration of the DNA damage response through genetic mutations or by transcriptional deregulation. Defects in DDR that result in genomic instability are considered enabling characteristics for cancer development (10,14). As a result of these defects, tumour cells are likely to conduct DNA repair somewhat differently than normal cells, possibly creating opportunities for specific targeting in combination with radiation.

Finally, cellular contexts such as oxygen availability (see Chapters 17 and 18) and metabolic state can also affect the lesion composition and/or the activity or abundance of proteins in the DDR. For example, increased numbers of cross links are formed after radiation under hypoxic conditions, requiring FA- and/or HR-directed repair. In addition, hypoxia leads to lower levels of HR proteins and mildly compromised repair capacity.

Although many molecular pathways can affect radiation response directly or indirectly, the highly radiosensitive phenotype of patients with mutations in genes like ATM, NBS and FA has taught us that the DDR is the strongest determinant of cellular and tissue radiation response.

## Key points

1. DNA is the critical target for radiation-induced cell killing.
2. Cells activate a DDR that consists of sensors, transducers and effectors.
3. Effector pathways include apoptosis, cell-cycle checkpoints and DNA repair.
4. DNA DSBs, in particular clustered complex DSBs, are the most important and difficult lesions to repair.
5. DSBs are repaired by HR and NHEJ processes.
6. DNA repair choice depends on the nature and location of the lesion, cell-cycle phase, cell type and micro-environmental conditions.

# ■ BIBLIOGRAPHY

1. Bartek J, Lukas C, Lukas J. Checking on DNA damage in S phase. *Nat Rev Mol Cell Biol* 2004;5:792–804.
2. Bernier J, Poortmans P. Clinical relevance of normal and tumour cell radiosensitivity in BRCA1/BRCA2 mutation carriers: A review. *Breast* 2015;24:100–106.
3. Ceccaldi R, Rondinelli B, D'Andrea AD. Repair pathway choices and consequences at the double-strand break. *Trends Cell Biol* 2016;26:52–64.
4. Chapman JD, Gillespie CJ. Radiation-induced events and their time-scale in mammalian cells. *Adv Radiat Biol* 1981;9: 143–198.
5. Citterio E. Fine-tuning the ubiquitin code at DNA double-strand breaks: Deubiquitinating enzymes at work. *Front Genet* 2015;6:282.
6. Deckbar D, Jeggo PA, Löbrich M. Understanding the limitations of radiation-induced cell cycle checkpoints. *Crit Rev Biochem Mol Biol* 2011;46:271–283.
7. Falck J, Coates J, Jackson SP. Conserved modes of recruitment of ATM, ATR and DNA-PKcs to sites of DNA damage. *Nature* 2005;434:605–611.
8. Fortini P, Dogliotti E. Base damage and single-strand break repair: Mechanisms and functional significance of short- and long-patch repair subpathways. *DNA Repair Amst* 2007;6:398–409.
9. Gibson BA, Zhang Y, Jiang H et al. Chemical genetic discovery of PARP targets reveals a role for PARP-1 in transcription elongation. *Science* 2016;353:45–50.
10. Goldstein M, Kastan MB. The DNA damage response: Implications for tumor responses to radiation and chemotherapy. *Annu Rev Med* 2015;66:129–143.
11. Goodarzi AA, Jeggo P, Lobrich M. The influence of heterochromatin on DNA double strand break repair: Getting the strong, silent type to relax. *DNA Repair (Amst)* 2010;9:1273–1282.
12. Goodhead DT. Energy deposition stochastics and track structure: What about the target? *Radiat Prot Dosimetry* 2006;122:3–15.
13. Grant EJ, Brenner A, Sugiyama H et al. Solid cancer incidence among the life span study of atomic bomb survivors: 1958–2009. *Radiat Res* 2017;187:513–537.
14. Hanahan D, Weinberg RA. Hallmarks of cancer: The next generation. *Cell* 2011;144:646–674.
15. Harper JW, Elledge SJ. The DNA damage response: Ten years after. *Mol Cell* 2007;28:739–745.
16. Kastan MB, Bartek J. Cell-cycle checkpoints and cancer. *Nature* 2004;432:316–323.
17. Le DT, Durham JN, Smith KN et al. Mismatch repair deficiency predicts response of solid tumors to PD-1 blockade. *Science* 2017;357:409–413.
18. Leuraud K, Richardson DB, Cardis E et al. Ionising radiation and risk of death from leukaemia and lymphoma in radiation-monitored workers (INWORKS): An international cohort study. *Lancet Haematol* 2015;2:e276–e281.
19. Lieber MR. The mechanism of human nonhomologous DNA end joining. *J Biol Chem* 2008;283:1–5.
20. Lomax ME, Folkes LK, O'Neill P. Biological consequences of radiation-induced DNA damage: Relevance to radiotherapy. *Clin Oncol (R Coll Radiol)* 2013;25:578–585.
21. Marples B, Wouters BG, Collis SJ, Chalmers AJ, Joiner MC. Low-dose hyper-radiosensitivity: A consequence of ineffective cell cycle arrest of radiation-damaged G2-phase cells. *Radiat Res* 2004;161:247–255.
22. Matsuoka S, Ballif BA, Smogorzewska A et al. ATM and ATR substrate analysis reveals extensive protein networks responsive to DNA damage. *Science* 2007;316:1160–1166.
23. Munro TR. The relative radiosensitivity of the nucleus and cytoplasm of Chinese hamster fibroblasts. *Radiat Res* 1970;42:451–470.
24. O'Driscoll M, Jeggo PA. The role of double-strand break repair – Insights from human genetics. *Nat Rev Genet* 2006;7:45–54.
25. Panier S, Boulton SJ. Double-strand break repair: 53BP1 comes into focus. *Nat Rev Mol Cell Biol* 2014;15:7–18.
26. Shiloh Y, Ziv Y. The ATM protein kinase: Regulating the cellular response to genotoxic stress, and more. *Nat Rev Mol Cell Biol* 2013;14:197–210.
27. Stucki M, Jackson SP. γH2AX and MDC1: Anchoring the DNA-damage-response machinery to broken chromosomes. *DNA Repair Amst* 2006;5:534–543.
28. Sullivan JM, Jeffords LB, Lee CL, Rodrigues R, Ma Y, Kirsch DG. p21 protects 'Super p53' mice from the radiation-induced gastrointestinal syndrome. *Radiat Res* 2012;177:307–310.
29. Sung JS, Demple B. Roles of base excision repair subpathways in correcting oxidized abasic sites in DNA. *FEBS J* 2006;273:1620–1629.
30. Tamulevicius P, Wang M, Iliakis G. Homology-directed repair is required for the development of radioresistance during S phase: Interplay between double-strand break repair and checkpoint response. *Radiat Res* 2007;167:1–11.
31. van Attikum H, Gasser SM. The histone code at DNA breaks: A guide to repair? *Nat Rev Mol Cell Biol* 2005;6:757–765.
32. Warters RL, Hofer KG, Harris CR, Smith JM. Radionuclide toxicity in cultured mammalian cells: Elucidation of the primary site of radiation damage. *Curr Top Radiat Res Q* 1978;12:389–407.
33. Wouters BG, Denko NC, Giaccia AJ, Brown JM. A p53 and apoptotic independent role for p21waf1 in tumour response to radiation therapy. *Oncogene* 1999;18:6540–6545.
34. Wouters BG, Giaccia AJ, Denko NC, Brown JM. Loss of p21Waf1/Cip1 sensitizes tumors to radiation by an apoptosis-independent mechanism. *Cancer Res* 1997;57:4703–4706.
35. Xu B, Kim ST, Lim DS, Kastan MB. Two molecularly distinct G(2)/M checkpoints are induced by ionizing irradiation. *Mol Cell Biol* 2002;22:1049–1059.
36. Zhang J, Powell SN. The role of the BRCA1 tumor suppressor in DNA double-strand break repair. *Mol Cancer Res* 2005;3:531–539.

# ■ FURTHER READING

37. Jeggo PA, Pearl LH, Carr AM. DNA repair, genome stability and cancer: A historical perspective. *Nat Rev Cancer* 2016; 16:35–42.

**3**

# Cell death after irradiation: How, when and why cells die

BRADLY G. WOUTERS

## 3.1 DEFINITIONS OF CELL DEATH

The successful use of radiation to treat cancer results primarily from its ability to cause the death of individual tumour cells. As discussed in Chapter 2, the biological consequences of irradiation, including cell death, are highly influenced by pathways within the DNA damage response (DDR) system. The DDR influences not only the sensitivity of cells to death following irradiation, but also the type of cell death that occurs, and the timing of when cell death occurs. Because the DDR differs among different types of normal and tumour cells (and likely even within different populations of tumour cells), the manifestation of cell death can also differ widely among different cell types.

It is important to define what is meant by cell death in the context of radiobiology and cancer therapy. For many years, little attention was paid towards differences in the mechanisms or types of cell death after irradiation or other cancer treatments. This was due in part because many of the pathways that influence cell death were unknown and because cell death is typically very hard to properly assess. Quantification is complicated by the fact that cells die at various times after irradiation, often after one or two trips around the cell cycle, and among surviving cells that continue to proliferate. As an alternative, researchers have focused on assessing clonogenic survival, which is operationally defined as the ability of a cell to survive, proliferate and form a colony of new cells (usually of at least 50) after irradiation. This is a much more robust and relevant parameter to assess radiation effect since any cell that retains proliferative capacity can cause failure to locally control the tumour (discussed in more detail in Chapters 4 and 5). Consequently, cell death in the context of radiobiology is generally equated with any process that leads to the permanent loss of clonogenic capacity. This is a rather wide inclusion criterion for cell death, and obviously does not have meaning when applied to terminally differentiated cell types that do not proliferate such as nerve and muscle cells. For these types of cells, it makes more sense to consider the specific types of cell death that lead to destruction of the cell, or to evaluate how radiation alters the function of these cells. Nonetheless, loss of reproductive capacity is a widely applicable definition for cell death in radiobiology and is highly relevant for proliferating cells, including those in tumours and in many of the normal tissues of relevance for radiotherapy.

## 3.2 HOW CELLS DIE

It is now clear that cells can die by many different mechanisms following irradiation. Increased attention to the mechanisms of cell death occurred following the discovery of a genetically 'programmed' form of cell death known as apoptosis. This form of cell death results in rapid and normally complete destruction and removal of the cell, and is considered as a 'choice' made by the cell itself often as a consequence of damage, stress or as a barrier against tumourigenesis. Furthermore, this pathway can be activated directly by the DDR, and is thus a strong determinant of radiation-induced cell death for certain cell types. Since the discovery of apoptosis, several other distinct mechanisms have been identified that can contribute to loss of reproductive capacity after irradiation including autophagy, senescence, necrosis and several other forms of cell death (8). Each of these pathways can be distinguished at the molecular and morphological levels (see Table 3.1) and each can potentially contribute to radiosensitivity in certain cell types and contexts. Importantly, the pathways that control these programmed forms of cell death are differentially activated in different tissue types, and are frequently altered in cancer. Consequently, differential activation of cell death pathways constitutes a main contributor to variation in radiation response among different cells, tumours and tissues.

In addition to these genetically controlled programs, a long recognized contributor to cell death after irradiation is mitotic catastrophe in which cells fail to complete mitosis correctly. Applying our definitions above, mitotic catastrophe can be considered a form of cell death of its own, the 'mitotic death', when it is severe enough to prevent mitosis completely or alter cell function sufficiently to prevent further proliferation. Mitotic catastrophe may also result in further chromosomal and DNA damage sufficient to activate the other forms of cell death.

Table 3.1 The characteristics of different types of cell death are described

| Type of cell death | Morphological changes | | | Biochemical features | Common detection methods |
|---|---|---|---|---|---|
| | Nucleus | Cell membrane | Cytoplasm | | |
| Apoptosis | Chromatin condensation; nuclear fragmentation; DNA laddering | Blebbing | Fragmentation formation of apoptotic bodies | Caspase dependent | Electron microscopy; TUNEL staining; annexin staining; caspase-activity assays; DNA-fragmentation assays; detection of increased number of cells in subG1/G0; detection of changes in mitochondrial membrane potential |
| Autophagy | Partial chromatin condensation; no DNA laddering | Blebbing | Increased number of autophagic vesicles | Caspase independent; increased lysosomal activity | Electron microscopy; protein-degradation assays; assays for marker-protein translocation to autophagic membranes |
| Necrosis | Clumping and random degradation of nuclear DNA. Generation of reactive oxygen species, or loss of membrane permeability | Swelling; rupture | Increased vacuolation; organelle degeneration; mitochondrial swelling | Caspase independent; increased forms of reactive oxygen species, lysosomal membrane rupture, plasma membrane rupture | Electron microscopy; nuclear staining (usually negative); detection of inflammation and damage in surrounding tissues; loss of membrane permeability |
| Senescence | Distinct heterochromatic structure (senescence-associated heterochromatic foci) | – | Flattening and increased granularity | SA-β-gal activity | Electron microscopy; SA-β-gal staining; growth-arrest assays |
| Mitotic catastrophe | Multiple micronuclei; nuclear fragmentation; dicentric chromosomes | – | – | Caspase independent (at early stage) abnormal CDK1/ cyclin B activation | Electron microscopy; assays for mitotic markers (MPM2); TUNEL staining |

Adapted from (12).

# Apoptosis

Apoptosis is a highly regulated form of cell death that can be initiated either as a result of conditions occurring within the cell itself (such as those after DNA damage) or from signals generated externally such as those from a surrounding tissue or immune cell (14). Apoptosis is an essential and normal part of many physiological processes including embryonic development, the immune system and maintenance of tissue homeostasis. Consequently, alterations in the control of apoptosis contribute to several human diseases including cancer.

Apoptosis is both morphologically and molecularly distinct from other forms of cell death (see Table 3.1). Morphologically it is characterized by membrane blebbing, condensation and digestion of the DNA into small fragments.

During this process, cellular contents are also fragmented into many membrane-enclosed apoptotic bodies, which *in vivo* are taken up by phagocytes. This prevents leakage of potentially damaging cellular proteins and destruction of tissue architecture that is a familiar feature of necrosis.

The molecular participants in the apoptotic pathway can be divided into two groups – the sensors and effectors. The sensor molecules are involved in making the decision to initiate apoptosis, whereas the effectors are responsible for carrying out that decision. Apoptotic cell death is characterized by the sequential activation of several different enzymes known as caspases. These proteins are initially expressed in an inactive form (procaspase) and are additionally kept in check by a family of inhibitor of apoptosis (IAP) proteins. Apoptosis begins following the activation of a 'sensor' caspase such as caspase 8 or 9, which generates the initial signal to induce apoptosis. These caspases subsequently activate a common set of other 'effector' caspases (e.g. caspase 3), which then cleave a large set of cellular proteins leading to the ultimate destruction of the cell.

Apoptosis that initiates from caspase 8 activation is termed the *extrinsic* pathway because it is normally activated upon the binding of an extracellular ligand and subsequent activation of a death receptor present in the cellular membrane. Examples of these death-inducing ligands include TNF, TRAIL and FAS ligand, which bind to the TNF receptor, TRAIL receptor and FAS, respectively. This extrinsic pathway of apoptosis is not induced by radiation to any significant degree, but is a candidate target for combining novel drugs with radiation.

Apoptosis that initiates from caspase 9 is termed the *intrinsic* pathway because it is activated within the cell in response to various forms of cell damage. The activation of caspase 9 is controlled in large part by the balance of pro- and anti-apoptotic proteins that reside in or near the mitochondria. Under normal conditions this balance is in favour of the anti-apoptotic factors (such as BCL2), and activation of caspase 9 is prevented. Conditions that alter this balance lead to release of cytochrome C and other molecules from the mitochondria into the cytoplasm resulting in formation of a structure known as the apoptosome, and subsequently activation of caspase 9. After irradiation, this balance can be tipped in favour of apoptosis due in part to p53 activation and induction of pro-apoptotic proteins such as BAX and PUMA.

Activation of apoptosis is highly dependent on the balance of the pro- and anti-apoptotic proteins and this balance varies widely among different cell types and tumours. This explains why irradiation causes apoptosis only in certain normal tissues, despite the fact that p53 is activated in response to DNA damage in nearly all normal cells. For example, fibroblast cells almost never undergo apoptosis despite demonstrating p53 and BAX induction. In these cells, induction of BAX is not sufficient to initiate release of cytochrome C and thus activation of caspase 9. These cells may have a larger proportion of anti-apoptotic molecules like those from the BCL2 family, or they may have higher levels of the IAP proteins which block caspase activation. Consequently, apoptosis plays little or no role in the radiosensitivity of these cell types. In contrast, other normal cells, such as lymphocytes and thymocytes, readily undergo apoptosis following irradiation. In these cells, p53 induction of BAX is sufficient to cause cytochrome C release from the mitochondria and induction of apoptosis. Thus, the importance of apoptosis and the genes controlling it such as p53 is highly context dependent.

In tumours, an additional mechanism for variation in apoptosis sensitivity arises from the fact that many of the genes that regulate apoptosis are frequently altered in cancer. For example, many tumours show loss of p53 function, and are thus unable to initiate apoptosis through this pathway. Apoptosis is an important cellular defence against cancer development and loss of apoptotic sensitivity is recognized as an essential hallmark of cancer. Consequently, apoptotic sensitivity is often reduced in cancer compared to normal tissues, although it can vary significantly among different tumours. Since radiation and other anticancer agents are capable of activating apoptosis, it has been widely suggested that apoptotic sensitivity is also an important contributor to radiosensitivity. However, this may or may not be correct, depending upon the relative importance of other forms of cell death.

## Autophagy

Autophagy is a term which literally means 'self-eating' and describes a process in which cells digest parts of their own cytoplasm in order to generate small macromolecules and energy. The molecular basis of autophagy and its relationship to cell survival mechanisms is an active area of current research. Autophagy is controlled by a large number of genes which initiate the formation of a double-membrane bound structure that grows and engulfs cytoplasmic components forming cytoplasmic filled vacuoles called autophagosomes (10). These fuse with lysosomes to initiate the degradation of the enclosed material into primary components and energy that can be used to fuel metabolism.

Autophagy is activated in response to several different situations, the best characterized of which occurs in response to growth factor or nutrient removal (starvation). This process is regulated by both the mammalian target of rapamycin (mTOR) kinase, which is a general sensor of nutrient status integrating upstream signalling pathways that sense energy levels, oxygen, and growth factor signalling, and by AMPK, which responds to low levels of ATP. In this situation, autophagy is thought to sustain overall survival during times of low nutrient environment by causing the limited digestion of cytoplasmic elements to sustain metabolic processes. As such, one would expect that autophagy promotes cell survival, rather than cell death.

However, in contrast to this pro-survival role, deregulated activation of autophagy can lead to a distinct form of cell death. Some aspects of this form of death are morphologically similar to apoptosis, although no caspase activation or DNA cleavage occurs. Autophagy also appears to function as a tumour suppressor, in much the same way that apoptosis does. The Beclin 1 gene is part of a complex required to initiate autophagy, and its loss leads to enhanced cancer development in mice. This gene is also altered in some human cancers, as are several tumour suppressors linked to autophagy including p53 and PTEN. These data suggest that autophagy acts in some way as a barrier to cancer formation, likely in part through its ability to promote cell death in transformed cells.

Autophagy activation has been observed following treatment with many anticancer agents including radiation, suggesting that it may be an important mechanism of cell killing by these agents (13). However, it is unclear to what extent autophagy represents an attempt by the cell for survival, or as an induced form of cell death. In most situations, autophagy is likely contributing to cell survival rather than death. There also appears to be some relationship between autophagy and apoptosis, because autophagy is more readily observed in cells with defects in apoptosis. Consequently, similar to what has been discussed for apoptosis, the contribution of autophagy to cell death is highly cell specific.

## Necrosis and other forms of direct cell death

It has been said that if apoptosis represents 'death by suicide', then necrosis is 'death by injury'. Necrosis has historically been considered to be an inappropriate or accidental death that occurs under conditions that are extremely unfavourable, such as those incompatible with a critical normal physiologic process. Examples of conditions that can activate necrosis include extreme changes in pH, energy loss and ion imbalance. Consequently, necrosis is generally thought of as an uncontrollable, irreversible and chaotic form of cell death. It is characterized by cellular swelling, membrane deformation, organelle breakdown and the release of lysosomal enzymes which attack the cell. These conditions can occur following infection, inflammation or ischaemia. Necrosis is also frequently observed in human tumours and can be induced following treatment with certain DNA damaging agents including radiation.

There is strong evidence that necrosis can also occur in a 'programmed' manner and constitute an alternative to apoptosis. Necroptosis refers to a specific form of programmed necrosis that is initiated by receptor-interacting protein kinase 3 (RIPK3) and other forms of programmed necrosis include the excitotoxicity of neurons. For example, induction of necrosis is dependent on cellular energy stores, such as NAD and ATP, and can be regulated by receptor signalling pathways. Furthermore, cell stress and cell signalling including oxidative stress, calcium levels and p53 activation have been shown to influence lysosomal membrane permeability. Permeabilization leads to intracellular acidification and release of various enzymes that can promote necrosis. Other distinct forms of non-apoptotic cell death that result from aberrant cell signalling have been identified. For example, ferroptosis is an iron-linked form of cell death that occurs when cells are unable to control iron-dependent reactive oxygen species generation. Although it is not clear how the cell controls necrosis, ferroptosis or other direct forms of programmed cell death following irradiation, the frequency with which this is observed varies among different cell types. This suggests that, just as for all the other forms of cell death, cellular pathways control the sensitivity of its activation.

## Senescence and 'indirect' cell death

*Cellular senescence* is the term given to the observation that over time normal cells permanently lose their ability to divide. These cells remain present, metabolically intact and may or may not display functional changes. Senescence was first described by Leonard Hayflick in 1965 in cultured primary cells that exhibit an initial period of exponential growth, followed by a permanent arrest termed *replicative senescence* or the *Hayflick limit* (9). Replicative senescence is associated with the aging process and correlates with the gradual shortening of telomeres at the ends of chromosomes during the exponential growth period.

In addition to this replicative form of senescence, 'premature' senescence can also be elicited by various cellular stresses such as those caused by oncogene activation or by radiation-induced DNA damage (3). In both situations, the cells enter a permanent cell-cycle arrest characterized morphologically by a flattened cytoplasm and increased granularity or biochemically by an increase in senescence-associated β-galactosidase expression. Senescence-inducing stresses typically do not induce shortening of the telomeres, but instead are controlled by a number of molecular pathways that are only partially understood. As is the case for replicative senescence, cells that undergo senescence after irradiation are not metabolically 'dead', but because they have permanently ceased proliferation are unable to contribute to tissue or tumour recovery.

The best understood part of accelerated senescence induction involves the activation of cell-cycle inhibitor proteins like those activated by the DDR system after radiation. In some cell types, a transient G1 checkpoint activation due to p53 induction of the p21 cyclin-dependent kinase inhibitor (CDKI) can lead to a secondary permanent arrest into G0 that is mediated by the CDKI p16 and the retinoblastoma tumour suppressor protein RB. This arrest may also be associated with chromatin changes and widespread gene silencing giving rise to senescent cells characterized by having increased areas of heterochromatin.

In much the same way as apoptosis, the propensity of different cell types and different tumours to undergo senescence is highly variable. Premature senescence occurs frequently in fibroblast cells after irradiation (which do not undergo apoptosis) and likely contributes in part to radiation-induced skin fibrosis. Both premature and replicative senescence also act as potential barriers to cancer development and, consequently, the pathways that control this process are frequently altered in cancer. However, it would appear that the pathways that control replicative and premature senescence are at least partially distinct since some tumour cells can be induced to undergo radiation-induced senescence although they have clearly acquired mechanisms to prevent replicative senescence. Nonetheless, the two pathways share some common features that may be altered during carcinogenesis. Consequently, there is a wide variation in the ability of cancer cells to initiate senescence after irradiation, depending upon the genetic changes within that individual cancer. Cells that enter senescence lose their ability to proliferate and thus would contribute to cell death as we have defined it (loss of clonogenic potential). Thus, while not a direct form of cell death, it does constitute cell loss from a cancer and is thus considered as an indirect form of cell death.

## Mitotic catastrophe

*Mitotic catastrophe* is a term that has evolved to encompass the type of cell death that results from, or following, aberrant mitosis. This is morphologically associated with the accumulation of multinucleated, giant cells containing uncondensed chromosomes and with the presence of chromosome aberrations and micronuclei. This process occurs when cells proceed through mitosis in an inappropriate manner due to entry of cells into mitosis with unrepaired or mis-repaired DNA damage. This is frequently the case in cells following irradiation, which often display a host of different types of chromosome aberrations when they enter mitosis. Death, as defined here by the loss of replicative potential, can occur simply from a physical inability to replicate and separate the genetic material correctly, or to the loss of genetic material associated with this process. This is determined in large part by the types of chromosome aberrations that may be present in irradiated cells.

In addition to acting as a mechanism of cell death, mitotic catastrophe can also serve as a trigger for other cell death pathways, independently of the initial damage cause by irradiation. Thus, mitotic catastrophe which results in cell fusion, polyploidy or failure to perform cytokinesis may subsequently lead to cell death by apoptosis, senescence, autophagy or necrosis. In this case, the attempt to undergo mitosis leads to the activation of the cell-death program, and not the initial DNA damage that was present prior to mitosis (4). The important distinction is that cell death is caused by the mitotic catastrophe, rather than as a direct cellular response to the initial DNA damage itself.

Several checkpoints in G2 and throughout mitosis exist to prevent mitotic catastrophe. These include two genetically distinct G2 checkpoints that are activated by the DDR following radiation-induced DNA damage (discussed in Chapter 2). Cells that show defects in checkpoint activation enter into mitosis prematurely and die through mitotic catastrophe. The failure to prevent entry into mitosis is thought to account for much of the enhanced radiosensitivity observed in ATM-deficient cells. Bypass of these checkpoints permits premature entry into mitosis even if the DNA has not been fully replicated or repaired, leading to an enhancement of mitotic catastrophe. Additional mitotic checkpoints ensure proper spindle assembly and attachment prior to cytokinesis. The spindle checkpoint is regulated by a number of different kinases, including the aurora kinases, polo kinases as well as the BUB1 and BUBR1 spindle checkpoint kinases. Deregulation of these kinases has been shown to lead to enhanced mitotic catastrophe. Many of the genes involved in the DDR and mitotic checkpoints are altered during cancer and consequently, the propensity to undergo mitotic catastrophe can also vary significantly among different tumours.

## 3.3 WHEN AND WHY CELLS DIE AFTER IRRADIATION

The relative importance of the different forms of cell death after irradiation is often debated and is of importance when considering approaches to predicting radiation response or when combining radiation with molecularly targeted agents. As outlined above, radiation has been demonstrated, in different cell types and circumstances, to induce all of the different known forms of cell death. Unfortunately, it is not possible to infer the importance of any particular cell death pathway simply by monitoring how a particular cell dies after being irradiated. Multiple cell death pathways may be activated within the same cell, but because a cell can die just once, the type of cell death that is observed will be that which occurs most rapidly and not necessarily that which is most sensitive to activation. For example, just because a cell dies by apoptosis after some given dose of radiation does not imply that it would not have died by some other pathway if apoptosis had been disabled. In this regard, it is perhaps less important to consider *how* cells die after irradiation, but rather *why* cells die after irradiation. For this consideration, it is possible to broadly classify cell death mechanisms into two classes, those that occur relatively soon after irradiation and before cell division, and those that occur comparatively late or after division and thus are linked to mitosis and mitotic catastrophe (Figure 3.1).

## Early cell death – pre-mitotic

In a small minority of cell types, cell death occurs rapidly, within several hours after irradiation (Figure 3.2) (5). This type of death, sometimes referred to as interphase death, is limited primarily to thymocytes, lymphocytes, spermatogonia and other cells in rapidly proliferating tissues such as those in hair follicles, in the small intestine and in developing embryos. Early cell death is also observed in some types of cancers that arise from these cell types, including lymphomas, and may explain the unexpected effectiveness of radiotherapy protocols used in the treatment of this disease (e.g. two fractions of 2 Gy). In solid tumours, this type of cell death is rarely observed.

Early cell death results primarily from activation of pathways in response to the initial cellular damage caused by irradiation. The best example of this is the induction of apoptosis that is initiated as part of the DDR. The DDR is activated within minutes of irradiation, and this leads to p53 activation and to the upregulation of pro-apoptotic proteins. Of course, the DDR also induces pro-survival pathways at the same time, including DNA repair pathways and cell-cycle checkpoints. However, in this case these pro-survival pathways are largely irrelevant because apoptosis is initiated regardless of whether repair takes place or not. In this case, activation of apoptosis is a direct result of the initial levels of damage put into the cell. Consequently, for this early form of apoptosis, the

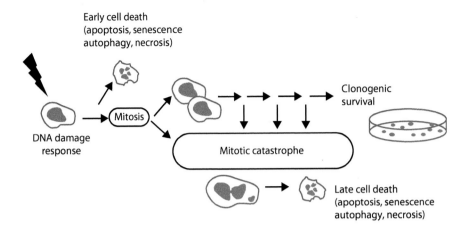

**Figure 3.1** Cell death following irradiation. DNA damage induced by irradiation elicits activation of the DNA damage response (see Chapter 2) which leads to induction of cell-cycle checkpoints and DNA repair. In certain rare cells, this response also induces apoptosis or other forms of cell death. However, in most cases cells only die after attempting mitosis. Remaining or improperly repaired DNA damage causes mitotic catastrophe which subsequently leads to cell death. Mitotic catastrophe and cell death can take place after the first attempt at cell division, or after several rounds of proliferation. Consequently, this form of cell death is considered late cell death.

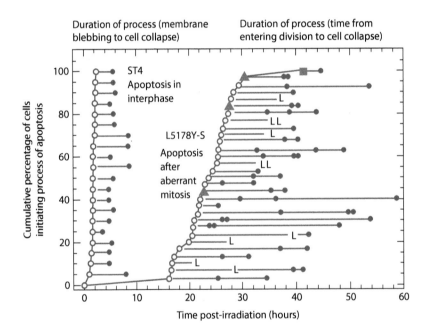

**Figure 3.2** Early and late forms of cell death. The ST4 lymphoid cells die rapidly by apoptosis prior to mitosis. L5178Y-S cells also die by apoptosis following irradiation, but only after attempting to complete mitosis. In this case, the initial DNA damage response is not sufficient to induce cell death and the cells die due to problems that occur during mitosis. (Data from (5).)

genes that regulate this process can significantly influence radiosensitivity. Loss of p53, for example, leads to a defect in apoptosis, loss of the early form of cell death, and an increase in radioresistance.

Early activation of cell death pathways can also occur in certain cell types as a result of damage caused to cellular structures other than the DNA. In endothelial cells that make up blood vessels, relatively high radiation doses (above 15 Gy) have been reported to induce apoptosis as a result of damage to the cellular membrane and the activation of an enzyme known as ceramide synthase (7). Endothelial cells contain very high amounts of this enzyme, and as a result after irradiation can produce large amounts of ceramide. As is the case for apoptosis induced by the DDR, ceramide-induced apoptosis results from pathways activated in response to initial damage caused by irradiation and is not sensitive to DNA repair and checkpoint pathways. Thus, for this form of cell death, the gene products that participate in the activation of apoptosis are important determinants of cellular radiosensitivity.

## Late cell death – post-mitotic

The vast majority of proliferating normal and tumour cells die at relatively long times after irradiation, usually after attempting mitosis one or more times (Figure 3.2). Time-lapse video microscopy has clearly demonstrated that following a transient delay (due to activation of checkpoints) most cells resume proliferation and progress through the cell cycle one, two or more times before eventually permanently ceasing proliferation (6). This has been known for more than 40 years and gave rise to the initial characterization of radiation-induced cell death as reproductive or mitotic cell death. In this case, cell death does not occur until after the cell attempts to divide.

In cells that die at long times of irradiation, the DDR activates both cell-cycle checkpoints and DNA repair systems that aid in the survival of the irradiated cells. In these cell types, the DDR is unable to induce apoptosis despite the fact that p53 or other pro death pathways may be induced. Instead, DNA repair is allowed to take place and will have a large influence on the outcome and radiosensitivity of the cell. Consequently, most proliferating cells from animal models and patients with defects in DNA double-strand break repair show uniformly large increases in sensitivity to radiation-induced cell death.

Although DNA repair and checkpoint pathways play important roles in determining cell survival, cell death at long times after irradiation takes place at times when the checkpoints are no longer active and when DNA repair processes have largely completed. The half-time for repair is approximately 2–4 hours for end joining and perhaps somewhat longer from homologous recombination. Thus, only a very small fraction of the initial DNA damage can be detected at times where cell death occurs. The signal for cell death in this case does not arise from the radiation-induced damage itself, but rather from the consequences of failure to properly complete mitosis. Mitotic catastrophe is therefore considered to be responsible for the majority of cell death in irradiated proliferating cells.

Why does irradiation cause proliferating cells to undergo mitotic catastrophe and cell death? This appears to result from the fact that although DDR pathways remove much of the initial damage caused by irradiation, they are unable to prevent some cells with DNA breaks or DNA rearrangements from entering mitosis. The consequences of incomplete or improper DNA repair become readily visible as chromosomes condense in metaphase as a series of different types of chromosome aberrations. The fate of cells harbouring chromosome aberrations is largely determined by the nature of the chromosome aberration itself (Figure 3.3) (1). Studies have demonstrated approximately equal numbers of reciprocal translocations and non-reciprocal translocations (a dicentric chromosome + acentric fragment) are formed after irradiation. Both of these types of aberrations result from misrepair in which chromosome ends are incorrectly ligated together in a largely stochastic process. However, whereas cells with dicentrics and acentric fragments all die, those with reciprocal translocations often survive. The presence of two centromeres in dicentric chromosomes prevents their separation at metaphase, and consequently leads to mitotic catastrophe and eventually cell death. Some cells with dicentric chromosomes may manage to complete mitosis, however, loss of genetic material present in the acentric fragment (which forms a 'micronuclei') in subsequent mitosis may lead to subsequent death at a later time. This explains the good correlation which has been

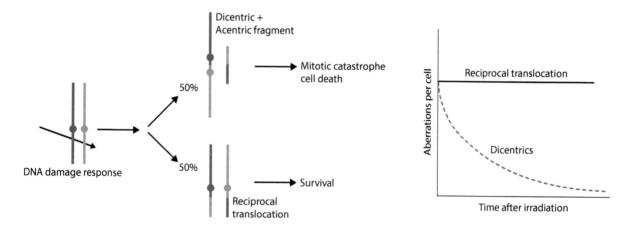

**Figure 3.3** Stochastic nature of cell death after irradiation. DNA repair processes frequently lead to events in which chromosomes are not repaired correctly. It has been shown that irradiated cells produce approximately equal amounts of reciprocal translocations and dicentrics. The broken chromosomes in these cases are ligated to each other in a random or stochastic manner. Formation of a dicentric chromosome prevents proper mitosis and leads to cell death, whereas a reciprocal translocation that does not involve an important region of the genome is stable (sometimes for many decades). Thus, a population of irradiated cells will have approximately equal numbers of both types of aberrations and over time the cells with dicentrics will be lost due to mitotic catastrophe-induced death. The initial amount of DNA damage and activation of the DNA damage response is the same in both types of cells but the outcome is very different. The outcome in this case is determined by the ability of the cells to avoid mitotic catastrophe. (Adapted from (1).)

observed between the formation of dicentric chromosomes or micronuclei formation and cell survival. Reciprocal translocations do not cause problems at metaphase, and thus do not cause mitotic catastrophe or cell death. In fact, these types of aberrations can be found in cells from people exposed to irradiation many years later.

As mentioned previously, cells that experience mitotic catastrophe may ultimately undergo a secondary form of programmed cell death such as apoptosis, autophagy, necrosis or senescence. In this case this secondary form of death is not the cause, but simply the method through which cells die. This has led to a great deal of confusion about the importance of various forms of cell death such as apoptosis as determinants of radiosensitivity. Whereas activation of apoptosis and other programmed cell death pathways are responsible for why cells die at early times after irradiation,

they are not similarly responsible for why cells die at late times after irradiation. As a result, alteration of a particular gene may dramatically alter the levels of radiation-induced apoptosis, without altering the overall ability of the cell to survive (15). In this case, cells are dying as the result of undergoing mitotic catastrophe and will die regardless of whether apoptosis is subsequently induced (Figure 3.4).

Although apoptosis or other programmed cell death pathways may not affect overall survival after irradiation, they can dramatically influence the rate at which cells die and thus the early response of tumours to treatment (2). Because apoptosis leads to rapid and complete destruction of the cell, tumours containing cells capable of undergoing apoptosis after mitotic catastrophe may shrink much faster than a similar tumour consisting of cells with the same overall radiosensitivity that do not similarly undergo apoptosis. For

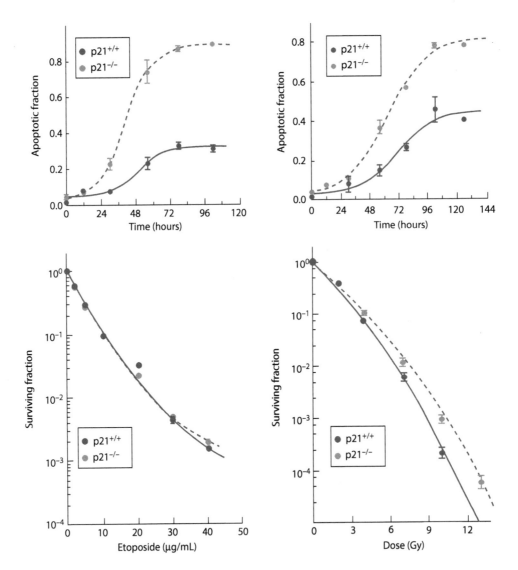

Figure 3.4 Discordance between assays of cell death and cell survival. The two cell lines differ only in the expression of the p21 cyclin-dependent kinase gene (CDKN1A). The p21 knockout cells show increased apoptosis after etoposide or irradiation (top panels) as compared to the p21 wild-type cells. However, when assessed by clonogenic survival, the p21 knockouts show a similar sensitivity to etoposide and a slight resistance to irradiation compared with the p21 wild-type cells. Here, apoptosis takes place after mitotic catastrophe and is just one mode of cell death that contributes to the loss of clonogenicity. (Adapted from (15).)

this reason, it is dangerous to make any conclusions about tumour radiosensitivity from initial changes in tumour size after treatment (Figure 3.5).

Time-lapse microscopy studies have demonstrated that in cells which experience mitotic catastrophe, both the timing and nature of cell death are highly variable (Figure 3.6) (5). As discussed earlier, a surviving cell is considered as one that can proliferate indefinitely. In tissue culture, this is quantified by the ability to form a colony of a certain size after irradiation (usually 50 cells). Conversely, cell death in this context means that eventually all progeny of an irradiated cell will die. An irradiated cell that is destined to die (not produce a colony) may, however, still proceed through mitosis multiple times. The resulting daughter cells can die at very different times after irradiation. For example, following the first mitosis, one of the cells may die and the other may proceed through DNA replication and mitosis to produce two more cells. Eventually these cells will die too, although they may or may not attempt mitosis multiple times. Furthermore, the type of cell death that each daughter

cell undergoes can be different. Consequently, a single irradiated cell can actually die through multiple modes of cell death. A similar situation also exists for irradiated cells that are destined to survive. These cells may also produce daughter cells with different survival potential. One daughter may die, while the other continues to proliferate and thus confers the status of 'survived' on the initially irradiated cell. Consequently, irradiated cells that die following cell division produce a pedigree of cells with different types that can only be tracked by time-lapse microscopy (6). Examples of cells destined for survival or death are shown in Figure 3.6. This figure underscores the many problems associated with trying to quantify or ascribe a particular form of cell death after irradiation and the importance of the clonogenic survival assay for determining the ultimate response of individually irradiated cells.

## 'Bystander' death

A much less understood type of cell death that has been described in response to irradiation is known as bystander-induced death (11). A number of experiments have challenged the widely held view that radiation kills cells exclusively by direct damage. The bystander effect describes a phenomenon in which cell death can occur in cells due to irradiation of neighbouring cells. Evidence for this effect has come from studies using high linear energy transfer $\alpha$-particles in which a larger fraction of cells die than are estimated to have been traversed. Supportive data have also been generated using microbeam irradiation, in which select cells or nuclei can be irradiated with particles (both $\alpha$-particles and protons have been used) or soft X-rays. In these experiments, irradiation of a select group of cells leads to increased cell death in the non-irradiated cells. In addition to cell death, bystander effects have also been observed for other known biological effects of irradiation including DNA damage, chromosomal aberrations, mutation, transformation and gene expression.

The precise mechanism or importance of bystander effects has not been determined and its observations have been largely limited to *in vitro* culture conditions. Some studies have shown that transfer of media from irradiated cells to non-irradiated cells can also cause the bystander effect. This would suggest that irradiated cells secrete factors which can be damaging to non-irradiated cells. Other experiments have shown that bystander effects are more easily observed when cells are physically connected to irradiated cells by gap junctions. This allows communication (transfer or molecules) directly between the cells. For example, irradiation may cause increased levels of long-lived reactive oxygen species which could be shared among irradiated and non-irradiated cells. The bystander effect is likely most important at low doses of radiation which cause damage to only a small number of cells, and may thus be of most relevance to risk estimation.

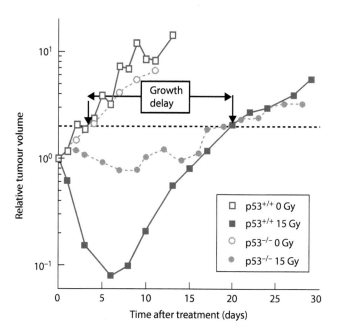

**Figure 3.5** Although the mode of cell death may not affect the overall number of cells that die, it can dramatically affect the timing of their death. In this tumour regrowth experiment from (2), tumours composed of p53 wild-type and knockout cells are irradiated and followed as a function of time. The unirradiated tumours grow at a similar rate. However, the p53 wild-type tumours undergo rapid apoptosis after irradiation and the tumours thus also shrink rapidly in size. The p53 knockout tumours do not undergo apoptosis and thus are considerably larger after irradiation during this first week. However, the total regrowth delay (measured when tumours reach twice their starting size) is identical for the two tumour types. This indicates that the total number of cells killed by irradiation is the same in both tumour types. In this case, apoptosis alters the speed at which the cells die, but does not affect the total number of initially irradiated cells that eventually will die.

Clonogenic unirradiated cell

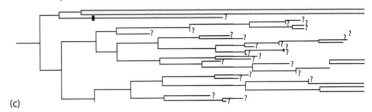

(a)

Clonogenic irradiated cell –
increased post-mitotic apoptosis

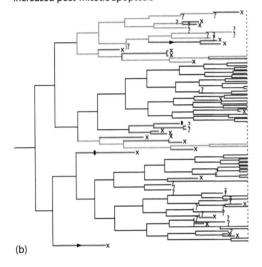

(b)

Clonogenic irradiated cell –
increased post-mitotic senescence

(c)

Non-clonogenic irradiated cell –
pre-mitotic apoptosis

(d) ————————————x

Non-clonogenic irradiated cell –
post-mitotic apoptosis

(e)

Non-clonogenic irradiated cell –
post-mitotic senescence

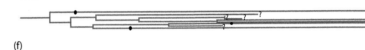

(f)

**Figure 3.6** Fate of several irradiated cells as a function of time (left to right) following exposure to radiation. (a) An unirradiated cell is shown as an example. Each cell division is indicated by a split of one line into two. After six or seven divisions, enough cell progeny have been created to produce a colony that can be scored as a survivor. The initial cell is thus said to be clonogenic. Two cells that survive irradiation and eventually form colonies are shown in (b) and (c). In (b), the first division produces two daughter cells that both progress to mitosis and divide, producing four cells. One of these four cells dies by apoptosis. Another one undergoes several more divisions but produces progeny which all eventually die. The other two cells both produce many surviving progeny which contribute to the long-term clonogenic potential of the initially irradiated cell. Note that many of the progeny die in this case even though the initial cell has 'survived'. In (c) the irradiated cell also is clonogenic. In this case, one of the first two daughter cells produces cells which all eventually undergo senescence. Irradiated cells that are non-clonogenic are shown in (d), (e) and (f). In (d), a cell dies by apoptosis prior to mitosis. In (e) cells die by apoptosis after completing two divisions and in (e) cells undergo senescence after undergoing one or more mitosis. (Adapted from (6).)

## Key points

1. Most cell death is controlled or programmed in some way.
2. Major death pathways include apoptosis, senescence, autophagy and necrosis.
3. Measuring one form of cell death (e.g. apoptosis) will not necessarily correlate with how many cells die.
4. The form of cell death may influence the rate at which cells die and thus tumour regression.
5. Most cell death after radiation occurs late in response to mitotic catastrophe and not from the initial response to damage.

■ BIBLIOGRAPHY

1. Brown JM, Attardi LD. The role of apoptosis in cancer development and treatment response. *Nat Rev Cancer* 2005;5:231–237.
2. Brown JM, Wouters BG. Apoptosis, p53, and tumor cell sensitivity to anticancer agents. *Cancer Res* 1999;59:1391–1399.
3. Campisi J, d'Adda di Fagagna F. Cellular senescence: When bad things happen to good cells. *Nat Rev Mol Cell Biol* 2007;8:729–740.
4. Chu K, Teele N, Dewey MW, Albright N, Dewey WC. Computerized video time lapse study of cell cycle delay and arrest, mitotic catastrophe, apoptosis and clonogenic survival in irradiated 14-3-3sigma and CDKN1A p21 knockout cell lines. *Radiat Res* 2004;162:270–286.

5. Endlich B, Radford IR, Forrester HB, Dewey WC. Computerized video time-lapse microscopy studies of ionizing radiation-induced rapid-interphase and mitosis-related apoptosis in lymphoid cells. *Radiat Res* 2000;153:36–48.

6. Forrester HB, Vidair CA, Albright N, Ling CC, Dewey WC. Using computerized video time lapse for quantifying cell death of X-irradiated rat embryo cells transfected with c-myc or c-Ha-ras. *Cancer Res* 1999;59:931–939.

7. Garcia-Barros M, Paris F, Cordon-Cardo C et al. Tumor response to radiotherapy regulated by endothelial cell apoptosis. *Science* 2003;300:1155–1159.

8. Green DR, Levine B. To be or not to be? How selective autophagy and cell death govern cell fate. *Cell* 2014;157: 65–75.

9. Hayflick L. The limited *in vitro* lifetime of human diploid cell strains. *Exp Cell Res* 1965;37:614–636.

10. Klionsky DJ. Autophagy: From phenomenology to molecular understanding in less than a decade. *Nat Rev Mol Cell Biol* 2007;8:931–937.

11. Mothersill C, Seymour CB. Radiation-induced bystander effects – Implications for cancer. *Nat Rev Cancer* 2004;4: 158–164.

12. Okada H, Mak TW. Pathways of apoptotic and non-apoptotic death in tumour cells. *Nat Rev Cancer* 2004;4:592–603.

13. Rubinsztein DC, Gestwicki JE, Murphy LO, Klionsky DJ. Potential therapeutic applications of autophagy. *Nat Rev Drug Discov* 2007;6:304–312.

14. Taylor RC, Cullen SP, Martin SJ. Apoptosis: Controlled demolition at the cellular level. *Nat Rev Mol Cell Biol* 2008;9: 231–241.

15. Wouters BG, Giaccia AJ, Denko NC, Brown JM. Loss of p21Waf1/Cip1 sensitizes tumors to radiation by an apoptosis-independent mechanism. *Cancer Res* 1997;57:4703–4706.

## ■ FURTHER READING

16. Ichim G, Tait SW. A fate worse than death: Apoptosis as an oncogenic process. *Nat Rev Cancer* 2016;16:539–548.

# Quantifying cell kill and cell survival

MICHAEL C. JOINER

## 4.1 CONCEPT OF CLONOGENIC CELLS

As explained in detail in Chapters 14 and 15, the maintenance of tissue size and therefore of tissue function in the normal renewal tissues of the body depends upon the existence of a small number of primitive 'stem cells' – cells that have the capacity to maintain their own numbers while at the same time producing cells that can differentiate and proliferate to replace the rest of the functional cell population. Stem cells are at the base of the hierarchy of cells that make up the haemopoietic and epithelial tissues.

Carcinomas are derived from such hierarchical epithelial tissues, and our ability to recognise this in histological sections derives from the fact that these tumours often maintain many of the features of differentiation of the tissue within which they arose. Well-differentiated tumours do this to a greater extent than anaplastic (poorly differentiated) tumours. It follows that not all the cells in a tumour are neoplastic stem cells: some have embarked on an irreversible process of differentiation. In addition, carcinomas also contain many cells that make up the stroma (fibroblasts, endothelial cells, macrophages, etc.). Stem cells thus may comprise only a small proportion of all the cells within a tumour.

When a tumour regrows after non-curative treatment, it does so because some neoplastic stem cells were not killed. We have therefore recognized that the key to understanding tumour response is to ask: How many stem cells are left? If we can eradicate the last neoplastic stem cell, then the tumour cannot regrow. It is difficult to reliably recognise true tumour stem cells *in situ*, and therefore, assays have been developed that allow them to be detected after removal from the tumour. These assays generally detect stem cells by their ability to form a cell colony within some growth environment. We therefore call these 'clonogenic' or 'colony-forming' cells – cells that form colonies exceeding about 50 cells within a defined growth environment. The number 50 represents five to six generations of proliferation. It is chosen in order to exclude cells that have a limited growth potential as a result of having embarked on differentiation, or having been critically, but not immediately lethally, damaged by therapeutic treatment.

Cells damaged by exposure to radiation may therefore not die immediately (see Chapter 3) and they may produce a modest family of descendants. This is illustrated in Figure 4.1. The growth of single mouse L-cells was observed microscopically and one selected colony was irradiated with 200 röntgens of X-rays at the four-cell stage (29). The röntgen is an old radiation unit, roughly equivalent to 1 cGy. Subsequent growth was carefully recorded and in the figure each vertical line indicates the lifetime of a cell from birth at mitosis to its subsequent division. The two irradiated cells on the left and the right of this figure produced continuously expanding colonies, although some daughter cells had long intermitotic times. The other two irradiated cells fared badly: they underwent a number of irregular divisions, including a tripolar mitosis. But note that at the end of the experiment cells are present from each of the original four cells: the difference is that two produced expanding colonies and the other two did not. The first two were 'surviving clonogenic cells' and the other two are usually described as 'killed' by radiation, since their regrowth is probably unimportant for clinical outcome. It would be more precise to say that two of the cells *lost their proliferative ability* as a result of irradiation.

Some cells fail to undergo even one division after irradiation. Interphase cell death can occur in many cell types at very high radiation doses, and at conventional therapeutic dose levels it is characteristic of lymphoid cells and some cells in the intestinal crypts. Although interphase cell death and apoptosis are related concepts (see Chapter 3), they are not synonymous for the same process. But the practical radiotherapeutic view is that it is loss of reproductive integrity that is the critical response to irradiation (either in tumour or normal tissue cells): this occurs within a few hours of irradiation through damage to the genome, and the subsequent metabolic and death processes are 'downstream' of this event.

## 4.2 CLONOGENIC ASSAYS

Clonogenic assays have formed the basis of cellular response studies in tumours, and also in some normal tissues. The basic idea is to remove cells from the tumour, place them in a defined growth environment and test for their ability to produce a sizeable colony of descendants. Many types of assay have been described; we illustrate the principle by a simple assay in tissue culture that is analogous to a microbiological assay.

A single-cell suspension of tumour cells is prepared and divided into two parts. One is irradiated and the other is kept as an unirradiated control. The two suspensions are then plated out in tissue culture under identical conditions, except

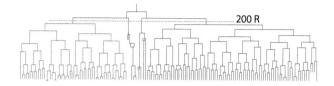

**Figure 4.1** Pedigree of a clone of mouse L-cells irradiated with a dose of 200 R (i.e. röntgens) at the four-cell stage, illustrating the concept of surviving and non-surviving clonogenic cells. (From (29), with permission.)

that since we anticipate that radiation has killed some cells, we will have to plate a larger number of the irradiated cells. We here envisage plating 100 control cells and 200 irradiated cells. After a suitable period of incubation, maybe 2 weeks, the colonies are scored (Figure 4.2). There are 40 control colonies, and we therefore say that the plating efficiency was 40/100 = 0.4. The plating efficiency of the treated cells is lower: 16/200 = 0.08. We calculate a surviving fraction as the ratio of these plating efficiencies:

$$\text{Surviving fraction} = \frac{PE_{treated}}{PE_{control}} = \frac{0.08}{0.4} = 0.2$$

thus correcting for the efficiency with which undamaged clonogenic cells are detected and for the different numbers of cells plated. Surviving fraction is often given as a percentage (20% in this case).

The above description started with a suspension of tumour cells. In order to measure *in vivo* cell survival, we take two groups of experimental tumours (often subcutaneously implanted tumours in mice), irradiate one and keep the other as a control, then at some time after irradiation we make cell suspensions from both groups and plate them out under identical conditions as before. The difference here is that the cells are irradiated under *in vivo* conditions.

Although colony assays have formed a central place in tumour radiobiology, they are not without artefacts. Bearing in mind that the numbers of cells plated will often differ between control and treated cultures, a key question is whether colony counts increase linearly with the number of cells plated. If they do not, then this will lead to errors in cell survival. The colonies in Figure 4.2 have been drawn to illustrate a feature

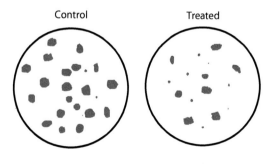

**Figure 4.2** The principle of measuring a cell surviving fraction (see text).

of colony assays that was mentioned in the previous section. Irradiation not only reduces the colony numbers, it also increases the proportion of smaller colonies: very tiny colonies represent clones that eventually die out; others may arise from cells that have suffered non-lethal injury that reduces colony growth rate. Very tiny colonies do not reach the accepted cut-off of 50 cells and so they are not counted, although their implications for the evaluation of radiation effects on tumours may be worthy of greater attention (23).

## 4.3 CELL SURVIVAL CURVES

A cell survival curve is a plot of surviving fraction $S$ against dose $D$ (of radiation, cytotoxic drug or other cell-killing agent). Figure 4.3a shows that when plotted on linear scales, the survival curve for cells irradiated in tissue culture is often reverse-sigmoid: there is a shoulder followed by a curve that asymptotically approaches zero survival. To indicate the sensitivity of the cells to radiation, we could just read off the dose that kills say 50% of the cells. This is sometimes called the ED50 (i.e. effect dose 50%). Sometimes ED90 is used. In doing this we need make no assumptions about the shape of the curve.

There are two reasons why cell survival curves are more usually plotted on a logarithmic scale of survival:

1. If cell killing is random, then survival will be an exponential function of dose, and this will be a straight line on a semi-log plot. Section 4.8 explains this in detail.
2. A logarithmic scale more easily allows us to see and compare the very low cell survivals required to obtain a significant reduction in tumour size, or even local tumour control.

Such a plot is illustrated in Figure 4.3b. The shapes of radiation survival curves and ways of describing their steepness are dealt with later in this chapter.

Note that for the data shown in Figure 4.3, radiation doses above 5 Gy reduce the survival of clonogenic cells to below 10%. Measurement of radiosensitivity in terms of the parameter $D_0$ (Section 4.8) is made on the exponential part of the survival curve, which in this case is above 5 Gy. These measurements are therefore made in a dose range where the surviving fraction is very low. Such $D_0$ values are relevant to the problem of exterminating the last few clonogenic cells, but if the cell population contains cells of differing radiosensitivity, these values may not be typical of the radiosensitivity of the bulk of the tumour cell population.

## 4.4 ASSAYS FOR THE SURVIVAL OF CLONOGENIC CELLS

Many techniques have been described for detecting colony formation by tumour cells and thus for measuring cell survival. They almost all require first the production of single-cell suspensions. This is usually not straightforward,

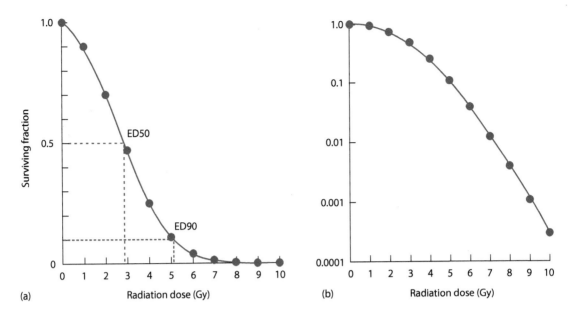

**Figure 4.3** A typical cell survival curve for cells irradiated in tissue culture, plotted (a) on a linear survival scale and (b) on a logarithmic scale.

because tumour tissues differ widely in the ease with which they can be disaggregated. Enzymes such as trypsin, collagenase and pronase are often used and some tissues can be disaggregated mechanically.

Such techniques can also be used for the assay of colony-forming cells in normal tissues, especially the haemopoietic tissues that can easily be sampled and made into cell suspensions. In addition, a variety of *in situ* assays for normal tissue stem cells have been described (21). The following are some of the principal assays that have been used for tumour cells.

### *In vitro* colony assays

Some tumour cells grow well attached to plastic tissue culture dishes or flasks. Others can be encouraged to do so by first laying down a feeder layer of lethally irradiated connective tissue or tumour cells. For cells that have been established as an *in vitro* cell line this often works well, but for studies on tumour samples taken directly from patients or animals it is commonly observed that normal tissue fibroblasts grow better than the tumour cells and often overgrow the cultures.

An alternative is to thicken the growth medium with agar or methylcellulose. This inhibits the growth of anchorage-requiring cell types, but many epithelial cells will still grow. An assay of this type is that of Courtenay and Mills (6) for human tumour cells. Agar cultures are grown in 15 mL plastic tubes overlaid with liquid medium that can regularly be replenished. The addition of rat red blood cells to the agar was found to promote the growth of a number of human tumour cell types. An important feature of the Courtenay-Mills assay was the use of a low oxygen tension (a gas phase of 90% nitrogen, 5% oxygen and 5% carbon dioxide) which enhanced the plating efficiency of human tumour cells.

It is noted that 5% ($\approx$40 mm Hg) is the oxygen tension approximating to venous blood.

### Spleen colony assay

Till and McCulloch (28) showed that when mouse bone marrow cells were injected intravenously into syngeneic recipients that had received sufficient whole-body irradiation to suppress endogenous haemopoiesis, colonies were produced in the spleen which derived from the stem cells in the graft. The colonies varied in morphology (erythroid, granulocyte or mixed) and these stem cells are therefore termed *pluripotent*. Their precise identity was not known and they are therefore often called *colony-forming units* (CFUs). Using this assay, Till and McCulloch obtained the first survival curve for bone marrow cells and found it to be very steep. The spleen colony assay has also been used for some types of mouse lymphoma cells.

### Lung colony assay

This is analogous to the spleen colony assay and is applicable to any transplanted mouse tumour that readily forms colonies in the lung following intravenous injection of a single-cell suspension. The cloning efficiency can often be increased by mixing the test cells with an excess ($\sim$10$^6$ per injection) of lethally irradiated tumour cells or plastic microspheres, which perhaps act by increasing the trapping of injected tumour cells in the lung. Not all the tumour cells grow: a few colonies per thousand tumour cells injected would be regarded as satisfactory. Although colonies are formed throughout the lung, they are usually scored only on the lung surface. The method was developed by Hill and

Stanley (11) on two experimental tumours and they give further experimental details.

## Limiting-dilution assay

This is a non-cloning assay that was used in early radiation cell survival studies and which for some experimental tumours has the advantage of high sensitivity. The principle of the method is to prepare a suspension of tumour cells and to make a large number of subcutaneous implants into syngeneic animals, covering a range of inoculum sizes and if possible spanning the level of 50% tumour takes. The animals, usually mice, are then observed for a long enough period to record nearly every tumour that can grow from a single-cell implant. Take-rate is plotted against inoculum size and the point of 50% takes is interpolated; this is usually called the 'TD50' cell number. The experiment is performed simultaneously on treated cells and control cells and the surviving fraction is given by the ratio of the TD50 values. The addition of an excess of lethally irradiated cells improves the take-rate; using this manoeuvre Steel and Adams (25) found a TD50 of one to three cells for the Lewis lung tumour and were thus able to measure cell survival down to $10^{-6}$. The method only works well in the absence of an immune response against the tumour grafts, a relatively uncommon situation especially with chemically and virally induced tumours.

## Short-term *in vitro* assays

Development of *in vitro* assays that yield a quicker result than a true clonogenic assay has arisen from the continuing efforts to develop reliable prediction of tumour response to treatment (see Chapter 21). A variety of assays have been exhaustively tested but their poor reliability and reproducibility in practice have often been a limit to their clinical usefulness. Three common pitfalls are as follows:

1. Biopsy samples of human tumours contain both tumour cells and normal connective-tissue cells; both may grow under the assay conditions and it may be difficult to distinguish colony formation by tumour cells.
2. If the method requires the production of single-cell suspensions, great care must be taken to exclude cell clumps, for these may preferentially give rise to scorable colonies.
3. Radiation-killed cells take time to die (e.g. Figure 4.1) and in a short-term assay they may be confused with genuine surviving tumour cells; therefore, the method may not easily distinguish between radiosensitive cells and cells that die rapidly after irradiation.

Many basic principles underlying the prediction of tumour response are dealt with in the book edited by Chapman et al. (4) and reviewed more recently by Coleman

et al. (5). Non-clonogenic assays for tumour cells include the following:

*The Micronucleus Test:* Tumour cells are cultured in the presence of cytochalasin-B which blocks cytokinesis, creates binucleate cells and thus allows nuclei that have undergone one post-treatment division to be identified. Micronuclei can be scored as small extranuclear bodies. Their frequency increases with radiation dose and gives a measure of radiation sensitivity (27). The reliability of the method is limited by the fact that diploid, polyploid and aneuploid cells may differ in their tolerance of genetic loss and therefore of micronucleus formation.

*Cell Growth Assays:* A variety of methods have been used to measure the growth of cultures derived from treated and control tumour specimens, thus to derive a measure of radiosensitivity or chemosensitivity. Incorporation of radioisotopes such as $^3$H-thymidine has been widely used. MTT is a tetrazolium salt (3-[4,5 dimethylthiazol-2-yl]-2,5-diphenyl tetrazolium bromide) that can be used to stain cell cultures and thus by a colorimetric assay to estimate the extent of growth (2,30). It can be used to evaluate growth in microtitre plates, and with careful attention to technical factors it can yield a measure of radiosensitivity. MTS (3-[4,5-dimethylthiazol-2-yl]-5-[3-carboxymethoxyphenyl]-2-[4-sulfonyl]-2H-tetrazolium) is a development of MTT and forms soluble formazans upon bioreduction by the cells. This has the advantage that it eliminates the error-prone solubilisation step which is required for the microculture tetrazolium assays which employ MTT (10). Such methods are vulnerable to the variable growth of fibroblasts and for studies on leukaemic cells it may be preferable to stain the cells differentially and analyse the cultures microscopically (1).

*DNA Damage Assays:* It is possible to measure DNA damage directly by antibody detection of foci of phosphorylated histone H2AX ($\gamma$H2AX) in the cell nucleus, using image cytometry or flow cytometry. It has been found that the rate of $\gamma$H2AX loss (a measure of DNA repair) correlates with cellular radiosensitivity measured with a clonogenic assay, although the relationship is by no means perfect (18). Moreover, the percentage of tumour cells that retain $\gamma$H2AX foci 24 hours after single or fractionated doses of radiation can correlate with cellular radiosensitivity (15,16) though this measurement does not have great accuracy or reproducibility which makes it of limited use clinically.

## Methods using precise cell counting

The methods so far described involve the plating of an aliquot of a cell suspension that *on average* will contain a known number of cells. The *actual* number of cells will vary according to Poisson statistics. For studies of the effects of low radiation doses (where the effects are small), greater statistical precision can be achieved by knowing *exactly* how many cells have been plated. This has been done using two principal methods. A fluorescence-activated cell sorter (FACS) allows counted numbers of cells to be plated into culture dishes (8). An alternative is to use a microscopic live cell recognition system (19) which allows the spatial coordinates of plated cells to be recorded; subsequently, the colony formation by each individual cell can be examined. Both of these methods give high precision in the initial region of a cell survival curve and their use led to the identification of low-dose hyper-radiosensitivity (HRS) (Section 4.14).

## 4.5 COMPARISON OF ASSAYS

Intercomparison of the results of assays of cell survival can provide an important check on their validity. This information can be valuable both at a practical and a fundamental level. At the practical level, it is logical to check a rapid short-term assay against the results of a more laborious but more reliable clonogenic assay. The more general question is whether assay of cell survival in two different growth environments does actually identify the same population of surviving tumour cells. It is usually cell survival *in situ* in the patient or in the experimental animal that we seek to determine, and to subject tumour cells to extraction procedures and to artificial growth environments might well produce artefacts. It is therefore reassuring that some careful comparisons between clonogenic assays *in vitro*, in the mouse lung and by subcutaneous transplantation, have demonstrated good agreement for mouse tumours (26).

## 4.6 DESCRIBING RELATIONSHIPS BETWEEN CELL SURVIVAL AND RADIATION DOSE

Research in experimental radiobiology encompasses studies across the cellular, animal and human levels. It deals at the fundamental level with the molecular, biochemical and biophysical nature of radiation damage. Descriptive models are therefore a necessary part of radiobiology research: they provide a framework in which to analyse, compare and discuss data and ultimately to assist in building up consistent theories of radiation action both *in vitro* and *in vivo*. Models and mathematics are also necessary to relate experimental studies to clinical cancer treatment with the aim of improving therapy. In the following sections, we explain the most important models that are used to describe and analyse the relationships between cell survival and radiation dose. It is important primarily to understand that no single model can describe all possible situations. Particularly, it is not possible to have one model which will describe response across the complete range of dose from very low to very high, unless that model is so complex as to make it of no practical use clinically because of the excessive uncertainty in model predictions.

## 4.7 A NOTE ON RADIATION RESPONSE AT THE MOLECULAR LEVEL

Radiation kills cells by producing secondary charged particles and free radicals in the nucleus which in turn produce a variety of types of damage in DNA. Evidence that damage to DNA is the primary cause of radiation cell killing and mutation is set out in Chapters 2 and 3. Each 1 Gy dose of low linear energy transfer (LET) radiation produces over 1000 base damages, about 1000 initial single-strand breaks and approximately 20–40 initial double-strand breaks (DSBs). Some lesions are more important than others and radiation lethality correlates most significantly with the number of residual, unrepaired DSBs several hours after irradiation. If cell kill is modified by changing LET, oxygen level, thiol concentration or temperature, then for a fixed radiation dose only the number of DSBs reliably correlates with the change in cell kill. Single-strand breaks, base damage and DNA-protein cross-links do not reflect the change in cell kill for all of these modifiers. The DNA DSB is therefore the most important type of cellular radiation damage. Just one residual DSB (or 'hit') in a vital section of DNA may be sufficient to produce a significant chromosome aberration and thus to sterilise the cell.

Despite this knowledge of how radiation actually kills cells, it has not been possible to translate this understanding at the molecular level directly into models which can be used simply and easily within daily clinical practice to describe, discuss and categorize the factors which govern the differences seen in response with dose. Cruder more general approaches have been more successful in this regard and are described in the following sections.

## 4.8 TARGET THEORY

A simple way of modelling how radiation kills cells is the idea that there may be specific regions of the DNA that are important to maintain the reproductive ability of cells. These sensitive regions could be thought of as specific targets for radiation damage so that the survival of a cell after radiation exposure would be related to the number of targets inactivated. There are two versions of this idea that have commonly been used. The first and simplest version is that just one hit by radiation on a single sensitive target would lead to death of the cell. This is called *single-target single-hit inactivation*, and it leads to the form of survival curve shown in Figure 4.4a. The survival curve is exponential (i.e. a straight line on a semi-logarithmic plot of cell surviving fraction $S$ against dose $D$). To derive an equation for this survival curve, Poisson statistics can be applied. The presumption is that during irradiation there are a very large number of hits on different cells taking place, but the probability ($p$) of the next hit occurring in a given cell is very small. Thus, for each cell,

$$p(\text{survival}) = p(0 \text{ hits}) = \exp(-D/D_0)$$

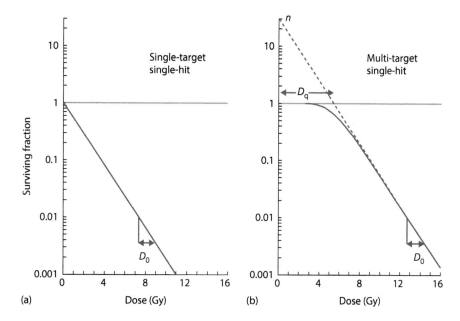

**Figure 4.4** The two most common types of target theory: (a) single-target inactivation and (b) multi-target inactivation.

where $D_0$ is defined as the dose that gives an average of one hit per target. A dose of $D_0$ Gy reduces survival from 1 to 0.37 (i.e. to $e^{-1}$), or from 0.1 to 0.037, etc. $D/D_0$ is the average number of hits per target (and in this case per cell). This is the reason why (e.g. in Figure 4.7) a scale of cell survival is sometimes labelled $-\log_e(S)$ or $-\ln(S)$: this is a scale of the natural logarithm of surviving fraction $S$ and in this model it is also the equivalent number of 'lethal lesions' per cell.

In this example (Figure 4.4a), $D_0 = 1.6$ Gy. Straight survival curves of this sort are usually found for the inactivation of viruses and bacteria. They may also be appropriate in describing the radiation response of some very sensitive human cells (normal and malignant) and also the radiation response at very low dose rates (see Chapter 13) and response to high LET radiations (see Chapter 6). This type of 'single-target single-hit' cell survival curve model is therefore valid outside of the 'target theory' framework. It describes the simple situation where if an individual cell receives an amount of radiation greater than $D_0$ then it will more likely die ($S < 37\%$), or an amount of radiation less than $0.5D_0$ it will more likely survive ($S > 60\%$).

For mammalian cells in general, their response to radiation is more usually described by 'shouldered' survival curves. To model this type of response, a more general version of target theory can be used called *multi-target single-hit inactivation*. In this extended target idea, the cell has $n$ sensitive targets rather than just a single target, and just one hit by radiation on each and every one of those $n$ targets is required for death of the cell. The shape of this survival curve is shown in Figure 4.4b. Again, the argument can be developed using Poisson statistics:

$$p(0 \text{ hits on a specific target}) = \exp(-D/D_0)$$

Thus,

$$p(\text{that specific target inactivated}) = 1 - \exp(-D/D_0)$$

As there are $n$ putative targets in the cell,

$$p(\text{all of } n \text{ targets inactivated}) = (1 - \exp(-D/D_0))^n$$

Thus,

$$p(\text{survival}) = p(\text{not all of } n \text{ targets inactivated})$$
$$= 1 - (1 - \exp(-D/D_0))^n \qquad (4.1)$$

Figure 4.4b shows that multi-target single-hit survival curves have an initial shoulder whose size can be indicated by the quasi-threshold dose ($D_q$). This is related to $n$ and $D_0$ by the following relation:

$$D_q = D_0 \log_e n \qquad (4.2)$$

For the example in Figure 4.4b, we have chosen $n = 30$ and $D_0 = 1.6$ Gy, giving $D_q = 5.4$ Gy. Such simple multi-target survival curves can be useful for describing the radiation response of mammalian cells at high doses, 'off the shoulder'. Such high doses (per fraction), even above 18 Gy, might now be given to patients using stereotactic body radiation therapy (SBRT), for example in early stage non-small cell lung cancer. Multi-target survival curves per se clearly do not describe the survival response well at lower more conventional clinical doses (per fraction) (e.g. 2 Gy).

## 4.9 A PROBLEM WITH TARGETS

The derivation of simple cell survival relationships in terms of targets and hits, particularly the straight survival curve shown in Figure 4.4a, is an intellectually attractive and still sometimes convenient idea, often within the context of high-LET radiations, and it dominated radiobiological thinking for a long time. The term '$D_0$' is still in common usage. Although descriptively useful, a key difficulty with this concept is that specific localized radiation targets, for example highly sensitive regions of the DNA, have not been identified for mammalian cells, despite considerable effort to search for them. Rather, what has emerged is the important role of all DNA strand breaks and their repair, with sites for such DNA damage being generally dispersed throughout the cell nucleus (see Chapter 2). An obvious shortcoming of the basic multi-target model is that, as shown in Figure 4.4b, it predicts a response that is flat for very low radiation doses. This is not supported by experimental data: there is overwhelming evidence for significant cell killing at low doses and for cell survival curves that have a finite initial slope. To take account of this, the multi-target model can be adjusted by adding an additional single-target component. The resulting equation for the survival curve is called the *two-component model*:

$$p(\text{survival}) = \exp(-D/D_1)$$
$$\times \left(1 - (1 - \exp(-D(1/D_0 - 1/D_1)))^n\right) \quad (4.3)$$

This type of survival curve is illustrated in Figure 4.5a. In addition to the parameters $n$, $D_0$ and $D_q$, this curve also has a parameter $D_1$ which fixes an initial slope (i.e. the dose required in the low-dose region to reduce survival from

1 to 0.37). In this example, $n = 30$ and $D_0 = 1.6$ Gy, and $D_1 = 4.6$ Gy. This type of curve can now more correctly predict finite cell killing in the low-dose region but it still has the drawback that the *change* in cell survival over the range 0 to $D_q$ occurs almost linearly. This implies that no sparing of damage should occur as dose per fraction is reduced below 2 Gy, which is usually not found to be the case either experimentally or in clinical radiotherapy (see Figures 9.1 and 9.2; Chapter 11). A way of overcoming this limitation would be to use a multi-target instead of single-target component as the initial slope. However, this would make the model far too complicated to be useful in comparing survival responses. It would require at least four parameters, and would be of little value in helping to understand the fundamental mechanisms determining radiation effect or in characterizing clinical responses.

## 4.10 THE LINEAR-QUADRATIC MODEL

The continually downward bending form of a cell survival can simply be fitted by a second-order polynomial, with a zero constant term to ensure that $S = 1$ at zero dose. This is exactly the formulation that is termed the linear-quadratic (LQ) model. Although we can regard this as based on pure mathematics (i.e. the simplest formula which can describe a curve), it has often been possible to usefully link radiobiological mechanisms to this model, most notably with the increase in number of dicentric or centric-ring chromosomes with dose (17). The formula for cell survival is

$$-\ln(S) = \alpha D + \beta D^2$$

$$p(\text{survival}) = \exp\left(-\alpha D - \beta D^2\right) \quad (4.4)$$

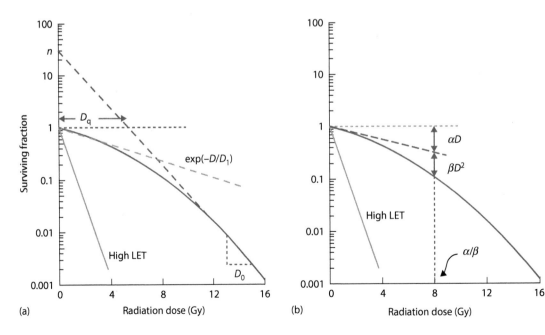

Figure 4.5 Models with non-exponential cell killing but a finite initial slope: (a) the two-component model and (b) the LQ model.

and the cell survival curve is drawn in Figure 4.5b. Although the shapes of the LQ model and the more complicated two-component model are superficially similar (compare Figures 4.5a and 4.5b), the simple LQ formula gives a better description of radiation response in the low-dose region (0–3 Gy): LQ survival curves are continuously bending with no straight portion either at low or high radiation doses. The shape (or 'bendiness') is determined by the value of $\alpha/\beta$.

Since the dimensions of the parameters are $\alpha$: $Gy^{-1}$ and $\beta$: $Gy^{-2}$, the dimensions of $\alpha/\beta$ are Gy: as shown in Figure 4.5b, this is the dose at which the linear contribution to damage ($\alpha D$ on the logarithmic scale) equals the quadratic contribution ($\beta D^2$). The response of cells to densely ionizing radiations like neutrons or $\alpha$-particles is usually a steep and almost exponential survival curve (see Figure 6.2). As shown in Figure 4.5, this would be explained in the two-component model by the ratio $D_1/D_0$ being near to 1, or in the LQ model by a very high $\alpha/\beta$ value.

As shown in Figure 4.5, the basic LQ model does not have a $D_0$ because the survival curve continuously bends downwards with increasing dose and so it is never completely straight. However, it is sometimes useful to be able to roughly convert between $\alpha$, $\beta$ and $D_0$ for example, if comparing two sets of research findings which have each been described with the different models. The precise mathematical description of $D_0$ is that it is the inverse of the first-order differential of $-\ln(S)$ with respect to dose. Applying this definition to the LQ model gives $D_0 = 1/(\alpha + 2\beta D)$. This formula shows that in the LQ model, the effective $D_0$ is not constant, but decreases with increasing dose.

The LQ model is widely used in both experimental and clinical radiobiology and generally works well in describing responses to radiation *in vitro* and also *in vivo*. What could be its mechanistic justification? One simple idea is that lethal dicentric or centric-ring chromosomes relate to the linear component ($\exp[-\alpha D]$) arising from a single electron track intersecting both of two adjacent chromosomes and the quadratic component ($\exp[-\beta D^2]$) arising from two independent electron tracks each intersecting one of two adjacent chromosomes (17). This interpretation is also supported by studies of the dose-rate effect (see Chapter 13) which show that as dose rate is reduced, cell survival curves become straight and tend to extrapolate the initial slope of the high dose-rate curve: the quadratic component of cell killing disappears, leaving only the linear component. This would be because at low dose rate, single-track events will occur farther apart in time and the probability of interaction between them in two adjacent chromosomes will be low. Although this interpretation of the LQ equation seems reasonable, the nature of the actual interactions between separate tracks is still a matter of some debate. Chadwick and Leenhouts (3) postulated that separate tracks might hit opposite strands of the DNA double helix and thus form a DSB. We now know that this is unlikely in view of the very low probability of two tracks interacting within the dimensions of the DNA molecule (diameter $\sim$2.5 nanometers) at a dose of a few grays. Interaction between more widely spaced regions of the complex DNA structure, or between DNA in different chromosomes, is a more plausible mechanism (see Chapter 2).

## 4.11 THE LETHAL, POTENTIALLY LETHAL DAMAGE MODEL

Curtis (7) proposed this model as a 'unified repair model' of cell killing. Ionizing radiation is considered to produce two different types of lesion: repairable (i.e. *potentially* lethal) lesions and non-repairable (i.e. lethal) lesions. The non-repairable lesions produce 'single-hit' lethal effects and therefore give rise to a linear component of cell killing ($= \exp[-\alpha D]$). The eventual effect of the repairable lesions depends on competing processes of repair and binary misrepair. This latter process leads to a quadratic component in cell killing. As shown in Figure 4.6, the model has two sensitivity parameters ($\eta_L$ determines the number of non-repairable lesions produced per unit dose, and $\eta_{PL}$ the number of repairable lesions). There are also two rate constants ($\varepsilon_{PL}$ determines the rate of repair of repairable lesions, and $\varepsilon_{2PL}$ the rate at which they undergo interaction and thus misrepair).

This model produces almost identical cell survival curves to the LQ equation, down to a survival level of perhaps $10^{-2}$ below which the relationship between $-\ln(S)$ and dose becomes more linear as dose increases. It can therefore be taken to provide one possible mechanistic interpretation of the LQ equation as well as more accurately modelling the response to high radiation doses or doses per fraction. It also correctly predicts that as dose rate is reduced, the probability of binary interaction of potentially lethal lesions will fall and parameter values can be found that allow the model accurately to simulate cell survival data on human and animal cells irradiated at various dose rates (see Chapter 13).

## 4.12 REPAIR SATURATION MODELS

Curtis' lethal, potentially lethal (LPL) model is an example of a lesion-interaction model which also incorporates repair processes. Figure 4.7a shows how this produces the

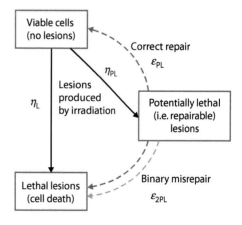

Figure 4.6 The LPL damage model of radiation action.

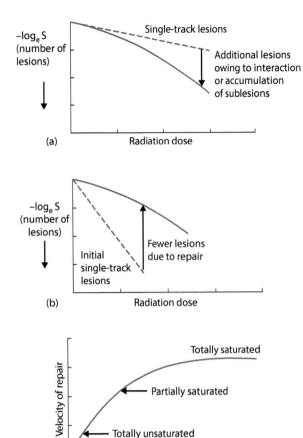

Figure 4.7 The contrast between lesion-interaction models and repair-saturation models: (a) the LPL model, (b) the effect of repair becoming less effective at higher radiation doses and (c) the basic concept of repair saturation. (Adapted from (9), with permission.)

downward-bending cell survival curve: the dashed curve indicates the component of cell killing that is due to single-track non-repairable lesions. It is the *extra* lethal lesions produced by the binary interaction of potentially lethal lesions which give the downward-bending curve.

Another class of models is the repair saturation models, which propose that the shape of the survival curve depends only on a dose-dependent rate of repair. Figures 4.7b and 4.7c demonstrate this idea. Only one type of lesion and

single-hit killing are postulated, and in the absence of any repair these lesions produce the steep dashed survival curve in Figure 4.7b. The final survival curve (solid line) results from repair of some of these lesions but if the repair enzymes become saturated (Figure 4.7c), there is not enough repair enzyme to bind to all damaged sites simultaneously and so the reaction velocity of repair no longer increases with increasing damage. Therefore, at higher doses (more lesions), there is proportionally less repair during the time available before damage becomes fixed; this will lead to more residual damage and to greater cell kill. The mechanisms of fixation of non-repaired damage are not understood but they may be associated with the entry of cells carrying such damage into DNA synthesis or mitosis. It should be noted that an alternative 'saturation' hypothesis, leading to the same consequence, is that the pool of repair enzymes is used up during repair, so that at higher doses the repair system is depleted and is less able to repair all the induced damage.

Table 4.1 illustrates how the basic conceptual difference between the lesion accumulation/interaction models such as Curtis' LPL and the dose-dependent repair models affects the interpretation of some radiobiological phenomena (9). Both types of models predict linear-quadratic cell survival curves in the clinically relevant dose region. They also provide good explanations of split-dose recovery (see Chapter 8), changing relative biological effectiveness (RBE) with LET (see Chapter 6) and the dose-rate effect (see Chapter 13). At present, radiation scientists are uncertain whether lesion interaction or repair saturation really exist in cells but it may well be that molecular and microdosimetric studies will eventually determine which explanation (maybe both) is correct.

## 4.13 THE LINEAR-QUADRATIC-CUBIC MODEL

The LQ model describes the cellular response to ionising radiation extremely well at doses less than ~5–6 Gy and is the preferred model to use in this dose range. However, at higher doses the survival response of cells is often found to more closely resemble a linear relationship between –ln(S) and dose, as described by the models based on target theory.

A simple way of adjusting the LQ model to account for the more linear response at higher doses is to add an additional term proportional to the cube of the dose, but opposite in

Table 4.1 Different interpretations of radiobiological phenomena by lesion-interaction and saturable-repair models

| | Explanation | |
| Observation | Lesion interaction | Repair saturation |
| --- | --- | --- |
| Curved dose-effect relationship | Interaction of sublesions | Saturation of capacity to repair sublesions |
| Split-dose recovery | Repair of sublesions (sublethal damage repair) | Recovery of capacity to repair sublesions |
| RBE increase with LET | More non-repairable lesions at high LET | High-LET lesions are less repairable |
| Low dose rate is less effective | Repair of sublesions during irradiation | Repair system not saturating |

Adapted from (9).

sign to the linear and quadratic terms. This is termed the linear-quadratic-cubic (LQC) model:

$$-\ln(S) = \alpha D + \beta D^2 - \gamma D^3$$

$$p(\text{survival}) = \exp(-\alpha D - \beta D^2 + \gamma D^3) \qquad (4.5)$$

A comparison of the LQ and LQC models is shown in Figure 4.8. By taking the second-order differential of $-\ln(S)$ with respect to dose, it can be shown that the survival curve can be straightened at dose $D_L$ by choosing $\gamma = \beta/(3D_L)$. In the example of Figure 4.8, the LQC curve becomes a straight line at a dose, $D_L$, of 18 Gy.

As with the two-component model, a disadvantage of the LQC model is the addition of a third parameter, but because the LQC model is a simple polynomial, it is nevertheless still more mathematically manageable than the target theory models. The LQC model is actually just a third-order polynomial approximation to the Curtis' LPL model, which also demonstrates a more linear relationship between $-\ln(S)$ and dose than predicted by the LQ model, at surviving fractions less than about $10^{-2}$. A particular caution in using this simple third-order polynomial approximation is that with increasing doses higher than $D_L$, the cell survival curve starts to bend back upwards so that eventually surviving fraction increases with increasing dose. This does not make sense biologically and serves to emphasize again that practically any useful model can predict successfully only over a defined range of dose and that outside of that dose range caution must be used with that model.

## 4.14 LOW-DOSE HYPER-RADIOSENSITIVITY

The LQ model and its mechanistic interpretations (Curtis' LPL and repair saturation) adequately describe cellular response to radiation above about 1 Gy. It has been difficult to make accurate measurements of cell killing by radiation below this dose, but this problem has been partially overcome by methods that determine exactly the number of cells 'at risk' in a colony-forming assay (Section 4.4). This can be achieved using a FACS to *plate* an exact number of cells or microscopic scanning to identify an exact number of cells *after* plating. Using such techniques, it can be shown that many mammalian cell lines, rodent and human, actually exhibit the type of radiation response shown in Figure 4.9 at doses less than 1 Gy. Below about 10 cGy, the cells show low-dose HRS which can be characterised by a slope ($\alpha_s$) that is considerably steeper than the slope expected by extrapolating back the response from high-dose measurements ($\alpha_r$). The transition (over about 20–80 cGy) from a sensitive to resistant response has been termed a region of increased radioresistance (IRR). This low-dose HRS was originally discovered *in vivo* using models of skin and renal damage in mice (12,13) and then subsequently shown to occur in mammalian cells *in vitro* first using V79 hamster fibroblasts (19). It has furthermore been demonstrated in

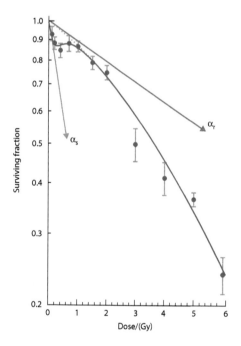

**Figure 4.9** Survival of asynchronous T98G human glioma cells irradiated with 240 kVp X-rays, measured using a cell-sorter protocol (24). Each data point represents 10–12 measurements. The solid line and dashed lines show the fits of the induced-repair (IndRep) model and LQ models, respectively. At doses below 1 Gy the LQ model, using an initial slope $\alpha_r$, substantially underestimates the effect of irradiation and this domain is better described by the IndRep model using a much steeper initial slope $\alpha_s$.

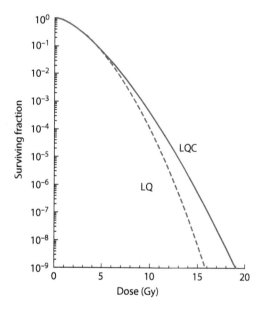

**Figure 4.8** Cell survival modelled with the LQ or LQC equations. In this example both equations model a cell-survival response with surviving fraction at 2 Gy (SF2) equal to 0.5, and an $\alpha/\beta$ value of 3 Gy. The value of $\gamma$ in the LQC model is given by $\gamma = \beta/(3D_L)$, where $D_L$ is the dose at which the curve becomes straight; here this dose has been chosen to be 18 Gy.

human lymphocytes using cytogenetic endpoints (22). It is due to an increase in the extent of DNA repair of the cells in the IRR region (14). This happens because a rapid cell-cycle arrest of cells, irradiated in the G2 phase of the cell cycle, only occurs when there are enough DNA DSBs to trigger phosphorylation of the ATM damage-recognition protein. This typically starts to happen only when the average dose exceeds about 10 cGy (20).

The LQ model can be modified to take account of this process and the result is called the *induced repair* (IndRep) model:

$$p(\text{survival})$$
$$= \exp(-\alpha_r D(1+(\alpha_s/\alpha_r -1)\exp(-D/D_c))-\beta D^2) \quad (4.6)$$

In this equation, $D_c$ is around 0.2 Gy and describes the dose at which the transition from the HRS response through the IRR response starts to occur. At very high doses ($D \gg D_c$), Equation 4.6 tends to a LQ model with active parameters $\alpha_r$ and $\beta$. At very low doses ($D \ll D_c$), Equation 4.6 tends to a LQ model with active parameters $\alpha_s$ and $\beta$. The IndRep model thus comprises two LQ models with different $\alpha$ sensitivities dependent on the dose given, merged into a single equation.

It has been proposed that this HRS phenomenon might be exploitable clinically, if it were practicable to deliver radiotherapy as a very large number of dose fractions each less than 0.5 Gy. The aim would be to take advantage of the extra radiosensitivity in the HRS region which could improve the response of tumours that are known to be resistant to radiotherapy at doses of 2 Gy per fraction.

---

### Key points

1. Tumour recurrence after treatment depends upon the survival of clonogenic cells, which may comprise only a small proportion of the total cells within the tumour.

2. Evaluation of the survival of clonogenic cells following treatment is an important aspect of experimental cancer therapy. In experimental situations this is relatively simple to perform, but for cells removed directly from human tumours great care is necessary in the selection and performance of the assays.

3. A number of different mathematical models adequately simulate the shape of cell-survival curves for mammalian cells.

4. Target theory proposes that a specific number of targets or DNA sites must be inactivated or damaged to kill the cell. This approach is only satisfactory if a component of single-hit killing is also introduced. So far it has not been possible to identify the location of these vital 'targets' within the cell nucleus.

5. Lesion-interaction models explain downward-bending cell-survival curves by postulating two classes of lesion. One class is directly lethal, but the other type is only *potentially* lethal and may be repaired enzymatically or may interact with other potentially lethal lesions to form lethal lesions.

6. Repair-saturation models also provide a plausible explanation of cell survival phenomena.

7. LQ equations model the shape of the cell survival curve very well at doses less than ∼5–6 Gy. At higher doses, it may be necessary to use LQC equations to model the more linear relationship between log(surviving fraction) and dose which is often seen.

8. The phenomenon of HRS at very low radiation doses illustrates that reactive molecular signalling and repair processes determine the balance between radiation cell killing and cell survival, and models which treat the cell only as a set of passive targets will be unlikely to describe the full spectrum of radiation response.

---

### ■ BIBLIOGRAPHY

1. Bosanquet AG. Correlations between therapeutic response of leukaemias and in-vitro drug-sensitivity assay. *Lancet* 1991;337:711–714.

2. Carmichael J, DeGraff WG, Gazdar AF, Minna JD, Mitchell JB. Evaluation of a tetrazolium-based semiautomated colorimetric assay: Assessment of radiosensitivity. *Cancer Res* 1987;47:943–946.

3. Chadwick KH, Leenhouts HP. A molecular theory of cell survival. *Phys Med Biol* 1973;18:78–87.

4. Chapman JD, Peters LJ, Withers HR (eds) *Prediction of Tumor Treatment Response.* New York, NY: Pergamon; 1989.

5. Coleman CN, Higgins GS, Brown JM et al. Improving the predictive value of preclinical studies in support of radiotherapy clinical trials. *Clin Cancer Res* 2016;22:3138–3147.

6. Courtenay VD, Mills J. An in vitro colony assay for human tumours grown in immune-suppressed mice and treated in vivo with cytotoxic agents. *Br J Cancer* 1978;37:261–268.

7. Curtis SB. Lethal and potentially lethal lesions induced by radiation – A unified repair model. *Radiat Res* 1986;106:252–270.

8. Durand RE. Use of a cell sorter for assays of cell clonogenicity. *Cancer Res* 1986;46:2775–2778.

9. Goodhead DT. Saturable repair models of radiation action in mammalian cells. *Radiat Res Suppl* 1985;8:S58–S67.

10. Goodwin CJ, Holt SJ, Downes S, Marshall NJ. Microculture tetrazolium assays: A comparison between two new tetrazolium salts, XTT and MTS. *J Immunol Methods* 1995;179:95–103.

11. Hill RP, Stanley JA. The lung-colony assay: Extension to the Lewis lung tumour and the B16 melanoma – Radiosensitivity of B16 melanoma cells. *Int J Radiat Biol* 1975;27:377–387.

12. Joiner MC, Denekamp J, Maughan RL. The use of 'top-up' experiments to investigate the effect of very small doses per fraction in mouse skin. *Int J Radiat Biol* 1986;49:565–580.

13. Joiner MC, Johns H. Renal damage in the mouse: The response to very small doses per fraction. *Radiat Res* 1988;114:385–398.

14. Joiner MC, Marples B, Lambin P, Short SC, Turesson I. Low-dose hypersensitivity: Current status and possible mechanisms. *Int J Radiat Oncol Biol Phys* 2001;49:379–389.

15. Klokov D, MacPhail SM, Banath JP, Byrne JP, Olive PL. Phosphorylated histone H2AX in relation to cell survival in tumor cells and xenografts exposed to single and fractionated doses of X-rays. *Radiother Oncol* 2006;80:223–229.

16. Koch U, Hohne K, von Neubeck C et al. Residual γH2AX foci predict local tumour control after radiotherapy. *Radiother Oncol* 2013;108:434–439.

17. M'Kacher R, Maalouf EE, Ricoul M et al. New tool for biological dosimetry: Reevaluation and automation of the gold standard method following telomere and centromere staining. *Mutat Res* 2014;770:45–53.

18. MacPhail SH, Banath JP, Yu TY, Chu EH, Lambur H, Olive PL. Expression of phosphorylated histone H2AX in cultured cell lines following exposure to X-rays. *Int J Radiat Biol* 2003;79:351–358.

19. Marples B, Joiner MC. The response of Chinese hamster V79 cells to low radiation doses: Evidence of enhanced sensitivity of the whole cell population. *Radiat Res* 1993;133:41–51.

20. Marples B, Wouters BG, Joiner MC. An association between the radiation-induced arrest of G2-phase cells and low-dose hyper-radiosensitivity: A plausible underlying mechanism? *Radiat Res* 2003;160:38–45.

21. Potten CS (ed.) *Stem Cells: Their Identification and Characterization*. Edinburgh: Churchill-Livingstone; 1983.

22. Seth I, Joiner MC, Tucker JD. Cytogenetic low-dose hyperradiosensitivity is observed in human peripheral blood lymphocytes. *Int J Radiat Oncol Biol Phys* 2015;91:82–90.

23. Seymour CB, Mothersill C. Lethal mutations, the survival curve shoulder and split-dose recovery. *Int J Radiat Biol* 1989;56:999–1010.

24. Short S, Mayes C, Woodcock M, Johns H, Joiner MC. Low dose hypersensitivity in the T98G human glioblastoma cell line. *Int J Radiat Biol* 1999;75:847–855.

25. Steel GG, Adams K. Stem-cell survival and tumor control in the Lewis lung carcinoma. *Cancer Res* 1975;35:1530–1535.

26. Steel GG, Stephens TC. Stem cells in tumours. In: Potten CS (ed.) *Stem Cells: Their Identification and Characterization*. Edinburgh: Churchill-Livingstone; 1983.

27. Streffer C, van Beuningen D, Gross E, Schabronath J, Eigler FW, Rebmann A. Predictive assays for the therapy of rectum carcinoma. *Radiother Oncol* 1986;5:303–310.

28. Till JE, McCulloch EA. A direct measurement of the radiation sensitivity of normal mouse bone marrow cells. *Radiat Res* 1961;14:213–222.

29. Trott KR. Relation between division delay and damage expressed in later generations. *Curr Topics Radiat Res Q* 1972;7:336–337.

30. Wasserman TH, Twentyman P. Use of a colorimetric microtiter (MTT) assay in determining the radiosensitivity of cells from murine solid tumors. *Int J Radiat Oncol Biol Phys* 1988;15:699–702.

## ■ FURTHER READING

31. Alpen EL. *Radiation Biophysics*. 2nd ed. San Diego, CA: Academic Press; 1998.

32. Douglas BG, Fowler JF. The effect of multiple small doses of X rays on skin reactions in the mouse and a basic interpretation. *Radiat Res* 1976;66:401–426.

33. Elkind MM, Sutton H. Radiation response of mammalian cells grown in culture. 1. Repair of X-ray damage in surviving Chinese hamster cells. *Radiat Res* 1960;13:556–593.

34. Elkind MM, Whitmore GF. *The Radiobiology of Cultured Mammalian Cells*. New York, NY: Gordon and Breach; 1967.

35. Potten CS (ed.) *Stem Cells: Their Identification and Characterization*. Edinburgh: Churchill-Livingstone; 1983.

36. Ward JF. The yield of DNA double-strand breaks produced intracellularly by ionizing radiation: A review. *Int J Radiat Biol* 1990;57:1141–1150.

# Radiation dose-response relationships

SØREN M. BENTZEN

## 5.1 INTRODUCTION

Clinical radiobiology is a field of medical research concerned with the relationship between a given physical absorbed dose of radiation in the range used for cancer therapy and the resulting biological response in a human as well as with the factors that influence this relationship. What is seen in clinical practice is a broad range of doses where the probability of a specific type of radiation response increases from 0% towards 100% with increasing dose (i.e. a dose-response relationship). Although the term *tolerance* is frequently used in a loose sense when discussing radiotherapy toxicity, it is important to realize that there is no dose below which the complication rate is exactly zero: there is no clear-cut tolerance dose, although of course the probability of a given effect may become very low as the dose tends to zero.

An endpoint is a specific biological event that may or may not have occurred at a given time after treatment. Endpoints are used to assess the effect of treatment; examples are overall survival, cause-specific survival, time to progression and various health states reflecting side effects of therapy. The idea of dose-response is almost built into our definition of a radiation endpoint: to classify a specific biological phenomenon as a radiation effect we would require that this phenomenon be never or rarely seen after zero dose and seen in nearly all cases after very high doses. Certain signs and symptoms occurring after radiation therapy are not specific radiation effects, for example erectile dysfunction (ED) after radiotherapy for prostate cancer. Some men will have ED before the commencement of radiotherapy; others may develop ED over time even without having been exposed to radiotherapy. In this case, a simple dose-incidence curve may not be the best way to quantify risk from radiation therapy. Alternative descriptions could be to quantify the *excess absolute risk* of ED as a function of dose and time or to analyse the change in erectile function score relative to the baseline value. In the latter case, it may be sensible to restrict the analysis to patients who had a level of erectile function at baseline. The present chapter will concentrate on endpoints that are specific expressions of radiation effects in order to simplify the presentation. The concept of dose-response relationships was introduced in Section 1.5 and various ways of characterizing normal tissue endpoints are discussed in Chapter 14.

With increasing radiation dose, radiation effects may increase in severity (i.e. grade), in frequency (i.e. incidence) or both. A plot of, say, average level of stimulated growth hormone secretion after graded doses of cranial irradiation in children may reveal a dose dependence, an example of severity increasing with dose. This type of model assumes that the average loss of growth hormone secretion is a reasonable way to quantify the effect of radiation therapy in the exposed population. For many normal tissue effects, however, the clinical observation is that some patients will experience the side effect while many will not. In such a case, the *probability* of expressing the effect, or the *incidence* of the side effect in a population of patients, is a more adequate quantitation of toxicity. In the above example this risk could be quantified, for instance, by a curve showing the proportion of children requiring growth hormone replacement therapy as a function of dose. Thus, the dependent variable in a dose-response plot is the incidence or probability of response as a function of dose (Figure 5.1). In this chapter, we concentrate on the latter type of dose-effect relationship – dose-incidence curves – and following the convention in the field, we restrict the terms *dose-response curve* or *dose-response relationship* to refer to this type of relationship.

Many of the key concepts in the quantitative description of dose-response relationships are fundamental to understanding the general principles of radiotherapy. Furthermore, they form the basis of most of the more theoretical considerations in radiotherapy. In the following, we keep the mathematics to a minimum but a few formulae are needed to substantiate the presentation. Interested readers may refer to Section 5.8 for a more concise description of some of the topics discussed in the preceding sections.

The dose on the *x*-axis of a dose-response plot will often be a transformed 'equivalent dose'; for example we may plot observed response as a function of EQD2 (Section 10.2) if multiple fraction sizes are used in the data set. Or we may adjust the dose for partial volume irradiation of an organ (Section 14.8). In order to simplify the presentation, we address the situation where a uniform dose is delivered to the organ at risk or the target volume. It should also be stressed that dose-response relationships are data-driven representations of empirical data. Thus, all the parameters in the following will in practice be estimated from clinical data and with confidence limits around the estimates. Analysis of

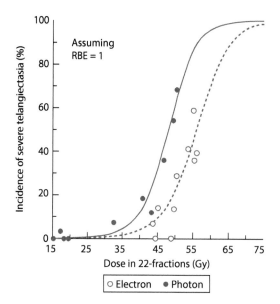

**Figure 5.1** Examples of dose-response relationships in clinical radiotherapy. Data are shown on the incidence of severe telangiectasia following electron or photon irradiation. (From (7), with permission.)

clinical data raises a number of methodological issues and some of these are discussed in Chapter 10.

## 5.2 MATHEMATICAL DESCRIPTION OF DOSE-RESPONSE RELATIONSHIPS

Empirical attempts to establish dose-response relationships in the clinic date back to the first decade of radiotherapy. A major advance in the field came in 1936 when the great clinical scientist Hermann Holthusen was the first to present a theoretical analysis of dose-response relationships and this became a major influence on the conceptual development of radiotherapy optimization. Holthusen (15) analysed clinical data on the incidence of skin telangiectasia and local control of skin cancer after graded prescribed doses of radiation. He demonstrated the sigmoid shape of dose-response curves both for normal tissue reactions and local tumour control. Holthusen noted the resemblance between these curves and the cumulative distribution functions known from statistics, and this led him to the idea that the dose-response curve simply reflected the cumulative distribution of clinical radioresponsiveness in a population of patients. In other words, if the probability of expressing a given toxicity of radiation therapy at, say, 60 Gy is 40%, the Holthusen interpretation is that 40% of cases have a radioresponsiveness corresponding to a 'tolerance dose' of ≤60 Gy. This remains one of the main interpretations of dose-response relationships and this has had a renaissance in recent years with the research interest in patient-to-patient variability in response to radiotherapy.

Radiation dose-response curves have a sigmoid (i.e. *S*-) shape, with the incidence of radiation effects tending to zero as dose tends to zero and tending to 100% at very large

doses. Many mathematical functions could be devised with these properties, but three standard formulations are used in the literature: the Poisson, the logistic and the probit dose-response models (10). In principle, it is an empirical problem to decide whether one model fits observed data better than the other. In reality, both clinical and experimental dose-response data are too noisy to allow statistical discrimination between these models and in most cases they will give similar fits to a data set. The situation where major discrepancies may arise is when these models are used for extrapolation of experience over a wide range of dose; see Bentzen and Tucker (10).

## The Poisson dose-response model

Munro and Gilbert (20) published a paper in 1961 in which they formulated *the target-cell hypothesis of tumour control*: 'The object of treating a tumour by radiotherapy is to damage every single potentially malignant cell to such an extent that it cannot continue to proliferate'. From this idea and the random nature of cell killing by radiation, they derived a mathematical formula for the probability of tumour cure after irradiation of 'a number of tumours each composed of N identical cells'. More precisely, they argued that this probability depends only on the average number of clonogens surviving per tumour. This was a compelling idea; also it tagged nicely on to Puck and Marcus' *in vitro* cell survival work published 5 years earlier (23).

Figure 5.2 shows a Monte Carlo (i.e. random number) simulation of the number of surviving clonogens per tumour in a hypothetical sample of 100 tumours with an average number of 0.5 surviving clonogens per tumour. In panel A, each tumour is represented by one of the squares in which the figure indicates the actual number of surviving clonogens, these numbers having been generated at random. The cured tumours are those with zero surviving clonogens. In this simulation, there were 62 cured tumours. The relative frequencies of tumours with 0, 1, 2,... surviving clonogens follow closely a statistical distribution known as the Poisson distribution, as shown in panel B. Many processes involving the counting of random, uncorrelated events are (approximately) Poisson distributed, for example the number of decaying atoms per second in a radioactive sample, the number of tumour cells forming colonies in a Petri dish or the number of typographical errors per page of a textbook.

According to the target cell hypothesis, the tumour cure probability (TCP) is equal to the probability of zero surviving clonogens in a tumour. This is the zero-order term of the Poisson distribution and if $\lambda$ denotes the average number of clonogens per tumour after irradiation this is simply

$$TCP = e^{-\lambda} \qquad (5.1)$$

Munro and Gilbert went one step further: they assumed that the average number of surviving clonogenic cells per tumour was a (negative) exponential function of dose. Under

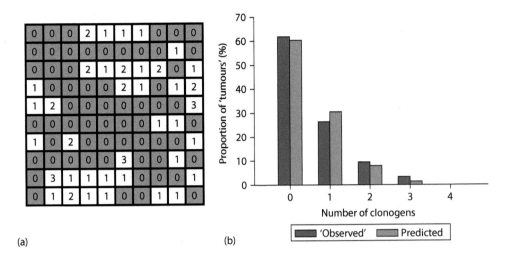

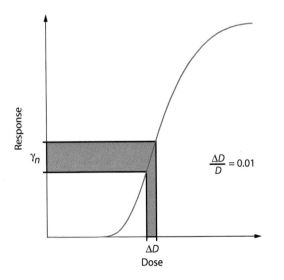

(a)                                                             (b)

**Figure 5.2** Simulation of a Poisson distribution. (a) The number of clonogens surviving per tumour in a hypothetical sample of 100 tumours. The average number was 0.5 surviving clonogens/tumour. The histogram (b) shows the proportion of tumours with a given number of surviving clonogens (black bars) and this is compared with the prediction from a Poisson distribution with the same average number of surviving clonogens (hatched bars).

these assumptions, they obtained the characteristic sigmoid dose-response curve (Figure 5.3). Thus, the shape of this curve could be explained solely from the random nature of cell killing (or clonogen survival) after irradiation: there was no need to assume variability of sensitivity between tumours.

The Poisson dose-response model derived by Munro and Gilbert became very influential in theoretical radiobiology. The simple exponential dose-survival curve was later replaced by the linear-quadratic model (Section 9.4) and thus we arrive at what for many years was considered the standard model of tumour control:

$$\text{TCP} = \exp[-N_0 \cdot \exp(-\alpha D - \beta d D)] \qquad (5.2)$$

**Figure 5.3** Geometrical interpretation of $\gamma$. A 1% dose increment ($\Delta D$) from a reference dose $D$ yields an increase in response equal to $\gamma$ percentage points. (From (2), with permission.)

Here, $N_0$ is the number of clonogens per tumour before irradiation and the second exponential is simply the surviving fraction after a dose $D$ given with dose per fraction $d$ according to the linear-quadratic model. Thus, when we multiply these two quantities we obtain the (average) number of surviving clonogens per tumour and this is inserted into the Poisson expression in Equation 5.1. $N_0$ can easily be expressed as a function of tumour volume and the clonogenic cell density (i.e. clonogens per cm³ of tumour tissue – assuming that this is constant as a function of tumour volume) and similarly it is easy to introduce exponential growth, with or without a lag time before accelerated repopulation, in this model (e.g. [5]). The theoretical attraction of the Poisson model is that the model parameters appear to have a biological or mechanistic interpretation. This, however, is much less of an advantage than it was thought to be 20 years ago. There are at least two reasons for this. First, the Poisson model is increasingly seen as an oversimplification of the complex cancer biology that has been uncovered in recent years; a tumour is not simply 'a bag of cells'. Consequently, the conceptual basis for the Poisson model has largely disappeared. Second, even if the underlying dose-response relationship did follow a Poisson model, model parameter estimates from an actual clinical data set will be strongly influenced by biological and dosimetric heterogeneity and therefore cannot be regarded as realistic measures of some intrinsic biological property of the tumour (1,5). Closed-form expressions of the Poisson dose-response model that takes patient-to-patient variability explicitly into account have been proposed (e.g. [13,24]), but this approach has only been used in a few analyses. The interest in the extensions of the Poisson model has cooled with the turn towards more pragmatic data-driven or 'statistical' approaches, see the following text.

In the heyday of the target-cell hypothesis (see Chapter 4), normal tissue toxicity was also hypothesized to be a consequence of target cell depletion in some putative cell population, and it was proposed to use the Poisson model to describe the corresponding dose-response relationship. More recent research has found that the radiation pathogenesis of normal tissue effects is considerably more complex than suggested by the simple target cell model (4) which again means that the Poisson model parameters have no simple interpretation in this situation.

In view of the above considerations for both tumour and normal tissue effects, most researchers have turned to 'statistical' dose-response models, flexible mathematical functions that offer a good empirical fit to clinical data from a large number of clinical and pre-clinical studies and provide flexibility in terms of incorporating other covariates in the model. Computer code for estimating the parameter of these models is available in many standard statistics software packages and this provides the further attraction of embedding the modelling within a larger statistical framework for parameter estimation and hypothesis testing.

## The logistic dose-response model

The logistic model is a convenient and flexible standard tool for estimating response probabilities after various graded exposures and is widely used in many areas of biology besides radiobiology. The idea of the model is to write the probability of an event ($P$) as

$$P = \frac{\exp(u)}{1 + \exp(u)} \tag{5.3}$$

where, when analysing data from fractionated radiotherapy, $u$ has the following form:

$$u = a_0 + a_1 \cdot D + a_2 \cdot D \cdot d + \cdots \tag{5.4}$$

Here, $D$ is total dose and $d$ is dose per fraction, and the representation of the effect of dose-fractionation in this way is, of course, reflecting the assumption of a linear-quadratic relationship between dose and effect. Additional terms, representing other patient or treatment characteristics, may be included in the model to test if they have a significant influence on the probability of effect. The coefficients $a_0$, $a_1$,... are estimated by logistic regression, a method that is available in many standard statistical software packages. The parameters $a_1$ and $a_2$ play a role similar to the coefficients $\alpha$ and $\beta$ of the linear-quadratic model. But note that there is no direct mechanistic interpretation of these parameters: $a_1$ is not an estimate of $\alpha$ and $a_2$ is not an estimate of $\beta$. What is preserved is the ratio $a_1/a_2$, which is an estimate of $\alpha/\beta$.

Rearrangement of Equation 5.3 yields the following expression:

$$u = \ln\left(\frac{P}{1-P}\right) \tag{5.5}$$

The ratio $P/(1 - P)$ is called the *odds* of a response, and the natural logarithm of this is called the *logit* of $P$. Therefore, logistic regression is also called *logit analysis*.

Often in applications of the logistic dose-response model, it is convenient to use $D_{50}$ and $\gamma_{50}$ directly as the model parameters, see Section 5.8.

## The probit dose-response model

Following Holthusen (15), it is attractive to fit a cumulative probability distribution directly to a set of dose-response data. Typically, the cumulative normal distribution is used and this leads to the *probit* dose-response model. Several authors have applied the probit dose-response model in analyses of the effect of dosimetric error on dose-response relationships (14,27). It was also the dose-response model embedded in Lyman's 1985 dose-volume-response model (19).

## 5.3 QUANTIFYING THE POSITION OF THE DOSE-RESPONSE CURVE

Several descriptors are used for the position of the dose-response curve on the radiation dose scale. They all have the unit of dose (Gy) and they specify the dose required for a given level of tumour control or normal tissue complications. For tumours, the most frequently used position parameter is the $\mathrm{TCD}_{50}$ (i.e. the radiation dose for 50% tumour control). For normal tissue reactions, the analogous parameter is the radiation dose for 50% response ($\mathrm{RD}_{50}$) or in case of rare (typically more severe) complications $\mathrm{RD}_5$, that is the dose producing a 5% incidence of complications.

## 5.4 QUANTIFYING THE STEEPNESS OF DOSE-RESPONSE CURVES

The most convenient way to quantify the steepness of the dose-response curve is by means of the '$\gamma$-value' or, more precisely, the normalized dose-response gradient (10,12). This measure has a simple interpretation: $\gamma$ is the increase in response probability in percentage points for a 1% increase in dose. (Note: an increase in response probability from, say, 10% to 15% is an increase of 5 percentage points, but a 50% relative increase.) Figure 5.3 illustrates the definition of $\gamma$ geometrically.

A more precise definition of $\gamma$ requires a little mathematics. Let $P(D)$ denote the response as a function of dose, $D$, and $\Delta D$ a small increment in dose, then the previous 'loose definition' may be written as follows:

$$\gamma \approx \frac{P(D + \Delta D) - P(D)}{(\Delta D / D) \cdot 100\%} \cdot 100\%$$
$$= D \cdot \frac{P(D + \Delta D) - P(D)}{\Delta D} = D \cdot \frac{\Delta P}{\Delta D} \tag{5.6}$$

The second term on the right-hand side is recognized as a difference-quotient and in the limit where $\Delta D$ tends to zero, we arrive at the formal definition of $\gamma$:

$$\gamma = D \cdot P'(D) \tag{5.7}$$

where $P'(D)$ is the derivative of $P(D)$ with respect to dose.

If we look at the right-hand side of Equation 5.6, we arrive at the approximate relationship

$$\Delta P \approx \gamma \cdot \frac{\Delta D}{D} \tag{5.8}$$

In other words, $\gamma$ is a multiplier that converts a relative change in dose into an (absolute) change in response probability. Most often we insert the relative change in dose in percent, and in that case P is the (approximate) change in response rate in percentage points.

Equation 5.8 is very useful in practical calculations (Chapter 10). For example, increasing the dose to a tumour from 66 to 68 Gy in a schedule employing 2 Gy dose per fraction corresponds to a 3% increase in dose: $(2/66) \cdot 100\%$. If we assume that the $\gamma$-value of the dose-response curve for local control of this type of tumour is 1.8 at the level of response seen after 66 Gy, then the estimated improvement in local control from Equation 5.8 is $1.8 \times 3.0 \approx 5.4$ percentage points.

Mathematically, Equation 5.8 corresponds to approximating the S-shaped dose-response curve by a straight line (the tangent of the dose-response curve). As discussed briefly, this will only be a good approximation over a relatively narrow range of doses; exactly *how narrow* depends on the response level and the steepness of the dose-response curve.

Clearly, the value of $\gamma$ depends on the response level at which it is evaluated: at the bottom or top of the dose-response curve a 1% increase in dose will produce a smaller increment in response than on the steep part of the curve. This local value of $\gamma$ is typically written with an index indicating the response level, for example $\gamma_{50}$ refers to the $\gamma$-value at a 50% response level. A compact and convenient way to report the steepness of a dose-response curve is by stating the $\gamma$-value at the level of response where the curve attains its maximum steepness: this can be shown to be at the 37% ($e^{-1}$) response level for the Poisson model and at the 50% response level for the logistic

and probit models. From this single value and a measure of the position of the dose-response curve, the whole mathematical form of the dose-response relationship is specified (10). In particular, the steepness at any other dose or response level can be calculated. Table 5.1 shows how the $\gamma$-value varies with the response level for logistic dose-response curves of varying steepness. Using this table, it is possible to estimate the relevant $\gamma$-value at, say, a 20% response level, the $\gamma_{20}$, if we know $\gamma_{50}$. As an example, for a dose-response curve with $\gamma_{50} = 2.5$, we find by linear interpolation of the relevant $\gamma_{20}$-values in Table 5.1, that $\gamma_{20} = 1.4$.

Table 5.1 also provides an impression of the range of response (or dose) where the simple linear approximation in Equation 5.8 will be reasonably accurate: if we extrapolate between two response levels where the $\gamma$-value changes markedly, the approximation of assuming a fixed value for $\gamma$ will not be precise.

## 5.5 CLINICAL ESTIMATES OF THE STEEPNESS OF DOSE-RESPONSE CURVES

Several clinical studies have found evidence for a significant dose-response relationship and have provided data allowing an estimation of the steepness of clinical dose-response curves. Clinical dose-response curves generally originate from studies where the dose has been changed while keeping either the dose per fraction or the number of fractions fixed. Under the assumption that the linear-quadratic model is a valid description of the dose-per-fraction effect, there is a further advantage of tabulating the $\gamma$-value at the steepest point of the dose-response curve: it is independent of the size of dose per fraction in the case of a dose-response curve generated using a fixed dose per fraction (2,12). Figure 5.4 shows clinical estimates of $\gamma_{37}$ for head and neck tumours estimated under the assumption of a fixed dose per fraction (2). Typical values range from 1.5 to 2.5. Thus, a simple rule of thumb is that, around the midpoint of the dose-response curve, for each percent increment in dose, the probability of controlling a head and neck tumour will increase by about two percentage points. Steepness estimates of dose-response curves for other tumour histologies were reviewed by Okunieff et al. (21), but it should be noted that data for other histologies are sparser than for the head and neck tumours.

Table 5.1 'Local' $\gamma_P$ values as a function of the response level for logistic dose-response curves of varying steepness

| $\gamma_{50}$ | Response level, $P$, % | | | | | | | | |
|---|---|---|---|---|---|---|---|---|---|
| | 10 | 20 | 30 | 40 | 50 | 60 | 70 | 80 | 90 |
| 1 | 0.2 | 0.4 | 0.7 | 0.9 | 1.0 | 1.1 | 1.0 | 0.9 | 0.6 |
| 2 | 0.5 | 1.1 | 1.5 | 1.8 | 2.0 | 2.0 | 1.9 | 1.5 | 0.9 |
| 3 | 0.9 | 1.7 | 2.3 | 2.8 | 3.0 | 3.0 | 2.7 | 2.1 | 1.3 |
| 4 | 1.2 | 2.3 | 3.2 | 3.7 | 4.0 | 3.9 | 3.5 | 2.8 | 1.6 |
| 5 | 1.6 | 3.0 | 4.0 | 4.7 | 5.0 | 4.9 | 4.4 | 3.4 | 2.0 |

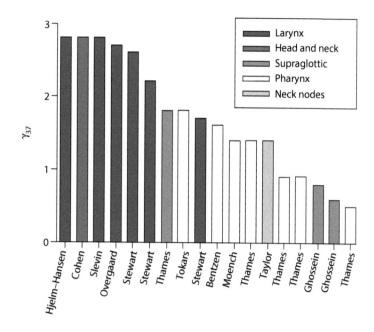

**Figure 5.4** Estimated $\gamma_{37}$ values from a number of studies on dose-response relationships for squamous cell carcinoma in various sites of the head and neck. (From (7), where the original references may be found.)

Also, some of the tabulated values are obviously outliers that cannot be taken as a realistic estimate of the steepness of the clinical dose-response curve. These extreme values must be explained by patient selection bias or errors in dosimetry.

Under the target cell hypothesis it can be shown (12) that the $\gamma_{37}$ of a Poisson dose-response curve for a fixed dose per fraction depends only on the number of clonogens that have to be sterilized to cure the tumour. As mentioned in Section 5.2, many tumour and treatment variables, for example tumour volume and overall treatment time, are thought to affect the (effective) number of clonogens to be sterilized. Therefore, in a multivariate analysis, $\gamma_{37}$ will depend on all the significant patient and treatment characteristics. Even then, we would roughly expect a value of $\gamma_{37} = 7$ for a homogenous population of tumours (26). Values this high are not seen in the clinic or even in transplantable mouse tumour models under highly controlled experimental conditions $\gamma_{37} \lesssim 4$ (17). The principal reason why dose-response curves in the lab and in the clinic are shallower than this theoretical limit is dosimetric and biological heterogeneity. The tendency for vocal cord tumours to have $\gamma_{37}$-values at the upper end of the interval seen for other head and neck sub-sites probably reflects the relatively lower heterogeneity among laryngeal carcinomas treated with radiotherapy. Other patient and treatment characteristics will influence both the position and the steepness of the dose-response curve.

Figure 5.5 shows $\gamma_{50}$-values for various normal tissue endpoints. Estimates are given both for treatment with a fixed dose per fraction and, where possible, also for treatment in a fixed number of fractions, namely 22. The estimates in the latter situation are considerably higher, which is as expected from the linear-quadratic model. The explanation is that when treating with a fixed number of fractions, increasing the dose leads to a simultaneous increase in dose per fraction, and this is associated with an increased biological effect per gray. This is another manifestation of the 'double-trouble' phenomenon discussed in Section 10.11. For further discussion, see Section 5.8.

Another observation from Figure 5.5 is that the dose-response curves for many late normal-tissue endpoints are steeper than typical dose-response curves for head and neck cancer. An exception is rectosigmoid complications after combined external-beam and intracavitary brachytherapy where a large dose-volume variability is present in a population of patients due to the steep gradients in the dose distribution from the intracavitary sources. Also, the lung data arise from a treatment technique where the dose to the lung tissue varies considerably from patient to patient. Thus, it is likely that dosimetric heterogeneity rather than intrinsic biological factors is the main cause of the relatively low steepness seen for these endpoints.

## 5.6 THE THERAPEUTIC WINDOW

As with any other medical procedure, prescription of a course of radiotherapy must represent a balance between risks and benefits (Section 1.6). The relative position and shape of the dose-response curves for tumour control and a given radiotherapy complication determine the possibility of delivering a sufficient dose with an acceptable level of side effects. This was compellingly illustrated by Holthusen (15), who plotted dose-response curves for tumour control and complications in the same co-ordinate system for two hypothetical situations: one favourable, that is with a wide therapeutic window between the two curves, and the other one less favourable. Figure 5.6 shows an example of how changing treatment parameters may affect the therapeutic window. For split-course treatment (Figure 5.6a) the

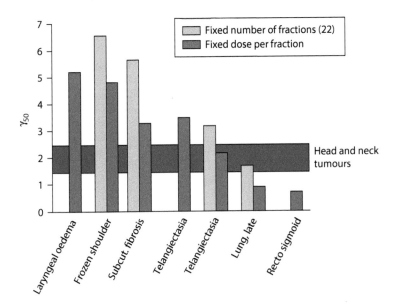

**Figure 5.5** Estimated $\gamma_{50}$ values for various late normal-tissue endpoints. Estimates are shown for treatment with a fixed dose per fraction and a fixed number of fractions. The shaded horizontal band corresponds to the typical $\gamma$ values at the point of maximum steepness for dose-response curves in head and neck tumours. Compare with Figure 5.4. (Data from (2,6) where the original references may be found.)

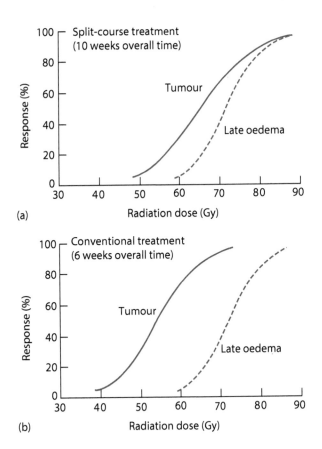

**Figure 5.6** Dose-response curves for local control of laryngeal carcinoma (full line) and late laryngeal oedema as estimated from the data by Overgaard et al. (22). Protraction of overall treatment time narrowed the therapeutic window. (From (6), with permission.)

tumour and oedema curves are closer together than for conventional treatment (Figure 5.6b), and the therapeutic window is therefore narrower. In practice, there will be several sequelae of clinical concern, and each of these will have its characteristic dose-response curve and will respond differently to treatment modifications. This complicates the simple strategy for optimization suggested by Figure 5.6.

Several suggestions are found in the literature for quantifying the effect of treatment modifications on the therapeutic window. Holthusen's proposal was to calculate the probability of uncomplicated cure, and this is still used frequently in the literature. The difficulty with this measure is that it gives equal weight to the complication in question and to tumour recurrence, which may often be fatal, and this is against common sense. A simple alternative, which is easy to interpret, is to specify the tumour control probability at isotoxicity with respect to a specific endpoint, as illustrated in Figure 1.3.

## 5.7 CLINICAL CONSIDERATIONS INVOLVING THE STEEPNESS OF DOSE-RESPONSE CURVES

### Accuracy requirements in radiation therapy

The $\gamma$-value is not only useful as a multiplier in converting from a dose change to a change in response but may also be used as a multiplier for converting an uncertainty in dose into an uncertainty in response. If the standard deviation of the absorbed-dose distribution in a population of patients is $\pm5\%$, a $\gamma$-value of 3 would yield an estimated $\pm15\%$

standard deviation on the response-probability distribution. Note that in this situation it is generally the $\gamma$-value for a fixed number of fractions that applies. Figure 5.5 shows that the high $\gamma$-values at the maximum steepness of the dose-response curve for normal tissues would yield a large variability in response probability for a $\pm 5\%$ variability in absorbed dose. This provides an indication of the precision required in treatment planning and delivery in radiotherapy.

## Patient-to-patient variability and stratification

Several modelling studies have shown that patient-to-patient variability in tumour biological parameters could strongly affect the steepness of the dose-response curve (1,8,26,29). Compelling support for this idea also comes from experimental studies (17). A direct illustration of the effect of inter-patient variability is obtained from an analysis of local tumour control in patients with oropharyngeal cancers (1). Analysing the data with the Poisson model yielded $\gamma_{37} = 1.8$. An analysis taking an assumed variability in tumour cell radiosensitivity into account allowed the dose-response curve to be broken down into a series of very steep curves, each of which would apply to a subpopulation of patients stratified according to intrinsic radiosensitivity (Figure 5.7). Clinical data on pathological response after radiotherapy, analysed by Levegrün et al. (18), showed how the dose-incidence curve got steeper when stratifying patients according to clinico-pathological risk group. Also for normal tissue effects, adjustment for patient-related risk factors leads to a steeper dose-response curve (e.g. [16]).

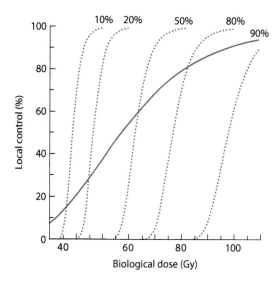

**Figure 5.7** Local control of oro-pharyngeal carcinoma as a function of the biological dose in 2 Gy fractions. Dotted lines are theoretical dose-response curves after stratification for intrinsic radiosensitivity. These represent dose-response relationships from five homogeneous patient populations with radiosensitivity equal to selected percentiles of the radiosensitivity distribution in the total population. (From (2), with permission.)

Viewing these curves in relation to Figure 5.6, it is clear that some of these subgroups could be expected to have a greater therapeutic window than others. If, by means of a reliable predictive assay, these subgroups could be identified prior to starting therapy, a substantial therapeutic benefit could be realized.

Another field where considerations of the steepness of the dose-response curves for tumours and normal tissue reactions play – or should play – a crucial role is in the design of clinical trials. For a discussion of this topic, see Bentzen (2).

## 5.8 SOME (SLIGHTLY) MORE ADVANCED TOPICS – OPTIONAL READING

Some potential readers of this chapter may enjoy a few extensions of all the above discussion – going one level deeper and requiring a little more math. These extensions are viewed as optional for an introductory course.

### A few simple relationships for the logistic dose-response curve

The logistic dose-response model can be parameterized in terms of $\gamma_{50}$ and $D_{50}$ as

$$P(D) = \frac{1}{1 + \exp\left[4 \cdot \gamma_{50} \cdot \left(1 - \frac{D}{D_{50}}\right)\right]} \tag{5.9}$$

If the responses at two dose levels are known, i.e. if we know two points on the dose-response curve, $(D_1, P_1)$ and $(D_2, P_2)$, then it is possible to estimate $\gamma_{50}$ and $D_{50}$ as

$$\gamma_{50} = \frac{D_1 \cdot \mathrm{logit}(P_2) - D_2 \cdot \mathrm{logit}(P_1)}{4 \cdot (D_2 - D_1)} \tag{5.10}$$

and

$$D_{50} = \frac{D_1 \cdot \mathrm{logit}(P_2) - D_2 \cdot \mathrm{logit}(P_1)}{\mathrm{logit}(P_2) - \mathrm{logit}(P_1)} \tag{5.11}$$

where the logit transformation is given by Equation 5.5.

Also, the relationship between $\gamma_{50}$ and the $\gamma$-value at any given response level $P$, $\gamma_P$, can be expressed analytically for the logistic dose-response relationship as

$$\gamma_P = P \cdot (1 - P) \cdot \left(4 \cdot \gamma_{50} - \ln\left(\frac{1 - P}{P}\right)\right) \tag{5.12}$$

### Mathematical form of the probit model

For completeness, we specify the mathematical form of the probit model. There are various parameterizations of this model, but the formulation here uses $\gamma_{50}$ and $D_{50}$ as the two free parameters to be estimated from a fit to dose-response data (10):

$$P(D) = \frac{1}{2} \cdot \left( 1 - \mathrm{erf}\left[ \gamma_{50} \cdot \sqrt{\pi}\left(1 - \frac{D}{D_{50}}\right)\right]\right) \quad (5.13)$$

where erf is the error function defined as

$$\mathrm{erf}(z) = \frac{2}{\sqrt{\pi}} \cdot \int_{0}^{z} \exp(-u^2)\,du \quad (5.14)$$

For parameterizations of the logit and Poisson models in terms of $\gamma_{50}$ and $D_{50}$ see Bentzen and Tucker (10).

## Steepness of a dose-response curve for a fixed number of fractions

Under the assumption of a linear-quadratic model of the effect of changing dose per fraction, it is possible to derive an analytic relationship between $\gamma_n$, the steepness of the dose-response curve for a fixed fraction number, and $\gamma_d$ the steepness for a fixed dose per fraction. This formula does not depend on the mathematical form of the dose-response relationship. It can be shown (3) that at a dose per fraction of $d_r$,

$$\gamma_n = \gamma_d \cdot \frac{(\alpha/\beta) + 2 \cdot d_r}{(\alpha/\beta) + d_r} \quad (5.15)$$

As both $\alpha/\beta$ and $d_r$ are positive numbers, $\gamma_n$ is always larger than $\gamma_d$. In the limit of very large dose per fraction, $\gamma_n$ has a limiting value of two times $\gamma_d$. In the limit of dose per fraction tending to zero $\gamma_n$ tends to $\gamma_d$. For more discussion of Equation 5.15 and its significance for dosimetric precision requirements in radiotherapy, see Bentzen (3).

## Modelling dose response for sub-clinical disease

The dose-response curve for control of sub-clinical disease does not range from 0 to 1 but rather from a level of control with no radiation, $P_0$, to 1 (30). For sub-clinical breast cancer, for example, $P_0$ is estimated from randomized controlled trials around 0.7, i.e. some 70% of women will have their loco-regional disease controlled by surgery alone (30). This gives rise to a dose-response curve of the following form:

$$P(D) = P_0 + (1 - P_0) \cdot \frac{1}{1 + \left(\dfrac{D}{D_{50}}\right)^{4 \cdot \gamma_{50m}}} \quad (5.16)$$

The last term corresponds to a logistic dose-response model with the logarithm of dose instead of dose itself as a carrier (10). This mathematical form ensures a horizontal asymptote of the dose-response curve as $D$ tends to zero. The apparent value of $\gamma$ in a mixed population of cases with and without sub-clinical disease at the time of treatment will be considerably lower than for gross disease. This should not be confused with the steepness parameter in the (unknown) sub-group with actual microscopic disease, $\gamma_{50m}$ in Equation 5.16.

## Analysing time-to-event data

Many endpoints of interest in radiation oncology require prolonged observation of the patient, specifically late adverse effects and tumour control (i.e. the event occurs after a latent period). This often gives rise to (right-)censored observations: at the time of analysis it is known for a proportion of cases that a given patient had not reached the endpoint at the time when he or she was last seen, but it is not known whether this will happen in the future. Statistical methods for analysing censored time-to-event data were developed in the 1950s and 1960s. Analysis of this kind of data without correction for latency and censoring may give rise to misleading results (11). For time-to-event endpoints where variability in observation time causes the dose-response relationship to become shallower, fitting a model with latent-time correction will recover a steeper underlying dose-response curve (25). Two main approaches have been used in the literature: one based on the semi-parametric Cox proportional hazards model and the other based on mixture models with a parametric latent time distribution (9,28). It is beyond the scope of this book to discuss these models in detail.

> ## Key points
>
> 1. There is no well-defined 'tolerance dose' for radiation complications or 'tumouricidal dose' for local tumour control: rather, the probability of a biological effect rises from 0% to 100% over a range of doses.
> 2. The steepness of a dose-response curve at a response level of $P$% may be quantified by the value $\gamma_P$, that is the increase in response in percentage points for a 1% increase in dose.
> 3. Dose-response curves for late normal tissue endpoints tend to be steeper (typical $\gamma_{50}$ between 2 and 6) than the dose-response curves for local control of squamous cell carcinoma of the head and neck (typical $\gamma_{50}$ between 1.5 and 2.5).
> 4. The steepness of a dose-response curve is higher if the data are generated by varying the dose while keeping the number of fractions constant ('double trouble') than if the dose per fraction is fixed.
> 5. Dosimetric and biological heterogeneity cause the population dose-response curve to be shallower.

# BIBLIOGRAPHY

1. Bentzen SM. Steepness of the clinical dose-control curve and variation in the in vitro radiosensitivity of head and neck squamous cell carcinoma. *Int J Radiat Biol* 1992;61:417–423.

2. Bentzen SM. Radiobiological considerations in the design of clinical trials. *Radiother Oncol* 1994;32:1–11.

3. Bentzen SM. Steepness of the radiation dose-response curve for dose-per-fraction escalation keeping the number of fractions fixed. *Acta Oncol* 2005;44:825–828.

4. Bentzen SM. Preventing or reducing late side effects of radiation therapy: Radiobiology meets molecular pathology. *Nat Rev Cancer* 2006;6:702–713.

5. Bentzen SM, Johansen LV, Overgaard J, Thames HD. Clinical radiobiology of squamous cell carcinoma of the oropharynx. *Int J Radiat Oncol Biol Phys* 1991;20:1197–1206.

6. Bentzen SM, Overgaard J. Clinical normal tissue radiobiology. In: Tobias JS and Thomas PRM, editors. *Current Radiation Oncology*. London: Arnold; 1996. pp. 37–67.

7. Bentzen SM, Overgaard M. Relationship between early and late normal-tissue injury after postmastectomy radiotherapy. *Radiother Oncol* 1991;20:159–165.

8. Bentzen SM, Thames HD, Overgaard J. Does variation in the in vitro cellular radiosensitivity explain the shallow clinical dose-control curve for malignant melanoma? *Int J Radiat Biol* 1990;57:117–126.

9. Bentzen SM, Thames HD, Travis EL et al. Direct estimation of latent time for radiation injury in late-responding normal tissues: Gut, lung, and spinal cord. *Int J Radiat Biol* 1989;55:27–43.

10. Bentzen SM, Tucker SL. Quantifying the position and steepness of radiation dose-response curves. *Int J Radiat Biol* 1997;71:531–542.

11. Bentzen SM, Vaeth M, Pedersen DE, Overgaard J. Why actuarial estimates should be used in reporting late normal-tissue effects of cancer treatment... now! *Int J Radiat Oncol Biol Phys* 1995;32:1531–1534.

12. Brahme A. Dosimetric precision requirements in radiation therapy. *Acta Radiol Oncol* 1984;23:379–391.

13. Fenwick JD. Predicting the radiation control probability of heterogeneous tumour ensembles: Data analysis and parameter estimation using a closed-form expression. *Phys Med Biol* 1998;43:2159–2178.

14. Herring DF. The consequences of dose response curves for tumor control and normal tissue injury on the precision necessary in patient management. *Laryngoscope* 1975;85:1112–1118.

15. Holthusen H. Erfahrungen über die verträglichkeitsgrenze für röntgenstrahlen und deren nutzanwendung zur verhütung von schäden. *Strahlenther Onkol* 1936;57:254–269.

16. Honore HB, Bentzen SM, Moller K, Grau C. Sensori-neural hearing loss after radiotherapy for nasopharyngeal carcinoma: Individualized risk estimation. *Radiother Oncol* 2002;65:9–16.

17. Khalil AA, Bentzen SM, Overgaard J. Steepness of the dose-response curve as a function of volume in an experimental tumor irradiated under ambient or hypoxic conditions. *Int J Radiat Oncol Biol Phys* 1997;39:797–802.

18. Levegrün S, Jackson A, Zelefsky MJ et al. Risk group dependence of dose-response for biopsy outcome after three-dimensional conformal radiation therapy of prostate cancer. *Radiother Oncol* 2002;63:11–26.

19. Lyman JT. Complication probability as assessed from dose-volume histograms. *Radiat Res Suppl* 1985;8:S13–S19.

20. Munro TR, Gilbert CW. The relation between tumour lethal doses and the radiosensitivity of tumour cells. *Br J Radiol* 1961;34:246–251.

21. Okunieff P, Morgan D, Niemierko A, Suit HD. Radiation dose-response of human tumors. *Int J Radiat Oncol Biol Phys* 1995;32:1227–1237.

22. Overgaard J, Hjelm-Hansen M, Johansen LV, Andersen AP. Comparison of conventional and split-course radiotherapy as primary treatment in carcinoma of the larynx. *Acta Oncol* 1988;27:147–152.

23. Puck TT, Marcus PI. Action of x-rays on mammalian cells. *J Exp Med* 1956;103:653–666.

24. Roberts SA, Hendry JH. Inter-tumour heterogeneity and tumour control. In: Dale R and Jones B, editors. *Radiobiological Modelling in Radiation Oncology*. London: British Institute of Radiology; 2007. pp. 169–195.

25. Ronjom MF, Brink C, Bentzen SM, Hegedus L, Overgaard J, Johansen J. Hypothyroidism after primary radiotherapy for head and neck squamous cell carcinoma: Normal tissue complication probability modeling with latent time correction. *Radiother Oncol* 2013;109:317–322.

26. Suit H, Skates S, Taghian A, Okunieff P, Efird JT. Clinical implications of heterogeneity of tumor response to radiation therapy. *Radiother Oncol* 1992;25:251–260.

27. Svensson H, Westling P, Larsson LG. Radiation-induced lesions of the brachial plexus correlated to the dose-time-fraction schedule. *Acta Radiol Ther Phys Biol* 1975;14:228–238.

28. Tucker SL, Liu HH, Liao Z et al. Analysis of radiation pneumonitis risk using a generalized Lyman model. *Int J Radiat Oncol Biol Phys* 2008;72:568–574.

29. Webb S, Nahum AE. A model for calculating tumour control probability in radiotherapy including the effects of inhomogeneous distributions of dose and clonogenic cell density. *Phys Med Biol* 1993;38:653–666.

30. Yarnold J, Bentzen SM, Coles C, Haviland J. Hypofractionated whole-breast radiotherapy for women with early breast cancer: Myths and realities. *Int J Radiat Oncol Biol Phys* 2011;79:1–9.

# Linear energy transfer and relative biological effectiveness

## MICHAEL C. JOINER, JAY W. BURMEISTER AND WOLFGANG DÖRR

## 6.1 INTRODUCTION

Modern radiotherapy is usually delivered using linear accelerators producing X-rays with energies of 4–25 MV which have generally superseded therapy with lower energy $^{60}$Co or $^{137}$Cs $\gamma$-rays.

X-rays and $\gamma$-rays are uncharged electromagnetic radiations, physically similar in nature to radio waves or visible light except that their wavelength is less than 10 picometers ($10^{-12}$ m) so that the individual photons ('packets' of energy) are energetic enough to ionize molecules in tissues that they penetrate. This ionization results in the biological effects seen in radiotherapy. These X- and $\gamma$-rays all have roughly the same biological effect per unit dose, although there is a small dependence on the energy with lower energies being slightly more effective. The biological damage produced by high-energy photon beams is the result of ionizations by energetic electrons set in motion by photon interactions. Accordingly, the biological effects from beams of energetic electrons are similar to that from high-energy photon beams. While one could therefore refer to conventional radiotherapy as 'particle therapy', this terminology generally refers to another class of radiotherapy which is being increasingly adopted. The term *particle therapy* typically refers to radiotherapy using protons, neutrons, $\alpha$-particles, fully stripped carbon ions or even heavier ions.

These particles may have a greater biological effect per unit dose compared with conventional X- and $\gamma$-rays and the basis for this greater biological effect is described within this chapter. Charged particles have, in addition, very different depth-dose absorption profiles compared with uncharged particles (i.e. neutrons) or conventional electromagnetic radiations (X- and $\gamma$-rays) and this enables more precise dose distributions to be achieved in radiotherapy (see Chapter 25). This chapter explains the basic physical characteristics of absorbed dose deposition and the ensuing effects on the radiobiology of these different types of radiation used in cancer therapy.

## 6.2 MICRODOSIMETRY

It is possible to build up a picture of the submicroscopic pattern of ionizations produced by radiation within a cell nucleus using special techniques for measuring ionization in very small volumes, and/or with computer simulations: this is the field of microdosimetry. Figure 6.1 shows examples of microdosimetric calculations of ionization tracks from $\gamma$-rays or $\alpha$-particles passing through a cell nucleus (5). At the scale of the cell nucleus, the $\gamma$-rays deposit much of their energy as single isolated ionizations or excitations and much of the resulting DNA damage is efficiently repaired by enzymes within the nucleus (see Chapter 2). About 1000 of these sparse tracks are produced per gray of absorbed radiation dose. The $\alpha$-particles produce fewer tracks but the intense ionization within each track leads to more severe damage where the track intersects vital structures such as DNA. At the low doses of $\alpha$-particle irradiation that are encountered in environmental exposures, only some cells will be traversed by a particle and many cells will be unexposed.

*Linear energy transfer* (LET) is the term used to describe the density of ionization in particle tracks. LET is the average energy per unit distance (usually given in keV $\mu m^{-1}$) deposited by a charged particle. In Figure 6.1, the $\gamma$-rays have a LET of about 0.3 keV $\mu m^{-1}$ and are described as 'low-LET' radiation. The $\alpha$-particles have a LET of about 100 keV $\mu m^{-1}$ and are an example of 'high-LET' radiation.

Why are neutrons described as 'high-LET' radiation when they are uncharged particles? Neutrons do not interact with the orbital electrons in the tissues through which they pass and they do not directly produce ionization. They do, however, interact with atomic nuclei from which they eject slow, densely ionizing protons and other particles (Figure 6.2). This secondary production of knock-on particles confers high LET and the resulting DNA damage may involve several adjacent base pairs and is much more difficult or even impossible for a cell to repair; this is the reason why neutrons and heavy charged particles will produce greater cell kill than X-rays for the same dose delivered.

Figure 6.3 further illustrates high-LET through the presentation of the lineal energy spectrum of charged particles produced by a high-energy therapeutic neutron beam (3). This spectrum was measured using a tissue equivalent proportional counter simulating a 1 $\mu m$ diameter

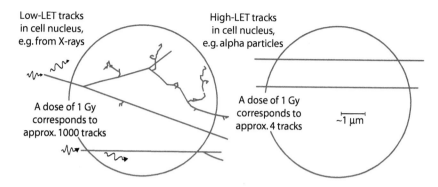

**Figure 6.1** The structure of particle tracks for low-LET radiation (left) and $\alpha$-particles (right). The circles indicate the typical size of mammalian cell nuclei. Note the tortuous tracks of low-energy secondary electrons, greatly magnified in this illustration. (From (5), with permission.)

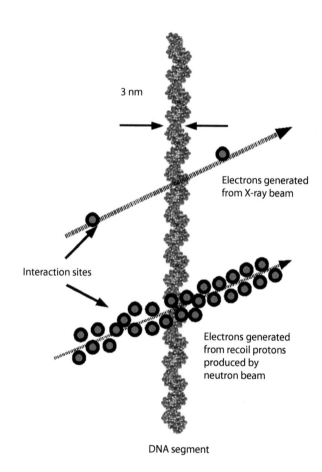

**Figure 6.2** The greater DNA damage caused by the higher density of charged particles following irradiation with neutrons compared with photons.

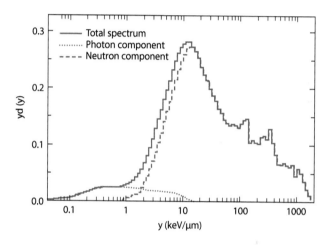

**Figure 6.3** Total, photon and neutron LET spectra in the Wayne State University/Karmanos Cancer Center therapeutic fast neutron therapy beam measured with a tissue equivalent proportional counter simulating a 1 µm site diameter. (From (3), with permission.)

information lies in the fact that the biological effects of radiation are strongly dependent upon the LET.

## 6.3 BIOLOGICAL EFFECTS DEPEND UPON LET

As LET increases, radiation produces more cell killing per gray. Figure 6.4 shows the survival of human T1g kidney cells plotted against dose for eight different radiations, with LET varying from 2 keV µm$^{-1}$ (250 kVp X-rays) to 165 keV µm$^{-1}$ (2.5 MeV $\alpha$-particles). As LET increases, the cell-survival curves become steeper, they also become straighter with less shoulder, which indicates either a higher ratio of lethal to potentially lethal lesions (in lesion-interaction models; Chapter 4) or that high-LET radiation damage is less likely to be repaired correctly (in repair saturation models; Chapter 4). In the linear-quadratic description, these straighter cell-survival curves have a higher $\alpha/\beta$ value, thus higher LET radiations usually give responses with higher

site in tissue and is therefore an example of experimental microdosimetry. The area under the curve represents the absorbed dose and the total absorbed dose is separated into a photon component, made up of recoil electrons from photon interactions, and a neutron component, made up of recoil protons up to approximately 150 keV µm$^{-1}$, recoil $\alpha$-particles up to approximately 400 keV µm$^{-1}$, and heavier recoil particles at higher LET values. The utility of such

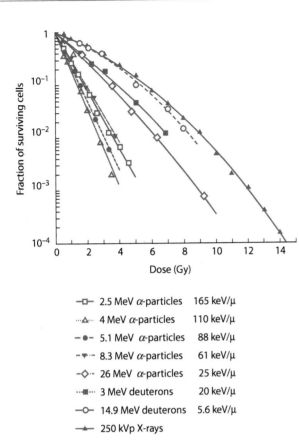

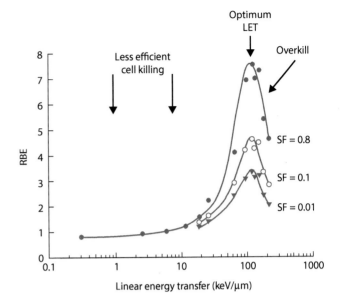

Figure 6.5 Dependence of RBE on LET and the phenomenon of overkill by very high LET radiations. RBE has been calculated from Figure 6.3 at cell surviving fraction (SF) levels of 0.8, 0.1 and 0.01. (From (1), with permission.)

Figure 6.4 Survival of human kidney cells exposed *in vitro* to radiations of different LET. (From (1), with permission.)

$\alpha/\beta$. For a particular particle, LET generally increases with decreasing particle kinetic energy. However, notice that 2.5 MeV $\alpha$-particles are less efficient compared with 4 MeV $\alpha$-particles even though they have a higher LET; this is due to the phenomenon of *overkill* shown in Figure 6.5.

The *relative biological effectiveness* (RBE) of a radiation under test (e.g. a high-LET radiation) is defined as

$$\text{RBE} = \frac{\text{Dose of reference radiation}}{\text{Dose of test radiation}} \quad (6.1)$$

to give the same biological effect. The reference low-LET radiation is commonly 250 kVp X-rays or $^{60}$Co $\gamma$-rays since these radiations are usually available whenever RBE is being evaluated. Figure 6.5 shows RBE values for the T1g cells featured in Figure 6.4. RBE has been calculated at cell survival levels of 0.8, 0.1 and 0.01, illustrating the fact that RBE is not constant but depends on the level of biological damage and hence on the dose level. RBE also depends on LET, and rises to a maximum at a LET of about 100 keV $\mu m^{-1}$, then falls for higher values of LET due to overkill. For a cell to be killed, enough energy must be deposited in the DNA to produce a sufficient number of double-strand breaks (see Chapter 4). Sparsely ionizing, low-LET radiation is inefficient because more than one particle may have to pass through the cell to produce enough DNA double-strand

breaks. Densely ionizing, very high-LET radiation is also inefficient because it deposits more energy per cell, and hence produces more DNA double-strand breaks than are actually needed to kill the cell. These cells are 'overkilled', meaning that a larger amount of dose is deposited in each cell than is necessary for cell kill, leading to a reduced biological effectiveness per unit dose. Radiation of optimal LET deposits the right amount of energy per cell which produces just enough DNA double-strand breaks to kill the cell. This optimum LET is usually around 100 keV $\mu m^{-1}$ but it does vary between different cell types and also depends on the spectrum of LET values in the radiation beam as well as the mean LET.

Figure 6.5 also shows that the increase in RBE begins to occur at approximately 10 keV $\mu m^{-1}$. This LET value is the unofficial 'dividing line' between 'low-LET' and 'high-LET' radiation. Returning to Figure 6.3, one can see that the vast majority of the photon absorbed dose in a fast neutron therapy beam, for example, is delivered below 10 keV $\mu m^{-1}$, where the RBE is unity, while the relatively low-energy protons generated in this neutron beam span from approximately 1 keV $\mu m^{-1}$ to 150 keV $\mu m^{-1}$. Using this kind of information, one could weight the absorbed dose by the estimated RBE based on the LET spectrum of the absorbed dose. Such an RBE-weighted absorbed dose would be much more predictive of biological effects than the simple measurement of energy deposited per unit mass.

As LET increases, the oxygen enhancement ratio (OER) (Section 17.1) decreases. The measurements shown as an example in Figure 6.6 were also made with cultured T1g cells of human origin (1). The sharp reduction in OER occurs

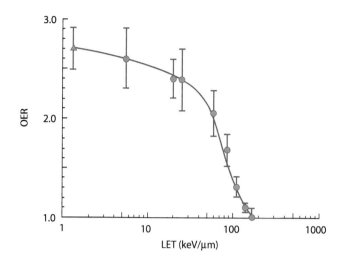

**Figure 6.6** The OER decreases with increasing LET. Closed circles refer to monoenergetic $\alpha$-particles and deuterons and the triangle to 250 kVp X-rays. (From (1), with permission.)

over the same range of LET as the sharp increase in RBE (Figure 6.5).

## 6.4 RELATIVE BIOLOGICAL EFFECTIVENESS DEPENDS ON DOSE

As indicated in Figure 6.5, the RBE is higher if measured at lower radiation doses, corresponding to higher levels of cell survival (less effect). Figure 6.7 shows in more detail the RBE for test doses of 4 MeV $\alpha$-particles plotted against a reference dose of 250 kVp X-rays, for the T1g human cells irradiated *in vitro*. The data points were derived from Figure 6.4 by reading off from the $\alpha$-particle survival curve the dose required to achieve the same cell survival as obtained for each X-ray

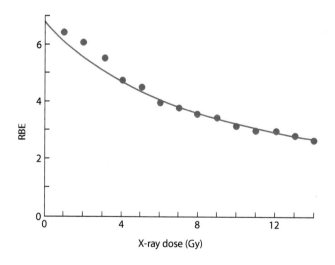

**Figure 6.7** RBE of 4 MeV $\alpha$-particles increases with decreasing dose for cell lines irradiated *in vitro*. RBE values were calculated from the cell survival data shown in Figure 6.4. The full line is calculated as described in the text.

dose evaluated. The RBE for the 4 MeV $\alpha$-particles increases with decreasing dose because the low-LET X-ray survival response is more curved and has a bigger shoulder compared with the high-LET survival response. If linear-quadratic equations are used to model both the low-LET (reference) and the high-LET (test) responses, RBE can be predicted mathematically as a function of the reference dose ($d_R$) or the test dose ($d_T$) using formulae containing the $\alpha/\beta$ values and the ratio $\alpha_T/\alpha_R$ (6). The formulae are

$$RBE = \frac{K + \sqrt{K^2 + 4Kd_R(1 + d_R/V)/C}}{2(1 + d_R/V)} \quad (6.2)$$

$$RBE = \frac{-V + \sqrt{V^2 + 4VKd_T(1 + d_T/C)}}{2d_T} \quad (6.3)$$

where $K = \alpha_T/\alpha_R$, $V = \alpha/\beta$ for the reference radiation and $C = \alpha/\beta$ for the test radiation.

In Figure 6.7, the solid line shows the prediction of Equation 6.2 which gives RBE as a function of the reference dose, in this case X-rays.

RBE can also be measured *in vivo*. In normal tissues this is done by comparing the relationships between damage and dose for both high- and low-LET radiations. This can be done for any endpoint of damage, including tissue breakdown or loss of tissue function. As an example, Figure 6.8a shows the results of experiments to study the loss of renal function in mice after external-beam radiotherapy. This was done by measuring the increased retention of $^{51}$Cr-radiolabelled ethylenediamine tetra-acetic acid (EDTA) in the plasma at 1 hour after injection; normally functioning kidneys completely clear this substance from the body within this time. For the high-LET radiation, in this example, neutrons produced by bombarding beryllium with 4 MeV deuterons, designated d(4)-Be, fractionation makes almost no difference to the tolerance dose but for X-rays a much higher total dose is required to produce renal damage when the treatment is split into 2, 5 or 10 fractions. This difference in the fractionation response for high- and low-LET radiations *in vivo* could be interpreted as reflecting the shape of survival curves for putative target cells in the tissue: almost straight for neutrons, and downwards-bending for X-rays (Figure 6.4). Practically, as shown in Section 9.4, this is expressed in the different $\alpha/\beta$ values derived directly from the relationships between isoeffective total dose and dose per fraction *in vivo* for the high- and low-LET radiations: high-LET with a high $\alpha/\beta$ and low-LET with a low $\alpha/\beta$. In this *in vivo* situation, RBE values themselves are calculated from the ratio of X-ray to neutron total doses required to produce the same biological effect in the same number of fractions. This is plotted against X-ray dose per fraction in Figure 6.8b. It can be seen that *in vivo*, RBE increases with decreasing dose per fraction in the same way as RBE increases with decreasing single dose for cells *in vitro* shown in Figure 6.7. *In vivo*, RBE versus dose can also be modelled using Equations 6.2 and 6.3. The solid line in Figure 6.8b shows the mathematical fit of Equation 6.2 to

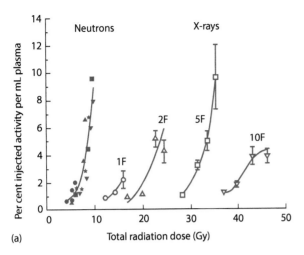

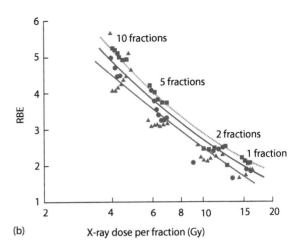

**Figure 6.8** The RBE for kidney damage increases with decreasing dose per fraction. RBE values are derived from graphs similar to panel (a), which shows dose-effect curves for $^{51}$Cr-EDTA clearance following irradiation with 1, 2, 3, 5 and 10 fractions of neutrons or 1, 2, 5 and 10 fractions of X-rays. The RBE values in panel (b) were obtained with various renal-damage endpoints: isotope clearance (circles), reduction in haematocrit (squares); increase in urine output (triangles). (From (7), with permission.)

the data, from which it is possible to obtain $\alpha_{\text{Neutrons}}/\alpha_{\text{Xrays}}$, and $\alpha/\beta$ for X-rays and for neutrons, directly from these RBE versus dose-per-fraction data and hence calculate a predicted RBE at any value of dose per fraction.

## 6.5 THE RADIOBIOLOGICAL BASIS FOR HIGH-LET RADIOTHERAPY

We have seen that the differential radiosensitivity between poorly oxygenated (more radioresistant) and well-oxygenated (more radiosensitive) cells is reduced with high-LET radiations (Figure 6.6). Therefore, tumour sites in which hypoxia could be a problem in radiotherapy (some head and neck tumours, and cervix cancers, for example) might benefit from high-LET radiotherapy in the same way as from chemical hypoxic-cell sensitisers (see Section 17.5).

Treatment of tumours that have lower X-ray $\alpha/\beta$, for example prostate and breast, might also benefit radiobiologically from using high-LET radiotherapy under some conditions, because of higher RBE. However, in this situation, the actual benefit obtained from high-LET radiation will always depend also on the treatment plan because of the requirement to adequately spare late-responding tissues which also have low $\alpha/\beta$ values.

The effect of low-LET radiation on cells is strongly influenced by their position in the cell cycle, with cells in the S-phase being more radioresistant than cells in G2 or mitosis (see Chapter 8). Cells in the stationary (i.e. plateau) phase also tend to be more radioresistant than cells in active proliferation. Both of these factors act to increase the effect of fractionated radiotherapy on more rapidly cycling cells compared with those cycling slowly or not at all, because the rapidly cycling cells which survive the first few fractions are statistically more likely to be caught later in a sensitive phase and so be killed by a subsequent dose, a process termed *cell-cycle resensitisation*.

This differential radiosensitivity due to cell-cycle position is considerably reduced with high-LET radiation (4) and is a reason why we might expect high-LET radiotherapy to be beneficial in some slowly growing, X-ray resistant tumours.

A further biological rationale for high-LET therapy is based on the observation that the range of radiation response of different cell types is reduced with high-LET radiation compared with X-rays. This is shown in Figure 6.9, which compares the *in vitro* response of 20 human cell lines to photon and neutron irradiation (2). This reduced range of response affects the benefit expected, which is the balance between tumour and normal tissue responses. Thus, if tumour cells are already more radiosensitive to X-rays than the critical normal-cell population, high-LET radiation should not be used since this would reduce an already favourable differential. Possible examples are seminomas, lymphomas and Hodgkin disease. However, if the tumour cells are more resistant to X-rays than the critical normal cells, high-LET radiation might reduce this difference in radiosensitivity and thus would effectively 'sensitise' the tumour cell population relative to a fixed level of normal tissue damage. High-LET radiation would be advantageous in this case.

Some quantitative examples of the translation of high-LET into high RBE are provided here. For proton therapy, the LET remains relatively low for the majority of the particle tracks in tissue. This is a consequence of the very high energies required to reach deep-seated tumours. Near the end of the particle track (within the Bragg peak), the LET becomes significantly greater than 10 keV $\mu$m$^{-1}$ and thus the RBE becomes greater than unity. Since clinical application of proton therapy generally utilizes a spread-out Bragg peak, which is the summation of multiple beams of different energy, the region of increased RBE is 'smeared' over the target volume and the resulting clinical RBE is generally taken to be approximately 1.1 (see review article by Paganetti [8]). In contrast, neutron therapy

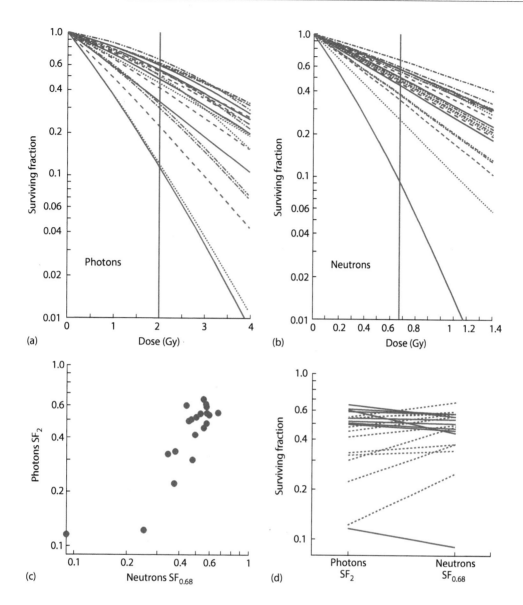

**Figure 6.9** Response of 20 human tumour cell lines to (a) 4 MVp photons, or (b) p(62.5)-Be neutrons. The vertical lines show the photon (2 Gy) and neutron (0.68 Gy) doses that give the same *median* cell survival; the average RBE is therefore $2/0.68 = 2.94$. (c) The range of cell survival at the reference neutron dose of 0.68 Gy ($SF_{0.68}$) is less than the range of cell survival at a photon dose of 2 Gy ($SF_2$). In 9/20 of the cell lines neutrons gave lower cell survival than photons at these doses (d).

sets in motion low-energy recoil protons throughout the irradiated region and thus has a significantly larger RBE than proton therapy. This RBE is relatively constant as a function of position in a particular tissue type within the treated volume but can vary significantly between different tissue types due to various factors such as oxygenation, cell cycle effects, etc. These variations can be greater than a factor of 2 as illustrated in Figure 6.9. Similar findings were reported subsequently by Warenius et al. (10) who compared 30 different cell lines irradiated *in vitro* with both X-rays and neutrons. RBE estimation for carbon and heavier ions is even more challenging, since it depends not only on cell sensitivity but on depth as well. RBE values and their variability with cell type similar to that from neutron therapy are observed for lower-energy carbon ions

in the spread-out Bragg peak (9). In addition, variations on the order of a factor of 3 may be observed as a function of particle energy (i.e. as a function of depth within the patient). These data illustrate some of the relative difficulties involved in the clinical application of high-LET/high-RBE radiotherapy. In Chapter 25, we summarise the clinical experience with high-LET radiations.

## Key points

1. X- and $\gamma$-rays are sparsely ionizing radiations with a low LET. Some particle radiations (e.g. neutrons, $\alpha$-particles or heavy ions) have a high LET.

2. High-LET radiations are *biologically* more effective per gray than low-LET radiations. This is measured by the RBE. For most high-LET radiations at therapeutic dose levels, RBE is in the range of 2–10.

3. RBE increases as the LET increases up to about 100 keV $\mu m^{-1}$, above which RBE decreases because of cellular overkill. The OER also decreases rapidly over the same range of LET.

4. RBE increases as the dose is reduced *in vitro*, or the dose *per fraction* is reduced *in vivo*. In late-responding tissues, this increase occurs more rapidly with decreasing dose per fraction than in early responding tissues.

5. Heavy particles such as He, C and Ne ions, have a high LET and in addition they have improved physical depth-dose distributions.

6. Proton beams provide the best improvement in dose distribution for the lowest cost; however, their RBE averaged over a whole treatment volume is similar to low-energy photons.

## ■ BIBLIOGRAPHY

1. Barendsen GW. Responses of cultured cells, tumours and normal tissues to radiations of different linear energy transfer. *Curr Topics Radiat Res Q* 1968;4:293–356.

2. Britten RA, Warenius HM, Parkins C, Peacock JH. The inherent cellular sensitivity to 62.5 MeV(p-Be) neutrons of human cells differing in photon sensitivity. *Int J Radiat Biol* 1992;61:805–812.

3. Burmeister J, Kota C, Maughan RL, Waker AJ. Miniature tissue-equivalent proportional counters for BNCT and BNCEFNT dosimetry. *Med Phys* 2001;28:1911–1925.

4. Chapman JD. Biophysical models of mammalian cell inactivation by radiation. In: Meyn RE and Withers HR, editors. *Radiation Biology in Cancer Research*. New York, NY: Raven Press; 1980. pp. 21–32.

5. Goodhead DT. Spatial and temporal distribution of energy. *Health Phys* 1988;55:231–240.

6. Joiner MC. A comparison of the effects of p(62)-Be and d(16)-Be neutrons in the mouse kidney. *Radiother Oncol* 1988;13:211–224.

7. Joiner MC, Johns H. Renal damage in the mouse: The effect of d(4)-Be neutrons. *Radiat Res* 1987;109:456–468.

8. Paganetti H. Relative biological effectiveness (RBE) values for proton beam therapy. Variations as a function of biological endpoint, dose, and linear energy transfer. *Phys Med Biol* 2014;59:R419–R472.

9. Suzuki M, Kase Y, Yamaguchi H, Kanai T, Ando K. Relative biological effectiveness for cell-killing effect on various human cell lines irradiated with heavy-ion medical accelerator in Chiba (HIMAC) carbon-ion beams. *Int J Radiat Oncol Biol Phys* 2000;48:241–250.

10. Warenius HM, Britten RA, Peacock JH. The relative cellular radiosensitivity of 30 human *in vitro* cell lines of different histological type to high LET 62.5 MeV (p→Be+) fast neutrons and 4 MeV photons. *Radiother Oncol* 1994;30:83–89.

## ■ FURTHER READING

11. Alpen EL. *Radiation Biophysics*. 2nd ed. San Diego, CA: Academic Press; 1998.

12. Conference Proceedings. Nordic conference on neutrons in research and cancer therapy, *Conference Proceedings*. Linkoping, April 29–30, 1993. *Acta Oncol* 1994;33:225–327.

13. Engenhart-Cabillic R, Wambersie A (Eds). Fast neutrons and high-LET particles in cancer therapy. In *Recent Results in Cancer Research*, Vol. 150. New York, NY: Springer-Verlag; 1998.

14. Goodhead DT. The initial physical damage produced by ionizing radiations. *Int J Radiat Biol* 1989;56: 623–634.

15. *International Commission on Radiation Units and Measurements*. ICRU Report 36–Microdosimetry. Bethesda, MD: International Commission on Radiation Units and Measurements; 1983.

16. Noda K, Furukawa T, Fujisawa T et al. New accelerator facility for carbon-ion cancer-therapy. *J Radiat Res (Tokyo)* 2007;48(Suppl. A):A43–A54.

17. Suit H, DeLaney T, Goldberg S et al. Proton vs carbon ion beams in the definitive radiation treatment of cancer patients. *Radiother Oncol* 2010;95:3–22.

18. Wambersie A, Auberger T, Gahbauer RA, Jones DT, Potter R. A challenge for high-precision radiation therapy: The case for hadrons. *Strahlenther Onkol* 1999;175(Suppl. 2): 122–128.

19. Wambersie A, Richard F, Breteau N. Development of fast neutron therapy worldwide. Radiobiological, clinical and technical aspects. *Acta Oncol* 1994;33:261–274.

20. Withers HR, Thames HD, Jr., Peters LJ. Biological bases for high RBE values for late effects of neutron irradiation. *Int J Radiat Oncol Biol Phys* 1982;8:2071–2076.

# Physics of radiation therapy for the radiobiologist

## JAY W. BURMEISTER AND MICHAEL C. JOINER

## 7.1 INTRODUCTION

Radiation oncology is an extraordinarily interdisciplinary field. The realms of clinical radiation oncology, medical physics and radiobiology are thoroughly intertwined within both clinical practice and research. To fully utilize the knowledge acquired in one of these disciplines, one must have a solid understanding of the theory and practices involved in the others. The purpose of this chapter is to provide a broad overview of the fundamental physical processes and technical procedures involved in radiotherapy in its modern state. Our purpose in introducing this chapter is that a better understanding of the theory and practices involved in radiotherapy physics along with uncertainties involved in the process should help the radiobiologist better interpret clinical data and will provide a stronger background from which to develop and apply radiobiological models.

## 7.2 RADIATION INTERACTION FUNDAMENTALS FOR RADIATION THERAPY

The concept that cell damage was due to discrete events of ionizing radiation imparted to specific biological targets was first suggested in the 1920s (2,3). Investigations over the following several decades forged the path for understanding the mechanism of radiation-induced reproductive cell death and in 1956, it was postulated that two chromosome breaks could interact provided they were within roughly a micrometre of one another (13). However, it was not until 1970 that experimental verification confirmed the nucleus as the principal target for radiation-induced cell inactivation (15). We now know that the biological effects of radiation result principally from damage to the DNA. To make further predictions and/or models to represent the effects of radiation on cells, it is valuable to have an understanding of radiation interaction mechanisms and their effects at the level of the DNA. Thus, the discussion of the physics of radiation therapy should start at the level of radiation interactions.

Radiation therapy utilizes high-energy charged and uncharged particles for the purposes of eliminating neoplastic disease. Since the cell damage we are interested in is either direct or indirect damage resulting from

ionization caused by the radiation, we do not discuss sources or interactions of non-ionizing radiation. Specifically, we discuss high energy photons, neutrons, electrons and light ions. Charged particles and uncharged particles interact very differently, so we treat them separately. Uncharged particles interact through a relatively small number of catastrophic interactions. As such, they do not slow down gradually as charged particles generally do. Charged particles interact constantly with their surroundings through the Coulomb force. The slowing down of charged particles in matter can be visualized as a sort of 'friction-like' process since it is generally a cumulative effect of many small interactions at a distance. However, charged particles can also have catastrophic interactions as we discuss. Interaction probabilities for both charged and uncharged particles are generally dependent upon energy, particle type and medium which they are traversing. Here we briefly discuss both the interaction mechanisms and some of the factors that influence the interaction probabilities.

Photons and neutrons are examples of uncharged particles. In large part, uncharged particles either interact in a medium and are absorbed or scattered out of the radiation beam, or they continue through the medium without interaction. As a result, the mean energy of a narrow beam of monoenergetic uncharged particles passing through a medium does not change significantly. Since the number of particles remaining in the beam is decreasing and the probability for interaction for each particle remains the same, the number of particles attenuated from the beam per unit depth gradually decreases as a function of depth. This results in an exponentially decreasing number of particles remaining in the beam, and this exponential attenuation is commonly observed by beams of uncharged particles as a function of depth. This is analogous mathematically to the exponential decrease in the number of radioactive nuclei in a sample as a function of time, since the number of radioactive nuclei is decreasing but the probability of decay for each nucleus per unit time remains constant. The mean energy of a beam of polyenergetic uncharged particles will change as a function of depth due to preferential absorption, since the lower-energy particles will be more easily attenuated from the beam. This phenomenon is referred to as 'filtration' and creates a 'harder' beam which has a higher mean energy. Once sufficient hardening has taken place, the mean energy of the beam remains relatively constant with depth, and we observe a relatively exponential decrease in the number of particles in the beam as a function of depth.

## Photon interactions

There are five main interaction mechanisms for high-energy photons used for radiation therapy purposes. These include the photoelectric effect (PE), Compton interaction, pair production (PP), Rayleigh (coherent) scatter, and photodisintegration. In PE, the photon is completely absorbed and gives its energy to a bound atomic electron which leaves the atom with the energy of the incident photon minus the binding energy by which it was bound to the atom. PE cannot occur with a free (unbound) electron and the PE interaction probability increases with binding energy, thus it is higher for inner shell electrons and increases with increasing atomic number. PE is the dominant photon interaction mechanism at low energies and for high atomic number absorbers. PE is in large part responsible for the excellent contrast between bone and soft tissue for diagnostic energy X-ray imaging, since the PE interaction probabilities are far higher in bone than in soft tissue due to the higher binding energies of electrons in the higher atomic number elements in bone.

In the Compton interaction, the photon is scattered and gives part of its energy to a recoil electron. Interaction probabilities for the Compton interaction depend on the number of electrons available with which to interact. The number of electrons per unit mass is given by $N_A Z/A$ where $N_A$ is Avogadro's number (number of atoms per mole), $A$ is the atomic weight (mass per mole) and $Z$ is the atomic number (number of protons or electrons per atom). For low atomic number materials, the ratio $Z/A$ (and thus the number of electrons per unit mass) is roughly constant as a function of atomic number with the exception of hydrogen. As a result, the number of Compton interactions per unit mass is roughly independent of the atomic number. For high atomic number materials, the ratio $Z/A$ gradually decreases with increasing atomic number due to the increase in neutron-to-proton ratio in the nucleus. The number of electrons per unit volume is, of course, given by the number of electrons per unit mass times the density. Therefore, more Compton interactions will take place in a given volume of a higher-density medium. However, the absorbed dose is the energy deposited per unit mass. Thus, in the case of Compton interactions, the absorbed dose will be related to the number of interactions per unit mass (proportional to $Z/A$), the amount of energy given to electrons in those interactions and the amount of energy deposited by those electrons in the mass of interest.

Megavoltage energy photons are required to effectively reach deep-seated targets within the body, and the Compton interaction is the dominant interaction mechanism in this domain. One can use a radiotherapy treatment beam of megavoltage photons to image patients prior to treatment; however, the bone/soft tissue contrast will be far lower than when using kilovoltage diagnostic energy photons. In the megavoltage (Compton) domain, we are essentially only viewing the density difference between different tissues since the Compton interaction probability per unit mass is roughly independent of atomic number. In the kilovoltage (PE) domain, we are viewing not only density differences between different tissues but also large differences in interaction probability as a function of the atomic number of the tissue.

In PP, the photon is absorbed in the nuclear Coulomb field, and an electron/positron pair is created. The threshold energy below which this interaction cannot take place is approximately the rest mass energy of the electron/positron pair (1.022 MeV). When the positron meets an electron, they annihilate, converting their rest mass into energy and generating two oppositely directed photons with this energy in order to conserve momentum. PP is the dominant interaction mechanism for high energies and high atomic number absorbers.

In Rayleigh (coherent) scatter, the photon only changes direction and does not impart any energy to the medium. Since it does not deposit energy and thus does not contribute to the absorbed dose, this interaction mechanism is of relatively little importance here. In photodisintegration, the photon enters and excites the nucleus which then emits one or more nucleons. This interaction occurs at high energies, but its interaction probability is significantly lower than competing interactions such as PP. Its principal significance is that it can eject photoneutrons from the nucleus. These neutrons may have significantly higher biological effectiveness than the photons in the beam as we discuss later. As a result, the photoneutron interaction mechanism may be of significance in particular situations even though it occurs with much lower frequency than competing interactions. Two examples of this possible significance are the potential risk of radiation-induced cancer resulting from neutron irradiation of sensitive tissues in a patient's body during radiotherapy, and the choice of shielding materials and thicknesses required around a radiotherapy treatment vault to protect against radiation exposure from neutrons. Total photon interaction probabilities represent the aggregate probability of all of these interactions combined.

## Neutron interactions

Neutrons are uncharged and therefore also exhibit exponential attenuation in matter. Neutrons interact through elastic (scatter) and inelastic (absorption) interactions with nuclei in the matter. The amount of energy retained by the neutron and imparted to the nucleus or ejected nucleons is dependent upon the angle of the scattered neutron and the mass of the nucleus. The elastic collisions can be imagined as billiard ball–like collisions. As is intuitive, a neutron can impart essentially all of its energy to a proton since they have roughly equal mass. The heavier the nucleus, the smaller is the amount of energy the neutron can impart to it. As a result, interaction with hydrogen nuclei is the dominant mechanism of energy deposition in tissue for high-energy neutrons. Low-energy neutrons have much less energy to impart in elastic collisions. Since some neutron absorption reactions release significant amounts of energy resulting from changes in rest mass, these often become the dominant mechanism of energy deposition for low-energy neutrons in matter. Since they absorb more energy from the neutron per interaction, materials with low atomic number are best for shielding against neutrons, in contrast to photons for which high atomic number materials are the most efficient for shielding within a given thickness.

## Energy deposition by uncharged particles

The deposition of energy by uncharged particles is a two-step process. The first step is the transfer of energy from uncharged to charged particles. The amount of energy per unit mass transferred from uncharged to charged particles is referred to as the KERMA (kinetic energy released per unit mass). The second step is the deposition of that energy by the charged particles, typically through many small Coulomb interactions. While photons set in motion electrons in matter, neutrons set in motion protons and other recoil nuclei or nuclear fragments in matter. Thus, the energy in a photon beam is ultimately deposited by the interactions of secondary electrons while the energy in a high-energy neutron beam is ultimately deposited primarily by the interactions of secondary protons and other nuclei or fragments. For low-energy neutrons, the dominant energy deposition mechanism depends on the types and relative likelihood of the various scattering and absorption reactions. For example, if the primary mechanism of neutron interaction is an absorption reaction that emits a gamma ray, the energy may be deposited primarily by secondary electrons set in motion by those gamma rays.

## Electron interactions

Electrons and other charged particles traversing a medium interact primarily through many small Coulomb force interactions. However, it is possible that an electron traveling through a medium can collide with an atomic electron or a nucleus. The many small Coulomb interactions in which electrons generally participate result in a gradual deposition of the electron's kinetic energy over the pathlength of the particle. When an electron traveling through a medium strikes an atomic electron in that medium, it can transfer a significant amount of energy in the collision, thus creating another energetic electron. The struck electron in this case is referred to as a delta ray. When an electron interacts with the atomic nucleus, its trajectory is deflected giving rise to a 'bremsstrahlung' X-ray which has energy equal to the kinetic energy lost by the electron in the interaction. It is

this interaction which is used to generate high-energy X-rays for imaging and radiotherapy purposes. One can visualize the relative likelihood of each of these potential interactions by considering the scale of the constituents of matter. The nuclear diameter is on the order of femtometres ($\sim 10^{-15}$ m), while the atomic electron orbitals and interatomic spacing are on the order of tenths of nanometres ($\sim 10^{-10}$ m). To illustrate this scale difference, if the nucleus were the size of a baseball, the typical atomic electron would be on the order of 2 miles away. Therefore, the vast majority of matter is empty space. The likelihood that an electron traveling through matter will collide with another electron is very small, and the likelihood that it will collide with a nucleus is even smaller. As a result, the efficiency of X-ray production is relatively low. Moreover, the distance and trajectory of any individual electron in matter are strongly dependent upon the relative proximity of this trajectory to atomic electrons, nuclei or both. Since electrons are relatively light, their trajectory is easily deflected by close interactions with other electrons or nuclei. Consequently, they scatter a great deal and travel in tortuous paths through matter.

## Light ion interactions

Many light ions have been used for radiotherapy, most commonly protons, helium and carbon ions. The term *heavy ion radiotherapy* is often used to distinguish between proton therapy and other ions, and in this context simply means radiotherapy using ions heavier than the proton. Here we use the terminology *light ions* to include protons and the heavier ions that have been used for radiotherapy since all of these ions are relatively light with respect to most other nuclei. Since they are charged particles by definition, these ions interact through the Coulomb force in much the same way as electrons. The major difference is that since they are thousands of times heavier than electrons, their trajectory is generally not significantly affected by these interactions. Consequently, unlike a beam of electrons in which the electrons scatter through tortuous paths in matter, light ions travel relatively straight paths, and all gradually slow down together at roughly the same depth in the matter. The amount of energy lost per unit distance by charged particles is called the stopping power. The stopping power is affected by the particle type (including its charge), its energy and the medium in which it is traveling. One can relatively easily show that for a light ion passing (and interacting with) an electron, the energy transfer is proportional to the square of the charge of the particle, and inversely proportional to the kinetic energy of the particle. As a result, multiply charged ions have significantly higher stopping power, and the stopping power also increases significantly when the particle velocity becomes small. Thus, near the end of a charged particle's track, it will deposit more energy per unit distance and thus more absorbed dose. Electrons also share this dependency for collisional energy loss and have an increase in stopping power near the end of their track. However, since all light ions in a beam reach the end of their tracks in close proximity to one another, the aggregate result is a significant increase in the absorbed dose from this beam near the end of the particle range. This significant increase in dose is referred to as a Bragg peak. Even though electrons interact in much the same way as light ions, they do not all slow down together at the same depth in matter. Since the electrons come to rest over a wide range of depths, they do not create an aggregate increase in dose at a particular depth and therefore do not exhibit a Bragg peak.

The stopping power also has an effect on the relative biological effectiveness (RBE) of the radiation. Particles with low stopping power produce relatively sparsely ionizing tracks and create relatively simple damage in and around the DNA. Conversely, particles with very high stopping power have very densely ionizing tracks and can create much more complex damage in the DNA that is much more difficult to repair. Particles with high stopping power may therefore have a biological advantage in that they are more efficient in killing cells. This may be advantageous when treating cells that have a high repair capacity. Experimental evidence indicates that the RBE of radiation begins to increase once the stopping power is higher than approximately 10 keV $\mu m^{-1}$ (see Chapter 6). Electrons do not reach this stopping power in tissue until they have slowed down to on the order of tens of keV, at which point they have almost no remaining range and very little energy left to deposit. Even protons do not reach this stopping power in tissue until they are below about 5 MeV at which their range is only a fraction of a millimetre. As a result, neither electrons nor protons offer a significant advantage in terms of RBE. In contrast, the stopping power of carbon ions in tissue is greater than 10 keV $\mu m^{-1}$ even at several GeV; thus, they have a higher RBE for their entire range in the patient. Since the dose in a photon beam is deposited by electrons, photon therapy also provides no advantage in RBE. However, while dose in a beam of high-energy neutrons is deposited largely by recoil protons, many of these protons have relatively low energy (on the order of a few MeV) and thus have a higher RBE. Proton therapy does not provide a significant advantage in RBE since the energy of the protons must be very high in order to penetrate to the target; however, neutron therapy can be thought of as generating a low-energy proton distribution at depth and by this mechanism is able to provide a significant advantage in RBE. A uniform RBE value of 1.1 is generally applied to absorbed doses in proton radiotherapy. This RBE value is an average for conventionally fractionated delivery and is similar for both existing *in vitro* and *in vivo* data. However, there is significant variation in this value between different cell lines and different tissues, and for different fractionation regimens. These variations, along with the rapid change in stopping power near the end of the proton track, mean that even though proton radiotherapy does not have a significantly higher RBE than conventional photon radiotherapy, there are still potentially significant uncertainties in the assignment of an RBE as a function of tissue type and location in the beam.

The major advantage of photons is their penetrating capability which allows them to reach deep-seated tumours. Since they are exponentially attenuated, there is a higher dose deposited for a given photon beam upstream from the target and a finite amount of dose deposited to all tissues downstream from the target regardless of the thickness of the patient. The major advantage of electron beam therapy is that the electrons have a relatively well-defined range, and while it is not possible to predict with any accuracy where any individual electron will come to rest, one can say with certainty that no electrons can penetrate farther than a particular depth. This depth in tissue may be estimated in centimetres as roughly half of the energy of the electron beam in MeV. Very little dose is deposited in an electron beam past this depth. Once all of the electrons in the beam have been stopped, the only remaining dose component is a small tail of bremsstrahlung radiation produced by the electron beam. The major advantage of neutron therapy is the high linear energy transfer (LET), or energy deposited per unit distance, of the charged particles generated by the neutrons in tissue. This large energy per unit distance results in more complex damage at the level of the DNA resulting in increased RBE. The ability of cells to repair this complex damage is limited, thus allowing neutron therapy to potentially be more effective in the treatment of certain radioresistant tumours. The major advantage of proton therapy is that the Bragg peak allows greater dose deposition in the target than in tissues proximal to the target and almost no dose deposited to tissues distal to the target. Carbon ion therapy has both the physical dose-shaping advantages resulting from the Bragg peak and the RBE advantages resulting from the higher stopping power. Carbon ion beams have sharper penumbra than proton beams and have a steeper fall-off at the distal edge of the Bragg peak; however, they have a small tail of dose past the Bragg peak resulting from fragmentation of target nuclei and the carbon ions themselves. These factors, along with considerations of cost to produce these beams and the relative complexity of treatment and associated uncertainties in absorbed dose and RBE, go into the clinical choice of particle type for a particular treatment.

## 7.3 RADIATION DOSIMETRY

The absorbed dose is the quantity most closely correlated with biological effects of ionizing radiation. Absorbed dose is defined as the amount of energy deposited per unit mass. The SI unit is the gray which is equal to 1 J kg$^{-1}$. In a charged particle beam this energy is deposited through Coulomb interactions with the medium as the particles come to rest. In a beam of uncharged particles, the energy of the particles is first transferred to charged particles through interaction and then deposited by the charged particles as they slow down. Since the KERMA in a photon or neutron beam represents the amount of energy transferred from uncharged particles to charged particles, it is clearly related to the number and energy of uncharged particles in the beam and their probability for interaction. Specifically, KERMA is equal to the energy fluence (the energy per unit area carried by the beam of particles) times the mass energy absorption coefficient (which includes both the probability for interaction and the average fraction of the uncharged particle's energy transferred in these interactions). KERMA is directly related to the absorbed dose. If all charged particles deposited all of the energy they receive at the spot they received it, then KERMA would be identical to the absorbed dose. Of course, the charged particles carry that energy over their path as they come to rest. In a beam of megavoltage photons, for example, the secondary electrons travel largely in the direction of the incident beam and carry this energy on the order of centimetres as one would estimate from the electron range rule of thumb introduced earlier. So while the number of photons in the beam, and thus the KERMA, decrease exponentially, the absorbed dose is deposited by the electrons set in motion when these photons interact. Thus, at any given depth, the absorbed dose will be greater than or equal to the energy given to electrons at that depth since the dose is deposited by electrons set in motion upstream where there were more photons in the beam. Assuming that the number of electrons in the beam when incident upon a patient is small, the dose at the surface of the patient is therefore also small. The dose then builds up as the number of electrons set in motion by photon interactions increases, then begins to decrease past this buildup region due to the decrease in the number of photons in the beam. The depth of this 'buildup' region is related to the distance the electrons travel while depositing their dose. For megavoltage photons, this is on the order of centimetres, and thus the skin dose to the patient will be significantly less than the maximum dose in the beam. This is advantageous in radiotherapy in reducing skin reactions from treatment. Conversely, the buildup region in a kilovoltage diagnostic energy photon beam will be very small (on the order of hundredths of a millimetre) and therefore the skin receives essentially the maximum dose in the beam.

Exposure is another quantity historically used for the measurement of radiation. Exposure represents the amount of charge per unit mass produced when radiation ionizes air. Its significance is due to the fact that the measurement of charge from the ionization of air is the most common method of measuring radiation. The practical mechanisms of radiation detection and dosimetry, while of great importance to radiological physics, are beyond the scope of this chapter.

With the foundational physical principles for radiation interaction and dosimetry set forth, we proceed into the discussion of the practical physical, clinical and radiobiological aspects of radiation therapy in its current state. This discussion begins with the process of 'simulation' in which we gather information about the patient's disease and anatomy which are required to generate a treatment plan. The next phase is the creation of the treatment plan, which includes not only the planning techniques, but also methods used to evaluate the quality of the treatment plan prior to

proceeding to the delivery of treatment. Finally, we discuss the processes involved in radiation therapy delivery during which we will be able to more clearly evaluate the effects of and uncertainties resulting from each of the decisions and techniques involved in the preceding processes.

## 7.4 RADIATION THERAPY SIMULATION

The radiotherapy process begins with the 'treatment simulation' or 'simulation' procedure, originally designed to simulate the treatment beam orientation and acquire images to be used for beam shaping and verification of field placement on the patient during treatment. Today, most patients receive 'virtual simulation' or 'CT simulation' meaning that volumetric imaging information is acquired from computed tomography (CT), and the process of selection of beam orientations and beam shapes is performed virtually within a computerized treatment planning system without the patient present. Image information gathered during the simulation process is used not only to delineate target and normal tissue structures but also to verify the correct setup of the patient for subsequent treatment.

Target and normal tissue structures are delineated using image data gathered during simulation (typically a CT scan) and potentially other imaging studies. Magnetic resonance (MR), positron emission tomography (PET) and single photon emission computed tomography (SPECT) imaging techniques provide additional information for structure delineation and may be used in conjunction with CT imaging. MR imaging provides better soft tissue differentiation than CT, while PET and SPECT can provide metabolic and functional information useful in differentiating tumours from normal tissue. Other molecular imaging techniques may prove to be valuable sources of additional information and the potential ability to image tumours or metastases at very early stages.

Since the treatment plan will be created for the spatial orientation of anatomical structures at the time of simulation, great care must be taken to ensure that this spatial orientation is preserved throughout the course of treatment. Patient immobilization is therefore an extremely important part of the simulation and treatment process. Immobilization devices and techniques must be stable, reproducible and comfortable enough to keep the patient in the same position for long treatment setup and delivery procedures. While patient motion can be minimized during simulation and treatment using appropriate immobilization techniques, physiological motion is more problematic. It is possible to minimize respiratory motion through abdominal compression, breath holding or breathing control techniques; however, it is also common to evaluate respiratory motion and incorporate it into the treatment plan. This is often accomplished through the use of 4DCT, where the '4D' denotes the three spatial dimensions and time. A 4DCT scan uses a device to track patient respiration and all acquired image data are binned according to the respiratory phase at the time of acquisition. From these data, a three-dimensional CT data set can be reconstructed sequentially for each individual respiratory phase, and an aggregate 4DCT scan including all phases can be viewed like a movie loop to assess anatomical motion as a function of respiration. This information can then be used to identify the motion of target and normal tissue structures with respiration or to perform respiratory gated treatment. In respiratory gated treatment, a stable region of the respiratory cycle is chosen, generally at end exhalation, during which the treatment will be delivered. Target and normal tissue structures are delineated only in the chosen phases of the respiratory cycle, and the treatment beam is turned on during these phases and remains off during the remainder of the cycle. This requires a device in the treatment room that is capable of monitoring the respiratory cycle.

Patient motion has a tremendous influence on the treatment planning and plan evaluation processes. This influence clearly also extends into the potential incorporation of biological information in these processes. A great deal of research has been performed on the application of biological models to the evaluation of radiotherapy treatment plan quality with the idea that these models could not only potentially predict outcome but could then also be used to optimize the treatment plan for predicted outcome. Treatment plans are often evaluated based on dosimetric information calculated within the treatment planning system, and biological models are then applied to these dosimetric data. One must always be mindful that the CT data on which these calculations are performed represent a snapshot of the patient at the time of simulation, and these dose calculations may not necessarily be representative of what the patient receives from any individual treatment fraction. These calculations may or may not attempt to incorporate respiratory motion and cannot incorporate day-to-day variations in patient setup, changes in patient size and shape such as weight loss or gain during treatment or other physiological factors such as rectal and bladder filling. Attempts to modify the patient's treatment plan to account for changes in size and shape of anatomical structures at the time of treatment are termed *adaptive radiotherapy* and are discussed later.

The simulation procedures discussed thus far describe the processes for external beam radiotherapy. Similar processes also exist for brachytherapy procedures. Prior to a permanent prostate seed implant, a transrectal ultrasound is performed to determine the size and shape of the prostate. This process is referred to as a 'volume study'. The resulting series of transverse ultrasound images is then used to create the treatment plan. Similarly, patients receiving temporary implants will typically undergo a CT and/or MRI simulation to determine the location of the applicator or catheters and to generate an image data set on which the treatment plan will be created and the dose distribution calculated. For some patients, only this single three-dimensional data set will be used, and the same plan will be delivered each day. For other patients, a new image data set will be acquired

prior to each treatment and a new plan generated. These patients essentially have a simulation performed for each treatment fraction.

In summary, treatment simulation is the first step in the radiotherapy process during which critical information necessary to create the treatment plan will be acquired. Any attempt to correlate treatment plan information with patient outcome is dependent upon the degree to which the spatial orientation of the patient's anatomy during simulation is preserved throughout the course of radiotherapy.

## 7.5 RADIOTHERAPY TREATMENT PLANNING

### Target delineation

Once imaging data have been acquired and transmitted to the treatment planning system, the next step in the process is the delineation of target and normal tissue structures. Target delineation is a subjective process dependent upon the image type and quality along with the planner's contouring skill and knowledge of radiological anatomy. How this delineation is performed has a profound impact on the radiotherapy treatment plan. In addition, differences in this process can hinder our ability to accumulate data from multiple institutions in an effort to draw statistical inferences in the comparison of different radiotherapy techniques. As a result, several reports have been issued, notably by the International Commission on Radiation Units and Measurements (ICRU), aimed at standardizing the processes of prescribing and reporting radiotherapy treatment (e.g. [1,4–7]). These reports provide standard definitions of volumes to be delineated and/or reported such that results from multiple institutions can be either objectively compared or accumulated to provide greater statistical strength. The definitions include the gross tumour volume (GTV) which includes 'the gross demonstrable extent and location of the malignant growth', the clinical target volume (CTV) which 'contains a demonstrable GTV and/or subclinical microscopic malignant disease, which has to be eliminated', and the PTV which includes the CTV along with 'a margin for variations in tissue position, size, and shape, as well as for variations in patient position and beam position, intrafractionally and interfractionally'. In addition, a margin called the internal margin (IM) has been defined which is added to the CTV 'to compensate for expected physiologic movements and variations in size, shape, and position of the CTV during therapy', and the internal target volume (ITV) has been proposed to 'represent the volume encompassing the CTV and Internal Margin'. A margin to 'account for uncertainties in patient positioning and alignment of the therapeutic beams during treatment planning and through all treatment sessions' has been developed and termed the setup margin (SM). Figure 7.1 shows the relationship between these volumes and margins. They are depicted here within three scenarios, labelled A, B and C. Scenario A represents the simple 'linear' addition of the margins, resulting in the largest global safety margin. In the case that such a global

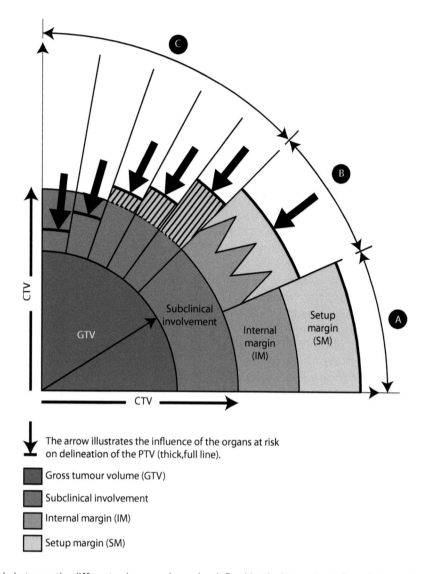

The arrow illustrates the influence of the organs at risk on delineation of the PTV (thick,full line).

Gross tumour volume (GTV)

Subclinical involvement

Internal margin (IM)

Setup margin (SM)

Figure 7.1 The relationship between the different volumes and margins defined by the International Commission on Radiation Units and Measurements (ICRU) in different clinical scenarios. (A), (B) and (C) represent clinical scenarios described in the text. (Reproduced from (5), with permission.)

safety margin is so large that it prevents necessary sparing of surrounding normal tissue, and individual uncertainties are known, these uncertainties may be added in quadrature, represented by scenario B. Finally, scenario C illustrates a spectrum of global safety margins representing clinical cases in which critical normal tissue structures are in varying proximity to the GTV. The choice of global margin size is thus a clinical decision made for an individual treatment plan and may vary with the parameters of that plan. A quantity analogous to the PTV but surrounding each organ at risk (OAR) is defined and termed the *planning organ at risk volume* (PRV). Finally, treated volume (TV) and irradiated volume (IV) are defined as a 'volume enclosed within a specified isodose envelope' where the isodose value for the TV is defined to be appropriate to achieve the purpose of treatment, while the isodose value for the IV is defined as a dose that is considered significant in relation to normal tissue tolerance (see also Figure 16.1).

While the GTV is a visible or palpable structure, the CTV is a clinical concept and relies on the clinician's understanding of disease spread and microscopic extent. Further, the PTV is a geometrical concept used to assure that the entire CTV receives the prescribed dose for each treatment fraction. The extent of the PTV depends on the accuracy and reproducibility of the patient immobilization and target localization processes, and the magnitude of the margin required for the PTV relies on the specific equipment and processes used for immobilization, localization and treatment. Aspects such as mechanical accuracy of equipment, capabilities for pre-treatment image guidance and physiological processes in close proximity to the treatment region have significant bearing on the extent of the PTV margin. Even aspects of the treatment not commonly associated with uncertainties in structure localization can affect this margin. For example, the amount of time required for treatment delivery can have an effect since longer treatment times may be associated with greater probability for patient movement due to discomfort and/or physiological processes such as rectal or bladder filling. Thus, the delivery technique can actually affect the amount of normal tissue irradiated by increasing the necessary size of the PTV margin. PRVs for each OAR are identified in a manner analogous to the identification of the PTV for the target volume.

The acquisition of 4DCT information is necessary to accurately assess the effects of respiratory motion on nearby structures. This allows the evaluation of the extent of the ITV for targets that move with respiration. For non-gated treatments, the ITV includes the full excursion of the target throughout the entire respiratory cycle. This can be evaluated by contouring the target in each phase of respiration or generated computationally within the imaging and/or treatment planning software. An example is the maximum intensity projection (MIP) which, for a 4DCT, represents an image in which each volume element in the image represents the maximum density recorded in that volume element throughout the entire 4DCT data set. Since a MIP does not represent the actual patient anatomy, it is only useful as a tool to identify the excursion of targets or anatomical structures with respiration and cannot be used for the calculation of the delivered dose distribution. One must use caution when estimating the full excursion of the target using such reconstructed representations. One must also exercise caution in interpreting the dose distribution calculated using a single static CT data set or on CT data extracted from a particular phase of the 4DCT data. Unless the treatment is gated, anatomical structures will be moving during treatment delivery and thus calculation of the delivered dose on a static snapshot image of the patient's anatomy will not be representative of what is actually delivered to the patient. While it is theoretically possible, it would be extremely difficult to calculate the actual delivered dose distribution since one would need to correlate the location of each volume element of tissue with the delivered dose as a function of time and accumulate the dose to each volume element throughout the course of treatment. As a result, the application of radiobiological models to correlate delivered dose statistics with outcome is limited by the uncertainties involved in the dose calculations in situations like this. Once all structures are identified, the process of creating the treatment plan begins.

## Brachytherapy treatment planning

For brachytherapy, the planning process is largely dependent upon whether the sources will be placed permanently or temporarily, and if temporarily, whether it is an interstitial or intracavitary treatment. For permanent implants, a relatively large number of low activity sources will be relatively uniformly spaced throughout the target volume. The initial planning involves determining how and where the sources will be placed. For example, for a prostate seed implant with individual seeds, the planner determines how many needles will be used and how many seeds will be placed and at what location using each needle. There is clearly a trade-off between the number of seeds and needles and the uniformity of the dose distribution. Since the placement of needles and seeds in the operating room will not exactly match the planned locations, dose distributions and plan data will be generated for the actual placement location of the seeds. This is referred to as a 'post-treatment plan' and is commonly performed using a CT scan of the distribution of seeds in the patient after the swelling from the procedure has diminished. Initial swelling after the procedure deforms the size and shape of the target volume and would result in a misestimate of the dose delivered to the target during the duration of the implant.

Temporary implants are either delivered interstitially through surgically implanted catheters or performed as intracavitary treatments using a standard applicator. For interstitial delivery, the planner will choose the number of catheters necessary to provide the desired dose distribution. Once these have been surgically implanted, the patient will receive a CT scan to determine the exact location of the catheters. Metal wires with fiducial markers allow the physicist to determine the location and length of each catheter as well as potential radioactive source dwell positions along it. The planning process involves determining the number and location of dwell positions and the amount of time the source should remain at each of these positions. For intracavitary treatments, the clinician determines the size of the applicator optimal to treat the target along with any other modifiers such as caps, tissue retractors and/or packing. Each of these modifiers changes the orientation of local anatomical structures with respect to the radioactive source locations. This is done to either make the dose distribution more uniform in a target tissue or reduce the dose to an organ at risk. Intracavitary applicators are placed for each day of treatment and then removed when treatment is complete. If it is necessary to know the exact location of the applicator with respect to the patient's anatomy on that particular day, a volumetric image data set is acquired using CT or MR imaging after placement of the applicator and a new plan is generated for each treatment day. An example is the treatment of cervical cancer, during which it is common to evaluate the target dose along with dose to the rectum, bladder, sigmoid colon and small bowel for the orientation of the source dwell positions with respect to the patient's anatomical structures on each treatment day.

## External beam radiotherapy treatment planning

External beam radiotherapy generally involves the delivery of a number of beams irradiating the treatment target but entering and exiting the patient through different areas. In a photon beam incident upon a patient, the absorbed dose 'builds up' as electrons are set in motion by photon interactions and then deposit their energy through Coulomb interactions. It then begins to decrease exponentially along with the number of photons in the beam. As a result, the maximum dose in the beam occurs at a depth dictated by the distance these secondary electrons travel in the incident beam direction while depositing their energy. For megavoltage photon beams, this is on the order of 1–3 cm, which is much closer to the surface of the patient than most treatment targets. In such cases, the tissue proximal to the target receives a higher dose from an external beam than the target itself. By delivering the dose to the target through several different treatment beams, one can 'spread out' the dose to the normal tissues since each beam passes through the target but enters and exits the patient through different volumes of normal tissue.

Beam selection is the first step in the creation of a treatment plan for external beam radiotherapy. Traditionally, individual external beams are selected to avoid entry and/ or exit through critical normal tissue structures. Parallel beams of radiation have traditionally been used to make the dose distribution more uniform throughout the target. However, when creating plans that will use inverse planning for intensity modulated radiation therapy (IMRT), beams are generally equally spaced rather than opposed. This is done to provide greater flexibility in the inverse planning optimization process. When selecting a treatment beam, the computerized treatment planning system (TPS) creates a beam's-eye-view of the patient reconstructed using the acquired CT data. This allows the planner to view the patient's anatomy from the perspective of the treatment beam, analogous to the way beam simulation was performed on patients using a conventional X-ray simulator. In the latter, an X-ray image of the patient was taken creating a beam's-eye-view upon which the clinician would draw the desired treatment field shape. In 'virtual simulation', this process is performed virtually in the TPS. The clinician then determines the treatment field shape for each beam using the beam's-eye-view.

In traditional simulation using an X-ray simulator, images were acquired in each beam orientation. Similar images, called 'portal images', taken at the treatment unit prior to treatment were then compared to the simulation images to verify the accuracy of the patient positioning. When using CT simulation, the beams are chosen after the simulation is complete; thus, one does not acquire image information for individual beams during simulation. Computerized treatment planning systems are able to generate digitally reconstructed radiographs (DRRs) from the patient's CT image data set to use for pre-treatment localization in a manner analogous to that described above. Alternatively, the full CT data set can be used along with volumetric image data acquired prior to treatment to evaluate the accuracy of the patient setup and anatomical orientation in three dimensions.

It should be mentioned that in helical or arc treatment delivery techniques such as TomoTherapy and volumetric arc therapy, the planner is not required to explicitly choose beam angles as the planning system evaluates the possible beam directions and chooses beam intensities at each angle based on a plan optimization process. In addition, when using inverse planning optimization techniques for IMRT, the planner is not required to explicitly choose the field size and shape or create a margin for penumbra as this is performed by the TPS in the optimization process. These issues are discussed further in the discussion of inverse planning and plan optimization processes.

Due to geometric considerations and radiation scatter, the edges of the treatment beam are not sharp but rather have a penumbral region in which the radiation intensity gradually falls off. Since the treatment field dimensions are defined by the full width at half maximum of the beam profile, a field shaped such that the collimator edges match the target cross section in the beam's-eye-view would be expected to deliver approximately 50% of the dose at the edge of the treatment field that it delivers at the centre of the field. As a result, the field is expanded to be larger than the cross section of the target to account for this penumbra, such that the edges of the field receive roughly the same dose as the centre of the field. Thus, the size of the treatment field in the beam's-eye-view is significantly larger than the visible disease in that view due to the addition of the CTV margin for clinically occult disease spread, the PTV margin for immobilization and localization uncertainties, and the additional field width to account for the beam penumbra.

While rectangular field shapes may be created using two sets of perpendicular jaws which can define the edges of the treatment beam, most targets require irregularly shaped fields. Castblocks formed from Wood's metal (also known as Lipowitz's alloy) were used to create custom field shapes but these have been nearly universally replaced by the multi-leaf collimator (MLC) which uses two opposed sets of narrow (on the order of several millimetres to a centimetre wide) attenuating leaves to shape the field. MLC shapes can be created for each treatment field and set remotely from outside the treatment room without the need to enter the room to change the field block. Some manufacturers replace one of the sets of jaws with a MLC while others add the MLC as a tertiary field-shaping device in addition to the two sets of perpendicular jaws.

Once the number and orientation of treatment beams are chosen, beam weighting and ancillary devices such as wedges and/or compensators may be used to modify the treatment fields to improve certain characteristics of the treatment plan, for example, to make the dose distribution more uniform. Evaluation of the quality of the treatment plan is performed using the dose distribution calculated by the TPS. As such, one must calculate the dose distribution prior to making modifications to improve the treatment plan. Traditional treatment planning for three-dimensional conformal radiation therapy (3DCRT) is an iterative process in which beam orientations and weights, field shapes and beam modifiers are chosen; the dose distribution is calculated; and then these parameters are modified to better match the desired characteristics of the treatment plan. This process is repeated until the planner is satisfied that the plan either meets the desired treatment goals or cannot be significantly improved beyond its current state. Reviewing the dose distribution in every CT slice throughout the patient is a time-consuming task. It can also be a subjective process. A variety of metrics have been developed to assist in evaluating the quality of the complex dose distribution calculated for a particular treatment plan. The most popular method to distil the large amount of three-dimensional dose information into a more manageable quantity is the dose volume histogram (DVH), which can incorporate all dose values for each calculated volume element for each structure into a single plot. DVHs can be presented in differential or cumulative form. The differential DVH represents the volume of a structure that receives a dose within a specified interval as a function of dose. The cumulative DVH, which is almost universally used in radiotherapy, represents the volume of a structure that receives greater than or equal to a certain dose as a function of dose. An example of a cumulative DVH is shown in Figure 7.2.

One should exercise caution in the use of the cumulative DVH to evaluate plan quality. While the DVH allows simple two-dimensional visualization of the characteristics of the three-dimensional dose distribution within each structure, it eliminates the spatial dose information. Thus, while one can visualize how much of a structure gets more or less than a particular dose, one cannot visualize where those high-dose or low-dose regions are within the structure. In addition, the DVH is dependent upon the simulation process. If a longitudinal structure extends out of the patient volume imaged in simulation, the DVH will not represent the entire structure but only the portion of the structure that the planner was able to, or chose to, contour. Also, the size of an individual volume element in the image data can influence the way the image data are distributed into the individual structures and thus numerically influence the DVH.

The number of iterations in the previously described planning process depends heavily on the skills and experience of the planner. This process is now sometimes referred to as 'forward planning' since the planner chooses characteristics of the treatment beams and then calculates appropriate quantities for plan evaluation. This is in contrast to 'inverse planning' in which the goals of the planner for plan evaluation purposes are set forth first, and the TPS uses computerized optimization techniques to adjust the characteristics of the treatment beams in the attempt to meet these goals.

## Inverse planning and plan optimization

The introduction of the inverse planning process was a result of the development of IMRT. In IMRT, the intensity as a function of position throughout each treatment field is variable and independent of the intensity at any other position within the field. To attempt to calculate an optimum intensity pattern, one must first define the resolution of this pattern, often referred to as a 'fluence map' or 'intensity map', as well as a set of potential intensity levels. When one considers a typical number of treatment beams of typical size and a reasonable intensity map resolution and number of intensity levels, the size of solution space for this computational problem becomes enormous. The problem cannot be solved analytically or in an intuitive iterative process such as that performed in forward planning. One must enlist computational help and optimization algorithms to successfully and efficiently search this solution space. In order for a computational system to help search for an optimum solution, the system must have specific instructions as to what characteristics of a plan are desirable so that it can effectively search for these characteristics. This can present a problem since evaluation of a radiotherapy treatment plan is generally a subjective process. There is no simple way to tell an algorithm that a complex dose distribution 'looks good'. Distilling the three-dimensional dose distribution into simpler quantities such as DVHs facilitates easier plan evaluation and optimization. Inverse planning is the process of specifying the plan characteristics, generally cumulative DVHs for each structure, and allowing computer algorithms to optimize the fluence maps in an attempt to meet these characteristics as closely as possible.

Even after distilling the dose data into a single plot for each structure, creating the best treatment plan is not a straightforward or objective process. Priorities for various aspects of each DVH and/or preferences for meeting DVH goals for one structure over another depend on the individual planner, patient, treatment site and treatment regimen. Inverse planning algorithms incorporate an objective function or 'cost' function to allow the planner's priorities to be incorporated into the optimization process. Failure to meet the specified planning goals for individual structures increases the magnitude, or 'cost', of the objective function and the amount of the increase is determined by parameters that can be varied by the planner. The planner therefore has the ability to input specific priorities quantitatively into the

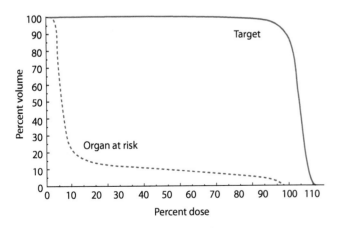

Figure 7.2 Sample cumulative DVH illustrating the characteristics of a typical target and organ at risk.

optimization process. Now the algorithm has a clear and simple goal, to minimize the objective function. A variety of optimization techniques are used within treatment planning systems to perform this task. The inverse planning process can also be an iterative process in that the plan can be evaluated after optimization, planning goals and priorities are adjusted, and optimization performed again in an effort to modify the plan characteristics to better suit the desires of the planner.

The term *optimization* may not be appropriate for the inverse planning process in its current state. While we may be able to computationally minimize, or at least find a local minimum in solution space for, a limited set of dose constraints and priorities using an objective function, the resulting treatment plan should not be considered 'optimum' in any clinical sense. Indeed, the vast majority of IMRT treatment plans currently delivered to patients (and termed *optimized*) take only physical dose information into account. It is difficult to conceive of any realistic approach to true plan optimization which does not incorporate the radiobiological aspects of the physical absorbed dose.

## 7.6 TREATMENT PLAN EVALUATION

Radiotherapy treatment plan evaluation has traditionally been a complex and subjective process due to the multiplicity of plan characteristics that are often of interest. Objective assessment of plan quality is difficult and quantitative assessment obligates the planner to find ways to distil the large amount of plan information into more manageable forms. While the DVH is the simplest and most common data reduction method, care must be taken when using DVH data for plan comparison since it inherently eliminates spatial dose information. One can distil the treatment plan data further and derive tumour control probability (TCP) and normal tissue complication probability (NTCP) if the appropriate models and model data are available. Some have even distilled the entire set of plan data into a single biological score. Here we provide a brief discussion of current plan evaluation techniques and an examination of methods by which biological information may be incorporated into these processes. More detailed and comprehensive reviews of models used for predicting effects of inhomogeneous dose distributions in normal tissues have been given by Yorke (18) and Kong et al. (10).

## TCP and NTCP models

Many early models incorporating biological information into radiotherapy plan evaluation and optimization focused on the attempt to predict TCP and NTCP. While the quantitative results provided by TCP and NTCP models have very large uncertainties and thus will not predict either quantity with tremendous accuracy, they are useful in terms of plan ranking and therefore may be useful in plan optimization and evaluation. A simplistic and brief description of TCP and NTCP models is presented here. A much more comprehensive analysis of the use of NTCP and TCP data for treatment planning have been presented by Jackson and Yorke (8). Obviously, one would like to maximize the TCP and minimize the NTCP. Since real dose-response data have complex characteristics and large uncertainties, it is useful to create simplistic models which provide a reasonably accurate fit to the clinical data.

## TCP models

Two types of TCP models are typically used, namely, phenomenological models (which are a simplistic mathematical representation, but not based on underlying physical principles) and mechanistic models (which attempt to model the real clinical situation of eradication of all tumour cells). Clinical data show that TCP has a sigmoidal relationship with dose. In the application of phenomenological models, this shape may be characterized by $D_{50}$ (which characterizes the position of the TCP curve) and $\gamma_{50}$ (which characterizes the slope of the TCP curve at $D_{50}$). The most common phenomenological method is the logistic model, introduced in Equation 5.9. An alternate way to express this relationship is

$$\text{TCP}(D) = \frac{1}{(1 + (D_{50}/D)^{4 \cdot \gamma_{50}})} \tag{7.1}$$

where $D$ is the prescription dose. The question then arises, 'What happens if the target dose is non-uniform?' This will be addressed later with the development of the $D_{\text{eff}}$, $V_{\text{eff}}$, and equivalent uniform dose concepts.

Alternatively, mechanistic models can be based on the premise that TCP is achieved when all clonogenic cells are destroyed. As shown in Chapter 5, if a population of $N_0$ clonogenic cells is irradiated to give, on average, a surviving fraction S of clonogens, the probability that there are no surviving clonogens can be calculated using Poisson statistics, leading to the Poisson dose-response model:

$$\text{TCP} = \exp(-N_0 S) \tag{7.2}$$

where S depends on tumour biology as well as total dose, dose per fraction, LET, etc. The linear-quadratic model is often used to calculate S as a function of dose, $D$, and dose per fraction $d$:

$$S(D, d) = \exp\left(-\alpha D\left(1 + \frac{d}{(\alpha/\beta)}\right)\right) \tag{7.3}$$

In this formula, $\alpha$ can also be expressed by the SF2, the surviving fraction obtained after a single dose of 2 Gy, as

$$\alpha = \frac{-\ln(\text{SF2})}{2 + 4/(\alpha/\beta)} \tag{7.4}$$

See Chapter 9 for details.

## NTCP models

NTCP is more difficult to quantify than TCP in the sense that one must specify the specific complication type. Clinical NTCP data can also be characterized by a sigmoidal relationship with dose, with a $\gamma_{50}$ similar to that described for TCP. Another complexity pertaining to NTCP calculation is the difficulty in specifying the dose received by normal tissue structures since such structures generally receive very heterogeneous dose distributions. The position of the NTCP curve is typically specified by the whole volume tolerance dose for $q\%$ complications, $TD(q,1)$, where the '1' indicates that the whole volume is irradiated to that dose. A common phenomenological NTCP model is the LKB (Lyman Kutcher Burman) model, which assumes that the tolerance dose increases inversely as a power of $(n)$ of the partial volume irradiated (11,12,14). This may be written as

$$TD(q,v) = TD(q,1) \cdot v^{-n} \qquad (7.5)$$

where $v$ is the fractional volume irradiated. We observe large partial volume effects from some normal tissue structures and very small effects from others. We should expect this based on the tissue architecture as we discuss later in the discussion of mechanistic NTCP models. For example, $n$ will be approximately 1 for lung, meaning that we observe a doubling of the tolerance dose when we irradiate only 50% of the structure. Conversely, $n$ will be approximately 0.1 for spinal cord, indicating that we will observe less than a 10% increase in tolerance dose when we irradiate only 50% of the structure.

Unfortunately, real clinical dose distributions do not yield the 'all or nothing' scenarios described above (i.e. only a certain fraction of the structure is 'irradiated' and that fraction receives a uniform dose of radiation while the rest receives none). While one may often be safe in assuming a relatively homogeneous irradiation of the target, normal tissue structures will nearly always receive a very heterogeneous dose distribution. For this reason, one cannot simply apply whole organ tolerance data to a typical RT plan and must find ways to simplify the inhomogeneous dose distribution. The LKB model employs a reduction scheme to find a homogeneous dose level or volume which would yield the same complication rate as the inhomogeneous distribution. If we consider an inhomogeneous structure irradiation, we may apply Equation 7.5 to each subvolume and calculate an effective whole volume dose which would yield the same effect as the real inhomogeneous dose distribution. We may thus calculate an effective dose, termed $D_{\text{eff}}$, given by

$$D_{\text{eff}} = \left( \sum_i v_i (D_i)^{1/n} \right)^n \qquad (7.6)$$

and an effective volume, $V_{\text{eff}}$, given by

$$v_{\text{eff}} = \sum_i v_i \left( \frac{D_i}{D_{\text{ref}}} \right)^{1/n} \qquad (7.7)$$

Thus, we have two options for converting the real physical DVH into a single dose and single volume value to be used in the Lyman model for NTCP calculation. These may be referred to as the Kutcher-Burman (KB) dose reduction scheme. The irregularly shaped real DVH may be converted into a rectangular shape (one dose value, one volume value) with either

1. Length $D_{\text{eff}}$ and height $V_{100}$ (tall and thin rectangular DVH)
2. Length $D_{\text{max}}$ and height $V_{\text{eff}}$ (short and wide rectangular DVH)

In other words, we can say that the real dose distribution is biologically equivalent to an effective dose $D_{\text{eff}}$ given to the entire organ *or* a dose $D_{\text{max}}$ given to an effective volume $V_{\text{eff}}$. It should be noted that the same DVH reduction formalism may be used for TCP as well when there exists significant non-uniformity in the target dose.

The LKB model incorporates the KB dose reduction scheme and the power law partial volume relationship into the Lyman NTCP model (14). The Lyman model uses a probability integral to generate a smooth sigmoidal curve of the NTCP curve as a function of the absorbed dose, $D$, in a partial volume $v$:

$$NTCP(D,v) = \frac{1}{\sqrt{2\pi}} \int_{-\infty}^{u(D,v)} e^{(-x^2/2)} dx \qquad (7.8)$$

where

$$u = \frac{D - D_{50}(v)}{m \cdot D_{50}(v)}, \quad D_{50}(v) = \frac{D_{50}(1)}{v^n} \qquad (7.9)$$

$D_{50}(1)$ is the uniform dose producing a 50% incidence of the specific endpoint if the whole organ is receiving this dose. The parameter $m$ is the inverse slope of the NTCP curve at 50% complications (i.e. smaller $m$ values correspond to steeper curves). The volume exponent, $n$, is always between 0 and 1 and the larger the value, the more pronounced is the volume effect.

A simpler NTCP calculation can be performed similar to the logistic TCP model:

$$NTCP(D) = \frac{1}{(1 + (D_{50}/D)^{4 \cdot \gamma_{50}})} \qquad (7.10)$$

where a calculated generalized equivalent uniform dose (gEUD) and gEUD$_{50}$ (see below for definition of gEUD) can be used in place of the $D$ and $D_{50}$.

There are two mechanistic NTCP models based on tissue architecture, namely, the serial (critical element) and parallel (critical volume) models. These models assume that complications arise from impairment of organ function carried out by functional sub-units (FSUs). These FSUs are assumed to be damaged independently, and their functional organization determines their dose volume response. In the serial model, FSUs are assumed to be organized in a linear chain; thus, damage to one FSU impairs the function of the whole organ and the tolerance dose will not depend greatly on the volume of the structure receiving this dose. In the parallel model, FSUs are assumed to function independently of one another; thus, one would expect to observe much larger variations in tolerance dose with changes in the volume of the structure receiving this dose. This kind of functional information is necessary when choosing between rival plans whose normal structure DVHs cross over one another. It answers the classic question of whether, for a particular organ, it is better to give 'a lot to a little, or a little to a lot'.

A popular NTCP model utilizing these concepts is the relative seriality model (9), where the tissue response in an inhomogeneous field is given by

$$P = \left[ 1 - \prod_i [1 - P(D_i)^s]^{1/v_i} \right]^{1/s} \qquad (7.11)$$

where the response probability is given by

$$P(D) = \frac{1}{(1 + (D_{50} / D)^{4 \cdot \gamma_{50}})} \qquad (7.12)$$

and $s$ is the 'relative seriality'. A small $s$ indicates a strong volume effect and as $s$ approaches unity, the model reduces to the serial architecture model.

## Equivalent uniform dose

Attempts to include biological information in the process of treatment plan optimization and evaluation have often made use of the equivalent uniform dose (EUD) (16). The EUD is relatively easily calculated and provides a value in the dose domain, which is more familiar and useful to the planner. Additionally, EUD provides a single value representative of the absorbed dose distribution to the structure, thus making plan comparison easier than analysing several parameters of a cumulative dose volume histogram (cDVH) or the complex characteristics of a dose distribution. The original concept of EUD was defined only for targets and was based on cell survival predicted by the linear-quadratic model. It is given by

$$EUD = \frac{D_{ref} \cdot \ln \left[ \frac{1}{N} \sum_{i=1}^{N} (SF2)^{Di/D_{ref}} \right]}{\ln(SF2)} \qquad (7.13)$$

Additional modification is necessary to incorporate the effects of cell proliferation and other complications to the simple model of Equation 7.13. The generalized EUD (gEUD) was later introduced as a phenomenological model which could be applied to both tumours and normal tissues. The obvious advantages of EUD, particularly in its generalized form (gEUD), make this a common choice as an optimization parameter for radiotherapy treatment plans. The gEUD is given by the following equation:

$$gEUD = \left( \frac{1}{N} \sum_{i=1}^{N} D_i^a \right)^{1/a} \qquad (7.14)$$

where $D_i$ is the dose in voxel $i$, $N$ is the number of voxels in the ROI (region of interest) and $a$ is the volume parameter which is related to the seriality of the organ under consideration (17). Mathematically, Equation 7.14 is what is referred to as the 'generalized mean' value. For target structures (tumours), $a < 1$; therefore, the EUD is dominated by the lowest dose values. For parallel organs at risk, $a = 1$; therefore, the EUD is appropriately the mean dose. Finally, for serial organs at risk, $a > 1$; therefore, the EUD is dominated by the maximum dose values. It should be observed that the gEUD is analogous to $D_{eff}$ where $a = 1/n$.

One drawback of traditional radiotherapy plan evaluation or optimization using DVHs (also with the use of most TCP and NTCP models or gEUD) is that they inherently eliminate all spatial information about the dose distribution. In traditional 3DCRT, one might be safe in assuming that any cold spots observed in the target DVH exist in the periphery of the target. However, with the very heterogeneous dose distributions produced by IMRT, the cold spot could potentially be right in the centre of the gross disease. Parenthetically, this result is due to the implicit assumption within DVH and gEUD analysis that all subvolumes of the target carry the same significance in terms of tumour control. This is an unfounded and questionable assumption, and the ability to retain spatial information in plan optimization may be of value for this reason.

## Dose calculations in treatment planning systems

A wide variety of dose calculation techniques have been used within commercial computerized treatment planning systems. These can be broadly divided into correction-based and model-based techniques. In correction-based techniques, radiation beam characteristics are measured in simple geometric arrangements (typically a large tank of water), and corrections are applied to predict the dose distribution within the complex geometric arrangement represented by patient treatment. Model-based techniques are capable of calculating dose distributions from first principles without first reconstituting the measured data in water. Measured data for model-based techniques are used only to tune the beam model which is then propagated into the patient image data. Commercial treatment planning systems generally use model-based calculations as these perform better in complex situations in the presence of significant heterogeneities. The convolution/superposition model is a commonly employed model-based technique which uses two essential components. One component represents the energy deposited in the medium by the interactions of the primary beam at that location, and the other represents the energy deposited around the interaction site following interaction of the primary beam. The latter represents the pattern of spread of scattered radiation for the radiation beam and medium of interest. Another important model-based algorithm is the Monte Carlo technique. This technique is a random sampling method which simulates the statistical fate of a large number of particles traversing the medium of interest. Given information about the incident radiation beam and the medium, one can determine probabilities for the distance the particle will travel before interaction; the type of interaction it undergoes; the new direction and energy of the particle after interaction; and the type, energy and direction of any new particles resulting from the interaction. Using a random number generator, one can then calculate a 'history' for each particle incident on the medium and, by accumulating this information for a large number of particle histories, can calculate the resulting predicted dose distribution. The Monte Carlo method is the most accurate calculation method. Its utility is limited only by the amount of time it takes to calculate a dose distribution with sufficient accuracy.

Any attempt to correlate quantitative treatment plan metrics with patient outcome is inextricably linked to the accuracy of the dose calculations within the TPS. The accuracy of these dose calculations depends on a variety of factors including uncertainties in target delineation, organ motion, treatment delivery accuracy and the calculation models themselves. Radiobiological models utilizing this dose information are therefore also constrained by these uncertainties and results of these models must be interpreted with a full understanding of both the uncertainties in the parameters used in the radiobiological models as well as those arising in the calculation of dose to the patient.

## 7.7 TREATMENT DELIVERY

A variety of processes and platforms are available for the delivery of radiotherapy. These may be initially divided into brachytherapy and external beam radiotherapy.

### Brachytherapy delivery

The delivery procedure for permanent brachytherapy implants involves surgical implantation of radioactive seeds in the target volume. This is most commonly done for the treatment of prostate cancer, during which seeds are implanted via transperineal needles under transrectal ultrasound guidance. Typically either I-125 or Pd-103 seeds are used. I-125 decays by electron capture and with the resulting emission of a 35.5 keV $\gamma$-ray from the daughter Te-125 nucleus along with several other lower-energy characteristic X-rays and internal conversion photons. Pd-103 also decays by electron capture with the emission of characteristic X-rays with an average energy of 21 keV. The primary difference between these two sources is their half-life, 59.4 days for I-125 and 17.0 days for Pd-103. Since the dose will be deposited much faster by Pd-103, there is a biological difference in the absorbed dose delivered by the two sources for a permanent implant.

Delivery for temporary brachytherapy implants is typically performed using an afterloading device, although some facilities still use radioactive sources manually loaded into applicators. In manual loading, the clinician is physically present during loading and places the sources manually with the help of tools to keep the sources at a safe distance. In contrast, the term *afterloading* refers to the process of automated movement of the source to its intended dwell positions once the applicator(s) are connected to the afterloading device using transfer tubes through which the source travels from its safe into the applicator inside the patient. Staff members are not physically present with the patient while this process takes place due to the very high dose rate involved. For this reason, this type of brachytherapy is often referred to as high dose rate (HDR) brachytherapy. Conversely, permanent seed implants and manually loaded temporary implants, which have much lower source activities, are referred to as low dose rate (LDR) brachytherapy. Ir-192 is the primary source used for afterloading devices. It emits a complicated spectrum of photons with a mean energy of 380 keV. Prior to the delivery of the radiation, imaging studies are performed to assure that the applicator and/or catheters are in their intended position with respect to the patient's anatomy. For some types of treatment, a single image data set is acquired and a single plan generated which will be used throughout the course of treatment. Pre-treatment imaging checks for these treatments are used to verify the constancy of the locations of the applicators and/or catheters with respect to one another and the patient's anatomy. For other types of treatment, an image data set is acquired prior to each treatment fraction, then a new plan is generated, evaluated, and delivered to the patient. In the latter case, the complete process of simulation, planning and delivery is performed independently for every treatment fraction.

### External beam radiotherapy delivery

External beam radiotherapy is generally delivered using a high-energy electron linear accelerator, two examples of which are shown in Figure 7.3. These linear accelerators or 'linacs' use microwaves to accelerate electrons down an

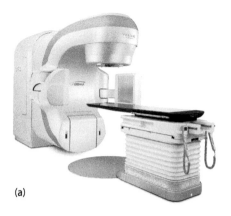
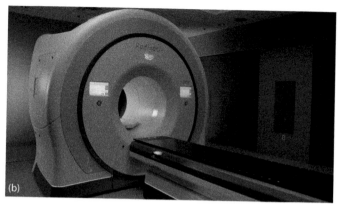

Figure 7.3 (a) Varian 'TrueBeam' C-arm linear accelerator treatment unit. (b) TomoTherapy 'Radixact' rotational treatment unit. ([a] Image courtesy of Varian Medical Systems, Inc. All rights reserved. [b] Image used with permission from Accuray, Incorporated.)

evacuated waveguide. These high-energy electrons, typically 5–20 MeV, can then be extracted out to treat the patient directly with electrons or used to bombard a target to generate high-energy X-rays. Among commercially available linacs, while there are many major similarities, there are unique features of particular devices such as different delivery mechanisms, different pre-treatment imaging devices, ability to track target motion, etc. Ions for ion therapy are accelerated using a number of different devices including cyclotrons, synchrotrons and synchrocyclotrons. While the details of the technology involved in external beam radiotherapy delivery are beyond the scope of this chapter, we discuss a few aspects of delivery which have a bearing on the radiobiological characteristics of the treatment.

Most external beam radiotherapy treatments are delivered using traditional C-arm linacs. In this design, the accelerating waveguide is oriented horizontally, and the radiation beam is extracted out perpendicularly to the accelerating waveguide. The acceleration and beam extraction systems are contained inside a gantry that can rotate around the patient so that the beam can be aimed at the patient from any direction. The lengths of traditional accelerating waveguides, which are on the order of a meter, necessitate the perpendicular extraction system. If one were to extract the beam out in the direction of acceleration, the gantry would be much larger in diameter and would require a much larger treatment room. Newer, higher-frequency accelerators allow a much shorter accelerator structure and allow extraction in the acceleration direction while still allowing a relatively small gantry diameter (<2 meters). One such compact accelerator is attached to an industrial robot in the CyberKnife treatment unit. A compact accelerator is mounted on a slip-ring gantry such as that used for CT scanners in both the TomoTherapy and Vero treatment units. In C-arm linacs, the electron beam is turned toward the patient after acceleration but before striking the photon target.

As one would expect from conservation of momentum, most bremsstrahlung photons produced by very high-energy electrons are generated traveling in roughly the same direction as the incident electron beam. Megavoltage bremsstrahlung photon beams are said to be 'forward peaked' as their intensity is highest in the direction of the incident electron beam. As a result, it is most efficient to generate the photons when the electrons are traveling toward the patient. This is in contrast to bremsstrahlung generation in a diagnostic X-ray tube in which we extract the photons out in a direction perpendicular to the direction of the accelerated electrons. This 'reflection target' design is necessitated by the fact that most low-energy diagnostic photons would be absorbed by a target thick enough to dissipate the heat generated in producing a clinically useful photon fluence. Thus, one cannot efficiently extract them out in the direction of the incident electrons. The reflection target is facilitated in this case by the fact that there are a significant number of photons generated in this perpendicular direction. Conversely, high-energy bremsstrahlung photons are both very forward directed and very penetrating, thus necessitating the use of a 'transmission target'.

Traditional linacs were designed to produce a 'flat' beam, meaning a beam with uniform intensity in a plane perpendicular to the beam direction. To accomplish this, they use a flattening filter which is thicker in the centre than in the periphery to preferentially absorb the centre of the beam due to the strong forward peaking. However, for IMRT, it is inefficient to flatten the beam only to modulate its intensity again afterward. As a result, many treatment units offer both flattened and unflattened beams or are designed with no flattening filter. Removal of the flattening filter results in a much higher dose rate which allows much faster treatment delivery. Reducing delivery time reduces the effects of gradual intrafraction motion due to physiological processes such as bladder or rectal filling or to 'settling' of the patient, but can significantly increase the dosimetric consequences of spurious patient movement such as coughing. This increased dose rate may have radiobiological consequences in addition to reducing delivery time.

Linacs also have beam monitoring and beam-shaping devices downstream from the beam extraction system. The beam monitoring devices measure the amount of radiation emitted from the linac and allow the delivery of carefully calibrated doses of radiation to the patient. Beam-shaping devices include both collimation jaws, which define an entire field edge, and multi-leaf collimators (MLCs). Some accelerators have both jaws and MLCs while others replace one jaw with a MLC. The MLC is the mechanism most often used to create the modulation used in IMRT. Typical leaf widths are on the order of 5 mm, which dictates the resolution of the fluence map in the direction perpendicular to leaf motion. IMRT delivery using a MLC is performed using either static (or 'step and shoot') delivery or dynamic (or 'sliding window') delivery. In static delivery, the MLC moves to a set shape and then the beam turns on, delivers the programmed amount of radiation and turns off again prior to shaping the next treatment segment. In dynamic delivery, the leaves move across the aperture while the beam is on with varying distance between opposing leaves dictated by the desired intensity of the radiation at that location for that field. MLC leaf motion and positional accuracy play a major role in the accuracy of IMRT delivery since small deviations in leaf position are significantly more important for the very small apertures used in IMRT compared to the relatively large fields used for traditional radiotherapy in which the entire field is treated with one open and 'flattened' beam.

The number of beams chosen affects the quality of the treatment plan as a larger number of beams generally allows greater conformity of the prescription dose to the target and less dose to any particular volume of normal tissue. However, larger numbers of beams result in a larger volume of normal tissue being exposed to a significant amount of radiation as more tissue is traversed by beams as they enter or exit the patient. Some treatment units allow 'rotational' delivery in which radiation is delivered throughout an entire arc around the patient, which can result in greater conformity of the radiation dose distribution to the target. Common examples include TomoTherapy and volumetric modulated arc therapy (VMAT). TomoTherapy, literally meaning 'slice therapy', employs a fan beam of radiation directed into the patient in a helical manner as the linac rotates around the patient and the treatment couch moves through the treatment unit bore. In VMAT, a traditional C-arm gantry can deliver an intensity modulated treatment using the MLC during continuous rotation of the gantry in an arc around the patient. Since

this is delivered by a 'cone beam' of radiation rather than a 'fan beam', the entire target volume may be treated in a single arc as opposed to the helical delivery of TomoTherapy, resulting in faster delivery. However, these two delivery types are radiobiologically equivalent in terms of dose rate. Even though VMAT can treat the entire treatment volume quicker, a particular volume element of tissue in the patient passes through the 'slice' of radiation in TomoTherapy (receiving almost all of its dose during this period) in about the same time as a VMAT delivery.

Another collimation mechanism is called the 'cone'. The cone is a long circular extension which collimates the beam as close to the patient as possible, thus decreasing the size of the penumbra and allowing sharper dose fall off outside the target. Cones are typically used for linac-based stereotactic radiosurgery (SRS). A competing modality for SRS is the Gamma Knife, shown in Figure 7.4a, which consists of a large number of Co-60 sources arranged in a hemispherical array around the patient and focused at the centre of the unit. The patient is rigidly immobilized at the centre of the unit and a motorized collimation system provides collimation sizes of 4, 8, and 16 mm corresponding to the diameter of a 'shot' of radiation delivered through the collimation system. The treatment plan is made up of individual shots which cumulatively produce the desired dose distribution. Since the Gamma Knife has no rotating gantry, its mechanical accuracy can exceed that of a linac. However, it is limited to treating intracranial and cervical spine targets. The CyberKnife, shown in Figure 7.4b, consists of a compact linac mounted on an industrial robot and a non-invasive image guidance system. It offers a greater number of potential beam angles, can treat regions anywhere within the body, and can perform target tracking using the robotic delivery system.

External beam radiotherapy generally involves the delivery of a number of beams irradiating the treatment target from different directions. The gantry, collimator and treatment couch are all designed to rotate to allow flexibility in the direction in which the radiation beams can be delivered. The point at which the axes of rotation of the gantry, collimator and couch intersect is called the 'isocenter'. If the target is placed at the isocenter then any combination of gantry, collimator or couch angles will

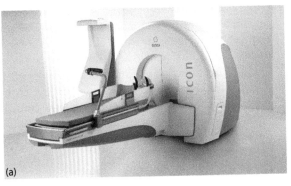
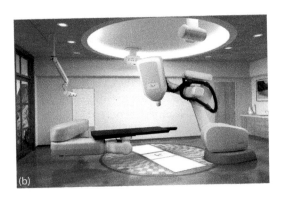

Figure 7.4 (a) Gamma Knife radiosurgery treatment unit. (b) CyberKnife robotic radiosurgery treatment unit. ([a] Image courtesy of Elekta. [b] Image used with permission from Accuray, Incorporated.)

result in a beam traversing the target volume provided the beam is shaped with the collimator to match the target cross section in the beam's eye view. As such, most treatments are delivered 'isocentrically' to avoid the requirement of moving the patient between successive treatment fields. Generally, a set of lasers is mounted in the room and used to indicate the location of the isocenter for patient positioning and alignment.

Other types of accelerators such as cyclotrons, synchrotrons and synchrocyclotrons are used to generate the high-energy particle beams for light ion radiotherapy. In addition, such high-energy particle beams can be used to bombard a target to generate a high-energy neutron beam for neutron radiotherapy. The physical aspects of these accelerators and particle beams are beyond the scope of this chapter. The reader is referred to Chapter 25 for a discussion of the clinical and radiobiological aspects of hadron therapy.

## Image-guided radiotherapy

Patients are generally given external reference marks on their body and/or their immobilization device during simulation, and those fiducial marks are used in the treatment planning process to determine the geometrical relationship between internal anatomy and external reference marks. Patients can then be aligned in the treatment room using the lasers and external reference marks. However, this assumes that the internal anatomy is exactly the same as it was at the time of simulation. Since the patient's internal anatomy is likely not exactly the same as at the time of simulation, we must either account for these potential changes in determining the size of our PTV margins or evaluate the anatomy on the treatment couch immediately prior to treatment. Most delivery platforms now incorporate an integrated mechanism for pre-treatment image guidance. This provides more accurate localization of the target prior to treatment thus allowing smaller PTV margins during the planning process.

Early image guidance processes used 'localization' films to determine whether the bony anatomy appeared to be in the correct location with respect to the treatment field prior to treatment by comparison with simulation films or digitally reconstructed radiographs (DRRs). Electronic portal imaging devices (EPIDs) were later developed to allow the immediate acquisition of a digital image of the patient without the need for processing a film. However, film and EPIDs provide only spatial orientation of bony anatomy, and soft tissue can move with respect to the bony anatomy. Thus, other techniques were developed to allow the localization of soft tissue. Ultrasound localization systems were developed which allow the visualization of soft tissue and can localize soft tissue structures with respect to the isocenter of the treatment unit. Internal fiducial markers were also used to facilitate soft tissue localization using plane radiographic systems. These can be implanted during surgical resection or implanted specifically for radiotherapy such as transrectal implantation of marker seeds for localization of the prostate.

Most radiotherapy treatment units have image guidance systems to allow acquisition of volumetric image information of the patient on the treatment couch. This has been accomplished using a CT on rails which images the patient on the treatment couch separate from the treatment unit but is generally performed now using cone beam CT using on-board imaging systems. Cone beam CT uses a diagnostic X-ray tube and flat panel imager mounted opposite one another and perpendicular to the gantry and EPID to gather planar imaging information using the full 'cone beam' rather than a 'fan (or slit) beam' like a traditional diagnostic CT. In this manner, a full set of volumetric CT data can be acquired using a single rotation of the gantry. In contrast, TomoTherapy uses its fan beam and a CT detector to acquire a megavoltage CT using the detuned treatment beam. These systems allow pre-treatment verification of patient localization and evaluation of the size, shape and orientation of anatomical structures. Image-guided radiotherapy (IGRT) is necessary to achieve the greatest conformity when using conformal treatment techniques such as IMRT. Without IGRT, PTV margins must be larger and result in dose distributions that are less conformal to the treatment target and include more normal tissue.

The ability to visualize anatomical changes immediately prior to treatment now allows us to treat significantly less normal tissue; however, we must be careful not to be 'too conformal' by overestimating our target delineation, localization and immobilization capabilities. While reducing the size of the PTV will result in less normal tissue toxicity, it also increases the possibility for a geometric miss of part of the treatment target through overestimation of our capabilities in one aspect of the treatment process. The result would be a reduction in tumour control which may not only be difficult to detect but may not be statistically demonstrated for a significant amount of time. Thus, acute toxicity rates would be expected to be reduced with results observed relatively quickly, but the long-term consequences of missing part of the tumour would not be observed until much later. If we assume the patient's anatomy to consist of rigid structures that move around but do not change shape or move with respect to one another, we should expect IGRT to allow the delivery of a dose distribution very close to what we expect from the treatment planning system calculations. However, organs do deform and move with respect to one another both between treatment fractions and potentially even during treatment.

## Adaptive radiotherapy/deformable image registration

The concept of adaptive radiotherapy (ART) represents the process of adapting the treatment plan to match changes in the patient's anatomy. A wide variety of adaptive radiotherapy techniques have been implemented or proposed, from adjusting target margins based on daily pre-treatment imaging and offline re-planning of the treatment accordingly, to re-simulating and re-planning the patient's treatment after weight loss, to the possibility of online re-planning after pre-treatment imaging. Early efforts toward ART involved the use of multiple cone beam CT data sets to determine a statistical PTV expansion based on observed variations in the patient's anatomical structure. This and other similar techniques are referred to as 'off-line' ART since the data are evaluated and adaptations to the patient's treatment plan are implemented between treatment fractions rather than while the patient is on the treatment couch. With our current ability to rapidly acquire volumetric imaging data and calculate treatment plans, we have the capability to implement on-line ART. A new treatment plan based on the patient's anatomy imaged immediately prior to treatment could be calculated and delivered for each treatment fraction. Several complications arise from such a scenario, including the difficulty in calculating the total dose as a function of position for the entire course of radiotherapy. The fact that the patient could be treated with a different treatment plan and parts of the patient's anatomy are at different locations and in different orientations with respect to one another for each treatment fraction make it extremely difficult to calculate a total dose distribution within the patient for the whole course of treatment. To do this requires deformable image registration. Deformable image registration systems attempt to correlate regions of the patient's anatomy between multiple image data sets. If this is accurately performed, the absorbed dose in each individual volume element can be accumulated for the course of therapy to determine what that volume element received for the course of therapy. This process results in interesting radiobiological consequences for volume elements in high-dose gradients which may receive large doses from some fractions and small doses from others. Performing such calculations for physical absorbed dose is very challenging and comes with significant uncertainty. The uncertainties become even larger when one attempts to include radiobiological information in the prediction of the effects of such ART treatments.

## Stereotactic radiosurgery/stereotactic body radiation therapy

Radiosurgery refers to the delivery of radiotherapy in a single fraction, as opposed to conventional fractionated radiotherapy. The reader is referred to Chapters 9, 10 and 11 for discussion of the concepts of hypofractionation. Stereotaxis refers to the localization of an internal anatomic structure through the use of a coordinate system based on a rigid external frame and/or internal imaging capabilities. Stereotactic radiosurgery (SRS) therefore describes the use of stereotactic techniques for the accurate direction of radiation beams to a target for single fraction radiotherapy. It has most commonly been used for intracranial lesions, for example using the Gamma Knife which has traditionally utilized a stereotactic frame affixed to the patient's skull and

CT and/or MR images to localize the target with respect to the frame. Recently, these techniques have been commonly applied to extracranial sites, a treatment called stereotactic body radiotherapy (SBRT). Since the name SBRT does not contain information about the fractionation scheme, it is not completely descriptive of the technique. SBRT has also often been referred to as stereotactic ablative radiotherapy (SAbR) to indicate its use as an ablative treatment like SRS. While not explicitly contained within the name, the term SBRT implies a hypofractionated, ablative treatment, delivered in one to five treatment fractions. As such, SRS and SBRT rely on different therapeutic and radiobiological principles than conventional fractionated radiotherapy. While conventional radiotherapy relies on fractionation to achieve a beneficial therapeutic ratio between normal tissue and tumour, ablative treatments are designed to eliminate targeted tissue. Ablative treatments therefore do not rely on hallmark radiobiological principles such as repair, reoxygenation, redistribution and repopulation. Such high doses of ablative radiotherapy require greater accuracy and precision than conventional radiotherapy. Targets must be very well defined. Generally, multimodality imaging techniques are used to define the target, and the GTV is essentially the same as the CTV. Treatment margins are made as small as possible through stereotactic localization and pre-treatment image guidance.

SRS is commonly delivered using a Gamma Knife, Cyberknife, or modified linac utilizing conical collimators to provide the sharpest possible dose falloff at the edges of the treatment beam. A stereotactic frame is typically used for treatment using either technique. SBRT is deliverable on many radiotherapy treatment platforms, with the primary requirements including very high geometric accuracy and suitable capabilities for pre-treatment image guidance. Specialized immobilization systems are commonly used for SBRT which not only provide accurate and reproducible immobilization but also often provide a means for management of respiratory motion. Treatment planning considerations are different in that portions of organs containing treatment targets will receive very high doses and the uniformity of the dose within the target is not considered as important as in conventional radiotherapy. Since the prescription dose is very large, the dose gradient outside the target must be very steep. In general, a large number of non-overlapping beams are used for SRS and SBRT to suitably spread out the dose distribution around the target in order to reduce the possibility of normal tissue toxicity. Dose-response relationships for the large doses per fraction employed for SRS and SBRT are much different than those for conventional radiotherapy and are not nearly as well understood. A commonly cited example of these differences is the significant number of cases of severe skin toxicity which have resulted from the use of an insufficient number of beams to spread out the surface dose in SBRT treatments. The process of collection and characterization of dose-response data for SBRT treatments is still far from mature. Another point of concern is the accuracy of treatment planning algorithms in calculating dose distributions for the very small beams typically used for SRS and SBRT, particularly in low-density tissues such as the lung. One must assure that the treatment planning system is suitably commissioned and its accuracy verified for such applications.

## 7.8 SUMMARY

We have discussed the fundamental aspects of radiotherapy physics at a relatively basic level. For readers who wish to gain a more in-depth perspective, there exist a variety of texts which treat these aspects in much greater detail. While the physical principles involved in radiotherapy remain relatively constant, the technology used for the clinical processes described here is rapidly evolving. Understanding how these advances in technology affect the radiobiological characteristics of radiotherapy is critical for predicting and assessing the efficacy of therapy as illustrated in several previously described clinical situations. For example, more complicated delivery processes can result in longer treatment delivery times and more heterogeneous dose distributions, both as a function of position in the patient and from fraction to fraction even at the same position in the patient. Better imaging and target localization may allow dose escalation or changes in fractionation schedules, and the use of different modalities may result in different RBE for the treatment. All of these situations result in changes in the radiobiological characteristics of the treatment and underscore the need for the disciplines of physics, biology and clinical radiation oncology to work together in the development of new treatment techniques.

New computational, imaging and delivery technology allows us to not only deliver more accurate treatments, but also to acquire much more accurate and much larger quantities of data regarding the radiation dose we deliver. The assessment of this data and its effect on patient outcome continues to contribute to our understanding of the principles of radiobiology and how they influence the success of radiation therapy. Thus, for the foreseeable future, radiation therapy will remain a particularly multidisciplinary specialty with its efficacy largely dependent upon our ability to synergistically combine our clinical, physics and biology knowledge.

## Key points

1. The DNA is the critical target for radiation inactivation of cells.
2. Specific radiation interaction mechanisms determine the amount and distribution of energy deposited in a medium.
3. Uncharged particles (such as photons and neutrons) interact through a small number of catastrophic interactions.
4. Charged particles (such as electrons and ions) interact through many small Coulomb interactions and less frequent catastrophic interactions.
5. Energy deposited by uncharged particles is first given to charged particles and then deposited along the tracks of those charged particles.
6. The absorbed dose (SI unit Gy = J kg$^{-1}$) is the quantity most closely correlated with biological effects of ionizing radiation.
7. The amount of energy loss per unit distance in a charged particle track is determined by the particle type, particle energy and medium it is traversing, and relative density of ionizing events influences the biological effectiveness of the radiation dose.
8. The radiotherapy process begins with 'treatment simulation', in which a patient is positioned optimally for radiotherapy and immobilized for the most accurate and reproducible treatment setup. Imaging data acquired during simulation are used to identify important target and normal tissue structures, for the creation of the treatment plan, and for the calculation of the distribution of absorbed dose from the treatment plan.
9. The treatment planning process includes delineation of target and normal tissue structures, determination of the method of treatment, appropriate number of radiation beams or radiation sources and their locations, as well as the evaluation of the distribution of absorbed dose in the target and normal tissue structures.
10. The DVH is a common data reduction technique in which the fractional volume of a structure receiving greater than or equal to a particular dose is plotted as a function of dose. Using the DVH, the planner can assess characteristics of the three-dimensional dose distribution in a simple two-dimensional plot.
11. IMRT is the process of modulating the intensity of each radiation beam in a plane perpendicular to the beam axis to produce highly conformal dose distributions. Inverse planning is generally used to create complex IMRT plans. In the inverse planning process, the goals of the treatment plan are first conveyed to the treatment planning system and an objective or 'cost' function is used to guide the system to produce a plan which meets the planning goals as closely as possible.
12. There are many techniques for radiotherapy plan evaluation including evaluation of DVHs and the calculation of many quantitative biological indices such as TCP, NTCP, EUD, gEUD, etc.
13. Radiotherapy is delivered via external beams, typically generated by a linear accelerator, or via brachytherapy, in which radioactive sources are placed inside the body either temporarily or permanently.

14. Modern external beam radiotherapy delivery systems have the capability to image the target and normal tissue structures immediately prior to treatment to allow more accurate and precise delivery of the radiation dose distribution.

15. Specialized equipment, including linacs, robotic delivery systems, gamma radiosurgery units and particle therapy systems are used in external beam radiotherapy to attempt to achieve optimal physical dose distribution characteristics. Specialized treatment regimens such as radiosurgery, ablative radiotherapy and high LET therapy, are often employed in the attempt to optimize the biological aspects of radiotherapy.

## ■ BIBLIOGRAPHY

1. Aaltonen P, Brahme A, Lax I et al. Specification of dose delivery in radiation therapy. Recommendation by the Nordic Association of Clinical Physics (NACP). *Acta Oncol* 1997;36(Suppl. 10):1–32.

2. Crowther JA. Some considerations relative to the action of X rays on tissue cells. *Proceedings of the Royal Society of London Series B Containing Papers of a Biological Character* 1924;96:207–211.

3. Dessauer F. Some effects of radiation I. *Zeitschrift Fur Physik* 1923;12:38–47.

4. International Commission on Radiation Units and Measurements (ICRU). Prescribing, recording and reporting photon beam therapy. ICRU Report 50. *J ICRU* 1993;os26.

5. International Commission on Radiation Units and Measurements (ICRU). Prescribing, recording and reporting photon beam therapy (supplement to ICRU report 50). ICRU Report 62. *J ICRU* 1999;os32.

6. International Commission on Radiation Units and Measurements (ICRU). Prescribing, recording, and reporting electron beam therapy. ICRU Report 71. *J ICRU* 2004;4.

7. International Commission on Radiation Units and Measurements (ICRU). Prescribing, recording, and reporting photon-beam intensity-modulated radiation therapy (IMRT). ICRU Report 83. *J ICRU* 2010;10.

8. Jackson A, Yorke E. NTCP and TCP for treatment planning. In: *A Practical Guide to Intensity-Modulated Radiation Therapy*. Madison, WI: Medical Physics; 2003. pp. 287–320. Copyright to Memorial Sloan-Kettering Cancer Center.

9. Kallman P, Agren A, Brahme A. Tumour and normal tissue responses to fractionated non-uniform dose delivery. *Int J Radiat Biol* 1992;62:249–262.

10. Kong FM, Pan C, Eisbruch A, Ten Haken RK. Physical models and simpler dosimetric descriptors of radiation late toxicity. *Semin Radiat Oncol* 2007;17:108–120.

11. Kutcher GJ, Burman C. Calculation of complication probability factors for non-uniform normal tissue irradiation: The effective volume method. *Int J Radiat Oncol Biol Phys* 1989;16:1623–1630.

12. Kutcher GJ, Burman C, Brewster L, Goitein M, Mohan R. Histogram reduction method for calculating complication probabilities for three-dimensional treatment planning evaluations. *Int J Radiat Oncol Biol Phys* 1991;21:137–146.

13. Lea DE. *Actions of Radiations on Living Cells*. 2nd ed. Cambridge: Cambridge University Press; 1956.

14. Lyman JT. Complication probability as assessed from dose-volume histograms. *Radiat Res Suppl* 1985;8:S13–S19.

15. Munro TR. The relative radiosensitivity of the nucleus and cytoplasm of Chinese hamster fibroblasts. *Radiat Res* 1970;42:451–470.

16. Niemierko A. Reporting and analyzing dose distributions: A concept of equivalent uniform dose. *Med Phys* 1997;24:103–110.

17. Niemierko A. A generalized concept of equivalent uniform dose (EUD). *Med Phys* 1999;26:1100 (abstract).

18. Yorke ED. Modeling the effects of inhomogeneous dose distributions in normal tissues. *Semin Radiat Oncol* 2001;11:197–209.

## ■ FURTHER READING

At a level required for practice as a radiation oncologist:

19. McDermott PN and Orton CG. *The Physics & Technology of Radiation Therapy*. Madison, WI: Medical Physics Publishing; 2010.

At a level required for practice as a radiation therapy physicist:

20. Khan FM. *The Physics of Radiation Therapy* (4th Ed.). Philadelphia, PA: Lippincott, Williams, and Wilkins; 2010.

21. Hendee WR, Ibbott GS, Hendee EG. *Radiation Therapy Physics* (3rd Ed.). Hoboken, NJ: John Wiley and Sons; 2005.

# Tumour growth and response to radiation

## DANIEL ZIPS

## 8.1 TUMOUR GROWTH

### Introduction

The growth of primary and metastatic tumours determines the clinical course of malignant disease. Tumour growth results from a disturbed tissue homeostasis, driven by functional capabilities acquired during tumourigenesis. These acquired capabilities include self-sufficiency in growth signals, insensitivity to anti-growth signals, limitless proliferative potential, evading apoptosis and sustained angiogenesis (21). The speed of growth, or the *growth rate*, varies considerably between different tumours due to differences in cell proliferation and cell loss.

### Measuring the size and growth rate of tumours

Under experimental conditions, such as with transplanted tumour models, the size of the tumour can be precisely and repeatedly measured using simple callipers. In the clinical situation, precision and feasibility of tumour size measurement depend on the anatomical site and the imaging technology. For instance, only lesions of 5–10 mm or larger in diameter can be detected in the lung on chest radiographs. Advanced spiral computer tomography allows detection of nodules as small as 3 mm in diameter. From the dimensions of the lesion, the tumour volume ($V$) can be calculated:

$$V = \frac{\pi}{6} \times \text{Length} \times \text{Width} \times \text{Height}$$

For experimental tumour models, a calibration curve can be obtained by plotting $V$ against the weight of excised tumours (58). This procedure allows for uncertainties of external tumour volume determination resulting from, for example, irregular volumes and skin thickness.

The tumour burden and tumour growth rate can also be estimated by determination of biochemical tumour markers such as prostate specific antigen (PSA) in patients with prostate cancer (54). Serial measurement of the tumour volume permits estimation of the growth rate. The tumour volume doubling time (VDT), for example, can be calculated by the time required for the tumour to double its volume. In untreated experimental tumours, volume doubling times have been found to be in the same range as the doubling times of tumour cell number and clonogenic tumour cell number (31).

### Exponential and non-exponential growth

Starting from one cell, each cell division produces two offspring resulting in 2, 4, 8, 16, 32, etc. cells after subsequent cycles of cell division. Accordingly, this results in an exponential increase in cell number and volume with time which can be expressed as

$$V = \exp\left(\frac{\text{time} \times \ln 2}{\text{VDT}}\right)$$

Figure 8.1 illustrates that the majority of cell doublings take place before a tumour becomes detectable which, in most clinical situations, is when the cell number approaches about $10^9$. This cell number is equivalent to a tumour weight of about 1 gram and a volume of about 1 cm³. Exponential growth implies that under constant conditions, the logarithm of tumour volume increases linearly with time. This can be seen easily from tumour growth curves if volume or weight is plotted on a logarithmic scale and therefore tumour growth is conventionally plotted in this way. Consequently, deviations from exponential growth, variability in the growth rate among different tumours and effects of treatment can be easily visualized. In contrast, plotting tumour volume on a linear scale might lead to the erroneous impression that growth accelerates with increasing volume (Figure 8.2). Instead, the volume doubling time actually tends to decrease with increasing volume. This effect in large tumours is due to impairment in oxygen and nutrient supply resulting in a lower proportion of cycling cells, a prolongation of cell cycle and/or a higher cell death rate. Such progressively slowing tumour growth has often been described by the Gompertz equation:

$$V = V_0 \exp\left[\frac{A}{B}(1 - \exp(-B.t))\right]$$

Here $V_0$ is the volume at the arbitrary time zero and $A$ and $B$ are parameters that determine the growth rate. At very early time intervals ($t$ small) the equation becomes exponential:

$$V = V_0 \exp(A.t)$$

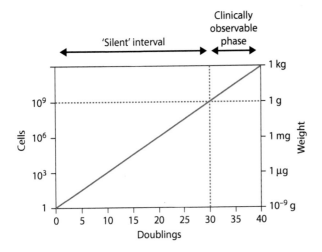

Figure 8.1 Relationship between the number of doublings from a single cell and the number of resulting cells in a tumour. To calculate the tumour weight, a cell number of $10^9$ per gram was assumed. The clinically observable phase represents a minor part in the history of the tumour. Tumour weight is plotted on a logarithmic scale. If the doubling time is constant, a straight line indicates exponential tumour growth.

At long time intervals, $\exp(-B.t)$ becomes small compared to 1.0 and the volume tends to a maximum value of $V_0\exp(A/B)$. The Gompertz equation is not a unique description of such growth curves. For a fuller discussion see Steel (58).

The volume doubling time of human tumours shows a considerable variability between tumours of different histology as well as between primary and metastatic lesions (58) (Table 8.1). For example, primary lung tumours double their volume every 2–6 months, whereas colorectal

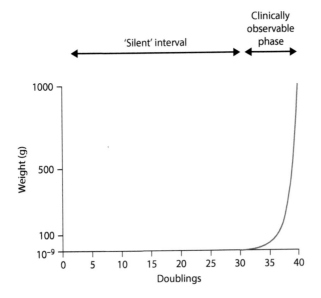

Figure 8.2 The same data as used for Figure 8.1 but tumour weight is plotted on a linear scale. This may lead to the erroneous impression that tumour growth accelerates during the clinically observable phase.

Table 8.1 VDTs for human tumours taken from a review of early data on the growth rate of human tumours

| Site and histology | Number of tumours measured | Mean VDT[a] (days) (confidence limits) |
|---|---|---|
| *Lung metastases* | | |
| Colon-rectum, adenocarcinoma | 56 | 95 [84–107] |
| Breast, adenocarcinoma | 44 | 74 [56–98] |
| Kidney, adenocarcinoma | 14 | 60 [37–98] |
| Thyroid, adenocarcinoma | 16 | 67 [44–103] |
| Uterus, adenocarcinoma | 15 | 78 [55–111] |
| Head and neck, squamous cell carcinoma | 27 | 57 [43–75] |
| Fibrosarcoma | 28 | 65 [46–93] |
| Osteosarcoma | 34 | 30 [24–38] |
| Teratoma | 80 | 30 [25–36] |
| *Superficial metastases* | | |
| Breast carcinoma | 66 | 19 [16–24] |
| *Primary tumours* | | |
| Lung, adenocarcinoma | 64 | 148 [121–181] |
| Lung, squamous cell carcinoma | 85 | 85 [75–95] |
| Lung, undifferentiated | 55 | 79 [67–93] |
| Colon-rectum | 19 | 632 [426–938] |
| Breast | 17 | 96 [68–134] |

Data from (58).

[a] Geometric mean.

carcinomas have been found to grow at a much slower rate with a mean VDT of about 2 years. In general, metastatic lesions tend to grow faster than primary tumours. In contrast to tumours in patients, model tumours in experimental animals usually grow much faster with doubling times in the order of days.

## The growth fraction and cell-cycle time in tumours

The net growth rate, or the VDT, of tumours results from the balance of cell production and cell loss. Cell production is determined by the proportion of cells in the compartment of actively dividing cells (growth fraction [GF]) and the time required to complete the cell cycle (cell-cycle time, $T_C$). Cells from the GF compartment move through the cell cycle and are distinguished from cells outside the cell cycle. Cells outside the cell cycle (in G0 phase) may enter the cell cycle (recruitment of temporarily resting cells) or remain permanently in the G0 phase (sterile or differentiated cells). Taking these parameters together, tumours grow fast if the GF is high, the cell-cycle time is short or the cell loss is low.

The GF can be measured in tumour biopsies, for example by immunohistochemistry, using a monoclonal antibody against the cell cycle–specific protein Ki-67. Human tumours vary considerably in their Ki-67 labelling index (i.e. the ratio of cells with positive staining for the Ki-67 protein divided by the total cell number) (Table 8.2). Clinical studies indicate a prognostic value for Ki-67 labelling in some tumour types including breast cancer, soft tissue tumours and lung cancer (10). Antibodies against different cell cycle–specific proteins also allow determination of the fractions of cells within the various phases of the cell cycle.

Determination of cell-cycle kinetics in tissues is more difficult than measuring the GF. In the past, pulsed or continuous infusion of tritiated thymidine, a radiolabelled nucleoside incorporated into the DNA during the S-phase, has been widely used to estimate the duration of the cell cycle ($T_C$) by the percent labelled mitosis method (46). With this method the $T_C$ for carcinomas was found to be widely scattered but averaged around 2 days (Table 8.3).

It is possible to rapidly determine the S-phase fraction and the duration of the S-phase from a single biopsy using a technique developed by Begg et al. (7). In this method, thymidine analogues, iododeoxyuridine (IdUrd) or bromodeoxyuridine (BrdUrd) are injected into a patient and are subsequently incorporated into the newly synthesized DNA in S-phase cells. A few hours after injection, a tumour biopsy is taken from which a single-cell suspension is prepared. This is stained with both a DNA-specific dye and a fluorescent-labelled antibody against BrdUrd or IdUrd. Using flow cytometry, the fraction of cells in the S-phase (labelling index, LI) and the duration of the S-phase ($T_S$) can be determined. Typical values for LI and $T_S$ are shown in Table 8.4. While in most tumours the S-phase duration is about 12 hours, or approximately 25% of $T_C$, the fraction of cells in the S-phase varies widely between the different tumours.

Molecular imaging, e.g. with radiolabelled fluorothymidine ($^{18}$F-FLT), can allow non-invasive assessment of tumour

**Table 8.2** Growth fractions determined by Ki-67 labelling for different human tumour types

| Tumour type and site | Mean/Median Ki-67 LI[a] (%) | Ki-67 LI[a] (% range) | Reference |
|---|---|---|---|
| Prostate | 8.5 | 1–28.4 | 61 |
| Central nervous system (meningioma) | 4.4 | 0–58 | 52 |
| Central nervous system (astrocytoma) | 21.5 | 0–47.3 | 47 |
| Head and neck | 27.8 | 8.2–80.8 | 51 |
| Colorectal | 37.2 | 18.9–71.4 | 36 |
| Breast | 31.6 | 0–99 | 64 |
| Lung (non-small cell) | 36.7 | 0–93 | 28 |
| Pancreas | 29.7 | 0.5–82.1 | 38 |
| Soft tissue sarcoma | 12 | 1–85 | 30 |
| Renal cell carcinoma | 11 | 0–43 | 20 |
| Bladder | 35 | 3–55 | 29 |
| Oesophagus | 33 | 6–95 | 53 |

[a] LI, labelling index.

**Table 8.3** Cell cycle time ($T_C$) for different human tumours determined by the percent labelled mitosis method

| Histology | Number of tumours measured | Mean $T_C$[a] (hours) [range] |
|---|---|---|
| Squamous cell carcinoma | 7 | 43.5 [14–217] |
| Adenocarcinoma | 5 | 34.9 [25–45] |
| Melanoma | 4 | 102 [76–144] |

Data taken from (39).

[a] Geometric mean.

proliferation *in vivo*. FLT is not incorporated into the DNA but it is phosphorylated by thymidine kinases (TK). While TK2 is expressed constitutively, TK1 activity is specifically regulated during the S-phase. As a result, metabolites of radiolabelled $^{18}$F-FLT (mono-, di- and triphosphates) are found preferentially in S-phase cells. The $^{18}$F tracer activity can then be detected by positron emission tomography (PET).

## The potential doubling time

The potential doubling time ($T_{pot}$) of a tumour is defined as the cell doubling time without any cell loss (58). $T_{pot}$ is determined by the GF and the cell cycle time ($T_C$):

$$T_{pot} = T_C \left( \frac{\ln 2}{\ln(\mathrm{GF}+1)} \right)$$

Using thymidine analogues and flow cytometry, the potential doubling time can be estimated by the duration of the S-phase ($T_S$) and by the fraction of cells within that phase (LI) (7,62):

$$T_{pot} = \frac{\lambda T_S}{\mathrm{LI}}$$

where $\lambda$ is a parameter which corrects for the non-rectangular age distribution of growing cell populations. This parameter usually lies between 0.7 and 1. Using this method, $T_{pot}$ for human tumours from different sites was found to vary between 4 and 34 days (Table 8.4). The differences in $T_{pot}$ are mainly attributed to the variability in LI between tumours, whereas $T_S$ appears to be relatively similar between tumours, with a value averaging about 12 hours.

To test the hypothesis that pre-treatment $T_{pot}$ reflects the effective doubling time during fractionated radiotherapy and thereby correlates with the repopulation rate of clonogenic tumour cells, treatment response of 476 patients with head and neck cancer was correlated with $T_{pot}$ and LI (6). However, multivariate analysis revealed that neither $T_{pot}$, nor LI, nor $T_S$ were statistically significant determinants of local tumour control. Thus, in this large multi-centre study, pre-treatment cell kinetic parameters measured by thymidine analogues

Table 8.4 Cell kinetic parameters of human tumours derived from *in vivo* labelling with iodo-deoxyuridine (IdUrd) or bromo-deoxyuridine (BrdUrd) and measured by flow cytometry

| Site | Number of patients | LI (%) | $T_S$ (h) | $T_{pot}$ (days) |
|---|---|---|---|---|
| Head and neck | 712 | 9.6 (6.8–20.0) | 11.9 (8.8–16.1) | 4.5 (1.8–5.9) |
| Central nervous system | 193 | 2.6 (2.1–3.0) | 10.1 (4.5–16.7) | 34.3 (5.4–63.2) |
| Upper intestinal | 183 | 10.5 (4.9–19.0) | 13.5 (9.8–17.2) | 5.8 (4.3–9.8) |
| Colorectal | 345 | 13.1 (9.0–21.0) | 15.3 (13.1–20.0) | 4.0 (3.3–4.5) |
| Breast | 159 | 3.7 (3.2–4.2) | 10.4 (8.7–12.0) | 10.4 (8.2–12.5) |
| Ovarian | 55 | 6.7 | 14.7 | 12.5 |
| Cervix | 159 | 9.8 | 12.8 | 4.8 (4.0–5.5) |
| Melanoma | 24 | 4.2 | 10.7 | 7.2 |
| Haematological | 106 | 13.3 (6.1–27.7) | 14.6 (12.1–16.2) | 9.6 (2.3–18.1) |
| Bladder | 19 | 2.5 | 6.2 | 17.1 |
| Renal cell carcinoma | 2 | 4.3 | 9.5 | 11.3 |
| Prostate | 5 | 1.4 | 11.7 | 28.0 |

Taken from (23,48).

*Notes:* Ranges (in parentheses) represent variations in median values between studies; ranges for individual tumours are considerably larger. Fraction of cells in S-phase (LI), duration of S-phase ($T_S$) and potential doubling time ($T_{pot}$) were taken from 23 and 48.

and flow cytometry have failed to predict outcome after radiotherapy.

## Cell loss in tumours

Taking typical values for human tumours (e.g. a GF of 32% and a $T_C$ of 2 days) results in $T_{pot}$ of 5 days. This time is obviously much shorter than the observed VDT of human tumours, which is usually in the order of months. The difference between VDT and $T_{pot}$ is explained by the high rate of cell loss in malignant tumours. The cell loss factor (CLF) can be calculated from

$$CLF = 1 - \frac{T_{pot}}{VDT}$$

Taking a VDT of 3 months and a $T_{pot}$ of 5 days, the CLF would be 95%. Examples of CLFs for human tumours are listed in Table 8.5. The high CLFs indicate that the vast majority of newly produced cells are lost from the GF, thus explaining the slow volume growth rate of many tumours. Cells are lost from the proliferative compartment when they enter the non-proliferative compartment (G0), for example by differentiation. The same occurs when they physically disappear from the viable tumour compartment by necrosis, apoptosis, metastasis and exfoliation or shedding. In solid tumours, necrotic cell loss due to insufficient oxygen and nutrient supply by the pathologic tumour vasculature appears to represent a major factor.

Transplanted tumours in experimental animals grow much faster than tumours in human patients. While $T_S$ is comparable with tumours in patients, experimental tumour models often exhibit a higher LI, shorter $T_{pot}$ and lower CLF. Cell-kinetic data obtained using these model systems must be therefore interpreted with caution in terms of their clinical relevance.

Table 8.5 Calculation of CLFs for human tumours based on labelling with radiolabelled thymidine (*) or thymidine analogues (**) and volume doubling times, in separate series

| Site | LI (%) | $T_{pot}$ (days) | VDT (days) | CLF (%) |
|---|---|---|---|---|
| Undifferentiated bronchus Ca[*,a] | 19.0 | 2.5 | 90 | 97 |
| Sarcoma[*,a] | 2.0 | 23.3 | 39 | 40 |
| Childhood tumours[*,a] | 13.0 | 3.6 | 20 | 82 |
| Lymphoma[*,a] | 3.0 | 15.6 | 22 | 29 |
| Head and neck[**,b] | 9.6 | 4.1 | 45 | 91 |
| Colorectal[**,b] | 13.1 | 3.9 | 90 | 96 |
| Melanoma[**,b] | 4.2 | 8.5 | 52 | 84 |
| Breast[**,b,c] | 3.7 | 9.4 | 82 | 89 |
| Prostate[**,b,d] | 1.4 | 28.0 | 1100 | 97 |

[a] From (58), calculations assume $T_S = 14$ h, $\lambda = 0.8$.

[b] LI, $T_S$, and $T_{pot}$ from 23 and 48; calculations assume $\lambda = 0.8$ (58).

[c] VDT values for pulmonary metastases from 57.

[d] VDT from PSA doubling times from 16,37,54.

## 8.2 TUMOUR RESPONSE TO RADIATION

### Introduction

Radiation effects on tumours under clinical as well as experimental conditions can be measured by different endpoints including local tumour control, tumour regrowth delay and tumour regression. Local tumour control is the aim of curative radiotherapy. Improvements in local tumour control after radiotherapy have been shown, in many clinical trials, to translate into the prolonged survival of cancer patients. Thus, local tumour control is conceptually the preferable endpoint for both clinical and experimental investigations on improving radiotherapy. A tumour is locally controlled when all of its clonogenic cells (i.e. cells with the capacity to proliferate and to cause recurrence after radiotherapy) have been inactivated. The probability of achieving local tumour control is radiation dose dependent and directly related to the number of surviving clonogenic tumour cells (see Chapter 5). Tumour regression is a non-specific endpoint to assay radiation response and the tumour regrowth delay assay is widely used in radiobiological experiments. Tumour regrowth delay increases with radiation dose but, due to inherent methodological limitations, it is difficult or impossible to accurately estimate cell kill.

## Clonogenic cell survival after irradiation

Radiotherapy is highly effective in killing clonogenic tumour cells. The quantitative relationship between radiation dose, inactivation of clonogenic cells and local tumour control is well established under clinical as well as experimental conditions (1,19,27,34,41,50,60,66,69). In fractionated radiotherapy, it has been demonstrated that the logarithm of surviving clonogenic tumour cells decreases linearly with total radiation dose. If the radiation dose is high enough to sterilize all cells capable of causing a recurrence, then local tumour control is achieved. This relationship is illustrated in Figure 8.3, which shows a theoretical clonogenic survival curve for the fractionated irradiation of a model tumour. This tumour has a diameter of about 3 cm, consisting of $10^{10}$ tumour cells with a clonogenic fraction of 10% (i.e. the tumour consists of $10^9$ clonogenic tumour cells). Assuming an intermediate radiation sensitivity, each fraction of 2 Gy inactivates 50% of the clonogenic cells. In other words, after a dose of 2 Gy then 50% of the clonogenic cells survive, after 4 Gy 25%, after 6 Gy 12.5%, and so on. This results in a linear decrease of the logarithm of surviving clonogen fraction as

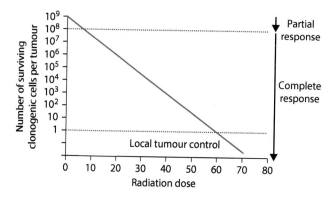

**Figure 8.3** Relationship between clonogenic cell survival, radiation dose and different endpoints to assay tumour response, assuming a tumour consisting of $10^9$ clonogenic cells and a surviving fraction after 2 Gy of 50%.

the dose increases and is depicted by the straight line in the log-linear plot in Figure 8.3. For this example, at doses higher than 60 Gy the number of surviving cells per tumour is less than 1 and local tumour control can be achieved. Clearly this is a simplification because it neglects, for instance, the possibility of changing radiosensitivity (maybe due to changes in tumour oxygenation) and of repopulation during fractionated radiotherapy (see Chapters 11 and 17). However, it demonstrates that response parameters such as partial or complete response, which are often used as clinical descriptors, are not robust endpoints for evaluating curative radiotherapy. It is obvious that a 'partial response is a complete failure' (L. Peters) of the treatment because the vast majority of clonogenic cells are presumably still alive. Even if we are unable to detect the tumour with clinical imaging (in a complete response) a large number of clonogenic tumour cells may have survived the treatment and may lead to a recurrence. Thus, in studies both on patients and on experimental animals, only by following-up treatment for long enough to detect all regrowing tumours, can it be precisely determined whether the given treatment was effective in sterilizing all clonogenic tumour cells.

## Local tumour control

If not a single tumour but a group of tumours (or patients) is considered, the probability of local tumour control (TCP) as a function of radiation dose can be described statistically by a Poisson distribution of the number of surviving clonogenic tumour cells (41). It describes the random distribution of radiation-induced cell kill within a population of clonogenic cells (see Chapter 5). As an illustration, one might imagine that a given radiation dose causes a certain amount of 'lethal hits' randomly distributed within the cell population. Some cells will receive one lethal hit and will subsequently die. Other cells will receive two or more lethal hits and will also die. However, some cells will not be hit, will therefore survive and subsequently cause a local failure. According to Poisson statistics, a radiation dose sufficient to inflict on average one lethal hit to each clonogenic cell in a tumour (number of lethal hits per cell $m$ equals 1) will result in 37% surviving clonogenic cells. The surviving fraction (SF) can be expressed as

$$SF = \exp(-m)$$

and the number of surviving clonogenic tumour cells ($N$) is

$$N = N_0 \times SF$$

where $N_0$ represents the initial number of clonogens. The TCP depends on the number of surviving clonogenic cells ($N$) and can be calculated as

$$TCP = \exp(-N) = \exp(-N_0 SF)$$

To illustrate the relationship between radiation dose, number of surviving clonogenic cells and TCP described by

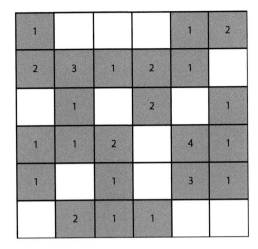

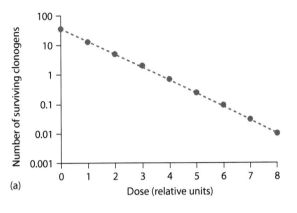

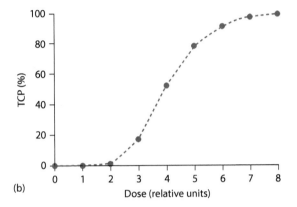

**Figure 8.4** A model tumour consisting of 36 clonogenic tumour cells (each square represents one clonogenic cell) after irradiation with a dose sufficient to inflict an average of one 'lethal hit' per clonogenic cell. Due to random distribution of the lethal hits among the tumour, some clonogenic cells received one (1), two (2), three (3) and four (4) lethal hits. These cells subsequently die (grey shadow). According to Poisson statistics (SF = exp[−$m$], see text) 37% of the clonogenic cells, i.e. a total of 13 cells, received no lethal hit and survived (white background). The TCP after this "treatment" can be calculated as TCP = exp(−13) = 2.3 × 10$^{-6}$. This means that only 1 out of 2.3 million tumours will be locally controlled in this situation. In Table 8.6 and Figure 8.5, the effects of higher radiation doses on SF and TCP are illustrated.

Poisson statistics, a model tumour consisting of 36 clonogenic cells is "treated" (Figure 8.4, Table 8.6). If the TCP is plotted as a function of dose (Figure 8.5), the resulting curve shows the typical sigmoid shape. The sigmoid shape of dose-response curves for local tumour control is supported by clinical observations and has been demonstrated in numerous experiments. Application of Poisson statistics implies

**Figure 8.5** The 'treatment effects' on the model tumour consisting of 36 clonogenic cells (compare Figure 8.4 and Table 8.6). Upper panel shows the number of surviving clonogens as a function of dose for a model calculation described in Table 8.6. The lower panel shows how the resulting tumour control probability (TCP) calculated from TCP = e$^{-N}$. Values for the number of surviving clonogens and TCP were taken from Table 8.6.

that, in a group of tumours with on average one surviving clonogenic cell per tumour, the local TCP equals 37%. A TCP of 50% results if, on average, 0.7 clonogenic tumour cells survive irradiation. Statistical models other than the Poisson equation, such as the logistic and probit equations, can also be used to describe dose-response relationships for local tumour control empirically (see Chapter 5).

The quantitative relationship between radiation dose, surviving fraction of clonogenic tumour cells and TCP forms the biological basis of local tumour control as a functional assay of clonogenic tumour cell survival after irradiation (1,19,27,41,50,60,66,69). In such studies, groups of transplanted tumours are irradiated with varying doses and during follow-up it is recorded whether a tumour has regrown (recurrence) or not (local control). In contrast to tumour volume measurement, which requires considerable training and is susceptible to inter-observer variability, the scoring of local recurrence or local control is simple and makes the tumour control assay very robust (for comparison with other assays see Table 8.7). The rates of local tumour control at each dose level (number of controlled tumours divided by number of total tumours) are obtained and

**Table 8.6** Relationship between radiation dose, fraction of surviving clonogenic tumour cells (SF) and local TCP according to Poisson statistics for the 'treatment' of a model tumour consisting of 36 clonogenic tumour cells

| Radiation dose (relative units) | Number of 'lethal hits' per clonogenic cell ($m$) | SF = e$^{-m}$ | Number of surviving clonogenic tumour cells ($N$ = SF × 36) | TCP = e$^{-N}$ |
|---|---|---|---|---|
| 1 | 36/36 = 1 | 37% | 13 | <0.0001% |
| 2 | 72/36 = 2 | 14% | 5 | 1% |
| 3 | 108/36 = 3 | 5% | 2 | 17% |
| 4 | 144/36 = 4 | 1.8% | 0.7 | 52% |
| 5 | 180/36 = 5 | 0.7% | 0.2 | 78% |
| 6 | 216/36 = 6 | 0.25% | 0.09 | 91% |
| 7 | 252/36 = 7 | 0.09% | 0.03 | 97% |
| 8 | 288/36 = 8 | 0.03% | 0.01 | 99% |

Table 8.7 Comparison of different experimental assays to measure radiation effects on tumours

| Assay | Advantages | Disadvantages | Comment |
|---|---|---|---|
| Local tumour control assay (TCD$_{50}$ assay) | • Depends only on inactivation of clonogenic cells<br>• All clonogenic cells are assayed<br>• Response evaluated *in situ*, i.e. in the original environment<br>• TCD$_{50}$ values can be easily obtained for comparisons with other tumour models or different treatments<br>• Data good for radiobiological modelling<br>• Endpoint scoring very simple | • Labour intensive and costly<br>• Sensitive to residual immune response of the host | • Most important assay for curative effects of radiotherapy |
| Excision assays | • Direct measurement of clonogen survival<br>• Not sensitive to host immune reaction (*in vivo*/*in vitro* assay)<br>• Less costly and labour intensive than TCD$_{50}$ assay | • Response not measured in the original environment<br>• Sensitive to effects from single cell preparation<br>• Cannot assess clonogen survival at low levels of surviving fractions (lung colony, *in vitro*/*in vivo*)<br>• Effects of prolonged treatments difficult or impossible to assess | • Standardized methods to assay clonogenic survival but more limitations than the TCD$_{50}$ assay |
| Tumour regrowth delay assay | • Response evaluated *in situ*, i.e. in the original environment<br>• Less costly and labour intensive than TCD$_{50}$ assay<br>• Specific tumour growth delay and the use of multiple radiation dose levels may allow conclusions on clonogenic cell kill and comparisons between different tumour models | • Reflects cell kill of the mass of non-clonogenic and clonogenic cells, proliferation, stromal reaction, inflammatory response<br>• Measures the effect only in a small range of tumour cell numbers<br>• Does not necessarily reflect inactivation of clonogenic tumour cells<br>• Sensitive to experimental manoeuvres without effects on tumour cell kill | • Standardized but non-specific endpoint, limited value for investigations of curative effects of radiotherapy |
| Tumour regression | • Response is evaluated *in situ*, i.e. in the original environment<br>• Less costly and labour intensive than other assays | • Reflects cell kill, proliferation, resorption of necrosis, stromal reaction, inflammatory response, oedema<br>• Measures the effect only in a small range of tumour cell numbers<br>• Sensitive to experimental manoeuvres without effects on tumour cell kill | • Highly unspecific endpoint, not suitable for investigations of curative effects of radiotherapy |

further analysed to calculate characteristic points on the dose-response curve. Mostly the TCD$_{50}$ (i.e. the radiation dose required to control 50% of the tumours) is reported (the local tumour control assay is therefore often called a TCD$_{50}$ assay). Results from a typical experiment are shown in Figure 8.6 and Table 8.8 in which FaDu human squamous cell carcinomas were transplanted into nude mice and irradiated with 30 fractions over 6 weeks. Total doses ranged from 30 to 100 Gy (dose per fraction ranged from 1 to 3.3 Gy) and six to eight tumours per dose level were treated. Local tumour control rates were determined 120 days after the end of

treatment. This follow-up period is sufficient for this tumour model to detect virtually all regrowing tumours. Careful observation in previous experiments, where animals were followed up until death (life span is about 2 years), revealed that 95% of all recurrent FaDu tumours occur within 60 days and 99% within 90 days after end of irradiation. The radiation dose-response curve for local tumour control exhibits a sigmoid shape with a threshold value. Below total doses of about 50 Gy no tumours are controlled, presumably due to the large number of clonogenic cells that survived the treatment. Above this threshold dose, local TCP increases

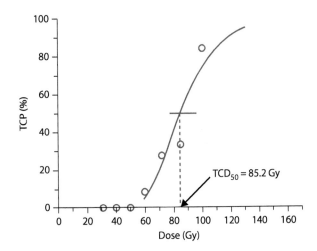

**Figure 8.6** Dose-response curve for local tumour control of FaDu human squamous cell carcinoma growing in nude mice. Tumours were treated with 30 fractions over 6 weeks. Total doses ranged from 30 to 100 Gy. Treatment started for all tumours at the same tumour volume. Each symbol represents the fraction of tumours locally controlled at a given dose level (see Table 8.8). The data were fitted using a Poisson-based model and the $\mathrm{TCD}_{50}$, i.e. the dose required to control 50% of the tumours locally, was calculated. In the experiment shown, the $\mathrm{TCD}_{50}$ is 85.2 Gy. The error bar represents the 95% confidence limit of the $\mathrm{TCD}_{50}$. (Data from (71).)

steeply with increasing dose. The data can be fitted using a Poisson-based statistical model and the $\mathrm{TCD}_{50}$ is calculated according to

$$\mathrm{TCD}_{50} = D_0 \times (\ln N_0 - \ln(\ln 2))$$

where $D_0$ reflects the intrinsic radiosensitivity of clonogenic cells (see Chapter 4) and $N_0$ is the number of clonogens before irradiation. The $\mathrm{TCD}_{50}$ value can be used to compare results obtained from different tumour models (Figure 8.7). The $\mathrm{TCD}_{50}$ assay has been used widely to investigate and quantify modifications in radiation sensitivity or number of clonogenic tumour cells (an example of a typical experiment is given in Figure 8.8) and the data evaluation and reporting of results are well established and standardized. The effect of treatment modifications on local TCP can be quantified by calculation of a dose modifying factor (DMF):

$$\mathrm{DMF} = \frac{\mathrm{TCD}_{50}\ (\text{without modification})}{\mathrm{TCD}_{50}\ (\text{with modification})}$$

DMF represents the relative reduction in radiation dose by a given treatment modification to achieve a certain level of TCP (isoeffect) compared to radiation without modification. In other words, DMF values larger than 1 indicate that the modification, for example by a new drug being tested, resulted in a greater sensitivity to radiation treatment.

Compared with other *in vivo* assays discussed in the following text, however, the $\mathrm{TCD}_{50}$ assay is time consuming and expensive. To design, perform and evaluate experiments using this local tumour control endpoint requires considerable technical knowledge and experience. Intercurrent death of animals may hamper adequate follow-up which needs to be sufficiently long enough to detect virtually all recurrences, i.e. mostly 4–6 months depending on the tumour line. Small variations in the number of surviving clonogenic cells after irradiation may cause dramatic differences in local TCP. Therefore, the $\mathrm{TCD}_{50}$ assay, particularly in xenograft models, is very sensitive to the host's immune reaction (49). Whether a tumour model evokes an immune response by the host must be therefore tested before local tumour control experiments are undertaken. Nevertheless, despite these drawbacks, the local tumour control assay remains the most relevant experimental method to determine survival of clonogenic tumour cells after irradiation in their environment of treatment. Importantly, the $\mathrm{TCD}_{50}$ assay is

**Table 8.8** Results from a typical $\mathrm{TCD}_{50}$ experiment

| Total dose (Gy) | Number of irradiated tumours | Number of locally controlled tumours | Number of censored animals (censoring interval in days) | Observed local control rates (%) | TCP (%)[a] |
|---|---|---|---|---|---|
| 30 | 11 | 0 | 0 | 0 | $13.4 \times 10^{-6}$ |
| 40 | 11 | 0 | 0 | 0 | $12.6 \times 10^{-3}$ |
| 50 | 11 | 0 | 0 | 0 | 0.6 |
| 60 | 12 | 0 | 1 (99) | 8.3 | 5.6 |
| 72.5 | 11 | 2 | 1 (119) | 27.3 | 24.1 |
| 85 | 12 | 2 | 2 (55–77) | 33.3 | 49.6 |
| 100 | 13 | 7 | 4 (51–116) | 83.9 | 74.1 |

*Note:* Human squamous cell carcinoma FaDu was transplanted subcutaneously into nude mice. At a diameter of about 7 mm, the tumours were irradiated with 30 fractions over 6 weeks. Total radiation doses ranged from 30 to 100 Gy. Local tumour control was evaluated 120 days after end of treatment. From the observed local control rates the tumour control probability (TCP) was calculated using the Poisson model. The dose required to control 50% of the tumours ($\mathrm{TCD}_{50}$) is 85.2 Gy (95% confidence limits 77–96 Gy).

[a] For calculations of TCP, censored animals were taken into account according to the method described by Walker and Suit (68).

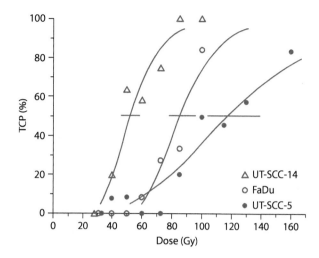

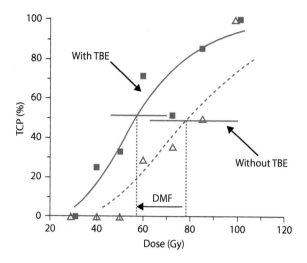

**Figure 8.7** Dose-response curves for local tumour control of three different human squamous cell carcinomas growing in nude mice. Tumours were treated with 30 fractions over 6 weeks with total doses from 30 to 160 Gy. Treatment started for all tumours at the same tumour volume. The data were fitted using a Poisson-based model and the $TCD_{50}$ values as well as their confidence limits were calculated. The three carcinomas show clear-cut differences in radiation sensitivity with UT-SCC-14 being the most sensitive, FaDu with intermediate sensitivity and UT-SCC-5 being the most resistant. The differences in radiation sensitivity can be quantified by comparing the $TCD_{50}$ values, i.e. 52.1 Gy (46; 59) for UT-SCC-14, 85.2 Gy (77; 96) for FaDu and 129.8 Gy (104; 207) for UT-SCC-5. (Data from (71).)

well standardized and the experimental endpoint is identical to the clinical endpoint used in curative radiotherapy.

## Excision assays

Alternative experimental methods to determine clonogenic survival after irradiation include the *in vivo/in vitro* assay, the endpoint dilution assay and the lung colony assay. These assays, introduced in Chapter 4, all require surgical excision of the tumours after irradiation *in situ* and the preparation of a single-cell suspension from the excised tumour using tryptic enzymes to disaggregate the tissue. For the *in vivo/in vitro* assay, different numbers of cells are seeded in culture flasks (26). After an incubation time of typically 7–21 days, the number of colonies is counted. A colony consists of at least 50 cells and is considered to derive from a single surviving clonogenic tumour cell. As in the classical *in vitro* colony-forming assay (see Chapter 4), the surviving fraction is calculated from the ratio of colonies counted to the number of cells seeded. For the lung colony assay, different numbers of cells derived from a tumour irradiated *in situ* are injected intravenously (typically via a tail vein) into groups of recipient mice. Usually around 10 days later, the number of tumour-cell colonies in the lungs is counted and the surviving fraction is calculated by comparison with lung colonies which grew from cells derived from

**Figure 8.8** FaDu human squamous cell carcinoma was transplanted either into unirradiated subcutaneous tissues or into pre-irradiated tissues of nude mice. Pre-irradiation of the transplantation site was performed to induce radiation damage to the supplying host tissues (tumour bed effect [TBE]) as an experimental model of impaired tumour angiogenesis. At a tumour diameter of about 6 mm, tumours of both groups (with TBE and without TBE/control) were treated with 30 fractions over 6 weeks with total doses from 30 to 100 Gy. Local tumour control rates were determined 120 days after the end of fractionated irradiation. The $TCD_{50}$ values were 56.6 Gy for the TBE group and 78.7 Gy for the control group. The effect of the pre-irradiation of the transplantation site on local tumour control after fractionated irradiation is given by the DMF of 1.4 ($TCD_{50,control}/TCD_{50,TBE}$). This indicates that the TBE improved local tumour control after fractionated irradiation (at the effect level 50%) by a factor 1.4. (Data from (72).)

unirradiated tumours. For the endpoint dilution assay ($TD_{50}$ assay), different numbers of cells from an irradiated tumour are inoculated into recipient animals and the frequency of tumour take (tumour growth) is scored.

Excision assays are less resource-consuming and give more rapid results than local tumour control assays. In the *in vivo/in vitro* assay, potential effects of the host immune system are also ruled out. However, a disadvantage of excision assays is that clonogen survival is not determined in the original environment of treatment. Furthermore, results may be affected by the disaggregation method used for single cell preparation, i.e. the influence of timing, chemicals, enzymes and mechanical stress. For colony assays (*in vivo/in vitro* assay and lung colony assay), extensive background information is necessary before the experiment can start: whether the cells form colonies, how many cells at a given radiation dose need to be plated or injected and how long to incubate before counting colonies. The maximum number of cells that can be plated in Petri dishes or injected intravenously is restricted, making it difficult to detect surviving fractions accurately below about $10^{-4}$. Thus, small but resistant subpopulations of clonogenic cells may be systematically overlooked particularly by colony assays. Furthermore, effects of prolonged treatment such as fractionated irradiations are difficult to assess by excision assays (26).

## Regression

To determine tumour regression, the volumes of treated and untreated tumours at a given time point are compared and the ratios for treated versus control tumours (T/C ratios) are reported. The magnitude of tumour regression depends upon radiation effects on the entire cell population in a tumour including malignant and non-malignant cells, for example, endothelial cells, fibroblasts and inflammatory cells. In addition, other factors such as oedema, resorption of dead cells and proliferation of surviving cells contribute to the tumour volume after radiation. These factors differ considerably between different tumours. Whereas tumour cell kill is radiation-dose dependent, resorption, oedema and proliferation may not be. From the notion that regression increases with radiation dose one can argue that for a given tumour model the magnitude of regression reflects the radiation dose-dependent tumour cell kill. Tumour volume measurements under experimental conditions are roughly limited to a range of $1.5 \times 10^7$ to $1.5 \times 10^9$ tumour cells (assuming $10^9$ cells/g tumour, compare Figure 8.1). Thus, even for a given tumour model, volume measurements only assay the radiation response of a very limited proportion of all tumour cells and the response of small and possibly resistant tumour cell populations cannot be detected. In summary, tumour regression is a highly non-specific parameter and of very limited value in describing and quantifying the effect of radiation on tumours.

## Tumour regrowth delay

This is a widely used assay which rapidly provides the researcher with data and can be applied in the laboratory or the clinic. The endpoint is the *time* to reach a certain tumour volume. Therefore, precise determination of tumour volume, e.g. by callipers for subcutaneously growing tumours, or by imaging methods, is essential. In experimental studies, groups of tumours are irradiated and one group of tumours is left unirradiated (control group). Then, the volume of each individual tumour is recorded over time and a growth curve is plotted (Figure 8.9). From this growth curve different parameters may be read, such as the time it takes for a tumour to grow (tumour growth time [TGT]) to five times the treatment volume ($\mathrm{TGT_{V5}}$). From the TGT values for individual tumours the average values for each treatment group ($\mathrm{TGT_{treated}}$) and of the control group ($\mathrm{TGT_{control}}$) are calculated. Tumour growth delay (TGD) is then calculated from

$$\mathrm{TGD} = \mathrm{TGT_{treated}} - \mathrm{TGT_{control}}$$

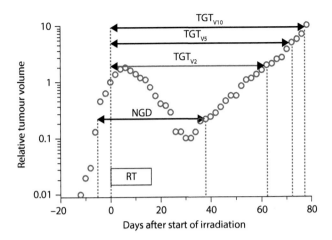

**Figure 8.9** Growth curve of an individual FaDu tumour treated with 15 fractions of 2 Gy. Tumour volume was calculated using the formula for a rotational ellipsoid ($V = [\pi/6]*a*b^2$) where $a$ is the longest tumour axis and $b$ is the axis perpendicular to $a$. The parameters $a$ and $b$ were measured every second day using callipers. The volume is plotted as relative to the volume at the start of treatment. During the initial phase of irradiation the volume increased and later decreased to reach to lowest relative volume (nadir) on day 30 after the start of treatment. After this regression the tumour regrew at a slower rate than before radiation (the regrowth curve is shallower than the growth curve before radiotherapy) indicating the tumour bed effect. From the growth curve, different parameters of the regrowth assay can be read: tumour growth time to reach twice, five times, and ten times the starting volume ($\mathrm{TGT_2}$, $\mathrm{TGT_5}$, $\mathrm{TGT_{10}}$). See text for explanation of NGD.

The specific growth delay (SGD) takes the growth rate of the tumour model into account and allows comparison between different tumour models or different treatments. SGD is calculated from

$$\mathrm{SGD} = (\mathrm{TGT_{treated}} - \mathrm{TGT_{control}}) / \mathrm{TGT_{control}}$$

or

$$\mathrm{SGD} = \mathrm{TGD} / \mathrm{VDT_{control}}$$

Tumour regrowth following irradiation depends upon the effect treatment has had on malignant and non-malignant cells. Radiation-induced damage to the host vascular connective tissues surrounding the tumour may result in a slower growth rate of irradiated tumours. This is named the *tumour bed effect*. As a consequence, SGD apparently increases with increasing tumour volume (Figure 8.9). To correct for the tumour bed effect, the parameter *net growth delay* has been suggested (5). Net growth delay (NGD) is defined as the time between when the regrowing tumour has reached twice its minimal volume (nadir) after treatment and the time at which the tumour had the same

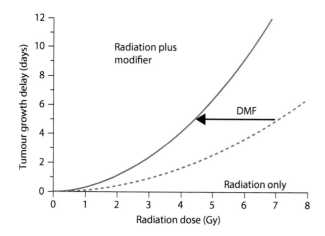

**Figure 8.10** Tumour growth delay after treatment at different radiation doses with and without a treatment modifier. The modifier results in a longer TGD per radiation dose. The effect of the modifier can be quantified as the DMF.

volume before treatment. An alternative would be to choose the endpoint size as low as possible.

TGD increases with radiation dose reflecting the dose-dependency of cell kill (Figure 8.10). The relationships found between radiation dose, the logarithm of surviving clonogenic tumour cells and the TGD suggest that the TGD is a surrogate parameter for clonogenic cell kill. However, there are several limitations. First, quantitative transplantation experiments revealed that the tumour growth rate decreases with decreasing numbers of inoculated cells (67). This suggests that at low levels of cell survival, TGD may not correlate well with the surviving number of clonogenic cells. Second, TGD depends on the radiation effect on the mass of non-clonogenic tumour cells. As a consequence, small variations in the population of clonogenic cells (number and/or sensitivity) may not be detected by the TGD assay. Third, the TGD reflects not only cell kill but also the growth rate of the regrowing tumour. Therefore, this assay is highly sensitive to variations in the proliferation rate including pharmacological manipulations. Thus, a longer TGD does not always mean a higher cell kill. The limitations of the TGD to precisely reflect clonogenic cell kill are underlined by the observation that results from TGD assays may not correlate with results obtained from local tumour control assays (3,32,42,73). The dissociation of volume-dependent endpoints and local tumour control has been observed in several experiments where molecular targeting compounds such as epidermal growth factor receptor (EGFR) inhibitors or anti-angiogenic drugs were combined with irradiation (2). This dissociation may be explained by the fact that these drugs are effective on the mass of non-clonogenic cancer cells, whereas the survival of the small proportion of clonogenic or cancer stem cells remains unaffected (compare Chapter 20). Solutions to this problem include performing confirmatory local tumour control experiments or possibly obtaining TGD at different radiation dose levels (dose-response relationship) as well as

calculating the growth delay per gray, i.e. the steepness of the dose-response curve (34).

To quantify and report the magnitude of effect caused by radiation modifiers on TGD, the DMF or the enhancement ratio (ER) have been used. The DMF is calculated as the ratio of radiation dose without and with modifier giving the same TGD, i.e. the ratio of isoeffective radiation doses. Thus, calculation of the DMF requires the investigation of multiple radiation dose levels and the construction of dose-response curves (Figure 8.10). Often, only one radiation dose level is investigated. In such situations the enhancement ratio (ER) has been used instead of DMF to describe the effect of the modifier. The ER is the ratio of TGD with or without modifier at a given radiation dose level. Both ER and DMF depend on the position and steepness of the dose-effect curves. ER might depend on the radiation dose and DMF might depend on the level of effect. In general, the interpretation of TGD, ER and DMF and their relevance for clonogenic tumour cell inactivation are complicated. Despite its apparent simplicity, the inherent methodological problems of the TGD assay (described previously), the lack of consensus about data evaluation and arbitrary procedural details limit its value in reliably quantifying the radiation response of clonogenic cells. It is therefore recommended to always test the conclusions from TGD assays by undertaking local tumour control studies, before introducing novel treatments into clinical radiotherapy.

## 8.3 FACTORS INFLUENCING LOCAL TUMOUR CONTROL

### Introduction

A number of factors can contribute to the probability of local tumour control after fractionated radiotherapy. These factors were summarized originally by Withers (70) as the 4 R's of radiotherapy: *recovery* from sublethal damage, cell-cycle *redistribution*, cellular *repopulation* and tumour *reoxygenation*. Steel and colleagues have suggested intrinsic cellular *radiosensitivity* as a fifth "R" to account for the different tolerance of tissues to fractionated irradiation (59).

### Recovery from sublethal damage

Most of the damage induced in cells by radiation is satisfactorily repaired. Evidence for this comes from studies of strand breaks in DNA, the vast majority of which disappear during the first few hours after irradiation (see Chapter 2). Further evidence for repair comes from the wide variety of recovery experiments that have been done, both on cell lines *in vitro* and on normal and tumour tissues *in vivo*. It is useful to draw a distinction between these two sources of evidence:

*Repair* – refers to the biochemical process by which the function of macromolecules is restored. Rejoining of DNA strand breaks provides some evidence for this, although the rejoining of a break does not necessarily mean that gene function is restored. Rejoining can leave a genetic defect (i.e. a mutation) and specific tests of *repair fidelity* are needed to detect this. The word *repair* is often loosely used as a synonym for cell-ular or tissue recovery.

*Recovery* – refers to the increase in cell survival or reduction in the extent of radiation damage to a tissue, when time is allowed for this to occur.

There are a number of experimental sources of evidence for recovery, including the following:

*Split-Dose Experiments.* The effect of a given dose of radiation is less if it is split into two fractions, delivered a few hours apart. This effect has been termed 'recovery from sublethal damage' (SLD), or 'Elkind recovery' (13). SLD recovery can be observed using various experimental endpoints: for instance using cell survival (Figure 8.11a), tumour growth delay (Figure 8.11c) or mouse lethality after irradiating a vital normal tissue (Figure 8.11d). The typical timing of split-dose recovery is shown in Figure 8.11a. Considerable recovery occurs within 15 minutes to 1 hour, and recovery often seems to be complete by roughly 6 hours but can be slower than this in some

normal tissues such as the spinal cord (Table 10.2). When the split-dose technique is applied to cycling cells (Figure 8.11a), there is usually a wave in the data caused by cell-cycle progression effects (see below).

*Delayed-Plating Experiments.* If cells are irradiated in a non-growing state and left for increasing periods of time before assaying for survival, an increase in survival is often observed (Figure 8.11b). During this delay the cells are recovering the ability to divide when called upon to do so. This has been termed 'recovery from potentially lethal damage' (PLD). The kinetics of PLD recovery and SLD recovery are similar.

*Dose Rate Effect.* Reduction in radiation damage as dose rate is reduced to around 1 Gy/hour is primarily due to cellular recovery (see Chapter 13).

*Fractionation.* The sparing effect of fractionating radiation treatment within a relatively short overall time is primarily due to recovery. This is therefore the main reason why isoeffect curves slope upwards as the fraction number is increased (Figures 9.1 and 9.2).

What is the relationship between all these various ways of detecting recovery? The damage induced in cells by ionizing radiation is complex, as are the enzymatic processes that immediately begin to repair it. The various types of 'recovery experiment' listed above evaluate this complex repair process in slightly different ways. For instance, the evaluation based on giving a second dose (i.e. SLD recovery) may be different

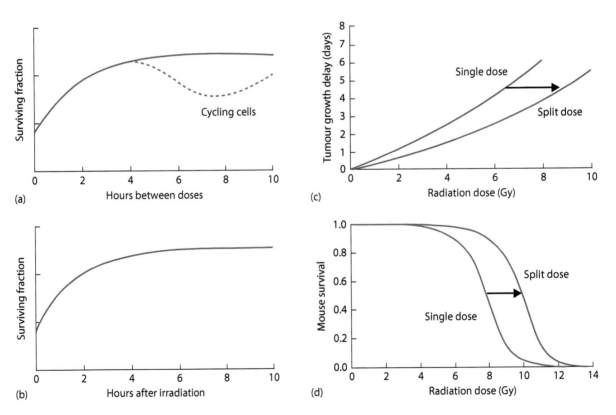

**Figure 8.11** Four ways of measuring recovery from radiation damage (see text). Panels (a), (c) and (d) show three types of split-dose experiment; (b) shows the result of a 'delayed-plating experiment'. The arrows indicate the measurement of ($D_2 - D_1$) values.

from that obtained by asking irradiated non-dividing cells to divide (i.e. PLD recovery).

## Variation of cell killing through the cell cycle, cell-cycle delay and redistribution

The radiosensitivity of cells varies considerably as they pass through the cell cycle. This has been studied in a large number of cell lines, using cell synchronization techniques and also fluorescence-activated cell sorting (FACS) to obtain cell populations in each cell-cycle phase. There is a general tendency for cells in the S-phase (in particular the latter part of the S-phase) to be the most resistant and for cells in very late G2 and mitosis to be the most sensitive. The reason for the resistance in S is thought to be due to homologous recombination, increased as a result of the greater availability of the undamaged sister template through the S phase, together with conformational changes in DNA facilitating easier access of repair complexes during replication. Sensitivity very late in G2 and into mitosis probably results from the fact that those cells have passed a final checkpoint in G2 which occurs within minutes of radiation exposure and allows cells in early G2 to repair their damage probably using homologous recombination (see Chapter 2). The work of Sinclair and Morton (56) is illustrated in Figure 8.12. They synchronized Chinese hamster cells at five different points in the cell cycle and performed cell survival experiments. The survival curves showed that it was mainly the shoulder of the curve that changed: there was little shoulder for cells in mitosis and the shoulder was greatest for cells in late S-phase.

The effect of this process on an asynchronous cell population is that it creates a degree of synchrony in the cells that survive irradiation. Immediately after a dose of X-rays, all the cells will still be at precisely the same point in the cell cycle as they were before irradiation, but some will have lost their reproductive integrity and it is the number that retains this which will tend to be greatest in the S-phase. With increasing time after irradiation the surviving clonogenic cells will show the same distribution over the cell cycle as before irradiation. This process is called *redistribution*. In the 1970s there was much interest in *synchronization therapy*. This was the attempt to exploit cell-cycle progression by treating with a second agent (usually a cytotoxic drug) at the optimum time interval after a priming treatment with drug or radiation. Although this approach to improving tumour therapy was thoroughly researched it proved in most cases to be disappointing. One possible reason for this is that tumours tend to be very heterogeneous from a kinetic point of view: cells move at very different speeds through the phases of the cell cycle and induced cell synchrony is therefore quickly lost and/or impossible to achieve for the whole tumour (58).

## Reoxygenation

This important factor influencing local tumour control and its clinical implications for modified fractionation are comprehensively described in Chapter 17.

## Repopulation

Each fraction during a course of fractionated radiotherapy reduces the total population of clonogenic tumour cells in a tumour, i.e. causes a depopulation of the clonogenic tumour cell compartment (Figure 8.3). In general, clonogenic cells that survive radiation can repopulate the tumour by proliferation and/or reduced cell loss. Repopulation of clonogenic tumour cells might occur during the course of fractionated radiotherapy and thereby reduce the efficacy of treatment. If a tumour has the capacity to repopulate, any prolongation of the overall treatment time results in a higher number of clonogenic tumour cells that needs to be inactivated and thereby requires a higher radiation dose required to achieve local tumour control. The time factor of fractionated radiotherapy (see Chapter 11) has been largely attributed to repopulation of clonogenic tumour cells during treatment (24,35,45,63). Accelerated repopulation describes a process that the net clonogen doubling time during or shortly after irradiation exceeds the clonogen doubling time in untreated tumours. Repopulation of clonogenic tumour cells during fractionated radiotherapy has been shown in a large variety of different experimental and clinical studies as described in Chapter 11 and reviewed by Baumann et al. (3). The results are most consistent for squamous cell carcinomas, but also for other tumour types evidence for a time factor is accumulating (see Table 10.3). The rate, kinetics and underlying radiobiological mechanisms of repopulation vary substantially between tumour types as well as between different tumour lines of the same tumour type. For example, FaDu human squamous cell carcinoma

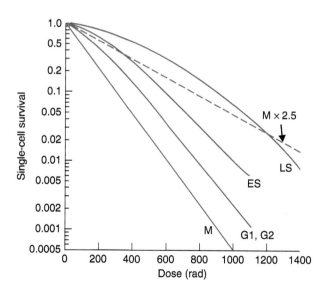

Figure 8.12 Variation of radiosensitivity through the cell cycle of Chinese hamster cells. (Adapted from (56).)

transplanted into nude mice repopulates rapidly with a dose of about 1 Gy recovered per day during fractionated irradiation (4).

The kinetics and radiobiological mechanisms of repopulation have been studied in an extensive series of experiments with fractionated irradiation given to human tumour xenografts either under clamp hypoxia or under normal blood flow conditions (45). A switch to rapid repopulation was observed after about 3 weeks of fractionated irradiation with the clonogen doubling time decreasing from 9.8 days during the first 3 weeks to 3.4 days thereafter (Figure 8.13). In this study, acceleration of repopulation was preceded by a decrease in tumour hypoxia after 2 weeks of fractionated irradiation suggesting that improved tumour oxygenation might trigger repopulation in tumours either by facilitating more proliferation and/or by reducing cell loss. Increased labelling indices for BrdUrd (S-phase fraction) and Ki-67 (growth fraction) during fractionated irradiation indicate that increased proliferation contributes directly to repopulation (44). Repopulation rate was found to be lower in tumours with increased cell loss, indirectly implying that decreased cell loss might also enhance repopulation (25). This latter concept was originally postulated by Fowler (17), i.e. that clonogens always proliferate at their maximum rate ('potential clonogen doubling time') but due to the limited supply of nutrients and oxygen, clonogens are pushed towards necrosis by the proliferative pressure from the cell layers close to supporting blood vessels. Once radiotherapy has killed off enough well-oxygenated tumour cells, the oxygen and nutrient supply improves and the spontaneous cell loss decreases. The effective doubling time of clonogens therefore

becomes shorter and shorter during treatment and eventually the *potential doubling time* of clonogens is 'unmasked'.

In contrast to this concept, it has been suggested, particularly for well-differentiated tumours, that an actively regulated regenerative response of surviving clonogens reminiscent of a normal epithelium represents the major mechanism of clonogen repopulation (11,22,35,65). Signalling via the epidermal growth factor receptor (EGFR) has been proposed as a potential molecular mechanism of this regulated regenerative response underlying repopulation (8,14,33,44,55), as described in Chapter 20.

## Tumour volume

Large tumours are more difficult to cure than small tumours. This has been known since the early years of radiotherapy (40). There are several explanations for this observation. First, tumour volume is proportional to the number of clonogens per tumour. Second, hypoxia is more pronounced in large than in small tumours. Third, in the clinical situation large tumours can often not be irradiated to curative doses because of the larger irradiated volume and limited tolerance of the adjacent normal tissues. Assuming a linear relationship between the number of clonogens and tumour volume, and other parameters, e.g. density, radiosensitivity and hypoxic fraction of clonogenic tumour cells all being equal, the relationship between the $TCP_2$ and the relative tumour volume ($V_{rel}$) can be described according to Dubben et al. (12) as

$$TCP_2 = TCP_1^{V_{rel}}$$

where $TCP_1$ represents the reference TCP when the relative tumour volume ($V_{rel}$) equals 1. If, for example, a $TCP_1$ of 50% (0.5) is chosen, then the relationship between relative tumour volume and TCP can be described with the function $TCP_2 = 0.5^{V_{rel}}$ (Figure 8.14). Over a wide range, the TCP decreases roughly linearly with the logarithm of tumour volume (or the number of clonogens), whereas at very low and very high TCPs the impact of tumour volume is less pronounced. Both experimental and clinical data lend support to this simple theory, indicating that tumour volume is indeed an important factor influencing local tumour control after radiotherapy (1,9,12). Yet, analysis of clinical data has also revealed that the effect of tumour volume on TCP is less than expected from Figure 8.14 (9). This is not surprising as the above-mentioned assumption that all other factors than volume are equal is not realistic in the clinical situation. Instead, patient-to-patient heterogeneity in a large variety of known and unknown determinants of local tumour control may interfere with the simple proportionality of TCP and tumour volume. However, as for other known prognostic factors in radiotherapy such as stage, age, histology, etc., tumour volume should be routinely measured and reported in clinical trials as well as included in data analyses.

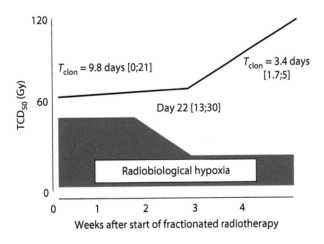

Figure 8.13 Rate, kinetics and underlying mechanism of repopulation of clonogenic tumour cells in FaDu squamous cell carcinoma growing in nude mice. As the result of repopulation, the tumour control dose ($TCD_{50}$) increases with time. Clonogenic FaDu tumour cells repopulate at a low rate during the first 3 weeks with an estimated clonogen doubling time ($T_{clon}$) of 9.8 days. After a switch around day 22, repopulation accelerates to a $T_{clon}$ of 3.4 days. In this tumour model the switch in repopulation is preceded by a decrease in radiobiological hypoxia. (Data from (45).)

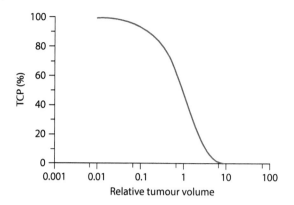

**Figure 8.14** Theoretical relationship of TCP and relative tumour volume according to Dubben et al. (12). A TCP of 50% (0.5) is arbitrarily chosen to correspond to a relative tumour volume of 1. The relationship is based on the assumption of a linear relationship between the number of clonogens and tumour volume and that all other parameters, e.g. density, radiosensitivity and hypoxic fraction of clonogenic tumour cells, are invariant.

## Tumour response to high doses per fraction

In addition to all the factors described above, other radiobiological mechanisms might contribute to local tumour control especially when single or large doses per fraction are used, e.g. in hypofractionation or radiosurgery. Thus, at doses per fraction more than 5 Gy, vascular effects may become important (18,43). Inflammatory and immunological responses triggered by large doses per fraction may also enhance the direct tumour cell killing from radiotherapy and generate abscopal effects on malignant cells outside the radiation target volume. Extensive clinical evaluation of these non-targeted effects is taking place (15), recognising that studying these effects in models of human tumours in animals may be compromised by the immune modification of the host animal necessary to grow the human tumour experimentally.

### Key points

1. Volume of growing tumours increases exponentially with time. Therefore, tumour volume should always be plotted on a logarithmic scale to facilitate evaluation of growth curves, comparison of growth rates among different tumours and judgment of treatment effects.
2. Growth rates vary among different tumours. Primary tumours tend to grow slower than metastatic lesions. A volume doubling time of 3 months is typical for many primary tumours.
3. Tumour growth rate is determined by the fraction of cycling cells (growth fraction [GF]), the cell cycle time ($T_C$) and the cell loss rate. Typical values for human tumours are 40%, 2 days and

90%, respectively. However, these parameters vary considerably between tumours and even among tumours of the same histological type.
4. Potential doubling time ($T_{pot}$) is the theoretical volume doubling time in the absence of cell loss. Therefore, the difference between the observed volume doubling time and the potential doubling time is explained by cell loss in tumours, which exceeds 90% in many histological types.
5. The faster growth of experimental tumours compared with tumours in patients results from a higher GF, a shorter $T_{pot}$ and a lower cell loss factor.
6. Response of tumours to radiation can be assayed using different endpoints including local tumour control, tumour regrowth delay and regression.
7. Local tumour control is the aim of curative radiotherapy and therefore conceptually the most relevant endpoint to assay radiation response.
8. Local tumour control is achieved when all clonogenic tumour cells, i.e. cells with the capacity to proliferate and to cause a local recurrence, are inactivated.
9. Ionizing irradiation is highly effective in inactivating clonogenic tumour cells. The logarithm of the number of surviving clonogenic tumour cells decreases linearly with total radiation dose during fractionated radiotherapy.
10. Response criteria such as partial response or complete response are not appropriate to describe the radiation response of clonogenic tumour cells.
11. Tumour regression is a non-specific parameter of very limited value to describe and quantify radiation effects in tumours.
12. The tumour regrowth delay assay is widely used in experimental radiotherapy. Methodological problems limit the value of this assay to accurately measure the survival of clonogenic tumour cells. Thus, confirmatory local tumour control experiments are recommended.
13. Different factors influence the probability of local tumour control (5 R's of fractionated radiotherapy).
14. Repopulation of clonogenic tumour cells represents a major cause of resistance to fractionated irradiation in certain tumour types. The rate, kinetics and underlying radiobiological mechanisms vary widely among different tumours.
15. Tumour volume is an important determinant of local tumour control.

## ■ BIBLIOGRAPHY

1. Baumann M, Dubois W, Suit HD. Response of human squamous cell carcinoma xenografts of different sizes to irradiation: Relationship of clonogenic cells, cellular radiation sensitivity *in vivo*, and tumor rescuing units. *Radiat Res* 1990;123:325–330.

2. Baumann M, Krause M, Hill R. Exploring the role of cancer stem cells in radioresistance. *Nat Rev Cancer* 2008;8: 545–554.

3. Baumann M, Krause M, Zips D et al. Selective inhibition of the epidermal growth factor receptor tyrosine kinase by BIBX1382BS and the improvement of growth delay, but not local control, after fractionated irradiation in human FaDu squamous cell carcinoma in the nude mouse. *Int J Radiat Biol* 2003;79:547–559.

4. Baumann M, Liertz C, Baisch H, Wiegel T, Lorenzen J, Arps H. Impact of overall treatment time of fractionated irradiation on local control of human FaDu squamous cell carcinoma in nude mice. *Radiother Oncol* 1994;32:137–143.

5. Beck-Bornholdt HP, Wurschmidt F, Vogler H. Net growth delay: A novel parameter derived from tumor growth curves. *Int J Radiat Oncol Biol Phys* 1987;13:773–777.

6. Begg AC, Haustermans K, Hart AA et al. The value of pretreatment cell kinetic parameters as predictors for radiotherapy outcome in head and neck cancer: A multicenter analysis. *Radiother Oncol* 1999;50:13–23.

7. Begg AC, McNally NJ, Shrieve DC, Karcher H. A method to measure the duration of DNA synthesis and the potential doubling time from a single sample. *Cytometry* 1985;6: 620–626.

8. Bentzen SM, Atasoy BM, Daley FM et al. Epidermal growth factor receptor expression in pretreatment biopsies from head and neck squamous cell carcinoma as a predictive factor for a benefit from accelerated radiation therapy in a randomized controlled trial. *J Clin Oncol* 2005;23: 5560–5567.

9. Bentzen SM, Thames HD. Tumor volume and local control probability: Clinical data and radiobiological interpretations. *Int J Radiat Oncol Biol Phys* 1996;36:247–251.

10. Brown DC, Gatter KC. Ki67 protein: The immaculate deception? *Histopathology* 2002;40:2–11.

11. Dorr W. Three A's of repopulation during fractionated irradiation of squamous epithelia: Asymmetry loss, acceleration of stem-cell divisions and abortive divisions. *Int J Radiat Biol* 1997;72:635–643.

12. Dubben HH, Thames HD, Beck-Bornholdt HP. Tumor volume: A basic and specific response predictor in radiotherapy. *Radiother Oncol* 1998;47:167–174.

13. Elkind MM, Sutton H. Radiation response of mammalian cells grown in culture. 1. Repair of X-ray damage in surviving Chinese hamster cells. *Radiat Res* 1960;13:556–593.

14. Eriksen JG, Steiniche T, Overgaard J. The influence of epidermal growth factor receptor and tumor differentiation on the response to accelerated radiotherapy of squamous cell carcinomas of the head and neck in the randomized DAHANCA 6 and 7 study. *Radiother Oncol* 2005;74:93–100.

15. Formenti SC. The pace of progress in radiation and immunotherapy. *Int J Radiat Oncol Biol Phys* 2016;95: 1257–1258.

16. Fowler JE, Pandey P, Braswell NT, Seaver L. Prostate specific antigen progression rates after radical prostatectomy or radiation therapy for localized prostate cancer. *Surgery* 1994;116:302–305.

17. Fowler JF. Rapid repopulation in radiotherapy: A debate on mechanism. The phantom of tumor treatment – Continually rapid proliferation unmasked. *Radiother Oncol* 1991;22:156–158.

18. Garcia-Barros M, Paris F, Cordon-Cardo C et al. Tumor response to radiotherapy regulated by endothelial cell apoptosis. *Science* 2003;300:1155–1159.

19. Gerweck LE, Zaidi ST, Zietman A. Multivariate determinants of radiocurability. I: Prediction of single fraction tumor control doses. *Int J Radiat Oncol Biol Phys* 1994;29: 57–66.

20. Haitel A, Wiener HG, Migschitz B, Marberger M, Susani M. Proliferating cell nuclear antigen and MIB-1. An alternative to classic prognostic indicators in renal cell carcinomas? *Am J Clin Pathol* 1997;107:229–235.

21. Hanahan D, Weinberg RA. The hallmarks of cancer. *Cell* 2000;100:57–70.

22. Hansen O, Overgaard J, Hansen HS et al. Importance of overall treatment time for the outcome of radiotherapy of advanced head and neck carcinoma: Dependency on tumor differentiation. *Radiother Oncol* 1997;43:47–51.

23. Haustermans KM, Hofland I, Van Poppel H et al. Cell kinetic measurements in prostate cancer. *Int J Radiat Oncol Biol Phys* 1997;37:1067–1070.

24. Hessel F, Krause M, Helm A et al. Differentiation status of human squamous cell carcinoma xenografts does not appear to correlate with the repopulation capacity of clonogenic tumour cells during fractionated irradiation. *Int J Radiat Biol* 2004;80:719–727.

25. Hessel F, Petersen C, Zips D et al. Impact of increased cell loss on the repopulation rate during fractionated irradiation in human FaDu squamous cell carcinoma growing in nude mice. *Int J Radiat Biol* 2003;79:479–486.

26. Hill RP. Excision assays. In: Kallman RF, editor. *Rodent Tumor Models in Experimental Cancer Therapy*. New York, NY: Pergamon Press; 1987. pp. 67–75.

27. Hill RP, Milas L. The proportion of stem cells in murine tumors. *Int J Radiat Oncol Biol Phys* 1989;16:513–518.

28. Hommura F, Dosaka-Akita H, Mishina T et al. Prognostic significance of p27KIP1 protein and ki-67 growth fraction in non-small cell lung cancers. *Clin Cancer Res* 2000;6:4073–4081.

29. Hoskin PJ, Sibtain A, Daley FM, Saunders MI, Wilson GD. The immunohistochemical assessment of hypoxia, vascularity and proliferation in bladder carcinoma. *Radiother Oncol* 2004;72:159–168.

30. Jensen V, Sorensen FB, Bentzen SM et al. Proliferative activity (MIB-1 index) is an independent prognostic parameter in patients with high-grade soft tissue sarcomas of subtypes other than malignant fibrous histiocytomas: A retrospective immunohistological study including 216 soft tissue sarcomas. *Histopathology* 1998;32:536–546.

31. Jung H, Kruger HJ, Brammer I, Zywietz F, Beck-Bornholdt HP. Cell population kinetics of the rhabdomyosarcoma R1H of the rat after single doses of X-rays. *Int J Radiat Biol* 1990;57:567–589.

32. Krause M, Hessel F, Zips D, Hilberg F, Baumann M. Adjuvant inhibition of the epidermal growth factor receptor after fractionated irradiation of FaDu human squamous cell carcinoma. *Radiother Oncol* 2004;72:95–101.

33. Krause M, Ostermann G, Petersen C et al. Decreased repopulation as well as increased reoxygenation contribute to the improvement in local control after targeting of the EGFR by C225 during fractionated irradiation. *Radiother Oncol* 2005;76:162–167.

34. Krause M, Zips D, Thames HD, Kummermehr J, Baumann M. Preclinical evaluation of molecular-targeted anticancer agents for radiotherapy. *Radiother Oncol* 2006;80:112–122.

35. Kummermehr J, Dorr W, Trott KR. Kinetics of accelerated repopulation in normal and malignant squamous epithelia during fractionated radiotherapy. *BJR Suppl* 1992;24: 193–199.

36. Lanza G, Jr., Cavazzini L, Borghi L, Ferretti S, Buccoliero F, Rubbini M. Immunohistochemical assessment of growth fractions in colorectal adenocarcinomas with monoclonal antibody Ki-67. Relation to clinical and pathological variables. *Pathol Res Pract* 1990;186:608–618.

37. Lee WR, Hanks GE, Corn BW, Schultheiss TE. Observations of pretreatment prostate-specific antigen doubling time in 107 patients referred for definitive radiotherapy. *Int J Radiat Oncol Biol Phys* 1995;31:21–24.

38. Linder S, Parrado C, Falkmer UG, Blasjo M, Sundelin P, von Rosen A. Prognostic significance of Ki-67 antigen and p53 protein expression in pancreatic duct carcinoma: A study of the monoclonal antibodies MIB-1 and DO-7 in formalin-fixed paraffin-embedded tumour material. *Br J Cancer* 1997;76:54–59.

39. Malaise EP, Chavaudra N, Tubiana M. The relationship between growth rate, labelling index and histological type of human solid tumours. *Eur J Cancer* 1973;9:305–312.

40. Miescher G. Röntgentherapie der Hautkarzinome. *Schweiz Med Wochenschr* 1929;II:1225.

41. Munro TR, Gilbert CW. The relation between tumour lethal doses and the radiosensitivity of tumour cells. *Br J Radiol* 1961;34:246–251.

42. Overgaard J, Matsui M, Lindegaard JC et al. Relationship between tumor growth delay and modification of tumor-control probability of various treatments given as an adjuvant to irradiation. In: Kallman RF, editor. *Rodent Tumor Models in Experimental Cancer Therapy*. New York, NY: Pergamon Press; 1987. pp. 128–132.

43. Park HJ, Griffin RJ, Hui S, Levitt SH, Song CW. Radiation-induced vascular damage in tumors: Implications of vascular damage in ablative hypofractionated radiotherapy (SBRT and SRS). *Radiat Res* 2012;177:311–327.

44. Petersen C, Eicheler W, Frommel A et al. Proliferation and micromilieu during fractionated irradiation of human FaDu squamous cell carcinoma in nude mice. *Int J Radiat Biol* 2003;79:469–477.

45. Petersen C, Zips D, Krause M et al. Repopulation of FaDu human squamous cell carcinoma during fractionated radiotherapy correlates with reoxygenation. *Int J Radiat Oncol Biol Phys* 2001;51:483–493.

46. Potten CS, Wichmann HE, Dobek K et al. Cell kinetic studies in the epidermis of mouse. III. The percent labelled mitosis (PLM) technique. *Cell Tissue Kinet* 1985;18: 59–70.

47. Rautiainen E, Haapasalo H, Sallinen P, Rantala I, Helen P, Helin H. Histone mRNA in-situ hybridization in astrocytomas: A comparison with PCNA, MIB-1 and mitoses in paraffin-embedded material. *Histopathology* 1998;32:43–50.

48. Rew DA, Wilson GD. Cell production rates in human tissues and tumours and their significance. Part II: clinical data. *Eur J Surg Oncol* 2000;26:405–417.

49. Rofstad EK. Local tumor control following single dose irradiation of human melanoma xenografts: Relationship to cellular radiosensitivity and influence of an immune response by the athymic mouse. *Cancer Res* 1989;49: 3163–3167.

50. Rofstad EK, Wahl A, Brustad T. Radiation response of human melanoma multicellular spheroids measured as single cell survival, growth delay, and spheroid cure: Comparisons with the parent tumor xenograft. *Int J Radiat Oncol Biol Phys* 1986;12:975–982.

51. Roland NJ, Caslin AW, Bowie GL, Jones AS. Has the cellular proliferation marker Ki67 any clinical relevance in squamous cell carcinoma of the head and neck? *Clin Otolaryngol Allied Sci* 1994;19:13–18.

52. Roser F, Samii M, Ostertag H, Bellinzona M. The Ki-67 proliferation antigen in meningiomas. Experience in 600 cases. *Acta Neurochir (Wien)* 2004;146:37–44; discussion.

53. Sarbia M, Bittinger F, Porschen R et al. The prognostic significance of tumour cell proliferation in squamous cell carcinomas of the oesophagus. *Br J Cancer* 1996;74: 1012–1016.

54. Schmid HP, McNeal JE, Stamey TA. Observations on the doubling time of prostate cancer. The use of serial prostate-specific antigen in patients with untreated disease as a measure of increasing cancer volume. *Cancer* 1993;71:2031–2040.

55. Schmidt-Ullrich RK, Contessa JN, Dent P et al. Molecular mechanisms of radiation-induced accelerated repopulation. *Radiat Oncol Investig* 1999;7:321–330.

56. Sinclair WK, Morton RA. X-Ray and ultraviolet sensitivity of synchronized Chinese hamster cells at various stages of the cell cycle. *Biophys J* 1965;5:1–25.

57. Spratt JS, Meyer JS, Spratt JA. Rates of growth of human neoplasms: Part II. *J Surg Oncol* 1996;61:68–83.

58. Steel GG. *The Growth Kinetics of Tumours.* Oxford: Oxford University Press; 1977.

59. Steel GG, McMillan TJ, Peacock JH. The 5Rs of radiobiology. *Int J Radiat Biol* 1989;56:1045–1048.

60. Suit HD, Sedlacek R, Thames HD. Radiation dose-response assays of tumor control. In: Kallman RF, editor. *Rodent Tumor Models in Experimental Cancer Therapy*. New York, NY: Pergamon Press; 1987. pp. 138–148.

61. Taftachi R, Ayhan A, Ekici S, Ergen A, Ozen H. Proliferating-cell nuclear antigen (PCNA) as an independent prognostic marker in patients after prostatectomy: A comparison of PCNA and Ki-67. *BJU Int* 2005;95:650–654.

62. Terry NH, White RA, Meistrich ML, Calkins DP. Evaluation of flow cytometric methods for determining population potential doubling times using cultured cells. *Cytometry* 1991;12:234–241.

63. Thames HD, Ruifrok AC, Milas L et al. Accelerated repopulation during fractionated irradiation of a murine ovarian carcinoma: Downregulation of apoptosis as a possible mechanism. *Int J Radiat Oncol Biol Phys* 1996;35:951–962.

64. Thor AD, Liu S, Moore DH, 2nd, Edgerton SM. Comparison of mitotic index, *in vitro* bromodeoxyuridine labeling, and MIB-1 assays to quantitate proliferation in breast cancer. *J Clin Oncol* 1999;17:470–477.

65. Trott KR, Kummermehr J. Rapid repopulation in radiotherapy: A debate on mechanism. Accelerated repopulation in tumours and normal tissues. *Radiother Oncol* 1991;22:159–160.

66. Trott KR, Maciejewski B, Preuss-Bayer G, Skolyszewski J. Dose-response curve and split-dose recovery in human skin cancer. *Radiother Oncol* 1984;2:123–129.

67. Urano M, Kahn J. Some practical questions in the tumor regrowth assay. In: Kallman RF, editor. *Rodent Tumor Models in Experimental Cancer Therapy*. New York, NY: Pergamon Press; 1987. pp. 122–127.

68. Walker AM, Suit HD. Assessment of local tumor control using censored tumor response data. *Int J Radiat Oncol Biol Phys* 1983;9:383–386.

69. Wheldon TE, Abdelaal AS, Nias AH. Tumour curability, cellular radiosensitivity and clonogenic cell number. *Br J Radiol* 1977;50:843–844.

70. Withers HR. *The Four R's of Radiotherapy*. New York, NY: Academic Press; 1975.

71. Yaromina A, Zips D, Thames HD et al. Pimonidazole labelling and response to fractionated irradiation of five human squamous cell carcinoma (hSCC) cell lines in nude mice: The need for a multivariate approach in biomarker studies. *Radiother Oncol* 2006;81:122–129.

72. Zips D, Eicheler W, Bruchner K et al. Impact of the tumour bed effect on microenvironment, radiobiological hypoxia and the outcome of fractionated radiotherapy of human FaDu squamous-cell carcinoma growing in the nude mouse. *Int J Radiat Biol* 2001;77:1185–1193.

73. Zips D, Hessel F, Krause M et al. Impact of adjuvant inhibition of vascular endothelial growth factor receptor tyrosine kinases on tumor growth delay and local tumor control after fractionated irradiation in human squamous cell carcinomas in nude mice. *Int J Radiat Oncol Biol Phys* 2005;61:908–914.

## ■ FURTHER READING

74. Kallman RF. *Rodent Tumor Models in Experimental Cancer Therapy*. New York, NY: Pergamon Press; 1987.

75. Steel GG. *The Growth Kinetics of Tumours*. Oxford: Oxford University Press; 1977.

# Fractionation: The linear-quadratic approach

## MICHAEL C. JOINER AND SØREN M. BENTZEN

## 9.1 INTRODUCTION

Major developments in radiotherapy fractionation have taken place during the past four decades and continue to do so, and these have grown directly out of increasing understanding in clinical radiation biology. The relationships between equieffective total dose and dose per fraction for late-responding tissues, early responding tissues and tumours provide the basic information required to biologically optimise radiotherapy according to the dose per fraction, number of fractions and tumour type, site and treatment plan.

A milestone in this subject was the publication first by Thames et al. (23) of a survey of isoeffect curves for various normal tissues, mainly in mice. Their summary is shown in Figure 9.1. Each of the investigations contributing to this chart was a study of the response of a normal tissue to fractionated radiation treatment using a range of doses per fraction. In order to minimise the effects of repopulation, this survey was restricted to studies in which the overall time was kept short by the use of multiple treatments per day, or 'where an effect of regeneration of target cells was shown to be unlikely'. This summary thus represents the influence of dose per fraction on response and mostly excludes the influence of overall treatment time. It was possible in each study, and for each chosen dose per fraction, to determine the total radiation dose that produced some defined level of normal tissue damage. These endpoints of tolerance differed from one normal tissue or experimental study to another. Each line in Figure 9.1 is an isoeffect curve determined in this way. The dashed lines show isoeffect curves for early responding tissues and the full lines are for late-responding tissues. Note that fraction number *increases* from left to right along the abscissa and, therefore, the dose per fraction scale *decreases* from left to right. The results of this survey show that the isoeffective total dose increases more rapidly with decreasing dose per fraction for late effects than for early effects. If the vertical axis is regarded as a tissue tolerance dose, it can be deduced immediately from this plot that using lower doses per fraction (towards the right-hand end of the abscissa) will tend to spare late reactions if the total dose is adjusted to keep the early reactions constant. A linear-quadratic framework, introduced in Chapter 4, can be used to describe this relationship between total

isoeffective dose and the dose per fraction in fractionated radiotherapy. The linear-quadratic (LQ) model thus creates a robust quantitative environment for considering the balance between early reactions, late reactions and effect on the target tumour as dose per fraction and total dose are changed. This has been one of the most important advances in radiobiology applied to therapy. In this chapter, we present the theoretical background and supporting data that have led to the almost universal adoption now of the LQ approach to describing radiation fractionation and we show the basic framework in which calculations can be made. Detailed examples of such calculations in a clinical radiotherapy setting are demonstrated practically in Chapter 10.

## 9.2 HISTORICAL BACKGROUND: LINEAR-QUADRATIC VERSUS POWER-LAW MODELS

Two specific examples of isoeffect plots for radiation damage to normal tissues in the mouse are shown in Figure 9.2: skin is an early responding tissue and kidney a late-responding tissue. In each case, the total radiation dose to give a fixed level of damage is plotted against dose per fraction and fraction number on a double-log plot. Note that the curve for kidney is steeper than that for skin.

The solid lines in Figure 9.2 are calculated by an equation based on the LQ model:

$$\text{Total dose} = \frac{\text{Constant}}{1 + d/(\alpha/\beta)} \tag{9.1}$$

where $d$ is the dose per fraction. See Section 9.4 for the derivation of this equation. The overall steepness and curvature of these lines are both determined by one parameter: the $\alpha/\beta$ value. For the skin data (Figure 9.2a), $\alpha/\beta$ is about 10. The units of $\alpha/\beta$ are grays, so the $\alpha/\beta$ value in this case is 10 Gy. For the kidney data $\alpha/\beta$ is about 3 Gy.

The LQ model fits these data very well and produces curves in this type of log-log plot. Also shown in Figure 9.2 are broken lines showing the fit of Ellis' historical nominal standard dose (NSD) model (7) to both data sets. NSD is an example of a simple power-law relationship between total dose and number of fractions, and it and it's derivatives such

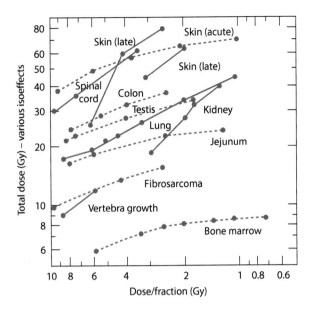

**Figure 9.1** Relationship between total dose and dose per fraction for a variety of normal tissues in experimental animals. The results for late-responding tissues (full lines) are systematically steeper than those for early responding tissues (broken lines). (From (23), with permission.)

as TDF ('time-dose-fractionation') were still used in many clinical centres until the 1980s. The equation for NSD is

$$\text{Total dose} = \text{NSD} \times N^{0.24} \times T^{0.11}$$

In these animal studies the overall treatment time ($T$) was constant. Power-law models like NSD and TDF give straight lines in this type of plot and fit the skin data well from 4 to 32 fractions but the data points fall below the broken line both for small and large dose per fraction. The discrepancy for doses per fraction of 1–2 Gy and >10 Gy is important in relation to both hyperfractionation and radical hypofractionation (Section 9.6). For late reactions, as illustrated by the kidney

data in Figure 9.2b, the NSD formula again does not fit as well as the LQ formula, even though the $N$ exponent has been raised from 0.24 to 0.35 in order to allow for the greater overall slope. A similar modification, but not necessarily by the same amount, must be made for all late-responding tissues if the NSD formulation is to be even approximately correct.

A crucial therapeutic conclusion is illustrated by these two sets of high-precision data. At both ends of the scale, in the region of large and small dose per fraction, power-law equations *overestimate* the actual tolerance dose (as shown by both experimental and clinical data). This means that all power-law models are *unsafe* in these regions, a conclusion that is well supported by clinical experience. At the present time it is strongly recommended that the LQ model should always be used, with a correctly chosen $\alpha/\beta$ value, to describe isoeffect dose relationships at least over the range of doses per fraction between 1 and 6 Gy. The LQ model is simple to use in clinical calculations and comparisons, and does not require the use of 'look-up tables'. Sections 9.4 through 9.8 and Chapter 10 provide a straightforward guide to LQ calculations.

## 9.3 POSSIBLE CELL-SURVIVAL INTERPRETATION OF THE LQ MODEL

What is an explanation for the difference between the fractionation response of early and late-responding tissues which is shown in Figures 9.1 and 9.2? Figure 9.3 shows hypothetical single-dose (one-fraction) survival curves for putative target cells in early and late-responding tissues, drawn according to the LQ equation (see Figure 4.5b). $E$ represents the reduction in cell survival (on a logarithmic scale) that is equivalent to tissue tolerance. The total dose that would need to be given in two fractions is obtained by drawing a straight line from the origin through the survival curve at $E/2$ and measuring the intersection of this line with the dose axis. As shown by the dashed line labelled 2

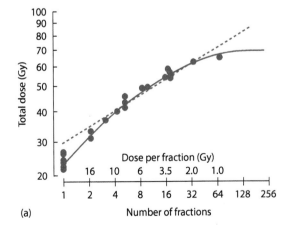

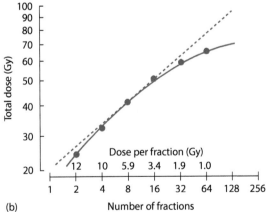

**Figure 9.2** Relationship between *total dose* to achieve an isoeffect and *number of fractions*. (a) Early reactions in mouse skin (6). (b) Late injury in mouse kidney (20). Note that the relationship for kidney is steeper than that for skin. The broken lines are NSD formulae fitted to the central part of each data set. The solid lines show the LQ model, from which the guide to the dose per fraction has been calculated.

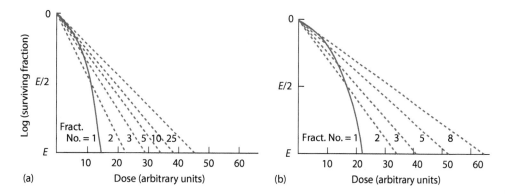

**Figure 9.3** Schematic survival curves for target cells in (a) early responding and (b) late-responding normal tissues. The abscissa is radiation dose on an arbitrary scale. (From (29), with permission.)

in panel A, a dose of around 11 Gy takes the effect down to E/2 and (with assumed constant effect per fraction) a second 11 Gy gives the isoeffect E: the total isoeffect dose is ~22 Gy. This compares with a single dose of ~14 Gy to give the same isoeffect E, shown by the solid line. The total dose for three fractions is obtained in the same way by drawing a line through E/3 on the survival curve, and similarly for the other fraction numbers. Because the late-responding survival curve (Figure 9.3b) is more 'bendy' (it has a lower $\alpha/\beta$ value), the isoeffective total dose increases more rapidly with increasing number of fractions compared with the early responding tissue where the survival curve bends less sharply.

## 9.4 THE LQ MODEL IN DETAIL

The surviving fraction ($SF_d$) of putative target cells after a dose per fraction $d$ is given in Section 4.10 as

$$SF_d = \exp\left(-\alpha d - \beta d^2\right)$$

Radiobiological studies have generally shown that each successive fraction in a multi-dose schedule is equally effective, so the effect ($E$) of $n$ fractions can be expressed as

$$E = -\log_e(SF_d)^n = -n\log_e(SF_d)$$
$$= n(\alpha d + \beta d^2) = \alpha D + \beta dD$$

where the total radiation dose $D = nd$. This equation can be rearranged into the following forms:

$$1/D = (\alpha/E) + (\beta/E)d \tag{9.2}$$

$$1/n = (\alpha/E)d + (\beta/E)d^2 \tag{9.3}$$

$$D = (E/\alpha)/(1 + d/(\alpha/\beta)) \tag{9.4}$$

The practical working of these equations may be illustrated by the results of careful fractionation experiments on the

mouse kidney (20). In these experiments, functional damage to the kidneys was measured by ethylenediamine tetra-acetic acid (EDTA) clearance up to 48 weeks after irradiation with 1–64 fractions. Figure 9.4 shows the response measured as a function of total radiation dose for each fraction number. To apply the LQ model to this example, we first measure off from the graph the total doses at some fixed level of effect (shown by the arrow) and then plot the reciprocal of these total doses against the corresponding dose per fraction. Equation 9.2 shows that this should give a straight line whose slope is $\beta/E$ and whose intercept on the vertical axis is $\alpha/E$. That this is true is shown in Figure 9.5a: the points well fit a straight line. This line cuts the $x$-axis at –3 Gy; it can be seen from Equation 9.2 that this is equal to $-\alpha/\beta$, thus providing a measure of the $\alpha/\beta$ value for these data. The relative contributions of $\alpha$ and $\beta$ to the $\alpha/\beta$ value can be judged by comparing the reciprocal total dose intercept ($\alpha/E$) and the slope of the line ($\beta/E$).

An alternative way of deriving parameter values from these data is to plot the reciprocal of the number of fractions against the dose per fraction as suggested by Equation 9.3.

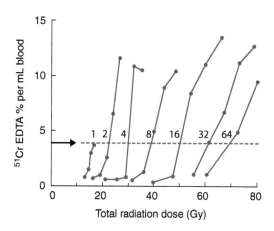

**Figure 9.4** Dose-response curves for late damage to the mouse kidney with fractionated radiation exposure. Damage is indicated by a reduction in EDTA clearance, curves determined for 1–64 dose fractions, illustrating the sparing effect of increased fractionation. (From (20).)

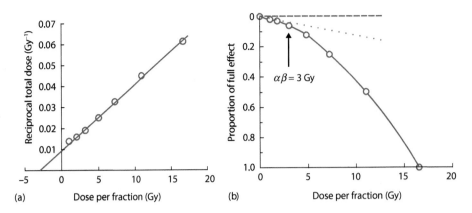

**Figure 9.5** The data of Figure 9.4 after two different transformations: (a) a reciprocal-dose plot according to Equation 9.2 and (b) transformation according to Equation 9.3 with the same data plotted as a proportion of full effect.

Figure 9.5b shows that this gives the shape of the putative target-cell survival curve with the $y$-axis proportional to $-\log_e(SF_d)$. (Statistical note: this method combined with nonlinear least-squares curve fitting is preferred over the linear-regression method shown in Figure 9.5a for determining $\alpha/\beta$, because the $1/n$ and the dose-per-fraction axes are independent.) Equation 9.4 shows the LQ model in the form used already to describe the relationship between total dose and dose per fraction (Figure 9.2).

A common clinical question is: 'What change in total radiation dose is required when we change the dose per fraction?' This can be dealt with very simply using the LQ approach. Rearranging Equation 9.4,

$$E/\alpha = D\left[1 + d/(\alpha/\beta)\right]$$

For isoeffect in a selected tissue, $E$ and $\alpha$ are constant. The first schedule employs a dose per fraction $d_1$ and the isoeffective total dose is $D_1$; we change to a dose per fraction $d_2$ and the new (unknown) total dose is $D_2$. $D_2$ is therefore related to $D_1$ by the following equation:

$$\frac{D_2}{D_1} = \frac{d_1 + (\alpha/\beta)}{d_2 + (\alpha/\beta)} \tag{9.5}$$

This simple LQ isoeffect equation was first proposed by Withers et al. (25). It has widely been found to be successful in clinical calculations.

## 9.5 THE VALUE OF $\alpha/\beta$

Exhaustive fractionation studies of the type analysed in Figures 9.2 and 9.4 have been made in animals. Table 9.1 summarises the $\alpha/\beta$ values obtained from many of these experiments. For early responding tissues which express their damage within a period of days to weeks after irradiation, $\alpha/\beta$ is in the range 7–20 Gy, while for late-responding tissues, which express their damage months to years after irradiation, $\alpha/\beta$ generally ranges from 0.5 to 6 Gy. It is important to recognise that $\alpha/\beta$ is not constant and its

value should be chosen carefully to match the specific tissue under consideration.

Values of $\alpha/\beta$ for a range of key human normal tissues and tumours are given in Tables 10.1 and 14.2. More human normal tissue data are available in the QUANTEC report (16). The fractionation response of well-oxygenated carcinomas of head and neck, and lung, are thought to be similar to that of early responding normal tissues. However, there is clear evidence that some human tumour types like prostate, breast, melanoma and sarcomas exhibit low $\alpha/\beta$ values, maybe with $\alpha/\beta$ even lower than for some late-responding normal tissues. Experimental animal tumour $\alpha/\beta$ values shown in Figure 9.6 were intercompared by Williams et al. (24). Values calculated from data obtained in experiments on rat and mouse tumours under fully radiosensitized conditions (marked 'miso' and 'oxic' in the figure) are plotted directly, and values calculated from fractionation responses under hypoxic conditions (marked 'clamp', 'anoxic' and 'hypoxic') are plotted after dividing by an assumed oxygen enhancement ratio (OER) of 2.7, because the $\alpha/\beta$ values for cells and tissues under anoxic and oxic conditions are in the same proportion as the OER. Error bars are estimates of the 95% confidence interval on each value. Such experiments assayed the effect of radiation either *in situ* by regrowth delay or local tumour control, or by excising the tumour from the animal and measuring the survival of cells *in vitro* (see Chapter 4). These early experimental tumour data also demonstrated a wide variation in $\alpha/\beta$ covering the full range shown by both early and late-responding normal tissues, just as in the more recent clinical data.

## 9.6 HYPOFRACTIONATION AND HYPERFRACTIONATION

Figure 9.7a shows the form of Equation 9.5. Curves are shown for two ranges of $\alpha/\beta$ values: 1–4 Gy and 8–15 Gy, which, respectively, can apply to late- and early responding tissues. It can be seen that when dose per fraction is increased above a reference level of 2 Gy, the isoeffective dose falls more rapidly for the late-responding tissues than for the early responses. Similarly, when dose per fraction is reduced below

**Table 9.1** Values of $\alpha/\beta$ for a variety of early and late-responding normal tissues in experimental animals

| Early reactions | | | Late reactions | | |
|---|---|---|---|---|---|
| | $\alpha/\beta$ | References | | $\alpha/\beta$ | References |
| *Skin* | | | *Spinal cord* | | |
| Desquamation | 9.1–12.5 | Douglas and Fowler (1976) | Cervical | 1.8–2.7 | van der Kogel (1979) |
| | 8.6–10.6 | Joiner et al. (1983) | Cervical | 1.6–1.9 | White and Hornsey (1978) |
| | 9–12 | Moulder and Fischer (1976) | Cervical | 1.5–2.0 | Ang et al. (1983) |
| *Jejunum* | | | Cervical | 2.2–3.0 | Thames et al. (1988) |
| Clones | 6.0–8.3 | Withers et al. (1976) | Lumbar | 3.7–4.5 | van der Kogel (1979) |
| | 6.6–10.7 | Thames et al. (1981) | Lumbar | 4.1–4.9 | White and Hornsey (1978) |
| *Colon* | | | | 3.8–4.1 | Leith et al. (1981) |
| Clones | 8–9 | Tucker et al. (1983) | | 2.3–2.9 | Amols, Yuhas (quoted by Leith et al. 1981) |
| Weight loss | 9–13 | Terry and Denekamp (1984) | *Colon* | | |
| *Testis* | | | Weight loss | 3.1–5.0 | Terry and Denekamp (1984) |
| Clones | 12–13 | Thames and Withers (1980) | *Kidney* | | |
| *Mouse lethality* | | | Rabbit | 1.7–2.0 | Caldwell (1975) |
| 30d | 7–10 | Kaplan and Brown (1952) | Pig | 1.7–2.0 | Hopewell and Wiernik (1977) |
| 30d | 13–17 | Mole (1957) | Rats | 0.5–3.8 | van Rongen et al. (1988) |
| 30d | 11–26 | Paterson et al. (1952) | Mouse | 1.0–3.5 | Williams and Denekamp (1984a,b) |
| *Tumour bed* | | | Mouse | 0.9–1.8 | Stewart et al. (1984a) |
| 45d | 5.6–6.8 | Begg and Terry (1984) | Mouse | 1.4–4.3 | Thames et al. (1988) |
| | | | *Lung* | | |
| | | | LD$_{50}$ | 4.4–6.3 | Wara et al. (1973) |
| | | | LD$_{50}$ | 2.8–4.8 | Field et al. (1976) |
| | | | LD$_{50}$ | 2.0–4.2 | Travis et al. (1983) |
| | | | Breathing rate | 1.9–3.1 | Parkins and Fowler (1985) |
| | | | *Bladder* | | |
| | | | Frequency, capacity | 5–10 | Stewart et al. (1984b) |

From (10); for references, see the original.

*Abbreviations:* $\alpha/\beta$ values are in grays. LD$_{50}$, dose lethal to 50%.

2 Gy, the isoeffective dose *increases* more rapidly in the late-responding tissues. Late-responding tissues are more sensitive to a change in dose per fraction and this could be interpreted as reflecting a greater curvature of an underlying survival curve for putative target cells (Section 9.3).

Since the change in total dose is greater for the lower $\alpha/\beta$ values, so is the potential for error if a wrong $\alpha/\beta$ value is used. The $\alpha/\beta$ values should therefore be selected carefully and always conservatively when doing calculations involving changing dose per fraction. Examples of the conservative

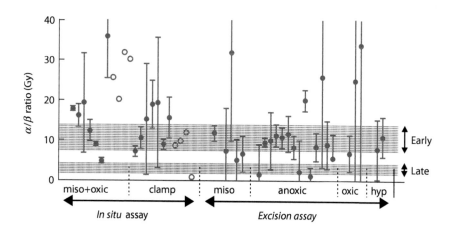

**Figure 9.6** Values of $\alpha/\beta$ for experimental tumours, determined under a variety of conditions of oxygenation (see text). The stippled areas indicate the range of values for early and late-responding normal tissues. (From (24), with permission.)

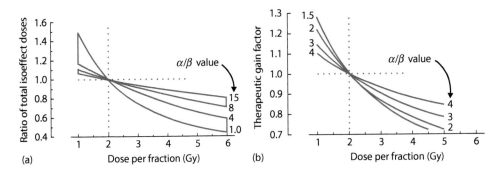

Figure 9.7 (a) Theoretical isoeffect curves based on the LQ model for various $\alpha/\beta$ values. The outlined areas enclose curves corresponding to early and late-responding normal tissues. (b) Therapeutic gain factors for various $\alpha/\beta$ values of normal tissue, assuming an $\alpha/\beta$ value of 10 Gy for tumours.

choice of $\alpha/\beta$ values and other radiobiological parameters are given in Chapter 10 (Examples 10.1, 10.3 and 10.10).

An increase in dose per fraction relative to 2 Gy is termed *hypo*fractionation and a decrease is *hyper*fractionation. (This use of terms may seem contradictory but it indicates that *hypo*fractionation involves fewer dose fractions and *hyper*fractionation requires more fractions.) We can calculate a therapeutic gain factor (TGF) for a new dose per fraction from the ratio of the relative isoeffect doses for tumour and normal tissue. An example is shown in Figure 9.7b where the tumour is taken to have an $\alpha/\beta$ value of 10 Gy. It can be seen from the figure that radiobiologically, hyperfractionation is predicted to give a therapeutic gain, and hypofractionation a therapeutic loss for tumours with high $\alpha/\beta$ value which could apply to head and neck and lung. Remember that we are assuming here that the new regimen is given in the same overall time as the 2 Gy regimen and that treatment is always limited by the late reactions. If an unacceptable increase in early normal tissue reactions prevented the total dose from being increased to the full tolerance of the late-responding tissues, the therapeutic gain for hyperfractionation would be less than shown in Figure 9.7b. In contrast, for tumours with low $\alpha/\beta$ values (e.g. breast, prostate – see Table 10.1) hyperfractionation should give little or no therapeutic gain and *hypo*fractionation could be a better radiobiological treatment strategy for these tumours particularly if improved treatment planning can also give more precise dose delivery. Note that hypofractionation may also be used as a convenient way of accelerating treatment, i.e. shortening the overall treatment time. Therefore, at least in some tumour types, this has led to shorter intensive schedules that compare favourably with more protracted schedules in terms of both tumour control and late normal tissue effects as discussed in Chapters 10 and 11.

## 9.7 EQUIVALENT DOSE IN 2 GY FRACTIONS (EQD2)

The LQ approach leads to various formulae for calculating isoeffect relationships for radiotherapy, all based on similar underlying assumptions. These formulae seek to describe a range of fractionation schedules that are isoeffective. The simplest method of comparing the effectiveness of schedules consisting of different total doses and doses per fraction is to convert each schedule into an equivalent schedule in 2 Gy fractions which would give the same biological effect. This is the approach that we recommend as the method of choice and can be achieved using a specific version of Equation 9.5:

$$\mathrm{EQD2} = D\frac{d+(\alpha/\beta)}{2+(\alpha/\beta)} \qquad (9.6)$$

where EQD2 is the total dose in 2 Gy fractions that is biologically equivalent to a total dose $D$ given with a fraction size of $d$ Gy, assuming a relationship between $D$ and $d$ which is defined by $\alpha/\beta$. Values of EQD2 may be numerically added for separate parts of a treatment schedule. They have the advantage that since 2 Gy is a commonly used dose per fraction clinically, EQD2 values will be recognised by radiotherapists as being of a familiar size. The EQD2 is identical to the normalised total dose proposed by Withers et al. (25), see also Maciejewski et al. (15).

## 9.8 INCOMPLETE REPAIR

The simple LQ description (Equations 9.1 through 9.6) assumes that sufficient time is allowed between fractions for complete repair of sublethal damage to take place after each dose. This allowed interval should be at least 8 hours but in some cases (e.g. spinal cord) may be as long as 1 day (see Chapter 10). If the interfraction interval is reduced below this value, for example when multiple fractions per day are used, the overall damage from the whole treatment is increased because the repair (or more correctly, recovery) of damage due to one radiation dose may not be complete before the next fraction is given, and there is then interaction between residual unrepaired damage from one fraction and the damage from the next fraction. As an example of this process, Figure 9.8 shows data from mouse jejunum irradiated with five X-ray

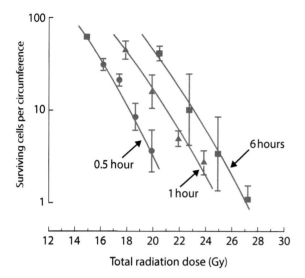

**Figure 9.8** Effect of inter-fraction interval on intestinal radiation damage in mice. The total dose required in five fractions for a given level of effect is less for short intervals, illustrating incomplete repair between fractions. (From (22), with permission.)

fractions in which the number of surviving crypts per gut circumference is plotted against total dose. A lower dose is needed to produce the same effects when the interfraction interval is reduced from 6 hours to 1 hour or 0.5 hour. This process is called *incomplete repair*.

The influence of incomplete repair is determined by the repair half-time ($T_{1/2}$) in the tissue. This is the time required between fractions, or during low dose-rate treatment, for half the maximum possible repair to take place. Incomplete repair will tend to reduce the isoeffective dose and corrections have to be made for the consequent loss of tolerance. This can be accomplished by the use of the incomplete repair model as introduced by Thames (21). In this model, the amount of unrepaired damage is expressed by a function $H_m$ which depends upon the number of equally spaced fractions ($m$), the time interval between them and the repair half-time. For

the purpose of tolerance calculations the extra $H_m$ term is added to the basic EQD2 formula; thus,

$$\text{EQD2} = D\frac{d(1+H_m)+(\alpha/\beta)}{2+(\alpha/\beta)} \qquad (9.7; \text{fractionated})$$

Once again, $d$ is the dose per fraction and $D$ the total dose. If repair from one day to the next is assumed to be complete, $m$ is the number of fractions *per day*. Values of $H_m$ are given in Table 9.2 for repair half-times up to 5 hours and for two or three fractions per day given with interfraction intervals down to 3 hours. Other values can be calculated using the formulae given in Appendix 9.1. Some clinical data sets have suggested even longer repair half-times for late reactions (4). In that case, repair cannot be assumed to be complete in the interval between the last fraction in a day and the first fraction the following day, and a more general version of the incomplete-repair LQ model must be used (12). Table 9.3 shows values of $T_{1/2}$ for some normal tissues in laboratory animals and the available values for human normal tissue endpoints are summarised in Table 10.2. (Advanced note: In several cases, experiments have indicated that repair has fast and slow components. The EQD2 equation above – and biologically effective dose [BED] and total effect [TE] formulae – have to be reformulated in a more complex form to take account of these cases (17).)

Figure 9.9 demonstrates the fit of the incomplete repair LQ model to data for pneumonitis in mice following fractionated thoracic irradiation with intervals of only 3 hours between doses (22). The endpoint was mortality, expressed as the $LD_{50}$. In these reciprocal-dose plots, incomplete repair makes the data bow upwards away from the straight line (dashed) which shows the pure LQ relationship that would be obtained when there is complete repair between successive doses, as would be the case with long time intervals between fractions. An estimate of the repair half-time can be found by fitting data of the type shown in Figures 9.8 and 9.9 with the incomplete repair LQ model and seeking the $T_{1/2}$ value that gives the best fit.

**Table 9.2** Incomplete repair factors: Fractionated irradiation ($H_m$ factors)

| Repair halftime (h) | Interval for $m=2$ fractions per day | | | | | | Interval for $m=3$ fractions per day | | | | |
|---|---|---|---|---|---|---|---|---|---|---|---|
| | 3 | 4 | 5 | 6 | 8 | 10 | 3 | 4 | 5 | 6 | 8 |
| 0.50 | 0.016 | 0.004 | 0.001 | 0.000 | 0.000 | 0.000 | 0.021 | 0.005 | 0.001 | 0.000 | 0.000 |
| 0.75 | 0.063 | 0.025 | 0.010 | 0.004 | 0.001 | 0.000 | 0.086 | 0.034 | 0.013 | 0.005 | 0.001 |
| 1.00 | 0.125 | 0.063 | 0.031 | 0.016 | 0.004 | 0.000 | 0.177 | 0.086 | 0.042 | 0.021 | 0.005 |
| 1.25 | 0.190 | 0.109 | 0.063 | 0.036 | 0.012 | 0.004 | 0.277 | 0.153 | 0.086 | 0.049 | 0.016 |
| 1.50 | 0.250 | 0.158 | 0.099 | 0.063 | 0.025 | 0.010 | 0.375 | 0.227 | 0.139 | 0.086 | 0.034 |
| 2.00 | 0.354 | 0.250 | 0.177 | 0.125 | 0.063 | 0.031 | 0.555 | 0.375 | 0.257 | 0.177 | 0.086 |
| 2.50 | 0.435 | 0.330 | 0.250 | 0.190 | 0.109 | 0.063 | 0.707 | 0.512 | 0.375 | 0.277 | 0.153 |
| 3.00 | 0.500 | 0.397 | 0.315 | 0.250 | 0.158 | 0.099 | 0.833 | 0.634 | 0.486 | 0.375 | 0.227 |
| 4.00 | 0.595 | 0.500 | 0.420 | 0.354 | 0.250 | 0.177 | 1.029 | 0.833 | 0.678 | 0.555 | 0.375 |
| 5.00 | 0.660 | 0.574 | 0.500 | 0.435 | 0.330 | 0.250 | 1.170 | 0.986 | 0.833 | 0.707 | 0.512 |

*Note:* Shaded cells: The approximation of complete overnight repair is less precise here and this affects the precision of biological dose estimates.

Table 9.3 Half-times for recovery from radiation damage in normal tissues of laboratory animals

| Tissue | Species | Dose delivery[a] | $T_{1/2}$ (hours) | Source |
|---|---|---|---|---|
| Haemopoietic | Mouse | CLDR | 0.3 | Thames et al. (1984) |
| Spermatogonia | Mouse | CLDR | 0.3–0.4 | Delic et al. (1987) |
| Jejunum | Mouse | F | 0.45 | Thames et al. (1984) |
| " | Mouse | CLDR | 0.2–0.7 | Dale et al. (1988) |
| Colon (early injury) | Mouse | F | 0.8 | Thames et al. (1984) |
| " " | Rat | F | 1.5 | Sassy et al. (1988) |
| Lip mucosa | Mouse | F | 0.8 | Ang et al. (1985) |
| " | Mouse | CLDR | 0.8 | Scalliet et al. (1987) |
| " | Mouse | FLDR | 0.6 | Stüben et al. (1991) |
| Tongue epithelium | Mouse | F | 0.75 | Dörr et al. (1993) |
| Skin (early injury) | Mouse | F | 1.5 | Rojas et al. (1991) |
| " " | Mouse | CLDR | 1.0 | Joiner et al. (unpublished) |
| " " | Pig | F | $0.4 + 1.2$[b] | van den Aardweg and Hopewell (1992) |
| " " | Pig | F | $0.2 + 6.6$[b] | Millar et al. (1996) |
| Lung | Mouse | F | $0.4 + 4.0$[b] | van Rongen et al. (1993) |
| " | Mouse | CLDR | 0.85 | Down et al. (1986) |
| " | Rat | FLDR | 1.0 | van Rongen (1989) |
| Spinal cord | Rat | F | $0.7 + 3.8$[b] | Ang et al. (1992) |
| " | Rat | CLDR | 1.4 | Scalliet et al. (1989) |
| " | Rat | CLDR | 1.43 | Pop et al. (1996) |
| Kidney | Mouse | F | 1.3 | Joiner et al. (1993) |
| " | Mouse | F | $0.2 + 5.0$ | Millar et al. (1994) |
| " | Rat | F | 1.6–2.1 | van Rongen et al. (1990) |
| Rectum (late injury) | Rat | CLDR | 1.2 | Kiszel et al. (1985) |
| Heart | Rat | F | >3 | Schultz-Hector et al. (1992) |

[a]  F = acute dose fractions, FLDR = fractionated low dose rate, CLDR = continuous low dose rate.

[b]  Two components of repair with different half-times.

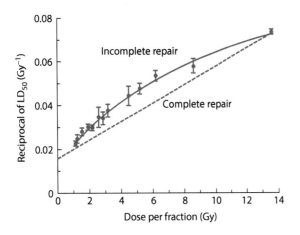

Figure 9.9 Reciprocal dose plot (compare Figure 9.5a) of data for pneumonitis in mice produced by fractionated irradiation; the points derive from experiments with different dose per fraction (and therefore different fraction numbers), always with 3 hours between doses. The upward bend in the data illustrates lack of sparing due to incomplete repair. (From (22), with permission.)

## Continuous irradiation

Another common situation in which incomplete repair occurs in clinical radiotherapy is during continuous irradiation. As described in Chapter 13, irradiation must be given at a very low dose rate (below about 5 cGy/h) for full repair to occur during irradiation. At the other extreme, a single irradiation at high dose rate may allow no significant repair to occur during exposure. As the dose rate is reduced below the high dose-rate range used in external-beam radiotherapy, the duration of irradiation becomes longer and the induction of DNA damage is continuously counteracted by repair, leading to an increase in the isoeffective dose. The corresponding EQD2 formula for continuous irradiation incorporates a factor $g$ to allow for incomplete repair:

$$\text{EQD2} = D\frac{d \cdot g + (\alpha/\beta)}{2 + (\alpha/\beta)} \quad \text{(9.8; continuous low dose-rate)}$$

where $D$ is the total dose (= dose rate × time). The parameter $d$ is retained, as in the equation for fractionated radiotherapy,

Table 9.4  Incomplete repair factors: Continuous irradiation (*g* factors)

| Repair half-time (h) | Exposure time (h) | | | | | | Exposure time (days) | | | | | | |
|---|---|---|---|---|---|---|---|---|---|---|---|---|---|
| | 1 | 2 | 3 | 4 | 8 | 12 | 1 | 1.5 | 2 | 2.5 | 3 | 3.5 | 4 |
| 0.5 | 0.6622 | 0.4774 | 0.3671 | 0.2959 | 0.1641 | 0.1130 | 0.0583 | 0.0393 | 0.0296 | 0.0238 | 0.0198 | 0.0170 | 0.0149 |
| 0.75 | 0.7517 | 0.5888 | 0.4774 | 0.3983 | 0.2339 | 0.1641 | 0.0861 | 0.0583 | 0.0441 | 0.0354 | 0.0296 | 0.0254 | 0.0223 |
| 1 | 0.8040 | 0.6622 | 0.5571 | 0.4774 | 0.2959 | 0.2115 | 0.1130 | 0.0769 | 0.0583 | 0.0469 | 0.0393 | 0.0338 | 0.0296 |
| 1.25 | 0.8382 | 0.7137 | 0.6165 | 0.5394 | 0.3504 | 0.2555 | 0.1390 | 0.0952 | 0.0723 | 0.0583 | 0.0488 | 0.0420 | 0.0369 |
| 1.5 | 0.8622 | 0.7517 | 0.6622 | 0.5888 | 0.3983 | 0.2959 | 0.1641 | 0.1130 | 0.0861 | 0.0695 | 0.0583 | 0.0502 | 0.0441 |
| 2 | 0.8938 | 0.8040 | 0.7276 | 0.6622 | 0.4774 | 0.3671 | 0.2115 | 0.1475 | 0.1130 | 0.0916 | 0.0769 | 0.0663 | 0.0583 |
| 2.5 | 0.9136 | 0.8382 | 0.7720 | 0.7137 | 0.5394 | 0.4269 | 0.2555 | 0.1803 | 0.1390 | 0.1130 | 0.0952 | 0.0822 | 0.0723 |
| 3 | 0.9272 | 0.8622 | 0.8040 | 0.7517 | 0.5888 | 0.4774 | 0.2959 | 0.2115 | 0.1641 | 0.1339 | 0.1130 | 0.0977 | 0.0861 |
| 4 | 0.9447 | 0.8938 | 0.8471 | 0.8040 | 0.6622 | 0.5571 | 0.3671 | 0.2693 | 0.2115 | 0.1739 | 0.1475 | 0.1280 | 0.1130 |

in order to deal with fractionated low dose-rate exposures. For a single continuous exposure $d = D$. This equation assumes that there is full recovery between the low dose-rate exposures; if not, the $H_m$ factor must also be added (see Appendix 9.1). Table 9.4 gives values of the *g* factor for exposure times between 1 hour and 4 days.

The simple LQ model has also been applied to, for example, permanent interstitial implants and to biologically targeted radionuclide therapy. The interested reader is referred to the book by Dale and Jones (26).

## 9.9 SHOULD A TIME FACTOR BE INCLUDED?

If the overall duration of fractionated radiotherapy is increased, there will usually be greater repopulation of the irradiated tissues, both in the tumour and in early reacting normal tissues. So far we have not discussed the change in total dose necessary to compensate for changes in the overall duration of treatment. Overall time was included in the historical NSD and TDF models but is not put into the basic LQ approach described above. The reason is because the time factor in radiotherapy is now perceived to be more complex than had previously been supposed. For example, Figure 9.10 shows that the extra dose needed to counteract proliferation in mouse skin does not become significant until about 2 weeks after the start of daily fractionation. In this and other situations, the time factor in the historical NSD formula (broken line: total dose $\propto T^{0.11}$) gives a false picture because it predicts a large amount of sparing if the overall time was increased from 1 to 12 days. These wrong historical time factors also underestimate the dose required to compensate for planned or un-planned gaps in treatment. Thus, a $T^{0.11}$ factor predicts only an 8% increase in total dose for a doubling of overall time, for example from 3.5 to 7 weeks. This would correspond to a 5.6 Gy increase in the total dose for a schedule delivering, say, 70 Gy to a squamous cell carcinoma of the head and neck. Clinical data summarized in Chapter 10 indicate that in this tumour type an additional dose of 16 Gy will actually be required to compensate for a 3.5 week prolongation of treatment time.

The use of the LQ model in clinical practice with no time factor is probably the best strategy for *late-reacting* tissues because any extra dose needed to counteract proliferation does not become significant until beyond the overall time of treatment, even up to 6 weeks. This is illustrated schematically in Figure 9.11 which compares the different effects of overall time in early and late-responding tissues. Attempts have been made to include time factors in the LQ model for early responding normal tissues and tumours, but such factors depend in a complex way on the dose per fraction and interfraction interval as well as on the tissue type, and have to take account of any delay in onset of proliferation which may depend in some way on these factors also. We therefore recommend considering the influence of changing overall time on radiotherapy as a separate problem from the effect of changing the dose per fraction which can be done in a straightforward way using

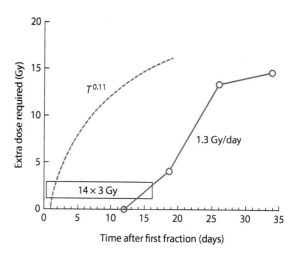

Figure 9.10 Extra dose required to counteract proliferation in mouse skin. Test doses of radiation were given at various intervals after a priming treatment with fractionated radiation. Proliferation begins about 12 days after the start of irradiation and is then equivalent to an extra dose of approximately 1.3 Gy/day. The broken line shows the prediction of the NSD equation. (Adapted from (5).)

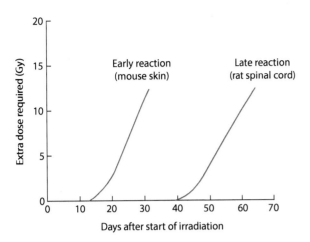

**Figure 9.11** The extra dose required to counteract proliferation does not become significant until much later for late-responding normal tissues such as spinal cord, beyond the 6 week duration of conventional radiotherapy. (From (9), with permission.)

the LQ model as described here. The practical approaches to handling changes in overall time are described in Chapters 10, 11 and 12.

## 9.10 ALTERNATIVE ISOEFFECT FORMULAE BASED ON THE LQ MODEL

Two other formulations that can be used for comparing schedules with differing doses per fraction are the concepts of extrapolated tolerance dose (ETD) introduced by Barendsen (1) and total effect (TE) described in Thames and Hendry (29). Both of these methods are biologically equivalent with the EQD2 concept, but are mentioned here because they have found presence in the literature.

### Extrapolated total dose or biologically effective dose

ETD and BED are mathematically identical. Fowler (10) preferred the term *BED*, because it can logically be understood to refer to levels of effect that are below normal tissue tolerance, whereas the term *ETD* implies the full tolerance effect. First, we must again define a particular isoeffect, or endpoint. Although the validity of the LQ approach to fractionation depends principally on its ability to predict isoeffective schedules successfully, there is an implicit assumption that the isoeffect has a direct relationship with a certain level of cell inactivation (or final cell survival, $[SF_d]^n$). However, the actual fraction of surviving cells associated with any isoeffect is unknown and it is customary to work in terms of a level of tissue effect, which we denote as $E$. From Equation 9.4,

$$E/\alpha = D\left[1 + d/(\alpha/\beta)\right] = \text{Biologically Effective Dose (BED)}$$

BED is a measure of the effect ($E$) of a course of fractionated or continuous irradiation; when divided by $\alpha$ it has the units of dose and is usually expressed in grays. Note that as the dose per fraction ($d$) is reduced towards zero, BED becomes $D = nd$ (i.e. the total radiation dose). Thus, BED is the theoretical total dose that would be required to produce the isoeffect $E$ using an infinitely large number of infinitesimally small dose fractions. It is therefore also the total dose required for a single exposure at very low dose rate (see Chapter 13). As with the simpler concept of EQD2, values of BED from separate parts of a course of treatment may be added in order to calculate the overall BED value. Dividing the right-hand side of Equation 9.6 by $\alpha/\beta$ gives a simple relationship between BED and EQD2 as

$$\text{BED} = \text{EQD2}\left(1 + \frac{2}{\alpha/\beta}\right)$$

For example, if $\alpha/\beta = 2$ as might be chosen for spinal cord, then BED is exactly twice the value of EQD2. Thus, a disadvantage of using BED as a measure of treatment intensity is that it is numerically much greater than any prescribable radiation dose of fractionated radiotherapy and is therefore more difficult to relate to everyday clinical practice. BED also rapidly increases and goes to infinity as $\alpha/\beta$ goes to zero, whereas EQD2 asymptotes towards $Dd/2$. These are the key reasons why we recommend the adoption of EQD2 which is also currently being encouraged by ICRU (3) adding an additional informational subscript to show the value of $\alpha/\beta$ used in the calculation, thus $\text{EQD2}_{\alpha/\beta}$.

### Total effect

The TE formulation is conceptually similar to BED and has also been used in the literature. In this case, we divide $E$ by $\beta$ rather than $\alpha$, to get

$$E/\beta = D[(\alpha/\beta) + d] = \text{Total Effect (TE)}$$

The units of TE are Gy$^2$, which again means that the TE values have no simple interpretation. The TE isoeffect formulae are similar to the EQD2 formulae except that the denominator $(2 + \alpha/\beta)$ is omitted. This has the computational advantage that division by this factor is done only for the final TE value and not for any intermediate calculations. However, it has the disadvantage that these intermediate results are not recognisable doses, and we recommend the EQD2 method instead as a means of making it easier to detect numerical errors in the calculation process.

## 9.11 LIMITS OF APPLICABILITY OF THE SIMPLE LQ MODEL, ALTERNATIVE MODELS

Uncritical application of the LQ model in clinical situations could potentially compromise the safety of a patient.

Extrapolation of experience from a standard regimen to a regimen using a considerably changed overall treatment time or dose per fraction should only be attempted with great care. This is partly because of a limited precision in the radiobiological parameters of the LQ model which will be 'blown up' when extrapolation between very diverse schedules is performed. But even if the parameters of the model were known with high precision, some limitations to the use of the LQ model are suggested by laboratory experiments.

At a dose per fraction of less than 1 Gy, the phenomenon of low-dose hyper-radiosensitivity (see Chapter 4) – if presenting in the particular critical normal tissue or tumour under consideration – would mean that using the standard LQ model could underestimate the biological effect of a given total dose. This could potentially affect the estimated biological effect of some intensity modulated radiation therapy dose distributions where a relatively large normal tissue volume may be irradiated with a dose per fraction in the hyper-radiosensitivity range (13). A modified form of the LQ formula has been developed (Equation 4.6) but the model parameters are not yet known with any useful precision for human tissues and tumours.

Also, at very high dose per fraction the mathematical form of the LQ model may not be correct. While the LQ survival curve represents a continuously bending parabola in a plot of the logarithm of surviving fraction versus dose, a number of *in vitro* and *in vivo* data sets suggest that the empirical survival curve asymptotically approaches a straight line. Several attempts have been made to extend the LQ model to high doses per fraction as well, all of them necessarily leading to the inclusion of at least one additional parameter in the model as described in Chapter 4, Section 4.13 (e.g. [11,14]). None of these models have found wider applications in the analysis of clinical data at least so far, the obvious limitation being that most clinical data sets have insufficient resolution to allow the estimation of three or more model parameters with useful certainty. It is difficult to give a specific dose per fraction beyond which the simple LQ model should not be used, but extrapolations beyond 6 Gy per fraction should be used cautiously.

## 9.12 BEYOND THE TARGET CELL HYPOTHESIS

The target cell hypothesis dominated much of radiobiological thinking for almost half a century. As described previously, this hypothesis has played a key role in developing the LQ formulae, yet LQ can now stand alone: the underlying explanation of LQ need only be that a quadratic equation is just the simplest way mathematically of describing the nonlinear relationship between total isoeffective dose and dose per fraction. More recently, the importance of damage processing and tissue remodelling in the pathogenesis of late effects have been recognized; see Chapter 14 and review by Bentzen (2). In addition, basic and clinical radiobiology studies have revealed non-targeted effects of ionizing radiation, such as the 'bystander' response induced in cells in the vicinity of a cell hit by ionizing radiation (19) and immune-mediated effects in patients (8). All of this has not restricted the clinical utility of the LQ formula. Equation 9.5 can usefully be viewed as an operational definition of $\alpha/\beta$ and a formula allowing practical correction for the change in biological effect per unit dose as a function of dose per fraction. The application of this formula therefore does not depend on a biological reality of 'target cells'. Chapter 10 pursues this more pragmatic or 'data-driven' approach to the LQ model in the clinic.

---

### Key points

1. The LQ model satisfactorily describes the relationship between total isoeffective dose and dose per fraction over the range of dose per fraction from 1 Gy up to 6 Gy. In contrast, power-law formulae can only be made to fit data over a limited range of dose per fraction.

2. The $\alpha/\beta$ value describes the *shape* of the fractionation response: a low $\alpha/\beta$ (0.5–6 Gy) is usually characteristic of late-responding normal tissues and indicates a rapid increase of total dose with decreasing dose per fraction and a survival curve for putative target cells that is significantly curved.

3. A higher $\alpha/\beta$ value (7–20 Gy) is usually characteristic of early responding normal tissues and rapidly proliferating carcinomas; it indicates a less significant increase in total dose with decreasing dose per fraction and a less curved cell-survival response for putative target cells.

4. The EQD2 formulae provide a simple and convenient way of calculating isoeffective radiotherapy schedules, based on the LQ model. Tolerance calculations always require an estimate of the $\alpha/\beta$ value to be included.

5. For interfraction intervals less than 24 hours, a correction may be necessary for incomplete repair. When using the EQD2 formulae to calculate schedules with multiple fractions per day or continuous low dose rate, an estimate of the repair half-time must also be included.

6. The basic LQ model is appropriate for calculating the change in total dose for an altered dose per fraction, assuming the new and old treatments are given in the *same overall time*. For late reactions it is usually unnecessary to modify total dose in response to a change in overall time, but for early reactions (and for tumour response) a correction for overall treatment time should be included. Although the effect of time on biological effect is complex, simple linear corrections have been shown to be of some value (see Chapters 10, 11 and 12).

## ■ APPENDIX 9.1: SUMMARY OF FORMULAE

*Basic equations:*

$$E = n(\alpha d + \beta d^2) = D(\alpha + \beta d)$$

$d$ = Dose per fraction
$D$ = Total dose
$n$ = Number of fractions

$$SF = \exp(-E) = \exp[-(\alpha + \beta d)D]$$

For schedules having the same $E$, i.e. isoeffective schedules,

$$\frac{D}{D_{ref}} = \frac{d_{ref} + (\alpha/\beta)}{d + (\alpha/\beta)} \quad \text{hence:} \quad EQD2 = D\frac{d + (\alpha/\beta)}{2 + (\alpha/\beta)}$$

*Incomplete repair correction:*

$$\phi = \exp(-\mu\Delta T) \quad \Delta T = \text{Interval between fractions}$$

$$H_m = \left(\frac{2}{m}\right) \cdot \left(\frac{\phi}{1-\phi}\right) \cdot \left(m - \frac{1-\phi^m}{1-\phi}\right)$$

$m$ = Number of fractions per day

$$EQD2 = D\frac{d(1 + H_m) + (\alpha/\beta)}{2 + (\alpha/\beta)}$$

*Low dose rate:*

$$\mu = \frac{\log_e 2}{T_{1/2}} \quad\quad T_{1/2} = \text{Repair half time}$$

$$g = 2[\mu t - 1 + \exp(-\mu t)]/(\mu t)^2 \quad t = \text{Exposure duration}$$

$$EQD2 = D\frac{d \cdot g + (\alpha/\beta)}{2 + (\alpha/\beta)}$$

*Incomplete repair between low dose-rate fractions:*

$$\phi = \exp(-\mu(t + \Delta T)) \quad \Delta T = \text{Interval between fractions}$$

$t$ = Exposure duration per fraction

$$g = 2[\mu t - 1 + \exp(-\mu t)]/(\mu t)^2$$

$$H_m = \left(\frac{2}{m}\right) \cdot \left(\frac{\phi}{1-\phi}\right) \cdot \left(m - \frac{1-\phi^m}{1-\phi}\right)$$

$m$ = Number of fractions per day

$$C = g + 2\frac{\cosh(\mu t) - 1}{(\mu t)^2} \cdot H_m$$

$$EQD2 = D\frac{d \cdot C + (\alpha/\beta)}{2 + (\alpha/\beta)}$$

For a full derivation of these equations, see Nilsson et al. (18).

## ■ BIBLIOGRAPHY

1. Barendsen GW. Dose fractionation, dose rate and iso-effect relationships for normal tissue responses. *Int J Radiat Oncol Biol Phys* 1982;8:1981–1997.
2. Bentzen SM. Preventing or reducing late side effects of radiation therapy: Radiobiology meets molecular pathology. *Nat Rev Cancer* 2006;6:702–713.
3. Bentzen SM, Dorr W, Gahbauer R et al. Bioeffect modeling and equieffective dose concepts in radiation oncology – Terminology, quantities and units. *Radiother Oncol* 2012;105: 266–268.
4. Bentzen SM, Saunders MI, Dische S. Repair halftimes estimated from observations of treatment-related morbidity after CHART or conventional radiotherapy in head and neck cancer. *Radiother Oncol* 1999;53:219–226.
5. Denekamp J. Changes in the rate of repopulation during multi-fraction irradiation of mouse skin. *Br J Radiol* 1973;46: 381–387.
6. Douglas BG, Fowler JF. The effect of multiple small doses of x-rays on skin reactions in the mouse and a basic interpretation. *Radiat Res* 1976;66:401–426.
7. Ellis F. Dose, time and fractionation: A clinical hypothesis. *Clin Radiol* 1969;20:1–7.
8. Formenti SC. The pace of progress in radiation and immuno-therapy. *Int J Radiat Oncol Biol Phys* 2016;95:1257–1258.
9. Fowler JF. The first James Kirk memorial lecture. What next in fractionated radiotherapy? *Br J Cancer Suppl* 1984;6:285–300.
10. Fowler JF. The linear-quadratic formula and progress in fractionated radiotherapy. *Br J Radiol* 1989;62:679–694.
11. Guerrero M, Li XA. Extending the linear-quadratic model for large fraction doses pertinent to stereotactic radiotherapy. *Phys Med Biol* 2004;49:4825–4835.
12. Guttenberger R, Thames HD, Ang KK. Is the experience with CHART compatible with experimental data? A new model of repair kinetics and computer simulations. *Radiother Oncol* 1992;25:280–286.
13. Honore HB, Bentzen SM. A modelling study of the potential influence of low dose hypersensitivity on radiation treatment planning. *Radiother Oncol* 2006;79:115–121.
14. Lind BK, Persson LM, Edgren MR, Hedlof I, Brahme A. Repairable-conditionally repairable damage model based on dual Poisson processes. *Radiat Res* 2003;160:366–375.
15. Maciejewski B, Taylor JM, Withers HR. Alpha/beta value and the importance of size of dose per fraction for late complications in the supraglottic larynx. *Radiother Oncol* 1986;7:323–326.

16. Marks LB, Ten Haken RK, Martel MK. Guest editor's introduction to QUANTEC: A users guide. *Int J Radiat Oncol Biol Phys* 2010;76(3 Suppl):S1–S2.

17. Millar WT, Canney PA. Derivation and application of equations describing the effects of fractionated protracted irradiation, based on multiple and incomplete repair processes. Part I. Derivation of equations. *Int J Radiat Biol* 1993;64:275–291.

18. Nilsson P, Thames HD, Joiner MC. A generalized formulation of the 'incomplete-repair' model for cell survival and tissue response to fractionated low dose-rate irradiation. *Int J Radiat Biol* 1990;57:127–142.

19. Prise KM, Schettino G, Folkard M, Held KD. New insights on cell death from radiation exposure. *Lancet Oncol* 2005;6: 520–528.

20. Stewart FA, Soranson JA, Alpen EL, Williams MV, Denekamp J. Radiation-induced renal damage: The effects of hyperfractionation. *Radiat Res* 1984;98:407–420.

21. Thames HD. An 'incomplete-repair' model for survival after fractionated and continuous irradiations. *Int J Radiat Biol Relat Stud Phys Chem Med* 1985;47:319–339.

22. Thames HD, Withers HR, Peters LJ. Tissue repair capacity and repair kinetics deduced from multifractionated or continuous irradiation regimens with incomplete repair. *Br J Cancer* 1984;49 (Suppl 6):263–269.

23. Thames HD, Withers HR, Peters LJ, Fletcher GH. Changes in early and late radiation responses with altered dose fractionation: Implications for dose-survival relationships. *Int J Radiat Oncol Biol Phys* 1982;8:219–226.

24. Williams MV, Denekamp J, Fowler JF. A review of alpha/beta ratios for experimental tumors: Implications for clinical studies of altered fractionation. *Int J Radiat Oncol Biol Phys* 1985;11:87–96.

25. Withers HR, Thames HD, Jr., Peters LJ. A new isoeffect curve for change in dose per fraction. *Radiother Oncol* 1983;1:187–191.

## ■ FURTHER READING

26. Dale RG, Jones B (eds.). *Radiobiological Modeling in Radiation Oncology.* London: British Institute of Radiology; 2007.

27. Joiner MC. The dependence of radiation response on the dose per fraction. In: McNally NJ (ed.). *The Scientific Basis for Modern Radiotherapy (BIR Report 19).* London: British Institute of Radiology; 1989. pp. 20–26.

28. Thames HD, Bentzen SM, Turesson I, Overgaard M, Van den Bogaert W. Time-dose factors in radiotherapy: A review of the human data. *Radiother Oncol* 1990;19:219–235.

29. Thames HD, Hendry JH. *Fractionation in Radiotherapy.* London: Taylor & Francis Group; 1987.

# The linear-quadratic approach in clinical practice

SØREN M. BENTZEN AND MICHAEL C. JOINER

## 10.1 INTRODUCTION: BIOLOGICAL EFFECT ESTIMATES ADJUSTING FOR DOSE-TIME-FRACTIONATION

As soon as relatively accurate dosimetry became available around 1910, it became clear that the biological effect of a given physical dose of ionizing radiation depends on how this dose is distributed over time. For many years, the differential response of tumours and normal tissues to changes in dose-time-fractionation appeared to be the most important means of improving the therapeutic ratio. Mathematical models – often referred to as bioeffect models – were first introduced in the 1920s with the aim of linking the probability of tumour control and normal tissue side effects to the dose of fractionated radiation delivered. As discussed in Chapter 9, the linear-quadratic (LQ) model was introduced around 1980 and this remains the model of choice for bioeffect estimation in radiotherapy. In the beginning, the use of the LQ model was conceptually linked to the target-cell hypothesis and to *in vitro* radiation cell survival curves. However, there is increasing evidence that many late effects, and even some early effects, of radiation therapy are not directly related to simple killing of a defined population of target cells (see Chapter 14, and [2]). The most prevalent current view is that the LQ approach represents an approximate, pragmatic method for converting dose-time-fractionation schedules into a dose that would produce the same probability of a given biological effect when delivered with a reference dose per fraction over a reference overall time (5). Consistent with this point of view, we use the notation $\alpha/\beta$ but refer to this quantity as the 'alpha-beta value' rather than the 'alpha-beta ratio': $\alpha/\beta$ is a single quantity estimated directly from dose-fractionation-response data rather than a ratio between two numbers. The $\alpha/\beta$ value is seen as a measure of *fractionation sensitivity*, rather than repair capacity, as often used in some of the older literature. The LQ model has shown to be useful over a range of dose per fraction, at least up to 6–7 Gy for a number of, mainly late, effects. Extrapolations outside the range of available data should be performed with the greatest care. Model parameters should ideally be estimated from clinical observations and their statistical precision should be taken into account when used to estimate the risks or benefits of a given schedule.

While the awareness has grown regarding the limitations to the LQ model and the dangers involved in using it uncritically, the application of this approach has also increased. There are several reasons for this. Intensity modulated radiation therapy (IMRT) represents a convenient way of delivering radiation therapy with varying dose per fraction to multiple target volumes in a single session. At the same time, IMRT and conformal radiotherapy generally lead to non-uniform dose distributions in normal tissues and organs, delivering dose with a varying dose per fraction to various critical structures – in contrast to parallel opposing field techniques that typically lead to partial organ irradiation with a dose per fraction close to the fraction size prescribed to the target volume. Finally, the realization that the fractionation sensitivity of at least some human tumours are in the same range as that typical of late normal tissue effects – in contrast to what was widely assumed when the LQ model was introduced in the 1980s – has renewed interest in the use of hypofractionation, that is prescriptions with fraction sizes larger than 2 Gy.

## 10.2 QUANTITATIVE CLINICAL RADIOBIOLOGY – THE LQ FRAMEWORK

Several, mathematically equivalent, methods have been devised for performing bioeffect calculations with the LQ model and these may be seen as special cases of a more general formalism (5), see also Chapter 9:

$$\text{EQDX}_{\alpha/\beta} = D\frac{d+(\alpha/\beta)}{X+(\alpha/\beta)} \tag{10.1}$$

where $X$ is a reference dose per fraction and $\alpha/\beta$ is an endpoint and radiation quality–specific parameter that describes the effect of a change in dose per fraction, i.e. the fractionation sensitivity of that endpoint. Note again that a *higher* $\alpha/\beta$ value indicates a *lower* sensitivity to dose per fraction in the sense that a smaller adjustment of total dose is needed to maintain equieffect. Throughout this chapter, the radiation quality considered will be megavoltage photons except when explicitly stated otherwise. The two choices of $X$ that dominate the field are $X = 2$ Gy or $X = 0$ Gy.

The latter choice gives rise to the BED formalism; here, we use $X = 2$ Gy, so the equieffective dose in 2 Gy fractions, EQD2. Depending on the context, it may be useful to add the $\alpha/\beta$ value used in the calculation of EQD2 informationally as an index, for example for $\alpha/\beta = 10$ Gy, and an EQD2 of 70 Gy, we would write $\text{EQD2}_{10} = 70$ Gy. It is not consistent with SI recommendations to change the unit Gy, e.g. to write $\text{EQD2} = 70 \text{ Gy}_{10}$. In other calculations, we may use a second index or perhaps omit the $\alpha/\beta$ value in order to indicate the value of other model parameters.

One key advantage of using 2 Gy as the reference fraction size in Equation 10.1 is that the EQD2 is immediately clinically relevant and is measured on the same scale where much of the clinical experience on dose-response relationships is available. The EQD2 values from various parts of a fractionation schedule may be added directly. The EQD2 is formally identical to the normalised total dose (NTD) proposed by Withers and colleagues, see also Chapter 9.

Large *in vivo* fractionation studies in the laboratory, mainly conducted in rodents in the 1980s, showed the ability of the LQ model to provide a close quantitative relationship between the equieffective doses for schedules applying varying dose per fraction. These studies also produced a number of $\alpha/\beta$ estimates for various normal tissue endpoints (see Table 9.1). In parallel with these experimental studies, a number of clinical studies have produced $\alpha/\beta$ estimates for human endpoints and these are summarised in Table 10.1.

Bioeffect calculations should be used only as guidance for clinical decision-making. All of the formulae applied here have a limited field of applicability, the model assumptions may be violated in some circumstances, relevant parameters may not be known for human tissues and tumours and the uncertainty in parameter estimates, even when these are available, may give rise to considerable uncertainty in the biological effect estimates. A (self-)critical and cautious attitude is recommended and the health and safety of patients should not be compromised by reliance on the result of calculations of the type described in this chapter. We advocate the use of clinical parameter estimates whenever possible. If no clinical estimates are available, we suggest using the values from experimental animal studies as a guidance, but be well aware of the fact that these may not be valid for the clinical endpoints of interest. The use of 'generic' values, say, 3 Gy for late effects and 10 Gy for tumours, should be seen as the least evidence-based approach. There is less and less reason to believe that these values are generalizable across a wider range of human normal tissue endpoints and tumour histologies. Therefore, calculations using these values may be seen as simply exploring the behaviour of the model, an exercise detached from the clinical reality that we should be studying.

Having said all this, a numerical estimate is often very useful when considering various therapeutic options and it is often possible to get an impression of how reliable such an estimate is, just by doing a simple calculation as illustrated in this chapter.

## 10.3 CHANGING THE DOSE PER FRACTION

The simplest case we consider is when the dose per fraction is changed without change in the overall treatment time and when incomplete repair between dose fractions is negligible. We use Equation 10.1 to convert a total dose $D$ delivered with dose per fraction $d$ into the equieffective dose in 2 Gy fractions:

$$\text{EQD2}_{\alpha/\beta} = D \frac{d + (\alpha/\beta)}{2 \text{ Gy} + (\alpha/\beta)}$$

Note that the only parameter in this formula is the $\alpha/\beta$ value, i.e. the fractionation sensitivity of the endpoint of interest. Any biological dose calculation will therefore start with the identification of the tumour or normal tissue endpoint of concern in the clinical situation. For a given fractionation schedule we may, for example, be interested in EQD2 for a squamous cell carcinoma of the lung and for lung fibrosis and we would then start by selecting appropriate $\alpha/\beta$ values for these two endpoints from Tables 9.1, 10.1 or 14.2.

### Example 10.1: Converting a dose into the equieffective dose in 2 Gy fractions

A patient with metastatic bone pain located to the fifth thoracic vertebra is considered for palliative radiotherapy using $1 \times 8$ Gy.

*Problem:* What is the equieffective dose in 2 Gy fractions for spinal cord?

*Solution:* First, we need to choose the value of $\alpha/\beta$. From Table 10.1 it is seen that the upper bound on $\alpha/\beta$ from human data is 3.5 Gy. Experimental animal studies (see Table 9.1) have produced estimates around 2 Gy. We choose $\alpha/\beta = 2$ Gy, insert the values for total dose, 8 Gy, as this is a single fraction, and dose per fraction, 8 Gy, in Equation 10.1 and get

$$\text{EQD2}_2 = 8 \text{ Gy} \cdot \frac{8 \text{ Gy} + 2 \text{ Gy}}{2 \text{ Gy} + 2 \text{ Gy}} = 20 \text{ Gy}$$

Thus, for an endpoint with $\alpha/\beta = 2.0$ Gy, a single 8 Gy fraction is equieffective to 20 Gy in 2 Gy fractions.

## 10.4 CHANGING THE TIME INTERVAL BETWEEN DOSE FRACTIONS

Multiple fractions per day schedules are associated with an increase in biological effect unless the interval between fractions is sufficiently long to allow full recovery between fractions. There are data to suggest that the characteristic half-time, $T_{1/2}$, of recovery is in the order of 4–5 hours for

Table 10.1 Fractionation sensitivity of human normal tissues and tumours

| Tissue/organ | Endpoint | $\alpha/\beta$ (Gy) | 95% CL (Gy) | Source |
|---|---|---|---|---|
| *Early reactions* | | | | |
| Skin | Erythema | 8.8 | [6.9; 11.6] | Turesson and Thames (1989) |
| | Erythema | 12.3 | [1.8; 22.8] | Bentzen et al. (1988) |
| | Dry desquamation | ~8 | N/A | Chogule and Supe (1993) |
| | Desquamation | 11.2 | [8.5; 17.6] | Turesson and Thames (1989) |
| Oral mucosa | Mucositis | 9.3 | [5.8; 17.9] | Denham et al. (1995) |
| | Mucositis | 15 | [−15; 45] | Rezvani et al. (1991) |
| | Mucositis | ~8 | N/A | Chogule and Supe (1993) |
| *Late reactions* | | | | |
| Skin/vasculature | Telangiectasia | 2.8 | [1.7; 3.8] | Turesson and Thames (1989) |
| | Telangiectasia | 2.6 | [2.2; 3.3] | Bentzen et al. (1990) |
| | Telangiectasia | 2.8 | [−0.1; 8.1] | Bentzen and Overgaard (1991) |
| | Telangiectasia | 3.8 | [1.8; 5.7] | Haviland et al. (2013) |
| Subcutis | Fibrosis | 1.7 | [0.6; 2.6] | Bentzen and Overgaard (1991) |
| Breast | Cosmetic change in appearance | 3.5 | [0.7; 6.4] | Haviland et al. (2013) |
| | Induration (fibrosis) | 4.0 | [2.3; 5.6] | Haviland et al. (2013) |
| | Breast oedema | 4.7 | [2.4; 7.0] | Haviland et al. (2013) |
| Muscle/vasculature/cartilage | Impaired shoulder movement | 3.5 | [0.7; 6.2] | Bentzen et al. (1989) |
| Nerve | Brachial plexopathy | <3.5[a] | N/A | Olsen et al. (1990) |
| | Brachial plexopathy | ~2 | N/A | Powell et al. (1990) |
| | Optic neuropathy | 1.6 | [−7; 10] | Jiang et al. (1994) |
| Spinal cord | Myelopathy | <3.3 | N/A | Dische et al. (1981) |
| Eye | Corneal injury | 2.9 | [−4; 10] | Jiang et al. (1994) |
| Bowel | Stricture/perforation | 3.9 | [2.5; 5.3] | Deore et al. (1993) |
| Bowel | Various late effects | 4.3 | [2.2; 9.6] | Dische et al. (1999) |
| Lung | Pneumonitis | 4.0 | [2.2; 5.8] | Bentzen et al. (2000) |
| | Lung fibrosis (radiological) | 3.1 | [−0.2; 8.5] | Dubray et al. (1995) |
| Head and neck | Various late effects | 3.5 | [1.1; 5.9] | Rezvani et al. (1991) |
| | Various late effects | 4.0 | [3.3; 5.0] | Stuschke and Thames (1999) |
| Supraglottic larynx | Various late effects | 3.8 | [0.8; 14] | Maciejewski et al. (1986) |
| Oral cavity + oroph. | Various late effects | 0.8 | [−0.6; 2.5] | Maciejewski et al. (1990) |
| *Tumours* | | | | |
| Head and neck | | | | |
|   Various | | 10.5 | [6.5; 29] | Stuschke and Thames (1999) |
|   Larynx | | 14.5[a] | [4.9; 24] | Rezvani et al. (1993) |
|   Vocal cord | | ~13 | 'Wide' | Robertson et al. (1993) |
|   Buccal mucosa | | 6.6 | [2.9; infinity] | Maciejewski et al. (1989) |
|   Tonsil | | 7.2 | [3.6; infinity] | Maciejewski et al. (1989) |
|   Nasopharynx | | 16 | [−11; 43] | Lee et al. (1995) |
| Lung (NSCLC, early) | | 8.2 | [7.0; 9.4] | Stuschke and Pöttgen (2010) |
| Skin | | 8.5[a] | [4.5; 11.3] | Trott et al. (1984) |
| Prostate[b] | | 2.7 | [1.6; 3.8] | Vogelius and Bentzen (2018)(26) |
| Breast | | 3.5 | [1.2; 5.7] | Haviland et al. (2013) |
| Oesophagus | | 4.9 | [1.5; 17] | Geh et al. (2006) |
| Melanoma | | 0.6 | [−1.1; 2.5] | Bentzen et al. (1989) |
| Liposarcoma | | 0.4 | [−1.4; 5.4] | Thames and Suit (1986) |

*Note:* Reference details are available from Søren Bentzen. See also (25) and Table 14.2 in this book.

[a] Re-analysis of original published data.

[b] Meta-analysis of randomized controlled trials of external beam therapy, more estimates are available from comparisons of outcome after brachytherapy versus external beam therapy. This analysis includes an adjustment for overall treatment time, see Table 10.3.

some human late endpoints (8) and possibly even longer for spinal cord and brain (14,20). This means that recovery will not be complete even with a 6–8 hour interval between fractions. In this situation it is necessary to modify the simple LQ model as described in Chapter 9:

$$EQD2_{\alpha/\beta} = D \frac{d \cdot g + (\alpha/\beta)}{2\,Gy + (\alpha/\beta)}$$

where g is called the Lea-Catcheside factor, it is a factor that effectively modifies the (apparent) dose per fraction. Equation 9.7 can be used under the assumption that recovery is complete in the long overnight interval, i.e. between the last fraction delivered in one day and the first fraction on the following day. Even this assumption starts to be problematic with recovery half-times of 4–5 hours. Guttenberger et al. (16) have derived a formula, where residual damage is allowed to accumulate throughout the fractionation course. Unfortunately, this formula is not easy to tabulate as it depends not only on the recovery half-time and the dose per fraction but also on the exact arrangement of dose fractions over time.

## Example 10.2: Incomplete recovery with multiple fractions per day

The Canadian RAPID trial (22) randomized 2135 women after breast-conserving surgery between three-dimensional conformal radiation therapy accelerated partial breast irradiation (APBI) versus standard whole breast irradiation (42.5 Gy in 16 or 50 Gy in 25 daily fractions with or without boost irradiation). The APBI schedule delivered 38.5 Gy in 10 fractions twice daily.

*Problem:* What is the equieffective dose in 2 Gy fractions for cosmetic outcome (change in breast appearance) of the APBI schedule for a 6 hour interval?

*Solution:* First, we need to choose the values of $\alpha/\beta$ and $T_{1/2}$. From Table 10.1 it is seen that $\alpha/\beta = 3.4$ Gy for change in breast appearance. There is no estimate of $T_{1/2}$ for this endpoint but from Table 10.2 we get $T_{1/2} = 4.4$ h for subcutaneous fibrosis, and we use this value in the following. We now use Equation 9.7:

$$EQD2 = D \cdot \frac{d \cdot \left(1 + H_m(T_{1/2}, \Delta T)\right) + (\alpha/\beta)}{2\,Gy + (\alpha/\beta)}$$

In this case, $m = 2$ and we use Table 9.2 to look up the values of $H_2$. For an interfraction interval of 6 hours, we see that $H_2$ is between 0.35 ($T_{1/2} = 4.0$ h) and 0.44 ($T_{1/2} = 5.0$ h). Interpolation between these values yields $H_2 = 0.39$ for $T_{1/2} = 4.4$ h and, therefore,

$$EQD2(T_{1/2} = 4.4\,h) = 38.5\,Gy \cdot \frac{3.85 \cdot (1 + 0.39)\,Gy + 3.4\,Gy}{2\,Gy + 3.4\,Gy}$$
$$= 62.4\,Gy$$

For a scenario with complete recovery between fractions, i.e. a recovery half-time much shorter than the interval, we get the 'standard' complete recovery version of Withers formula:

$$EQD2(T_{1/2} \ll 6\,h) = 38.5\,Gy \cdot \frac{3.85\,Gy + 3.4\,Gy}{2\,Gy + 3.4\,Gy} = 51.7\,Gy$$

Thus, incomplete recovery in this situation increases the EQD2 by 10.7 Gy. Clearly, this added effect will be moderated by the fact that the treated volume is reduced in the APBI arm of the trial.

As mentioned previously, this calculation assumes that the overnight interval is sufficiently long to assure complete recovery of sublethal damage. This assumption starts to break down when $T_{1/2}$ is 4.4 hours. A calculation using the formula of Guttenberger et al. (16) gives an EQD2 for the last week of twice daily treatment of 64.9 Gy (rather than 62.4 Gy as calculated above) for the 6 hour interval. Whether incomplete

Table 10.2 Recovery halftime ($T_{1/2}$) for human normal tissue endpoints

| Endpoint | Dose delivery[a] | $T_{1/2}$ (hours) | 95% CL (hours) | Source |
|---|---|---|---|---|
| Erythema, skin | MFD | 0.35 and 1.2[b] | ? | Turesson and Thames (1989) |
| Mucositis, head and neck | MFD | 2–4 | ? | Bentzen et al. (1996) |
| | FLDR | 0.3–0.7 | ? | Denham et al. (1995) |
| Laryngeal oedema | MFD | 4.9 | [3.2; 6.4] | Bentzen et al. (1999) |
| Radiation myelopathy | MFD | >5 | ? | Dische and Saunders (1989) |
| Skin telangiectasia | MFD | 0.4 and 3.5[b] | ? | Turesson and Thames (1989) |
| | MFD | 3.8 | [2.5; 4.6] | Bentzen et al. (1999) |
| Subcutaneous fibrosis | MFD | 4.4 | [3.8; 4.9] | Bentzen et al. (1999) |
| Temporal lobe necrosis | MFD | >4 | ? | Lee et al. (1999) |
| Various pelvic complications | HDR/LDR | 1.5–2.5 | ? | Fowler (1997) |

*Note:* Reference details are available from Søren Bentzen.

[a] MFD, multiple fractions per day; FLDR, fractionated low-dose rate irradiation; HDR/LDR, high dose-rate/low dose-rate comparison.

[b] Evidence of two components of recovery with different half-times.

recovery during the inter-fraction interval also affected the control of subclinical breast cancer is a question. Unfortunately, reliable recovery half-time estimates for tumours are lacking. We may also want to consider other normal tissue endpoints before making a final decision as to the safety of this schedule.

## 10.5 CONTINUOUS IRRADIATION

In brachytherapy, recovery takes place not only after irradiation but also during the application. In this case, the apparent dose per fraction is again modified by the Lea-Catcheside factor that is a function of the exposure time and the recovery half-time, $T_{1/2}$ (see Chapter 9). Depending on the detailed dose rates, the equieffective dose may depend strongly on $T_{1/2}$ for a given endpoint. As these half-times are usually not known with any useful precision from clinical data, great care should be taken when interpreting the results of bioeffect calculations for continuous irradiations.

### Example 10.3: Brachytherapy

There has been some interest in intraluminal brachytherapy combined with external beam radiotherapy for endobronchial cancer. Fuwa et al. (15) delivered external beam radiotherapy combined with intraluminal brachytherapy: typically two or three fractions of 5 Gy in 2.5 hours delivered using a thin catheter with a $^{192}$Ir wire, combined with an external beam dose of 52 Gy.

*Problem:* What is the equivalent dose in 2 Gy fractions, of 5 Gy in 2.5 hours for lung fibrosis assuming two different recovery half-times, $T_{1/2}$, of 1.5 hours and 5 hours?

*Solution:* From Table 10.1 we find the point estimate of $\alpha/\beta$ for lung fibrosis to be 3.1 Gy. We show here the calculation for $T_{1/2} = 5$ hours. We first calculate $\mu t$, where $t$ is the duration of one application:

$$\mu = \frac{\log_e 2}{T_{1/2}} \approx \frac{0.693}{5 \text{ h}} \approx 0.139 \text{ h}^{-1}$$

that is $\mu t$ becomes $0.139 \text{ h}^{-1} \cdot 2.5 \text{ h} = 0.348$. Next, we calculate $g$ (see Equation 13.2):

$$g = \frac{2 \cdot [\mu t - 1 + \exp(-\mu t)]}{(\mu t)^2}$$

$$= \frac{2 \cdot [0.348 - 1 + \exp(-0.348)]}{0.348^2} \approx 0.893$$

This value is inserted into Equation 9.8 (note that the total dose, $D$, in this case is equal to the dose per fraction, $d$ (i.e. the dose delivered in a single application of the brachytherapy):

$$EQD2_{5h} = D \frac{d \cdot g + (\alpha/\beta)}{2 + (\alpha/\beta)}$$

$$= 5 \text{ Gy} \cdot \frac{5 \times 0.893 \text{ Gy} + 3.1 \text{ Gy}}{2 \text{ Gy} + 3.1 \text{ Gy}} \approx 7.4 \text{ Gy}$$

For $T_{1/2} = 1.5$ hours, we get $g = 0.70$ and $EQD2_{1.5h} = 6.5$ Gy, that is roughly a 12% lower equivalent dose in 2 Gy fractions than we calculated for $T_{1/2} = 5$ hours.

Example 10.3 shows what we would also expect intuitively, that the effect of protracting the delivery of a dose fraction is reduced when the recovery halftime is longer (i.e. less recovery will take place *during* the irradiation). A 5 Gy fraction delivered with acute dose rate, that is assuming no recovery at all during delivery, which would be equivalent to a very long (infinite) $T_{1/2}$, would correspond to an EQD2 of 7.9 Gy for $\alpha/\beta = 3.1$ Gy.

## 10.6 CHANGING THE OVERALL TREATMENT TIME

Very often, two fractionation schedules will differ in overall treatment time. There are clinical data supporting that overall treatment time has very little, if any, influence on late radiation effects (7). However, for most tumour types and for early endpoints, the biological effect of a specific dose-fractionation will *decrease* if overall treatment time is *increased*. In other words, an extra dose will be needed to obtain the same level of effect in a longer schedule. This has traditionally been interpreted as the result of proliferation of target cells in the irradiated tissue or tumour, and attempts have been made to include this effect in the LQ model. Experimental animal studies have shown that this is a nonlinear effect as a function of time, in other words, the dose recovered per unit time will change as a function of the time since the initial trauma. At present, there is no generally accepted mathematical model describing this recovery over extended time intervals. Instead, the most pragmatic, non-mechanistic approach is to assume a constant dose in 2 Gy fractions recovered per day due to proliferation, $D_{prolif}$, with units of Gy/day, which may be a good approximation in a fairly narrow time interval around the overall time of the schedule from which it has been estimated. For minor changes in overall time, say, a 4 day protraction of a schedule, the simple estimate would then be that the EQD2 has to be reduced by $4 \times D_{prolif}$. Using this method, the isoeffective doses in 2 Gy fractions delivered over two different times, $t$ and $T$, will be related as

$$EQD2_T = EQD2_t - (T - t) \cdot D_{prolif} \qquad (10.2)$$

where the index now refers to the overall treatment time of the schedule. If required in the context, the reference to the $\alpha/\beta$ value may be included in the index as well. Note that if $T > t$ then $EQD2_T < EQD2_t$.

There is, however, one modification. For squamous cell carcinoma of the head and neck, the experience with strongly accelerated schedules such as the UK continuous hyperfractionated accelerated radiotherapy (CHART) (see Chapter 11) shows that the $D_{prolif}$ estimated from longer schedules does not apply all the way down to the 12 days of overall treatment time of the CHART schedule. This has led to a simple biphasic model, with a critical time, $T_k$ ($k$ for 'kick-off') below which it is assumed that $D_{prolif}$ is zero. Thus, Equation 10.2 becomes

$$EQD2_T = EQD2_t - \left[MAX(T, T_k) - MAX(t, T_k)\right] \cdot D_{prolif}$$

where $MAX(x,y)$ is the larger value of $x$ and $y$, in other words, only the days beyond $T_k$ are counted in the calculation. $T_k$ for head and neck squamous cell carcinoma is in the order of 21–24 days. Biologically, a biphasic curve may seem overly simplistic or even unrealistic; the reality, however, is that clinical data sets typically do not allow fitting a more complex relationship.

There is no simple rule specifying the maximum difference between the two times, $T$ and $t$, where this linear approximation is sensible. For a 1 week difference this is probably reasonable, whereas for a 3–4 week difference this would not be a reasonable assumption. Another concern is that $D_{prolif}$ may depend on the intensity of the schedule, in other words, a very short intensive schedule may give rise to an increased value of $D_{prolif}$. A serious limitation is that little is known about the value of $D_{prolif}$ for many tumours and normal tissue endpoints and that most of the currently published values only apply towards the end of a 6–8 week schedule. For tumours, the majority of available estimates are for squamous cell carcinoma of the head and neck, see Table 10.3. As previously mentioned, it appears safe to assume that $D_{prolif}$ is zero for late endpoints at least for overall treatment times up to 6–8 weeks. For early reactions, a linear correction is also applicable over a limited range of overall treatment times, see, for example Bentzen et al. (9), but at

least in rodent models there are data showing a considerably shorter $T_k$, in mucosa as short as 8 days.

## Example 10.4: Correcting for overall treatment time

The International Atomic Energy Agency (IAEA) ACC trial (23) was a randomised controlled trial delivering 66–70 Gy in 33–35 fractions with 6 versus 5 fractions per week for definitive treatment for head and neck squamous cell carcinoma (HNSCC) of the larynx, pharynx and oral cavity. The trial enrolled 908 patients from nine centres in Asia, Europe, the Middle East, Africa and South America. All patients received definitive radiotherapy without chemotherapy. The actual, observed median treatment time was 40 days in the accelerated (6 fractions per week) arm and 47 days in the conventional (5 fractions per week) arm.

*Problem:* What is the expected difference in biologically effective dose for HNSCC between the two arms of the trial?

*Solution:* From Table 10.3 we see that $D_{prolif}$ for HNSCC is about 0.7 Gy/day. There is no demonstrable difference in $D_{prolif}$ among the various sub-sites of the head and neck region. Noting that the treatment time in both arms of the trial is larger than $T_k$, we insert the median overall treatment time in Equation 10.2 and get

$$EQD2_{acc} = EQD2_{conv} - (40 - 47) \text{days} \cdot 0.7 \text{ Gy/day}$$
$$= EQD2_{conv} + 4.9 \text{ Gy}$$

Table 10.3 Values for $D_{prolif}$ from clinical studies

| Tissue | Endpoint | $D_{prolif}$ (Gy day$^{-1}$) | 95% CL (Gy day$^{-1}$) | $T_k$[b] (days) | Source |
|---|---|---|---|---|---|
| *Early reactions* | | | | | |
| Skin | Erythema | 0.12 | [−0.12; 0.22] | <12 | Bentzen et al. (2001) |
| Mucosa | Mucositis | 0.8 | [0.7; 1.1] | <12 | Bentzen et al. (2001) |
| Lung | Pneumonitis | 0.54 | [0.13; 0.95] | | Bentzen et al. (2000)[a] |
| *Tumours* | | | | | |
| Head and neck | | | | | |
| Larynx | | 0.74 | [0.30; 1.2] | | Robertson et al. (1998) |
| Tonsils | | 0.73 | | 30 | Withers et al. (1995) |
| Various | | 0.8 | [0.5; 1.1] | 21 | Robers et al. (1994) |
| Various | | 0.64 | [0.42; 0.86] | | Hendry et al. (1996)[a] |
| Breast | | 0.60 | [0.10; 1.18] | | Haviland et al. (2016) |
| Oesophagus | | 0.59 | [0.18; 0.99] | | Geh et al. (2005) |
| Non-small cell lung cancer | | 0.45 | N/A | | Koukourakis et al. (1996) |
| Medulloblastoma | | 0.52 | [0.29; 0.75] | 0 or 21 | Hinata et al. (2001) |
| Prostate | | 0.24 | [0.03; 0.44] | 52 | Thames et al. (2010) |

*Note:* Reference details are available from Søren Bentzen.

[a] Pooled estimate from a review of studies in the literature.

[b] $T_k$ is the assumed time for the onset of accelerated proliferation.

Thus, the EQD2 of the accelerated schedule is 4.9 Gy higher than that of the conventional schedule. This difference is constant irrespective of whether a dose of 66 Gy or 70 Gy was prescribed provided that the difference in overall treatment time remains 7 days.

If the two schedules in the IAEA ACC trial had employed doses per fraction that were different from 2 Gy, we would first have calculated their EQD2s before doing the time correction.

## 10.7 UNPLANNED GAPS IN TREATMENT

A problem, frequently encountered in radiotherapy practice, is the management of unscheduled treatment interruptions. Studies have shown that until 1990 about a third of all patients with HNSCC experienced one or more unplanned gaps in treatment leading to a protraction of overall treatment time of more than 6 days. These interruptions were typically due to patient-related factors (intercurrent disease, severe radiation reactions) or logistic factors (public holidays, treatment machine downtime, transport difficulties). The management of treatment gaps has been considered in some detail by a working party of the UK Royal College of Radiologists (17). The priority to avoid gaps or actively modify treatment after a gap is based on the strength of clinical evidence for a negative therapeutic effect of gaps in radiotherapy schedules. This evidence is strongest for SCC of the head and neck, non-small cell lung cancer and cancer of the uterine cervix, and it is therefore recommended that the remaining part of the treatment be modified in order to adjust for the unscheduled interruption. There is also some support for the importance of overall treatment time in SCC of the skin and vagina and in medulloblastoma. Less evidence exists for other radical treatments and there is no reason to believe that overall treatment time is a significant factor in palliative radiotherapy.

Treatment schedules may be adjusted by accelerating radiotherapy after the gap. In a planned schedule delivering one fraction per day, 5 days per week, this can be accomplished by giving more than five fractions per week, either as two fractions per day as in Example 10.2, or preferably by treating on Saturday and/or Sunday. The aim is to deliver the planned total dose, with the prescribed dose per fraction, in as near the planned overall time as possible. If two fractions per day are delivered, these should be separated by the maximum practical interval, at least 8 hours and preferably more. Note that with long repair half-times, incomplete repair between the dose fractions may require a dose reduction if the chance of late complications is kept fixed. Alternatively, it may be considered to deliver the remaining part of the treatment with *hypo*fractionation. Whether this type of adjustment will lead to increased late sequelae or decreased tumour control depends on the exact values of $\alpha/\beta$ for the relevant late normal tissue endpoints and the tumour type in question.

## Example 10.5: Change in fraction size, gap correction

A patient with colorectal cancer is planned to receive pre-operative radiotherapy with five times 5 Gy from Monday to Friday (e.g. [19]). The first two fractions are given as planned on Monday and Tuesday, but due to a machine breakdown, no treatment could be given on Wednesday. It is considered to deliver the isoeffective tumour dose by increasing the size of the two fractions to be given on Thursday and Friday, in order to finish as planned on Friday. We assume that $\alpha/\beta = 10$ Gy for colorectal cancer.

*Problem:* What is the required dose per fraction for the last two fractions? What is the accompanying change in the risk of rectal complications from this modified fractionation schedule?

*Solution:* The tumour EQD2 for the final three fractions originally planned is

$$\text{EQD2} = 15\,\text{Gy} \cdot \frac{5\,\text{Gy} + 10\,\text{Gy}}{2\,\text{Gy} + 10\,\text{Gy}} = 18.75\,\text{Gy}$$

We want to estimate the dose per fraction, $x$, so that delivering two fractions of this size gives an EQD2 of 18.75 Gy to the tumour:

$$\text{EQD2} = 2 \cdot x \cdot \frac{x + 10\,\text{Gy}}{2\,\text{Gy} + 10\,\text{Gy}}$$

In the following, we remember that $x$ will have the physical units of gray and start solving this quadratic equation:

$$18.75 = 2 \cdot x \cdot \frac{x + 10}{2 + 10} \Leftrightarrow$$
$$18.75 \times 12 = 2x^2 + 20x \Leftrightarrow$$
$$2x^2 + 20x - 225 = 0$$

The solution to a quadratic equation of the form '$ax^2 + bx + c = 0$' is

$$x = \frac{-b + \sqrt{b^2 - 4ac}}{2a}$$

(Note that only the positive root produces a physically meaningful dose). In the present case, we get

$$x = \frac{-20 + \sqrt{20^2 - 4 \times 2 \times (-225)}}{2 \times 2} = 6.7$$

Remember the unit: Gy. In other words, we would have to give fractions of 6.7 Gy on Thursday and Friday, a total of 13.4 Gy, to achieve the same tumour effect. This is of course less than the $3 \times 5$ Gy originally planned for Wednesday through Friday, and the reason for this is the larger effect per gray deriving from the increased dose per fraction in the modified schedule.

How will this affect the risk of bowel damage? From Table 10.1, we find $\alpha/\beta$ of 4 Gy. The EQD2 of the modified schedule to the bowel is now

$$\text{EQD2} = \left[ 10\,\text{Gy} \cdot \frac{5\,\text{Gy} + 4\,\text{Gy}}{2\,\text{Gy} + 4\,\text{Gy}} \right] + \left[ 6.7\,\text{Gy} \cdot 2 \cdot \frac{6.7\,\text{Gy} + 4\,\text{Gy}}{2\,\text{Gy} + 4\,\text{Gy}} \right]$$
$$= 38.9\,\text{Gy}$$

This value does not take the very short overall treatment time of 5 days into consideration and it is possible that such short schedules could involve an increased risk of consequential late reactions. Here, we only focus on the change in biological dose springing from the change in dose fractionation and we note that the overall treatment time is unchanged in the two schedules compared here. The originally planned five times 5 Gy corresponds to an EQD2 for bowel of about 37.5 Gy. Therefore, the risk of late bowel morbidity will be increased if this modification was implemented.

Clinically, one might be concerned about increasing dose per fraction from 5 to 6.7 Gy. Biologically, the validity of the LQ model at these large doses per fraction is still not documented for many types of clinical endpoints (see Chapter 9). It should also be noted, that if we use a lower $\alpha/\beta$, for example the 1.7 Gy estimated for fibrosis, the change in EQD2 for this endpoint is expected to be from 45 to 48.5 Gy. It could be considered to stick to 5 Gy per fraction and give the fifth fraction on Saturday or simply to accept a 3 day protraction, i.e. finishing on Monday. The concern about the prolongation of overall treatment time would be a possible loss of tumour control, but it could be argued that the overall treatment time would still be less than the kick-off time for accelerated repopulation, $T_k$, though admittedly, reliable estimates of $T_k$ are only available for squamous cell carcinoma of the head and neck, and we would have to assume that this is relevant for rectal cancer as well.

## 10.8 ERRORS IN DOSE DELIVERY

Dosimetric errors in delivering the prescribed dose per fraction made early in a treatment can be corrected by modifying the dose per fraction and total dose given subsequently to discovery of the error, using the LQ model to calculate the correcting doses which should be completed *within the same overall time* as originally prescribed. If the initial error was giving a larger dose per fraction than planned (a hypofractionated error), then the rest of the treatment should be *hyper*fractionated to compensate. If the initial error was giving a lower dose per fraction than planned (hyperfractionated), then the rest of the treatment should be *hypo*fractionated to compensate.

Joiner (18) showed how to calculate the dose per fraction used to bring the treatment back exactly to planned tolerance simultaneously for all tissues and tumour involved, following either hyperfractionated or hypofractionated errors made

initially, *without* the need to know any $\alpha/\beta$ values. Defining planned treatment as $p$ Gy per fraction to a total dose $P$ Gy, suppose the initial error is $e$ Gy per fraction given to a total of $E$ Gy. Using the LQ model to describe all isoeffect relationships between total dose and dose per fraction for the tumour and the normal tissues, then the compensating dose per fraction of $d$ Gy to a total dose of $D$ Gy are given by the simple formulae:

$$D = P - E \tag{10.3}$$

$$d = \frac{Pp - Ee}{P - E} \tag{10.4}$$

Notably, it can be seen that the total dose for the complete treatment (error plus compensation) remains as originally prescribed.

## Example 10.6: Error in the delivered dose per fraction at the beginning of treatment

A patient is planned to receive $35 \times 2$ Gy per fraction, with five fractions per week to an overall time of 7 weeks. By error, the treatments on each of the first two days are given as 4 Gy per fraction.

*Problem*: What is the dose per fraction that should be given in the remainder of the treatment, to exactly compensate for the initial error?

*Solution*: The total error dose ($E$) is 8 Gy, therefore, from Equation 10.3, the total compensating dose ($D$) is

$$70\,\text{Gy} - 8\,\text{Gy} = 62\,\text{Gy}$$

The dose per fraction used for the compensation, given by Equation 10.4, should be

$$\frac{70\,\text{Gy} \cdot 2\,\text{Gy} - 8\,\text{Gy} \cdot 4\,\text{Gy}}{70\,\text{Gy} - 8\,\text{Gy}} = 1.74\,\text{Gy}$$

This gives $62/1.74 = 35.6$ fractions for the compensating 62 Gy. Since an integral number of fractions must be given, the nearest compensating treatment is $36 \times 1.72$ Gy.

In this example, there are 33 weekday treatment days left to use in the original planned overall time, so three of the 1.72 Gy doses must be given on Saturdays, or using two fractions per day on three of the Fridays, in order not to extend overall treatment time. It must be noted that Equations 10.3 and 10.4 are only valid in the absence of incomplete recovery, therefore compensating treatments should not be scheduled in a way that would introduce significant incomplete repair. This favours using Saturdays to deliver the additional doses, or leaving the maximum possible time between two doses given on Fridays, but at least 8 hours.

## 10.9 RE-IRRADIATION

A specific problem in clinical practice is the radiotherapeutic management of patients with a new primary tumour or a loco-regional recurrence in an anatomical site that necessitates re-irradiation of a previously irradiated tissue or organ. Experimental animal data demonstrate that various endpoints differ markedly in their capacity for long-term recovery of radiation tolerance (see Chapter 23). Quantitative clinical data are sparse and it may not be safe to assume any particular value of the recovery in a clinical setting. The most reasonable approach is probably to use the LQ model to estimate the EQD2s for the normal tissue endpoints of concern without any explicit recovery assumed, and then to apply a clinical assessment of the re-irradiation tolerance based in part on the experience from animal experiments. Obviously, such an assessment would also include other clinical aspects like the life expectancy of the patient in relation to the latent period of late damage, and the prospects for long-term benefit from the re-treatment.

## 10.10 FROM CHANGE IN DOSE TO CHANGE IN RESPONSE RATE

Early papers on the use of the LQ model in biological dose calculations were all concerned with estimation of isoeffective doses. In practice, two dose-fractionation schedules will most often not produce exactly the same biological effect, and even if they are isoeffective with respect to a specific endpoint they will typically not be so with respect to other endpoints. In these situations, it is necessary to consider the steepness of the dose-response curve in order to estimate the associated change in the incidence of a clinical endpoint in going from one schedule to the other.

In the following, response probability refers to either a tumour control probability or a normal tissue complication probability. If the response probability is $R$ after a dose $D$, the change in this probability, in percentage points, after an increment in dose, $\Delta D$, is approximately

$$\Delta R \approx \frac{\Delta D}{D} \cdot 100\% \cdot \gamma_n \qquad (10.5)$$

where $\gamma_n$ is the local value of the normalised dose-response gradient (see Chapter 5), i.e. the value at a response probability of $n\%$, where $n$ is chosen approximately equal to $R$. The use of this formula is illustrated by the following example.

### Example 10.7: Converting from change in dose into change in response rate (I)

For the IAEA ACC trial (Example 10.4), we calculated that the acceleration in the six fractions per week arm corresponded to an effective 4.9 Gy dose increment. Assume that the local tumour control probability (T-position alone) in the two arms is around 40% (this is consistent with the actual observed control probability in the trial, see the following).

*Problem:* What is the expected increase in tumour control probability from the treatment acceleration?

*Solution:* First, we need to choose the value of $\gamma$. From Figure 5.4, we find that $\gamma_{50}$ is around 1.8 for head and neck cancer with a trend towards higher values for vocal cord tumours. From Table 5.1, we see that at the 40% control level, the $\gamma_{40}$ value is around 1.6. Using this value of $\gamma$ allows us to calculate the expected change in response:

$$\Delta R = \frac{4.9\,\text{Gy}}{66\,\text{Gy}} \cdot 100\% \cdot 1.6 = 11.9\%$$

For a patient treated with 70 Gy, $\Delta R$ is estimated at 11.2%. Thus, the local tumour control probability is expected to increase by about 11%–12%. The 5 year actuarial rate of local control observed in the trial was 46% in the accelerated group versus 33% in the conventional group (Figure 3a in Overgaard et al. [23]). Thus, the observed tumour control rate increased by 13%, in agreement with the expected increase calculated here. The statistical uncertainty in the observed 13% difference is not stated in the IAEA ACC report but a rough calculation based on the reported 95% confidence interval for the hazard ratio, suggests that the 95% confidence interval for the observed difference in local control between the arms is 5%–20%.

We may also revisit the effect of incomplete recovery in the RAPID trial.

### Example 10.8: Converting from change in dose to change in response rate (II)

For the RAPID trial (Example 10.2), we calculated that the effect of incomplete recovery between fractions in the accelerated partial breast irradiation arm was to increase the estimated EQD2 to 64.9 Gy. In the control arm, adverse cosmesis at 3 years was 17%.

*Problem:* What is the expected prevalence of adverse cosmesis at 3 years in the APBI arm if we assume that $\gamma_{50}$ for this endpoint is 2.2?

*Solution:* The $\gamma_{50}$ value above is that derived from the START trials. However, we first need to estimate the value at the 17% response level. We can obtain this value by interpolation in Table 5.1 or we can use Equation 5.12 and get $\gamma_{17} = 1.018$. Again, we can now estimate $\Delta R$:

$$\Delta R = \frac{14.9\,\text{Gy}}{50\,\text{Gy}} \cdot 100\% \cdot 1.018 = 30.3\%$$

This is likely to be an underestimate, as the simple linear extrapolation in the equation is not very accurate over this large a range of effect: the curve will get steeper as we approach the 50% response level, i.e. the increase in response will get larger.

The observed difference in the proportion of patients with adverse cosmesis at 3 years in the two arms of the RAPID trial was 19% with 95% confidence limits from 12% to 24%. Our estimate for $\Delta R$ is therefore outside the confidence interval from the trial estimate, but of course there is also uncertainty in the parameters we used for our calculation. A (kind) interpretation of this somewhat lower observed prevalence of adverse cosmesis compared to our previous rough estimate, would be that this could reflect the reduction of the treated volume in patients in the APBI arm of RAPID. A more detailed quantitative argument would require an NTCP model for change in breast appearance and more detailed data on the dose distribution in the APBI patients. For further discussion see Bentzen and Yarnold (10).

## 10.11 DOUBLE TROUBLE

Dosimetric hot spots receive not only a higher total dose but also a higher dose per fraction, a process referred to by Rodney Withers as 'double trouble' (see, e.g. [21]). The magnitude of this double-trouble effect depends on the fractionation sensitivity of the endpoint in question and will be a more pronounced effect for endpoints with a lower $\alpha/\beta$ value. A hot spot could arise due to internal and external inhomogeneities or due to the radiation field arrangement. A special case is in the match zone between two abutted fields, where depending on the geometrical matching technique used, a small tissue volume could be markedly over- or underdosed. Historically, match zone overdosage of the brachial plexus has been associated with an unacceptable incidence of radiation plexopathies in patients receiving postoperative radiotherapy for breast cancer (4). These problems can largely be avoided by using a more optimal treatment technique.

Clearly, the volume affected plays a major role when considering the clinical consequences of the double-trouble effect.

### Example 10.9: Double trouble

The UK FAST trial (1) randomised 915 women after breast conservation surgery between standard fractionation and two dose levels of a five-fraction regimen delivering 5.7 or 6.0 Gy fractions in 5 weeks, using three-dimensional dosimetry. The protocol allowed a hot spot of up to 107% of the prescribed dose.

*Problem:* What is the peak biologically equieffective dose in 2 Gy fractions in the hot spot for the endpoint of a late change in breast appearance relative to the EQD2 at the 100% isodose level in the $5 \times 6.0$ Gy arm of the trial?

*Solution:* This is a straightforward application of Withers' formula (Equation 10.1). For the late endpoint we get

$$EQD2 = 30\ \text{Gy} \cdot \frac{6.0\ \text{Gy} + 3.4\ \text{Gy}}{2\ \text{Gy} + 3.4\ \text{Gy}} = 52.2\ \text{Gy}$$

And for the hot spot, where the dose per fraction is $1.07 \times 6.0\ \text{Gy} = 6.42\ \text{Gy}$ and the total dose is $5 \times 6.42\ \text{Gy} = 32.1\ \text{Gy}$:

$$EQD2 = 32.1\ \text{Gy} \cdot \frac{6.42\ \text{Gy} + 3.4\ \text{Gy}}{2\ \text{Gy} + 3.4\ \text{Gy}} = 58.4\ \text{Gy}$$

If we take the ratio between these two doses, we see that while the absorbed dose in the hot spot is 7% higher than the prescribed dose, the EQD2 dose in the hot spot is 11.9% higher than the prescribed EQD2. This added biological effect from the higher dose *and* the higher dose per fraction is the double-trouble effect. Whether this overdosage affects breast appearance will depend critically on the volume affected and the magnitude of the volume effect for the endpoint in question. In the present clinical example, there are data documenting a marked volume effect for the endpoint of breast appearance after radiotherapy.

## 10.12 THE UNCERTAINTY IN BIOLOGICAL EFFECT ESTIMATES

An impression of the uncertainty in equieffective dose estimates may be obtained simply by varying the value of $\alpha/\beta$, $T_{1/2}$, $D_{\text{prolif}}$ or $\gamma_{50}$. The idea is simply to insert the lower and upper 95% confidence limits of the parameter in question and use these as 95% confidence limits for the biological effect estimate. This technique is only straightforward if we are concerned with uncertainty in a single parameter, say, uncertainty in $\alpha/\beta$. If we want to evaluate the effect of uncertainty in two parameters, for example $D_{\text{prolif}}$ and $\gamma_{50}$, it is necessary to use more advanced methods. It is *not* a good approximation simply to insert the lower and upper confidence limits for both parameters in the calculation.

### Example 10.10: Estimating uncertainty

We repeat the calculation in Example 10.9, but this time we use the confidence interval around the $\alpha/\beta$ value for change in breast appearance to get a confidence interval for the EQD2 in the hot spot.

*Problem:* What is the EQD2 with 95% confidence interval for the hot spot dose using the $\alpha/\beta$ value for change in breast appearance?

*Solution:* Table 10.1 gives $\alpha/\beta = 3.4$ Gy with 95% confidence limits 2.3 and 4.5 Gy. If we insert the lower limit on $\alpha/\beta$, we obtain the upper limit on the EQD2:

$$EQD2_{2.3} = 32.1\,Gy \cdot \frac{6.42\,Gy + 2.3\,Gy}{2\,Gy + 2.3\,Gy} = 65.1\,Gy$$

Similarly, for $\alpha/\beta = 4.5$ Gy, the upper 95% confidence limit for EQD2 in the hot spot becomes $EQD2_{4.5} = 53.9$ Gy. Thus, our best estimate of EQD2 for the hotspot is 58.4 Gy with 95% confidence limits 53.9 and 65.1 Gy.

Unfortunately, the width of the confidence interval in Example 10.10 is quite typical. Most $\alpha/\beta$ values for human normal tissue endpoints and tumours are known with a precision that does not allow very accurate predictions, in particular when we are considering relatively high dose per fraction. Perhaps it is worth noting that the accuracy in the estimate of the relative EQD2 in the hot spot versus the prescription is relatively less affected by this uncertainty in $\alpha/\beta$: the 11.9% we calculated in Example 10.9 has 95% confidence limits 11.3% and 12.4%. Intuitively, this is no surprise, as we vary $\alpha/\beta$ the value is obviously the same for the various dose levels in the breast.

Another useful principle when trying to mitigate the effect of uncertainty in $\alpha/\beta$ when performing equieffective dose calculations is to identify the main clinical concern and then select a value that would be conservative in terms of risk and benefit to the patient. In Examples 10.2 and 10.9, the main concern is the added risk of complications associated with the delivery of multiple fractions per day or the overdosage in the hotspot. In Example 10.5, the main concern is the possible increase of late effects after hypofractionation. In these cases, by assuming a *low* value for $\alpha/\beta$, we would err on the side of caution. If on the other hand, we want to estimate the added efficacy from hypofractionation in terms of local tumour control, it would be conservative, i.e. we would not be overestimating the benefit, if we assumed a relatively *high* value of $\alpha/\beta$ for the tumour. In both cases, low and high means relative to the 95% confidence interval or within a range of published values.

A final observation is that the confidence interval for $\alpha/\beta$ derived from animal studies is often narrower than for the corresponding human endpoint. This probably reflects that the number of subjects is often larger in the experimental studies and that dose and dose per fraction are varied more systematically and over a wider range of values. As mentioned previously, we would suggest that the full calculation, including the estimation of confidence limits, is done using the parameter estimates from the human data whenever possible, and that an independent calculation is done using the animal data.

## 10.13 SOME CURRENT ISSUES IN THE CLINICAL APPLICATION OF THE LQ MODEL

The question whether the LQ approach has been validated can only be addressed on an endpoint-by-endpoint basis. The LQ model has been applied to data sets from a lot of clinical studies, and there has in many cases been agreement between the predicted and observed study outcome. This gives some confidence in using the model to estimate the effects of changed dose fractionation in situations where there are clinical parameter estimates. Roughly, the dose per fraction, where use of the LQ model is supported by data, ranges from about 1 to 6–7 Gy or so. As mentioned in the introduction to this chapter, even then there is often a lack of appropriate parameter estimates, or the available estimates have wide 95% confidence limits. Parameter estimates for clinical endpoints remain relatively scarce. Some papers derive parameter values based on fixing one or more other parameters in the estimation. Clearly, these estimates become circular to some extent. While the clinical importance of low-dose hyper-radiosensitivity remains controversial, there is little empirical support from clinical studies for the use of the LQ model at dose per fraction of <1 Gy. This is an important issue as many IMRT techniques involve irradiation of large normal tissue volumes with dose fractions in this range. At the other end of the spectrum, techniques such as extra-cranial stereotactic body radiotherapy (SBRT) or intra-operative radiotherapy or high dose-rate brachytherapy may deliver dose fractions of 10 Gy or more. Again, there is little empirical evidence behind the use of the simple LQ model, or any of the proposed modifications of this model, in this high-dose range as reflected by conflicting views in the literature (e.g. [12,24]). In most cases, the dose fractionation issue is intertwined with the volume effect, and in practice it is difficult to separate these effects from clinical studies where patients receive roughly similar dose distributions. See also Chapter 16.

It should also be mentioned that a number of elegant formulations extending the LQ model have been developed, for example for internal emitters or permanent implants. Other formulations include relative biological effectiveness or oxygen enhancement ratio corrections, etc. The interested reader is referred to the book edited by Dale and Jones (2007) for an overview of many of these applications and refinements of the LQ model. From the perspective of clinical radiobiology, many of these models are over-parameterized in the sense that clinical data sets typically will not have sufficient structural resolution to allow estimation of all relevant model parameters, not to mention validating the model assumptions.

Do some tumours have low $\alpha/\beta$ values? Parameter estimates for malignant melanoma and liposarcoma from the late 1980s suggested that this might be the case, but this hypothesis has attracted considerable interest after Brenner and Hall (11) derived low $\alpha/\beta$ estimates for prostate cancer from a comparison between external beam and brachytherapy outcomes. Later studies comparing external-beam-only fractionation effects have provided further support for this idea (26) and recently this is supported by evidence from large, randomized controlled trials (13). There is also strong evidence that $\alpha/\beta$ for sub-clinical breast cancer may be around 4 Gy, i.e. considerably less than the often assumed 10 Gy, see the report from the UK START Trialists Group (3). A cautious attitude is that fractionation schedules designed to exploit these presumptive low $\alpha/\beta$ values for some cancer types should be tested in prospective clinical trials, as they could lead to major deviations from the established practice in a particular centre.

The final note here is that the move towards increasing use of combined modality therapy in many tumour types represents a further issue regarding the applicability of standard LQ modelling. The approach often taken is to perform bioeffect calculations for the radiation therapy part in isolation. This may produce valid results as long as the chemotherapy is strictly identical in the schedules being compared. However, this approach is also challenged by data suggesting that some cytotoxic and molecular targeted drugs actually modulate the dose-time-fractionation response (6). In this case, radiobiological parameters derived from radiation-alone studies may no longer be valid.

While the LQ approach 15 years ago appeared to be rather well established, a number of new developments – mainly driven by clinical and technology advances – have made bioeffect modelling an exciting and important area of clinical and experimental radiation research again.

---

## Key points

1. The LQ approach is the model of choice for bioeffect estimation in radiotherapy and can be used for a wide range of calculations.
2. The dose range where the LQ model is well supported by data is roughly 1–6 Gy per fraction. Extrapolations made outside this range should be done with extreme caution.
3. Clinical parameter estimates should be used in calculations whenever possible. If no clinical estimates are available, values from animal studies may be used as guidance but caution should be exercised in applying the results of such calculations to the clinical situation.
4. Estimates of uncertainty in LQ calculations should always be made, based on the uncertainty in the values of the parameters used in the calculation.
5. In combined modality therapy, it may not be valid to use parameters derived from studies using radiation alone.

---

■ BIBLIOGRAPHY

1. Agrawal RK, Alhasso A, Barrett-Lee PJ et al. First results of the randomised UK FAST Trial of radiotherapy hypofractionation for treatment of early breast cancer (CRUKE/04/015). *Radiother Oncol* 2011;100:93–100.
2. Bentzen SM. Preventing or reducing late side effects of radiation therapy: Radiobiology meets molecular pathology. *Nat Rev Cancer* 2006;6:702–713.
3. Bentzen SM, Agrawal RK, Aird EG et al. The UK Standardisation of Breast Radiotherapy (START) Trial A of radiotherapy hypofractionation for treatment of early breast cancer: A randomised trial. *Lancet Oncol* 2008;9:331–341.
4. Bentzen SM, Dische S. Morbidity related to axillary irradiation in the treatment of breast cancer. *Acta Oncol* 2000;39:337–347.
5. Bentzen SM, Dorr W, Gahbauer R et al. Bioeffect modeling and equieffective dose concepts in radiation oncology – Terminology, quantities and units. *Radiother Oncol* 2012;105:266–268.
6. Bentzen SM, Harari PM, Bernier J. Exploitable mechanisms for combining drugs with radiation: Concepts, achievements and future directions. *Nat Clin Pract Oncol* 2007;4:172–180.
7. Bentzen SM, Overgaard J. Clinical normal-tissue radiobiology. In: Tobias JS and Thomas PR, editors. *Current Radiation Oncology.* Vol 2. London: Arnold; 1995. pp. 37–67.
8. Bentzen SM, Saunders MI, Dische S. Repair halftimes estimated from observations of treatment-related morbidity after CHART or conventional radiotherapy in head and neck cancer. *Radiother Oncol* 1999;53:219–226.
9. Bentzen SM, Saunders MI, Dische S, Bond SJ. Radiotherapy-related early morbidity in head and neck cancer: Quantitative clinical radiobiology as deduced from the CHART trial. *Radiother Oncol* 2001;60:123–135.
10. Bentzen SM, Yarnold JR. Reports of unexpected late side effects of accelerated partial breast irradiation – Radiobiological considerations. *Int J Radiat Oncol Biol Phys* 2010;77:969–973.
11. Brenner DJ, Hall EJ. Fractionation and protraction for radiotherapy of prostate carcinoma. *Int J Radiat Oncol Biol Phys* 1999;43:1095–1101.
12. Brown JM, Carlson DJ, Brenner DJ. The tumor radiobiology of SRS and SBRT: Are more than the 5 Rs involved? *Int J Radiat Oncol Biol Phys* 2014;88:254–262.
13. Dearnaley D, Syndikus I, Mossop H et al. Conventional versus hypofractionated high-dose intensity-modulated radiotherapy for prostate cancer: 5-year outcomes of the randomised, non-inferiority, phase 3 CHHiP trial. *Lancet Oncol* 2016;17:1047–1060.
14. Dische S, Saunders MI. Continuous, hyperfractionated, accelerated radiotherapy (CHART): An interim report upon late morbidity. *Radiother Oncol* 1989;16:65–72.
15. Fuwa N, Ito Y, Matsumoto A, Morita K. The treatment results of 40 patients with localized endobronchial cancer with external beam irradiation and intraluminal irradiation using low dose rate (192)Ir thin wires with a new catheter. *Radiother Oncol* 2000;56:189–195.
16. Guttenberger R, Thames HD, Ang KK. Is the experience with CHART compatible with experimental data? A new model of repair kinetics and computer simulations. *Radiother Oncol* 1992;25:280–286.
17. Hendry JH, Bentzen SM, Dale RG et al. A modelled comparison of the effects of using different ways to compensate for missed treatment days in radiotherapy. *Clin Oncol* 1996;8:297–307.
18. Joiner MC. A simple alpha/beta-independent method to derive fully isoeffective schedules following changes in dose per fraction. *Int J Radiat Oncol Biol Phys* 2004;58:871–875.
19. Kapiteijn E, Marijnen CA, Nagtegaal ID et al. Preoperative radiotherapy combined with total mesorectal excision for resectable rectal cancer. *N Engl J Med* 2001;345:638–646.

20. Lee AW, Sze WM, Fowler JF, Chappell R, Leung SF, Teo P. Caution on the use of altered fractionation for nasopharyngeal carcinoma. *Radiother Oncol* 1999;52:207–211.

21. Lee SP, Leu MY, Smathers JB, McBride WH, Parker RG, Withers HR. Biologically effective dose distribution based on the linear quadratic model and its clinical relevance. *Int J Radiat Oncol Biol Phys* 1995;33:375–389.

22. Olivotto IA, Whelan TJ, Parpia S et al. Interim cosmetic and toxicity results from RAPID: A randomized trial of accelerated partial breast irradiation using three-dimensional conformal external beam radiation therapy. *J Clin Oncol* 2013;31:4038–4045.

23. Overgaard J, Mohanti BK, Begum N et al. Five versus six fractions of radiotherapy per week for squamous-cell carcinoma of the head and neck (IAEA-ACC study): A randomised, multicentre trial. *Lancet Oncol* 2010;11:553–560.

24. Sheu T, Molkentine J, Transtrum MK et al. Use of the LQ model with large fraction sizes results in underestimation of isoeffect doses. *Radiother Oncol* 2013;109:21–25.

25. Thames HD, Bentzen SM, Turesson I, Overgaard M, Van den Bogaert W. Time-dose factors in radiotherapy: A review of the human data. *Radiother Oncol* 1990;19:219–235.

26. Vogelius IR, Bentzen SM. Dose response and fractionation sensitivity of prostate cancer after external beam radiation therapy: A meta-analysis of randomized trials. *Int J Radiat Oncol Biol Phys* 2018;100:858–865.

## ■ FURTHER READING

27. Dale RG, Jones B, (eds.) *Radiobiological Modeling in Radiation Oncology.* London: British Institute of Radiology; 2007.

# Modified fractionation

MICHAEL BAUMANN, MECHTHILD KRAUSE AND VINCENT GRÉGOIRE

## 11.1 INTRODUCTION

Throughout the history of radiotherapy, the optimal distribution of dose over time has been a major issue, but the most important progress has been made in this area since the early 1980s. The relationships uncovered between total dose and fraction number for late versus early responding normal tissues and tumours provide the basic information required to optimise the dose per fraction in radiotherapy. More work still needs to be done particularly in a clinical setting to determine the exact time of onset, the rate and the mechanisms of repopulation in all tumours and normal tissues during radiotherapy, but enough is now known about *time factors* to support the important conclusions that (1) the overall duration of fractionated radiotherapy should not be allowed to extend beyond the originally prescribed time, (2) a reduced overall treatment time should be considered in a number of clinical situations and (3) inter-fraction time intervals should be made as long as possible in order to maximise the available benefit from fractionation schedules employing multiple fractions per day if these are warranted.

## 11.2 CONVENTIONAL FRACTIONATION

Conventional fractionation is the application of daily doses of 1.8–2 Gy and five fractions per week with a dose per week of 9–10 Gy. Depending on tumour histology, tumour size and localisation, total doses ranging from 40 to 70 Gy are given for macroscopic disease and lower doses when treating microscopic disease. These conventional fractionation schedules were developed on an empirical basis (15) and have been the mainstay of curative radiotherapy over the last decades in most institutions in Europe and the United States.

Radiosensitive tumours such as lymphomas and seminomas can be controlled with low doses of 45 Gy or even less, while for example *glioblastoma multiforme* is a very resistant tumour that is not controlled even after doses as high as 70 Gy. Most tumour types, including squamous cell carcinomas and adenocarcinomas, are of intermediate sensitivity. Small tumours, for example T1 or T2 carcinomas of the head and neck, are well controlled with acceptable normal tissue damage using conventional

fractionation and total doses between 60 and 70 Gy. However, local tumour control rates rapidly decline for larger tumours. As local tumour control increases with the total dose of radiotherapy, larger tumours could be better controlled by increasing the total dose of conventional fractionation above 70 Gy, say to doses between 80 and 100 Gy. Such dose escalation is currently being tested, e.g. for non-small cell lung cancer or carcinoma of the prostate. One constraint is that also the incidence and severity of normal tissue damage increase with increasing total doses (see Chapter 5). This was recognised as early as 1936 when Holthusen pointed out that the uncomplicated local tumour control rate initially increases with increasing dose but then falls again because of the steep increase in the incidence of normal tissue damage. Figure 11.1 is redrawn from one of Holthusen's papers: the frequency of 'uncomplicated tumour control' follows a bell-shaped curve. Once the optimum dose is established, further improvements in uncomplicated tumour control can only be achieved by either moving the dose-effect curve for local tumour control to lower doses or the curve for normal tissue damage to higher doses; the latter is the objective of hyperfractionated schedules (Section 11.3). High-precision radiotherapy is another option currently used in dose escalation protocols, reducing the volume of normal tissue irradiated to high dose and therefore also the probability of late normal tissue damage (see Chapters 16 and 22). As dose escalation using conventional fractionation is always associated with the prolongation of overall treatment time, some of the potential gain may be lost as a consequence of tumour-cell repopulation (see Section 11.4).

## 11.3 MODIFICATION OF DOSE PER FRACTION

### Hyperfractionation

Hyperfractionation is defined as the application of doses per fraction less than the 1.8–2.0 Gy given in conventional fractionation. The total number of fractions must be increased, hence the prefix *hyper*; usually two fractions are administered per day. The biological rationale of hyperfractionation is to exploit the difference between the small effect of dose per fraction on tumour control versus

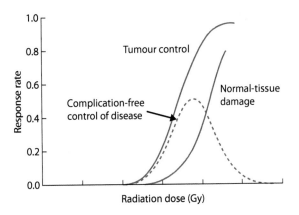

**Figure 11.1** Dose-response curves for tumour control and normal tissue damage. The uncomplicated local tumour control rate initially increases with increasing dose after which it falls again because of a steep increase of the incidence of normal tissue damage. (Adapted from (18).)

the larger effect of dose per fraction on the incidence and severity of late normal tissue damage. As pointed out in Chapter 9, this differential between tumours and late-responding normal tissues is thought to be caused by a different capacity of target cells in these tissues to recover from sublethal radiation damage between fractions.

In clinical practice hyperfractionation is usually applied to escalate the total dose compared with conventional fractionation, thereby aiming at improved tumour control rates without increasing the risk of late complications (see Figure 9.7). Dose-escalated hyperfractionation has been tested in two large multicentre randomized clinical trials on head and neck squamous cell carcinoma (EORTC 22791, RTOG 9003). The results of the EORTC trial are shown in Figure 11.2. The right-hand panel shows that hyperfractionated treatment with 70 fractions of 1.15 Gy (two fractions per day, 4–6 hours interval, total dose 80.5 Gy) produced a similar incidence of pooled grade 2 and 3 late tissue damage to a conventional schedule of 35 fractions of 2 Gy (70 Gy given in the same overall time of 7 weeks). However, the larger total dose in the hyperfractionated

treatment led to an increase of ~19% in long-term local tumour control (left-hand panel). Survival was non-significantly higher after hyperfractionation. In the RTOG trial (16), local tumour control was increased by 8% after hyperfractionation (68 fractions of 1.2 Gy, two fractions per day, 6 hours apart, total dose 81.6 Gy) compared with conventional fractionation using 2 Gy fractions to 70 Gy in the same overall time of 7 weeks. Overall survival was not significantly improved but the prevalence of grade III late effects was significantly increased after hyperfractionation. Both these clinical trials thus confirm the radiobiological expectation that local tumour control can be increased by dose-escalated hyperfractionation, thereby supporting a high average $\alpha/\beta$ value for squamous cell carcinoma of the head and neck (Table 10.1). However, while the EORTC trial supports the view that hyperfractionation allows the total dose to be increased without a simultaneous increase in late complications, the RTOG trial indicates that this is not always the case. The potential therapeutic gain from hyperfractionation has been extensively debated (2,5,6). Factors that contribute to an increased risk of late normal tissue damage when multiple fractions are applied per day are discussed in Section 11.5.

## Hypofractionation

This is the use of doses per fraction higher than 2 Gy; the total number of fractions is reduced, hence the prefix *hypo*. As explained in Chapter 9, Section 9.6, the radiobiological expectation is that hypofractionation will mostly *lower* the therapeutic ratio between tumours and late-responding normal tissues, compared with conventional fractionation given in the same overall time. This expectation depends on the $\alpha/\beta$ value for the tumour being considerably higher than for late-responding normal tissues; exceptions could therefore occur for tumours that have low $\alpha/\beta$ values, for example breast cancer, some melanomas, liposarcomas and potentially early stage prostate cancer (Table 10.1), and in these cases hypofractionation can be as good or even better than conventional fractionation. The best database exists for

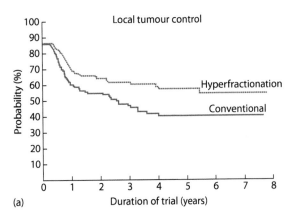
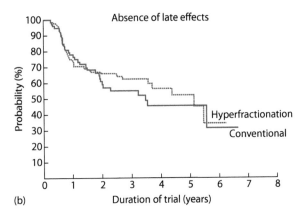

**Figure 11.2** Results of the EORTC (22791) trial of dose-escalated hyperfractionation. (a) Loco-regional tumour control (log rank, $p < 0.02$). (b) Patients free of late radiation effects, grade 2 or worse (log rank $p > 0.72$). (From (20), with permission.)

breast cancer. In four randomised phase III trials including a total of more than 5000 women with breast-conserving surgery (22,26,27,29), normofractionated radiotherapy with 50 Gy in 25 fractions within 5 weeks has been compared with different moderately hypofractionated schedules, applying total doses of 40–42.9 Gy with doses per fraction of 2.67–3.3 Gy in overall treatment times of 3 or 5 weeks. Despite the reduced total dose in the hypofractionated arms, local tumour control and survival were not different between normofractionated and hypofractionated radiotherapy, only the $13 \times 3$ Gy schedule led to higher recurrence rates as compared to the $13 \times 3.3$ Gy schedule (22). Acute and late toxicity were comparable after normo- and hypofractionated treatment, only on very late effects sufficient conclusions are not yet possible. The $\alpha/\beta$ value was estimated from these data to be 4.6 Gy (1.1–8.1 Gy) for breast cancer and 3.4 Gy (2.3–4.5) for normal breast tissue (26). The results of the above-mentioned studies allow the conclusion that hypofractionated dose-reduced radiotherapy is an equally effective and equi-toxic schedule compared to conventional fractionation in breast cancer at least for the patient population included in the trials (mostly low-risk patients). A different biology of more aggressive tumour types, e.g. in younger patients, cannot be ruled out, which would then turn the reduced total dose to a negative factor for treatment outcome. Also, caution is necessary when higher doses per fraction are applied, as for example 30 Gy in five fractions led to significantly higher toxicity as compared to normofractionated radiotherapy (1).

Single-dose irradiation or hypofractionation with only few large fractions are widely applied in palliative radiotherapy. These schedules use lower total doses than those applied in curative radiotherapy. For this reason, and because the patients have a limited life expectancy, late normal-tissue damage is of only minor concern. A number of randomised clinical trials have shown that symptom control after palliative hypofractionated schedules is comparable to that achieved with more highly fractionated schedules. For stereotactic radiotherapy of small tumours, e.g. in lung, where very steep dose gradients can be achieved and hence only very small volumes of surrounding normal tissue are at risk of radiation damage, single doses or hypofractionation with few large fractions are also frequently applied in clinical practice.

Moderate hypofractionation with doses per fraction up to approximately 3.5 Gy is routinely used for curative radiation therapy in many centres worldwide. To reduce the risk of late normal tissue damage in these schedules, slightly lower total doses are applied than for conventional fractionation. For tumours with a high $\alpha/\beta$ value, this decrease in total dose may well lead to a reduction in tumour control probability. However, some or all of this negative effect may be compensated by the shorter overall treatment times often used for this moderate hypofractionation (see Section 11.4). There is growing interest in the use of moderate hypofractionation to escalate total doses in the context of clinical trials of conformal radiation therapy.

For example, utilizing a field-in-field technique or intensity modulated radiotherapy (IMRT), a higher dose per fraction can be applied for boosting the macroscopic tumour while potential microscopic tumour extensions are treated at conventional doses per fraction. Such hypofractionated approaches for dose escalation avoid the necessity to prolong the overall treatment time and conserve treatment resources. However, these advantages have to be carefully weighed against the increased risk of late normal tissue injury, and clinical trials are therefore necessary to fully evaluate the therapeutic gain compared with standard approaches.

## 11.4 THE TIME FACTOR FOR FRACTIONATED RADIOTHERAPY IN TUMOURS

Starting in the 1970s, studies on experimental tumours were beginning to find that clonogenic cells proliferate rapidly after irradiation (see Chapter 8) so predicting that the ability of clinical radiotherapy to achieve local tumour control would decrease with increasing overall treatment time. Several experimental studies indicate that repopulation of clonogenic tumour cells accelerates at some point during fractionated radiotherapy (see Chapters 9 and 10). It should also be noted that other mechanisms such as long repair half-times or increasing radiobiological hypoxia during treatment might contribute to a detrimental effect of long overall treatment times on tumour control.

The possible existence of a time factor in clinical radiotherapy became widely acknowledged following a publication by Withers et al. (30) entitled 'The hazard of accelerated tumor clonogen repopulation during radiotherapy'. This review examined the correlation between tumour control and overall treatment time for squamous cell carcinomas of the head and neck and led to the diagram shown in Figure 11.3a: this shows the dose required to achieve tumour control in 50% of cases (i.e. $TCD_{50}$ values) plotted against the overall treatment time. The LQ model was used with an $\alpha/\beta$ value of 25 Gy to convert from the actual doses per fraction used in the various protocols into equivalent doses using 2 Gy per fraction (EQD2; see Chapter 9). The various studies also achieved different tumour control rates and it was therefore necessary to interpolate or extrapolate to the 50% control level. This required dose effect estimations, for example it was assumed that the dose to increase tumour control from 40% to 60% was 2.9 Gy. As can be seen from Figure 11.3a, this retrospective review of head and neck cancer data found that with increase of overall time a greater total radiation dose had been required to control these tumours. The other important conclusion was that there appeared to be an initial flat portion to this relationship (the 'dog-leg'); that is, for treatment times shorter than 3–4 weeks, tumour proliferation had little effect and that, as shown for experimental tumours, it also takes time for accelerated repopulation to be 'switched on' in human tumours. Withers et al. (30) concluded that for treatment times longer than

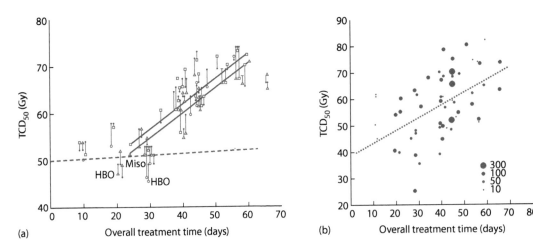

(a)    Overall treatment time (days)

(b)    Overall treatment time (days)

Figure 11.3 Tumour control dose (TCD$_{50}$) in head and neck cancer as a function of overall treatment time, normalised to a dose per fraction of 2 Gy. The same large set of clinical studies has been retrospectively summarised by (a) Withers et al. (30) and (b) Bentzen et al. (7). In panel (b) each point indicates the result of a particular trial, the size of the symbol indicating the size of the trial. There is a trend for the curative radiation dose to increase with overall treatment time, although the details of this association differ between the two studies.

4 weeks, the effect of proliferation was equivalent to a loss of radiation dose of about 0.6 Gy per day.

This publication gave rise to considerable debate. Subsequent analyses of the same clinical data by different authors (7,14) are shown in Figures 11.3b and 11.4. The analysis of Bentzen and Thames (7) made a different assumption about the steepness of dose-response curves: the dose to increase tumour control from 40% to 60% was taken to be 10.5 rather than 2.9 Gy, thought to be more clinically realistic. In addition, the data points in Figure 11.3b were drawn to indicate the size of the patient sample from which the estimate of TCD$_{50}$ had been made. Figure 11.3b suggests that the 'lag' period before commencement of repopulation may have been somewhat exaggerated by the plot shown in Figure 11.3a, although this issue is still actively discussed. Furthermore, the analysis by Dubben used the same radiobiological assumptions as the review by Withers et al. (30) and showed that the actual local tumour control rates could be replaced by random numbers without changing the conclusion of Figure 11.3a. As shown in Figure 11.4, the reason for this completely unexpected finding was a highly significant correlation between TCD$_{50}$ and the prescribed total dose (normalized to 2 Gy fractions). Dubben's conclusion was that the increase of TCD$_{50}$ with increasing treatment duration in Figure 11.3a reflects only dose-time prescriptions and that these data neither confirm nor exclude a time factor of fractionated radiotherapy. The comparison among these three analyses of the same data set is a good example of how difficult it is to draw reliable conclusions based on retrospective analyses of clinical data.

If we accept the data summarised in Figure 11.3b, the slope of the line indicates that 0.48 Gy per day is recovered during fractionated radiotherapy of head and neck squamous cell carcinoma. If we further accept that this effect is caused by repopulation and assume reasonable estimates of tumour cell radiosensitivity, we can deduce a clonogen doubling time of less than 1 week, similar to the values of

pre-treatment potential doubling times measured in human tumours (see Tables 8.4 and 8.5). The potential doubling time ($T_{pot}$) is a cell kinetic parameter that indicates the rate at which cells are proliferating in an untreated tumour. Although there is much uncertainty about this, it has been suggested that during treatment the rate at which clonogenic cells within the tumour repopulate may also resemble the $T_{pot}$ value. Thus, accelerated fractionation, which uses a reduced overall treatment time below the conventional 6–7 weeks, should increase tumour cure rates by restricting the time available for tumour cell proliferation. From Figure 11.3b, for example, the dose in a 5-week schedule would be effectively larger than that in a 7-week schedule by a factor $0.48 \times (7-5) \times 7 = 6.7$ Gy, or nearly 10% of a 70 Gy treatment.

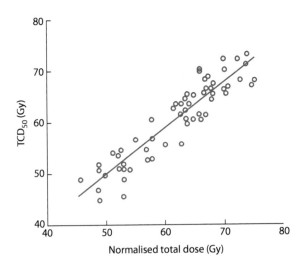

Figure 11.4 The clinical data shown in panels a and b of Figure 11.3 as reanalysed by Dubben (14). Tumour control dose is plotted against the prescribed total dose, normalised to a dose per fraction of 2 Gy. The positive trend in these data indicates a possible prescription bias.

## 11.5 CLINICAL EVALUATION OF ACCELERATED RADIOTHERAPY

Through the joint activities of radiation biologists and clinicians, accelerated fractionation schedules have been developed that aim to counteract the rapid repopulation of clonogenic cells during therapy (see Section 11.4). *Accelerated fractionation* is defined as a shortening of the overall treatment time or, more precisely, as an increase of the average dose per week above the 10 Gy given in conventional fractionation. *Early* normal tissue reactions are expected to increase using accelerated radiotherapy (see Chapter 12). In contrast, if recovery from sublethal radiation damage between fractions is complete (see Chapter 9), *late* normal tissue damage is expected to remain constant for accelerated fractionation schedules using 1.8–2 Gy fractions and total doses comparable to conventional fractionation. If the total dose and/or the dose per fraction is reduced (sometimes termed *accelerated-hyperfractionation*) late normal tissue damage could even decrease.

To test these ideas, many clinical trials of accelerated radiotherapy have been set up. Currently, 15 prospective randomised trials have been reported for head and neck, small cell or non-small cell lung cancer. Those trials, along with a meta-analysis (9) indicate that, for a given total dose, accelerated fractionation schedules are more effective in obtaining local tumour control than conventional fractionation schedules, or that the results are at least identical to conventional fractionation despite administering a reduced total dose in the accelerated arm. Overall, these studies on more than 7000 patients provide strong support for the existence of a significant time factor for tumours. In addition, retrospective data support the existence of time factors also for carcinoma of the cervix uteri and corpus uteri, prostate cancer, breast cancer and anal cancer (reviewed

in [11]). Recent re-analyses of randomised hypofractionation (and at the same time acceleration) trials in breast cancer support the existence of a time factor with a repopulation dose equivalent of 0.6 Gy/day for the endpoint of loco-regional recurrence (17). The following paragraphs describe some of the randomised trials of accelerated radiotherapy in more detail.

The continuous hyperfractionated accelerated radiotherapy (CHART) protocol, as an example of strongly accelerated fractionation, applies 36 fractions of 1.5 Gy over 12 consecutive days (including weekend), using three fractions per day with an interval of 6 hours between the fractions within each day. The total dose is reduced to 54 Gy compared with conventional therapy (here 60 Gy), in order to remain within the tolerance of acutely responding epithelial tissues. In the CHART head and neck trial, 918 patients were randomised between CHART and conventional fractionation in 2 Gy fractions to 66 Gy (13). Figure 11.5a shows that loco-regional tumour control was identical in both treatment arms. CHART used 12 Gy less than conventional therapy in an overall time reduced by 33 days. If this dose reduction is thought to just offset repopulation, this would correspond to 0.36 Gy per day lost through tumour cell proliferation, which is somewhat lower than the 0.48 Gy per day from the data in Figure 11.3b. This could be interpreted to mean that the lag period before onset of accelerated repopulation in head and neck carcinoma is longer than the 12 day duration of a course of CHART, but further data are required to confirm this. Overall patient survival was identical in both treatment arms (Figure 11.5b). As expected for accelerated radiotherapy, radiation mucositis was more severe with CHART; it occurred earlier but settled sooner. Unexpectedly, skin reactions were less severe and settled more quickly in the CHART-treated patients. For a number of late morbidities, a reduced severity was found

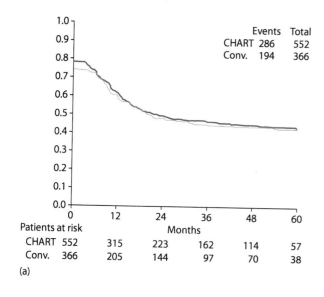

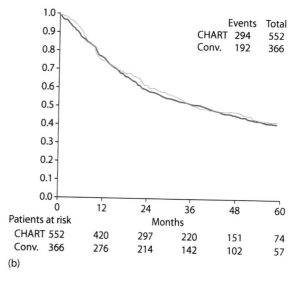

**Figure 11.5** Results of a phase III randomised trial of CHART in squamous cell carcinoma of the head and neck. (a) Probability of loco-regional tumour control. (b) Probability of overall survival of patients treated by CHART (bold line) and by conventional radiotherapy (solid line). (From (13), with permission.)

after CHART, but the magnitude of these differences would not allow a substantial increase in the total dose of CHART without increasing the risk of late damage over the rate observed for conventional fractionation. The overall conclusion is that CHART improved the therapeutic ratio in head and neck cancer by a small margin.

In the CHART Bronchus trial, 563 patients with non-small cell lung cancer were randomised between CHART (as described above) and conventional fractionation to 60 Gy in 2 Gy fractions (23,24). Despite the lower total dose, survival after 2 years was significantly increased by 9%, from 21% in the conventional arm to 30% in the CHART arm (Figure 11.6a). Exploratory analysis revealed that this was a consequence of improved local tumour control (Figure 11.6b) and, in squamous cell carcinoma, also a reduced incidence of distant metastases. Oesophagitis occurred earlier and reached higher scores in CHART patients, but symptoms also settled earlier and were of no major concern on longer follow-up. Pneumonitis was not decreased in the CHART arm. The overall conclusion of this study was that compared to conventional fractionation with 60 Gy, CHART offers a significant therapeutic benefit for patients with non-small cell lung cancer. Adapting the CHART protocol for 5 treatment days per week (CHART weekend-less = CHARTWEL), no significant difference in local tumour control and survival was detected between CHARTWEL to 60 Gy and conventional fractionation to 66 Gy in non-small cell lung cancer. However, CHARTWEL was, despite its lower total dose, more effective in larger primary tumours and after neoadjuvant chemotherapy (3,25), the latter supporting pre-clinical data on induction of repopulation by chemotherapy (see Section 11.6).

The DAHANCA 6&7 trial (21) provides an example of weakly accelerated radiotherapy. In the trial, 1476 eligible patients were randomly assigned five ($n = 726$)

or six ($n = 750$) fractions per week at the same total dose and fraction number (66–68 Gy in 33–34 fractions; 62 Gy to well-differentiated T1 glottic tumours). All patients, except those with glottic cancers, also received the hypoxic radiosensitizer nimorazole (see Chapter 17). Overall 5 year locoregional control rates were improved from 60% to 70% by accelerated fractionation ($p < 0.0005$). Disease-specific survival improved (73 versus 66% for six and five fractions, $p < 0.01$) but not overall survival. Acute but transient morbidity was significantly more frequent with six than with five fractions. The overall conclusion of this study is that shortening of overall treatment time by increase of the weekly number of fractions is beneficial in patients with head and neck cancer. Very importantly, the DAHANCA trial as well as some other clinical studies clearly show that not only large differences in overall treatment time but also a comparably small difference of only 1 week influences substantially the probability to achieve local tumour control.

In the EORTC 22851 trial (19), 512 patients with head and neck cancer received their treatment either conventionally in a median overall time of 54 days (1.8–2 Gy per fraction each day, total 35–40 fractions, 5 days per week) or accelerated in a median of 33 days (1.6 Gy per fraction three times per day, 4 hours minimum inter-fraction interval, total 45 fractions, 5 days per week, overall time allocated to 8 days radiotherapy, 12–14 days gap, 17 days radiotherapy). Patients who received the accelerated treatment showed an increase in loco-regional tumour control from 46% to 59% at 5 years (Figure 11.7a); there was no increase in survival compared with patients receiving conventional treatment. Early radiation effects, particularly mucositis, were much more pronounced in the accelerated arm. Thirty-eight percent of patients had to be hospitalised for acute toxicity compared with only 7% of the patients in the conventional arm. Figure 11.7b shows that grades 3 and 4 late damage (EORTC/RTOG scale) also occurred significantly more frequently

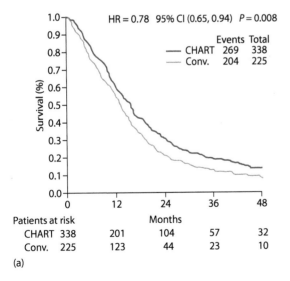

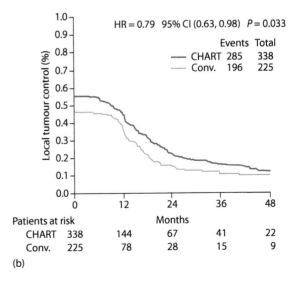

Figure 11.6 Results of a phase III randomised trial of CHART in non-small cell lung cancer. (a) Overall survival. (b) Local tumour control of patients treated by CHART or by conventional radiotherapy (CHART results are indicated by the heavier line). (From (24), with permission.)

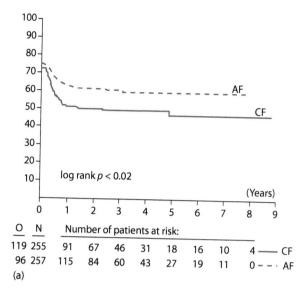

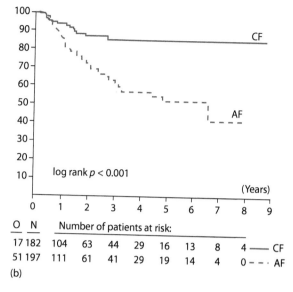

Figure 11.7 Results of the EORTC (22851) trial of accelerated fractionation. (a) Loco-regional tumour control (log rank $p < 0.02$). (b) Patients free of severe radiation effects, grade 3 and 4 (log rank $p < 0.001$). (From (19), with permission.)

after the accelerated fractionation than after conventional fractionation ($p < 0.001$). The probability of being free of severe late damage at 3 years was 85% in the conventional arm but only 63% in the accelerated arm. With increasing follow-up this difference is even increasing. Most of the difference in late effects has been attributable to late damage to connective tissues and mucosal sequelae.

In summary, accelerated fractionation has been shown in randomized clinical trials to counteract the time factor in head and neck and lung cancer. Some of the trials indicate an improved therapeutic ratio compared with conventional fractionation. However, one of the most intriguing biological observations from the clinical trials on accelerated fractionation is that sparing of late normal tissue morbidity compared to conventional fractionation was much less than anticipated. In fact, late damage in the EORTC trial was even higher than after conventional fractionation. Possible reasons for these unexpected findings are discussed in the following text.

## 11.6 TIME FACTOR FOR COMBINED RADIOCHEMOTHERAPY

Although there is sufficient evidence for a time factor when radiotherapy is applied alone (see Section 11.5), it is currently controversial whether and at which magnitude a time factor may also affect the results of radiochemotherapy. The current knowledge can be summarized as follows: If chemotherapy and radiotherapy are applied sequentially, a number of clinical data sets support the existence of an important time factor with the caveat that overall treatment time is here the time between onset of the first and end of the last treatment, i.e. for example between the first day of chemotherapy and the last day of radiotherapy (reviewed in [11]). In line with that, after induction, chemotherapy accelerated fractionation

appears to be more effective than conventional fractionation in non-small cell lung cancer (3,12).

If chemotherapy is applied simultaneously to radiotherapy, the situation is different: at least in head and neck cancer, simultaneous radiochemotherapy based on conventionally fractionated radiotherapy is superior to accelerated radiotherapy without chemotherapy, suggesting that repopulation during radiotherapy may at least in part be counteracted by simultaneous chemotherapy (8,10,11). This seems not to be true for small cell lung cancer, where improved survival has been shown after accelerated fractionation simultaneous to chemotherapy, compared to conventional fractionation (28). It is currently not clear what mechanisms underlie the different results. Besides the different tumour entities, for example, the specifics of radiotherapy or chemotherapy could be a reason.

## 11.7 COMPARISON BETWEEN HYPERFRACTIONATION AND ACCELERATED FRACTIONATION

Bourhis et al. (9) have reported a meta-analysis of hyperfractionation and accelerated radiotherapy in patients with head and neck tumours. This analysis included 15 randomized trials with a total of 6515 patients, all randomized between conventional radiotherapy and hyperfractionated or accelerated radiotherapy. The majority of patients had stage III or IV oropharyngeal or laryngeal squamous cell carcinoma and were monitored with a median follow-up of 6 years. Overall, a 3%–4% significant increase in overall survival (hazard ratio 0.92, $p < 0.003$) was found. Loco-regional control was significantly higher after altered fractionation (6.4% at 5 years, $p < 0.0001$ (Table 11.1). No effect was observed with altered fractionation on distant metastasis. The survival advantage was more pronounced

Table 11.1 Hazard ratio of altered fractionated radiotherapy versus conventional radiotherapy on overall population and by type of radiotherapy for locoregional, local, regional and metastatic control (number of patients = 7073)

| | Hyperfractionation | Accelerated radiotherapy (no dose reduction) | Accelerated radiotherapy (dose reduction) | Overall | P-value |
|---|---|---|---|---|---|
| Locoregional | 0.76 (0.66–0.89)[a] | 0.79 (0.72–0.87) | 0.90 (0.80–1.02) | 0.82 (0.77–0.88) | <0.0001 |
| Local | 0.75 (0.63–0.89) | 0.74 (0.67–0.83) | 0.83 (0.71–0.96) | 0.77 (0.71–0.83) | <0.0001 |
| Regional | 0.83 (0.66–1.03) | 0.90 (0.77–1.04) | 0.87 (0.72–1.06) | 0.87 (0.79–0.97) | <0.01 |
| Metastatic | 1.09 (0.76–1.58) | 0.93 (0.74–1.19) | 0.95 (0.68–1.32) | 0.97 (0.82–1.15) | >0.75 |

Reproduced from (9), with permission.

[a] 95% confidence intervals.

with hyperfractionation (8% at 5 years) than with accelerated fractionation (2% for regimens without dose reduction and 1.7% for regimens with dose reduction). Interestingly, the survival advantage observed with altered fractionation regimens is of the same order of magnitude seen with concomitant chemo-radiotherapy regimens (see Chapter 19), indicating that the debate on the relative merits of these two strategies is likely to continue.

## 11.8 SPLIT-COURSE RADIOTHERAPY

Intentional gaps in radiation therapy have sometimes been introduced in order to allow recovery of early responding normal tissues. However, if such gaps prolong the overall treatment time then local tumour control rates are expected to decrease. The DAHANCA 6&7 data (see Section 11.5), for example imply that even small prolongations of overall treatment times in the order of one or a few days should be avoided. If this is not possible, appropriate compensation has to be applied. Studies on experimental tumours suggest that, for a given overall treatment time, the magnitude of the time factor is the same for continuous fractionation or for fractionation protocols including gaps (4). This supports the current clinical guidelines for the compensation of unscheduled treatment gaps that are discussed in Chapter 10.

## 11.9 REASONS FOR INCREASED LATE NORMAL TISSUE DAMAGE AFTER MODIFIED FRACTIONATION

Hyperfractionation and accelerated radiotherapy both require multiple radiation treatments per day. In the case of hyperfractionation this is because application of only one small fraction per day would lead to very long overall treatment times. This would be unacceptable in view of the time factor for tumour-cell repopulation. In the case of accelerated radiotherapy, shortening the overall time but still giving one fraction per day would require an increase in dose per fraction; this would be expected to lead to an increase in late effects although hypofractionation is clinically useful in some situations (see Section 11.3).

A radiobiological constraint in giving multiple fractions per day is that the time interval between the fractions should not be too small because of incomplete repair (see Chapter 9). The damage inflicted by radiation is very largely repaired in most cell types, both normal and malignant (see Chapter 8.3). The repair of normal tissue stem cells is vital for their tolerance to radiation therapy. If fractions are given so close together that repair is incomplete, tissue tolerance will be reduced. Repair half-times for many tumours and normal tissues are in the region of 0.5–2 hours (Table 10.2). Assuming exponential decay of radiation damage, it takes six half-times for the damage to decay to 1/64, i.e. 1%–2% of its initial value. The problem is that, as shown in Table 10.2, some late-responding normal tissues appear to have long repair half-times. These tissues will therefore be especially disadvantaged by radiotherapy given with multiple fractions at a short inter-fraction interval; the therapeutic index will be impaired and the total radiation dose will have to be lowered in order to remain within tolerance. Most current schedules with multiple fractions per day employ inter-fraction times of at least 6 hours; in some situations even this gap may be too short.

Evidence on the clinical impact of incomplete repair comes from an analysis of data from the CHART head and neck trial (6). As noted previously, several late-damage endpoints were significantly reduced after CHART, compared with conventional treatment. The reduction was much less than expected on the basis of LQ calculations and analysis of these data yielded repair half-times in the range of 4–5 hours for laryngeal oedema, skin telangiectasia and subcutaneous fibrosis. This suggests that even 6 hours between dose fractions in schedules using multiple fractions per day may be too short for complete repair in some situations. Long repair half-times for late effects in human normal tissues therefore pose a significant problem for the development of novel fractionation schedules.

Consequential late effects (see Chapter 14) may also contribute to more than expected late morbidity after modified fractionation. Compared with conventional fractionation the dose per week is increased, both in accelerated radiotherapy and in hyperfractionation. This is expected to produce an increase in *early* normal tissue damage such as mucositis and more severe or more prolonged early damage may then lead to more pronounced consequential *late* effects.

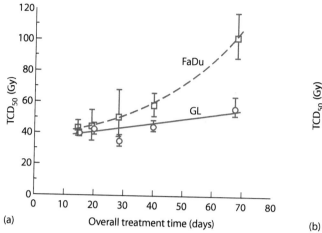 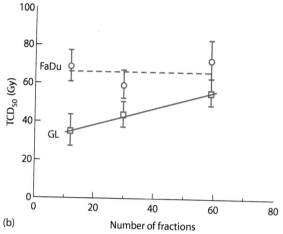

Figure 11.8 Tumour control dose in two experimental squamous cell carcinoma xenografts (FaDu, GL) as a function of overall treatment time for irradiation with 30 fractions (a) or as a function of number of fractions in a constant overall treatment time of 6 weeks (b). There are considerable differences in the response of these tumours to modification of the fractionation schedule. (See (4) sources.)

## 11.10 IS THE SAME MODIFIED FRACTIONATION SCHEDULE OPTIMAL FOR ALL PATIENTS?

Figure 11.8 summarises the results of experiments testing different modified fractionation schedules in two experimental squamous cell carcinomas xenografts in mice. After 30 fractions in FaDu tumours, the $TCD_{50}$ increased by roughly 0.6 Gy for each day of prolongation for overall treatment times up to 40 days but more steeply for longer times (panel a); this effect was much less pronounced (0.28 Gy per day) in GL squamous cell carcinomas. In contrast, when the number of fractions was increased from 12 to 60 in a constant overall treatment time of 6 weeks (panel b), the $TCD_{50}$ in FaDu tumours appeared to be constant while in GL tumours the $TCD_{50}$ increased with increasing fraction number. Both dose-escalated hyperfractionation and accelerated fractionation (using constant or reduced total doses) would be advantageous in human tumours that behave like FaDu. In contrast, for tumours like GL, dose-escalated hyperfractionation would at best yield identical control rates, while after accelerated fractionation with reduced total dose such tumours would do worse than with conventional radiotherapy. These results show that the response of experimental tumours to modified fractionation may be variable and it may well be that such heterogeneity also exists between tumours in patients.

Results from clinical studies always reflect the average effect of a treatment modification. For example, after the accelerated CHART treatment the local control rates of head and neck cancer were identical to those obtained after conventional fractionation with a 12 Gy higher total dose (see Section 11.5). Under the assumption of inter-tumour heterogeneity, this would mean that some tumours with a small time factor that would have been controlled after conventional treatment to 66 Gy recurred after CHART treatment because of the reduction in total dose. This negative effect may have been compensated by additional local control

achieved in tumours that showed greater repopulation and a more pronounced time factor, i.e. tumours in which the dose recovered per day was higher than the average value of 0.36 Gy. To further improve the results of modified fractionation, we need to identify subgroups of patients who are likely to benefit from a particular modification, and thus to individualise treatment. Considerable efforts have been made to develop predictive tests. First results suggest for non-small cell lung cancer that larger tumours and tumours pre-treated with chemotherapy are more sensitive to accelerated fractionation (25).

### Key points

1. *Hyperfractionation* is the use of a reduced dose per fraction over a conventional overall treatment time, employing multiple fractions per day. A therapeutic advantage is thought to derive from the more rapid increase in tolerance with decreasing dose per fraction for late-responding normal tissues than for tumours.
2. *Accelerated radiotherapy* is the use of a reduced overall treatment time with a conventional dose per fraction, achieved using multiple fractions per day. The aim is to reduce the protective effect of tumour-cell repopulation during radiotherapy.
3. *Hypofractionation* is the use of doses per fraction higher than 2 Gy, which will increase late-responding normal tissue damage compared with conventional fractionation. For palliation, hypofractionation is routinely applied, but also for certain curative situations hypofractionation is an option.
4. Multiple fractions per day should be given as far apart as possible and certainly not closer than 6 hours.

# ■ BIBLIOGRAPHY

1. Agrawal RK, Alhasso A, Barrett-Lee PJ et al. First results of the randomised UK FAST Trial of radiotherapy hypofractionation for treatment of early breast cancer (CRUKE/04/015). *Radiother Oncol* 2011;100:93–100.

2. Baumann M, Bentzen SM, Ang KK. Hyperfractionated radiotherapy in head and neck cancer: A second look at the clinical data. *Radiother Oncol* 1998;46:127–130.

3. Baumann M, Herrmann T, Koch R et al. Studygroup CH-B. Final results of the randomized phase III CHARTWEL-trial (ARO 97-1) comparing hyperfractionated-accelerated versus conventionally fractionated radiotherapy in non-small cell lung cancer (NSCLC). *Radiother Oncol* 2011;100:76–85.

4. Baumann M, Petersen C, Wolf J, Schreiber A, Zips D. No evidence for a different magnitude of the time factor for continuously fractionated irradiation and protocols including gaps in two human squamous cell carcinoma in nude mice. *Radiother Oncol* 2001;59:187–194.

5. Beck-Bornholdt HP, Dubben HH, Liertz-Petersen C, Willers H. Hyperfractionation: Where do we stand? *Radiother Oncol* 1997;43:1–21.

6. Bentzen SM, Saunders MI, Dische S. Repair halftimes estimated from observations of treatment-related morbidity after CHART or conventional radiotherapy in head and neck cancer. *Radiother Oncol* 1999;53:219–226.

7. Bentzen SM, Thames HD. Clinical evidence for tumor clonogen regeneration: Interpretations of the data. *Radiother Oncol* 1991;22:161–166.

8. Bourhis J, Lapeyre M, Tortochaux J et al. Accelerated radiotherapy and concomitant high dose chemotherapy in non resectable stage IV locally advanced HNSCC: Results of a GORTEC randomized trial. *Radiother Oncol* 2011;100:56–61.

9. Bourhis J, Overgaard J, Audry H et al. Hyperfractionated or accelerated radiotherapy in head and neck cancer: A meta-analysis. *Lancet* 2006;368:843–854.

10. Bourhis J, Sire C, Graff P et al. Concomitant chemoradiotherapy versus acceleration of radiotherapy with or without concomitant chemotherapy in locally advanced head and neck carcinoma (GORTEC 99-02): An open-label phase 3 randomised trial. *Lancet Oncol* 2012;13:145–153.

11. Bütof R, Baumann M. Time in radiation oncology – Keep it short! *Radiother Oncol* 2013;106:271–275.

12. De Ruysscher D, van Baardwijk A, Steevens J et al. Individualised isotoxic accelerated radiotherapy and chemotherapy are associated with improved long-term survival of patients with stage III NSCLC: A prospective population-based study. *Radiother Oncol* 2012;102:228–233.

13. Dische S, Saunders M, Barrett A, Harvey A, Gibson D, Parmar M. A randomised multicentre trial of CHART versus conventional radiotherapy in head and neck cancer. *Radiother Oncol* 1997;44:123–136.

14. Dubben HH. Local control, TCD50 and dose-time prescription habits in radiotherapy of head and neck tumours. *Radiother Oncol* 1994;32:197–200.

15. Fletcher GH. Regaud lecture: Perspectives on the history of radiotherapy. *Radiother Oncol* 1988;12:253–271.

16. Fu KK, Pajak TF, Trotti A et al. A Radiation Therapy Oncology Group (RTOG) phase III randomized study to compare hyperfractionation and two variants of accelerated fractionation to standard fractionation radiotherapy for head and neck squamous cell carcinomas: First report of RTOG 9003. *Int J Radiat Oncol Biol Phys* 2000;48: 7–16.

17. Haviland JS, Bentzen SM, Bliss JM, Yarnold JR, START Trial Management Group. Prolongation of overall treatment time as a cause of treatment failure in early breast cancer: An analysis of the UK START (Standardisation of Breast Radiotherapy) trials of radiotherapy fractionation. *Radiother Oncol* 2016;121:420–423.

18. Holthusen H. Erfahrungen über die verträglichkeitsgrenze für röntgenstrahlen und deren nutzanwendung zur verhütung von schäden. *Strahlenther Onkol* 1936;57:254–269.

19. Horiot JC, Bontemps P, van den Bogaert W et al. Accelerated fractionation (AF) compared to conventional fractionation (CF) improves loco-regional control in the radiotherapy of advanced head and neck cancers: Results of the EORTC 22851 randomized trial. *Radiother Oncol* 1997;44:111–121.

20. Horiot JC, Le Fur R, N'Guyen T et al. Hyperfractionation versus conventional fractionation in oropharyngeal carcinoma: Final analysis of a randomized trial of the EORTC cooperative group of radiotherapy. *Radiother Oncol* 1992;25:231–241.

21. Overgaard J, Hansen HS, Specht L et al. Five compared with six fractions per week of conventional radiotherapy of squamous-cell carcinoma of head and neck: DAHANCA 6 and 7 randomised controlled trial. *Lancet* 2003;362: 933–940.

22. Owen JR, Ashton A, Bliss JM et al. Effect of radiotherapy fraction size on tumour control in patients with early-stage breast cancer after local tumour excision: Long-term results of a randomised trial. *Lancet Oncol* 2006;7:467–471.

23. Saunders M, Dische S, Barrett A, Harvey A, Gibson D, Parmar M. Continuous hyperfractionated accelerated radiotherapy (CHART) versus conventional radiotherapy in non-small-cell lung cancer: A randomised multicentre trial. *CHART Steering Committee. Lancet* 1997;350:161–165.

24. Saunders M, Dische S, Barrett A, Harvey A, Griffiths G, Palmar M. Continuous, hyperfractionated, accelerated radiotherapy (CHART) versus conventional radiotherapy in non-small cell lung cancer: Mature data from the randomised multicentre trial. *CHART Steering Committee. Radiother Oncol* 1999;52:137–148.

25. Soliman M, Yaromina A, Appold S et al. GTV differentially impacts locoregional control of non-small cell lung cancer (NSCLC) after different fractionation schedules: Subgroup analysis of the prospective randomized CHARTWEL trial. *Radiother Oncol* 2013;106:299–304.

26. START Trialists' Group; Agrawal RK, Aird EG, Barrett JM et al. The UK standardisation of breast radiotherapy (START) trial A of radiotherapy hypofractionation for treatment of early breast cancer: A randomised trial. *Lancet Oncol* 2008;9:331–341.

27. START Trialists' Group; Agrawal RK, Aird EG, Barrett JM et al. The UK Standardisation of Breast Radiotherapy (START) Trial B of radiotherapy hypofractionation for treatment of early breast cancer: A randomised trial. *Lancet* 2008;371:1098–1107.

28. Turrisi AT, Kim K, Blum R et al. Twice-daily compared with once-daily thoracic radiotherapy in limited small-cell lung cancer treated concurrently with cisplatin and etoposide. *N Engl J Med* 1999;340:265–271.

29. Whelan TJ, Pignol JP, Levine MN et al. Long-term results of hypofractionated radiation therapy for breast cancer. *N Engl J Med* 2010;362:513–520.

30. Withers HR, Taylor JM, Maciejewski B. The hazard of accelerated tumor clonogen repopulation during radiotherapy. *Acta Oncol* 1988;27:131–146.

# ■ FURTHER READING

31. Baumann M, Bentzen SM, Dörr W et al. The translational research chain: Is it delivering the goods? *Int J Radiat Oncol Biol Phys* 2001;49:345–351.

32. Thames HD, Peters LJ, Withers HR, Fletcher GH. Accelerated fractionation vs hyperfractionation: Rationales for several treatments per day. *Int J Radiat Oncol Biol Phys* 1983;9:127–138.

33. Thames HD, Withers HR, Peters LJ, Fletcher GH. Changes in early and late radiation responses with altered dose fractionation: Implications for dose-survival relationships. *Int J Radiat Oncol Biol Phys* 1982;8:219–226.

34. Withers HR, Maciejewski B, Taylor JMG. Biology of options in dose fractionation. In: McNally NJ, editor. *The Scientific Basis of Modern Radiotherapy*. London: The British Institute of Radiology; 1989. pp. 27–36.

# Time factors in normal tissue responses to irradiation

## WOLFGANG DÖRR

## 12.1 INTRODUCTION

The response of normal tissues to therapeutic radiation exposure must be considered over a wide range of overall treatment durations from minutes, e.g. in stereotactic single-dose treatment, to many months to years such as in re-irradiation scenarios (Figure 12.1). Several distinct processes define the time factor for treatment-induced morbidity, differently in different (groups of) tissues. First, on a short scale of minutes to hours, incomplete *recovery* of sublethal damage may reduce the radiation tolerance of a tissue, particularly with regard to late radiation sequelae. Second, over a range of days to weeks, i.e. during a regular course of fractionated radiotherapy with varying overall treatment times, radiation-induced tissue regeneration (*repopulation*) may modulate the radiation tolerance. This radiation-induced compensatory response is seen in early responding tissues. Third, over a range of months to years, long-term *restoration* can occur in some tissues, which renders them more resistant to re-irradiation. In contrast, also long-term *progression* of the damage can occur – even at subclinical levels – in other tissues, which causes decreased re-irradiation tolerance with increasing time after the first treatment.

In this book, the impact of incomplete recovery within short time intervals is covered in the chapters on fractionation and the linear-quadratic approach (see Chapters 9 and 10). The changes in radiation tolerance that may occur in intervals that are clearly longer than the general duration of a radiotherapy course are discussed in Chapter 23 on retreatment tolerance. Therefore, this chapter focuses on the impact of repopulation processes on early radiation effects and their principal mechanistic basis.

*Repopulation* is the term used to describe the regeneration response of early reacting tissues to fractionated irradiation, which results in an increase in radiation tolerance with increasing overall treatment time. The biological basis of repopulation is a complex restructuring of the proliferative organisation of the tissue. A number of clinical and experimental observations do assist in illuminating the biological mechanisms underlying the repopulation processes. The majority of investigations have been performed in oral mucosa, representing a dose-limiting early side effect in head and neck cancer radiotherapy (e.g. [23]), which will hence be considered as a model for the description of radiation-induced repopulation also in other early responding normal tissues.

## 12.2 CLINICAL OBSERVATIONS

A number of clinical studies with accelerated radiotherapy protocols, i.e. with a shortened overall treatment time, have resulted in an aggravation of early radiation side effects. The most prominent example is the CHART head and neck trial, where a total dose of 54 Gy was administered in 36 fractions in only 12 days, compared with 66 Gy given in 33 fractions in 6.5 weeks in the control arm (4). A significant shift of oral mucosal effects towards more severe, confluent reactions was observed, resulting in an incidence of 73% with CHART versus 43% with the conventional fractionation. Similarly, the EORTC 22851 trial, comparing 72 Gy in 5 weeks with 70 Gy given conventionally in 7 weeks, resulted in a clear increase in the rate of confluent mucositis during as well as 6 weeks after the end of radiotherapy in the accelerated arm (18), although the difference in overall treatment time was only 2 weeks.

Oral mucositis heals in a certain proportion of patients receiving radiotherapy for head and neck cancer during the last treatment weeks – while this is a rare observation at earlier phases of the therapy – when doses below 2 Gy are administered (16). A less frequent incidence of healing of oral mucositis in patients treated with accelerated versus conventional fractionation was also reported by Wygoda et al. (29). These studies indicate a time delay before repopulation becomes effective. Furthermore, as this healing response occurs in a clearly smaller fraction of patients at doses >2 Gy, or weekly doses >10 Gy, these data show that the repopulation capacity is limited by the daily or weekly radiation dose.

Oral mucositis has also been studied in split course regimens (20). In a first radiotherapy treatment block with 32 Gy in 12 days, 90% of the patients developed confluent reactions. After a split of 9–13 days, which was introduced to allow for healing of mucositis, a second block of radiotherapy (34–38 Gy/12–14 days) was administered. None of the same patients developed confluent mucosal reactions in the second series, even despite the slightly higher dose. This again indicates that the onset of repopulation occurs within the first weeks after the start of radiotherapy, and then becomes highly effective.

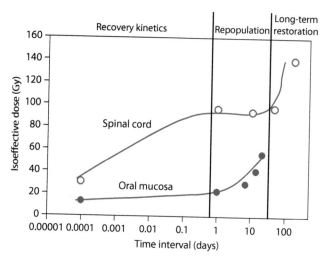

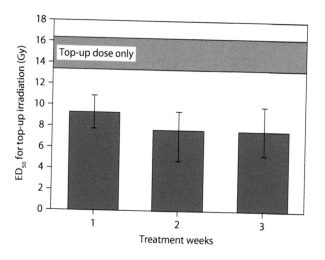

Figure 12.1 Changes in normal tissue tolerance with time. The figure compiles data for mouse oral mucosa (9,14), and for rat spinal cord (19,24). From the original data, isoeffective doses in 3 Gy fractions have been calculated using $\alpha/\beta$ values of 2 Gy for spinal cord and 11 Gy for oral mucosa. Note the log scale of the abscissa. At short durations of radiation exposure (<1 day), increasing completeness of recovery from sublethal damage increases tissue tolerance. At intermediate intervals from one day to several weeks, i.e. the duration of radiotherapy, tolerance increases by repopulation in early responding tissues like oral mucosa but not in late responding tissues like spinal cord. For long intervals clearly beyond the overall treatment time in radiotherapy, an increase in radiation tolerance by long-term restoration is seen in some (e.g. spinal cord), but not all late responding tissues.

## 12.3 EXPERIMENTAL OBSERVATIONS

The effects of changes in overall treatment time on normal tissue radiation tolerance have been studied in a number of early responding tissues, such as mouse epidermis, rat epidermis, pig epidermis, mouse lip mucosa and mouse tongue mucosa (6,17). One example is illustrated in Figure 12.2, in which oral mucosa was irradiated with 5 × 3 Gy/week over 1, 2 or 3 weeks (14), followed by graded test doses in order to assess the remaining radiation tolerance. Irradiation over 1 week clearly decreased the $ED_{50}$ (dose at which ulceration was expected in 50% of the animals) for the terminating test irradiation, which reflects the decrease in residual tissue tolerance by the fractionated dose. But – despite ongoing irradiation in weeks 2 and 3 – no further reduction in the test-$ED_{50}$ was found, indicating the onset of compensatory repopulation processes at the end of the first week.

In terms of changes in radiation tolerance during radiotherapy, a consistent pattern of the time course was found in most tissues studied (Figure 12.3): tolerance remained constant within the initial treatment period, and subsequently increased almost linearly. The time of onset of this increase was tissue dependent, at 5–7 days in mouse oral mucosa and skin, and 20–30 days in rat and pig skin (17).

Figure 12.2 Changes in mucosal radiation tolerance with overall treatment time. Mouse tongue mucosa was irradiated with 5 × 3 Gy/week over 1, 2 or 3 weeks, followed by graded test doses (14). Irradiation over 1 week decreased the $ED_{50}$ (dose at which mucosal ulceration occurs in 50% of the animals) from about 15 Gy in control animals to 9.3 Gy, the difference reflecting the biological effect of 5 × 3 Gy. Despite administration of a further 15 Gy per week, the $ED_{50}$ after 2 weeks was only slightly lower (7.7 Gy) and no further reduction was found after the third treatment week ($ED_{50} = 7.6$ Gy). Error bars indicate 95% confidence intervals.

The initial drop at short treatment intervals that was seen in some studies can be related to radiation-induced changes in the capacity for recovery of sublethal damage, which have been reported for these early responding tissues (8).

The capacity for repopulation, once the compensatory processes have started, was estimated by Dörr (6) in terms of the dose (expressed in the number of 2 Gy fractions) that was compensated per day. In human oral mucosa, 0.5–1.0 fractions are counteracted per day, thus confirming the clinical results on mucositis healing despite ongoing radiotherapy (see previous text). These experimental data indicate similar numbers – close to 1 fraction of 2 Gy per day – for most tissues, with a few possible exceptions, e.g. mouse epidermis (3), which might be related to the experimental design. In some experiments, where various weekly doses were applied (e.g. [15]), a dependence of the repopulation rate on the dose intensity (Gy per week) was observed.

In mouse oral mucosa, the functional measurements of radiation tolerance have been supplemented by detailed histological assessments of changes in mucosal cell density and proliferation (5,14). A reduction in cell number to approximately 70% occurred during the first week of daily fractionated treatment. Subsequently, constant to increasing cell numbers were found, despite continuing irradiation at the same dose intensity. In agreement, mucosal proliferation was significantly suppressed during the first week, but subsequently returned to subnormal to near normal values (5). Similar observations have been made in other tissues (25). In good accordance, in human oral mucosa a reduction

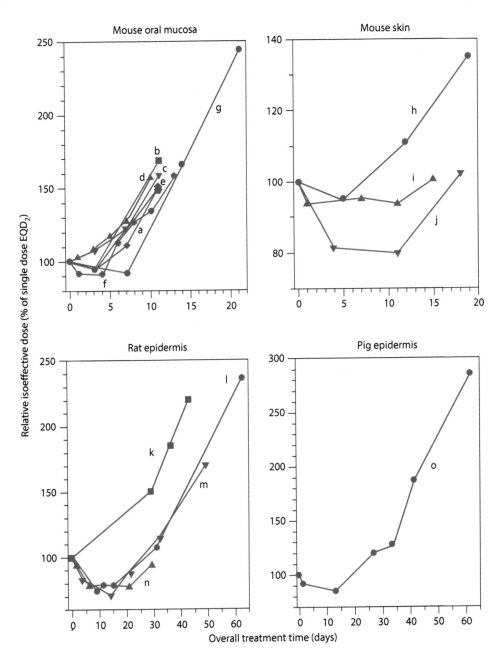

**Figure 12.3** Time course of repopulation: Experimental results. From reports in the literature of studies with variations in overall treatment time, the equieffective dose, EQD2$_{10\,Gy}$, has been calculated for the individual overall treatment times using an $\alpha/\beta$ value of 10 Gy. Note the different time scales of the abscissae. Treatment protocols and references are (a) 2 F (2); (b) 2 × 5 F (2); (c) 10 F (2); (d) 13 Gy + 1 F (14); (e) 10 Gy + 1 F (14); (f) 8 Gy + 1 F (Dörr and Spekl, unpublished); (g) 5 × 3 Gy/week (14); (h) 5 × 3 Gy/week (25); (i) 5 × 3 Gy/wk (3); (j) 2 F (1); (k) 5 × 3 Gy/week (27); (l) 10 F (21); (m) 3 F/week (21); (n) 5 F/week (21); (o) 2 F (26).

of cell production and consequently a steep decline in cell numbers were observed over the initial week of radiotherapy (12). Subsequently, proliferation rates were partially restored and cell depletion occurred significantly slower.

## 12.4 MECHANISMS OF REPOPULATION

Three important observations have been made in both clinical and experimental studies: (1) dose is compensated with increasing overall treatment time once repopulation has become effective; (2) the rate at which this compensation occurs is in the range of 5 × 2 Gy/week; and (3) the physiological loss of cells is counteracted once the lag phase before repopulation has ended, resulting in more or less constant cell numbers. In general, the mechanisms of repopulation that can explain these observations may be described by the following *3 A's*: asymmetry loss and acceleration of stem cell divisions, and abortive divisions of doomed cells (5).

## Asymmetry loss

According to the stem cell concept (see Chapter 14), the radiation tolerance of a tissue is defined by the number of tissue stem cells present at the time of irradiation, and their intrinsic radiosensitivity. Hence, radiation tolerance must decrease during fractionated irradiation according to the daily stem cell kill. This is clearly seen during the time lag before the onset of repopulation. However, after repopulation has started, the effect of at least part of the radiation dose is counteracted. This indicates that new stem cells must be produced that replace those sterilized by the irradiation.

In unperturbed turnover tissues, stem cells divide on average into one new stem cell and one differentiating cell (see Chapters 14 and 15). These divisions are called *asymmetrical*, as two different cells are generated. In this setting, the number of stem cells in each cell generation remains constant; it must be emphasized that this is independent of the proliferation rate. For additional production of new stem cells, as postulated on the basis of dose compensation during repopulation, at least a fraction of stem cell divisions must result in two stem cell daughters; this pattern is depicted as symmetrical division. Therefore, an *asymmetry loss* of stem cell divisions is one essential mechanism underlying repopulation in normal tissues. This loss can be complete, with two stem cell daughters from each division, or incomplete, with – on average – less than two, but more than one stem cell generated per stem cell division. A fraction of these divisions, presumably of cells with gross radiation-induced chromosomal damage, are abortive and can be observed histologically as abnormal mitotic figures (5), which in consequence result in bi- or multinucleate cells.

## Acceleration of stem cell proliferation

As illustrated earlier, human oral mucosa and also other tissues are able to compensate weekly doses of about five times 0.5 to 1.0 fractions of 2 Gy. For this to occur, assuming the surviving fraction of the stem cells after each radiation fraction to be about 0.5, five symmetrical divisions are needed within 7 days. This requires an average cell cycle time of 1.4 days if all divisions are symmetrical. Compared with cell-cycle times of at least 3.5 days in unperturbed tissue (5), this indicates clear *acceleration of stem cell proliferation* as the second mechanism of repopulation. Cell-cycle times must be even shorter if the asymmetry loss is incomplete, or if higher doses (associated with more stem cell kill) are compensated. The detailed interrelation between surviving fraction, number of symmetrical divisions between fractions and the proportion of symmetrical divisions is discussed by Dörr (5).

The degree to which the stem cell proliferation is accelerated is highly dependent on the radiation dose administered, i.e. on the daily or weekly stem cell kill (6). For example, in oral mucosa irradiated with 5 × 3.5 Gy/week, this dose was completely counteracted by repopulation in weeks 2 and 3 (14). However, during treatment with only 5 × 2.5 Gy/week, repopulation was exactly adjusted to just compensate this lower dose, despite the clearly higher regenerative capacity.

In the vast majority of tissues, no specific marker yet exists that would allow for the specific identification of stem cells. Therefore, cell kinetic studies can only assess proliferation of the entire cell population. After the lag phase of repopulation, i.e. after the initial treatment-associated cell kill, stem cells only comprise a minor fraction of the general population, and hence, such proliferation studies are not suitable to identify the acceleration at the stem cell level. However, in the intestinal crypts, which have well-defined localisation of the stem cell population, a significant shortening of the stem cell cycle time after irradiation has indeed been described (28), which reflects accelerated repopulation, albeit after single doses.

## Abortive divisions

After the onset of repopulation, the overall cell number in the tissue remains at a near constant, although reduced level that results from the lag phase. In contrast, it has been shown that differentiation and cell loss, e.g. at the surface of mucosal tissues, continue at a normal, physiological rate (11). Also, overall cell production, which can be directly measured, continues, which corresponds to the lack of change in cell numbers (10). Hence, the question arises, if this cell production can be based only on the surviving stem cells.

In unperturbed mucosa, with a relative stem cell number of 100%, the cells proliferate with a cell-cycle time of at least 3.5 days (10). A dose of 5 × 2 Gy during the first treatment week, before repopulation sets in, reduces the stem cell number to clearly below 10%. Hence, to result in the same number of cells as in untreated tissue, the remaining stem cells would have to proliferate with a cycle time of only a few hours (5,10). This is extremely unlikely on the basis of epithelial biology, which indicates a minimum cell-cycle time of 8–12 hours. Therefore, cells must be produced from other sources.

It has been shown *in vitro* (see Chapter 3) that "sterilized" cells can still undergo a limited number of divisions even after high doses of radiation. It can therefore be assumed, and indirectly concluded from experimental studies (11), that similarly *in vivo*, *abortive divisions* of sterilized or doomed cells can occur. This limited proliferative activity results in daughter cells that undergo near normal differentiation, and hence, counteract the ongoing cell loss. Quantitatively, in oral mucosa, the radiation-sterilized cells on average have to undergo two to three abortive divisions each in order to account for the cell production measured.

## 12.5 REGULATION OF REPOPULATION

The time at which repopulation processes become effective is tissue specific (Figure 12.3) and we may assume that it correlates with the turnover time of the tissue, and therefore the rate at which cells are lost. Reduced cell numbers may result in changes in intercellular communication or altered cell-matrix interactions, stimulating proliferation (see Chapter 14). This correlation between tissue turnover and lag time of repopulation, however, is only weak (6), and therefore other factors must also be important.

It has been demonstrated that the lag time before the start of repopulation is shorter, if the radiation dose is higher (6,14). This suggests that the rate at which stem cells are depleted may regulate the onset of repopulation. Autoregulatory processes within the stem cell compartment have also been suggested for intestinal crypts (22). The reduction in stem cell numbers can result in – still unidentified – intercellular signals, which eventually prevent the daughter cells of the stem cell divisions from undergoing differentiation, and thus effectively force them to remain in the stem cell compartment.

The regulation of the asymmetry loss is a very precise and rapidly responding mechanism. During short treatment breaks, even during weekends, the overall cell production clearly increases (18). However, the radiation tolerance of the tissue during these breaks remains almost constant, indicating that the cells that are produced are not stem cells (6). Hence, despite stimulated symmetrical stem cell divisions during the daily fractionated treatment, the stem cells quickly return to asymmetrical divisions if only one radiation fraction is missing at the start of the break.

Acceleration of stem cell divisions may be caused by overall cell depletion and also by impairment of the epithelial barrier function (10,25), which may increase the normal signals that physiologically regulate proliferation. This hypothesis is supported by increased proliferation rates after chemical ablation of superficial mucosal material, which has been observed in mice and humans, or after mechanical ablation ('tape stripping') in rodents. This increased proliferation rate, however, is not associated with increased tolerance to single-dose irradiation, i.e. increased stem cell numbers. This indicates that acceleration has occurred independently of the asymmetry loss. It must be assumed that sterilized cells initially continue to proliferate at nearly the rate of the stem cell divisions, before chromosomal damage accumulates and decreases the proliferation rate.

In combination with the asymmetry loss, e.g. by fractionated irradiation, artificially increased stem cell proliferation rates, however, may shorten the lag time before repopulation becomes effective. This has been demonstrated for chemical ablation in human oral mucosa (20). A similar mechanism has been suggested for the increase in mucosal radiation tolerance after administration of keratinocyte growth factor (KGF; Palifermin) in pre-clinical and clinical studies as reviewed by Dörr (7), and summarized in Chapter 24.

In conclusion (Figure 12.4), the asymmetry loss in the stem cell compartment is regulated independently of the acceleration of proliferation, presumably by autoregulatory processes on the basis of stem cell depletion. Acceleration of the stem cell divisions, in contrast, is controlled by

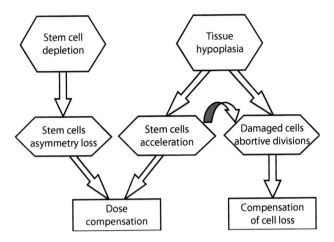

**Figure 12.4** Regulation of repopulation. Stem cell depletion, via autoregulatory processes, results in the loss of the division asymmetry of the stem cells. Tissue hypoplasia controls the acceleration of stem cell division and presumably also the rate of abortive division, which is indirectly also defined by the proliferation rate of the stem cells. Asymmetry loss and acceleration of stem cell division account for compensation of dose, while abortive divisions of sterilized cells counteract the overall cell loss to maintain tissue function.

overall tissue hypoplasia. The stem cell proliferation rate then translates into the initial rate of abortive divisions of sterilized cells, which subsequently decelerates with accumulation of damage. However, the doomed cells may also directly respond to paracrine signals released due to tissue hypoplasia.

## 12.6 CONSEQUENTIAL LATE EFFECTS

Consequential late effects are chronic normal tissue complications, which are influenced by the extent, i.e. severity and/or duration, of the *early* response in the same tissue or organ (13), as explained in Chapter 14. As the early response depends on the overall treatment time on the basis of repopulation processes, the same is therefore true for the corresponding consequential late effects. This has been demonstrated in experimental studies for intestinal fibrosis, and in clinical studies for skin telangiectasia, and for late (mucosa related) side effects after head and neck irradiation, as reviewed by Dörr and Hendry (13).

## 12.7 CONCLUSIONS

Repopulation processes that occur in early responding normal tissues follow a very complex biology. The major biological mechanisms are asymmetry loss and acceleration of stem cell division, as well as abortive divisions of sterilized cells. A number of parameters, which modulate the repopulation response, such as dose intensity (weekly dose), have been identified. However, the precise (molecular) regulatory mechanisms of tissue repopulation during fractionated radiotherapy still remain largely unclear. These regulatory signals would be attractive targets for biologically based modulation of radiation effects in early responding normal tissues, and thus also corresponding consequential late effects.

The convolution of all the underlying biology of repopulation also indicates that a time factor, in the sense of compensated dose, should be included in mathematical models of normal tissue complications (NTCP) only with great care and caution, if at all, as these models currently do not include the dominating repopulation-modifying factors.

---

## Key points

1. The radiation tolerance of typical early responding normal tissues increases with increasing overall treatment time. This also applies to the consequential component of late radiation effects.
2. This process is depicted as repopulation.
3. Repopulation starts after a tissue-specific lag time.
4. The biological basis is a complex restructuring of the proliferative tissue organisation.
5. This includes asymmetry loss and acceleration of stem cell proliferation.
6. Abortive divisions of doomed cells significantly contribute to cell production.
7. Tissue hypoplasia controls stem cell acceleration and abortive divisions, while the asymmetry loss is regulated by stem cell depletion.

---

## ■ BIBLIOGRAPHY

1. Ang KK, Landuyt W, Rijnders A, van der Schueren E. Differences in repopulation kinetics in mouse skin during split course multiple fractions per day (MFD) or daily fractionated irradiations. *Int J Radiat Oncol Biol Phys* 1984;10:95–99.
2. Ang KK, Xu FX, Vanuytsel L, van der Schueren E. Repopulation kinetics in irradiated mouse lip mucosa: The relative importance of treatment protraction and time distribution of irradiations. *Radiat Res* 1985;101:162–169.
3. Denekamp J. Changes in the rate of repopulation during multifraction irradiation of mouse skin. *Br J Radiol* 1973;46:381–387.
4. Dische S, Saunders M, Barrett A, Harvey A, Gibson D, Parmar M. A randomised multicentre trial of CHART versus conventional radiotherapy in head and neck cancer. *Radiother Oncol* 1997;44:123–136.
5. Dörr W. Three A's of repopulation during fractionated irradiation of squamous epithelia: Asymmetry loss, Acceleration of stem-cell divisions and Abortive divisions. *Int J Radiat Biol* 1997;72:635–643.
6. Dörr W. Modulation of repopulation processes in oral mucosa: Experimental results. *Int J Radiat Biol* 2003;79:531–537.
7. Dörr W. Oral mucosa: Response modification by keratinocyte growth factor. In: Nieder C, Milas L and Ang KK, editors. *Modification of Radiation Response: Cytokines, Growth Factors and Other Biological Targets.* Berlin: Springer-Verlag; 2003, pp. 113–122.
8. Dörr W, Brankovic K, Hartmann B. Repopulation in mouse oral mucosa: Changes in the effect of dose fractionation. *Int J Radiat Biol* 2000;76:383–390.
9. Dörr W, Breitner A, Kummermehr J. Capacity and kinetics of SLD repair in mouse tongue epithelium. *Radiother Oncol* 1993;27:36–45.
10. Dörr W, Emmendorfer H, Haide E, Kummermehr J. Proliferation equivalent of 'accelerated repopulation' in mouse oral mucosa. *Int J Radiat Biol* 1994;66:157–167.
11. Dörr W, Emmendorfer H, Weber-Frisch M. Tissue kinetics in mouse tongue mucosa during daily fractionated radiotherapy. *Cell Prolif* 1996;29:495–504.
12. Dörr W, Hamilton CS, Boyd T, Reed B, Denham JW. Radiation-induced changes in cellularity and proliferation in human oral mucosa. *Int J Radiat Oncol Biol Phys* 2002;52:911–917.
13. Dörr W, Hendry JH. Consequential late effects in normal tissues. *Radiother Oncol* 2001;61:223–231.
14. Dörr W, Kummermehr J. Accelerated repopulation of mouse tongue epithelium during fractionated irradiations or following single doses. *Radiother Oncol* 1990;17:249–259.
15. Dorr W, Weber-Frisch M. Effect of changing weekly dose on accelerated repopulation during fractionated irradiation of mouse tongue mucosa. *Int J Radiat Biol* 1995;67:577–585.
16. Fletcher GH, MacComb WS, Shalek RJ. *Radiation Therapy in the Management of Cancer of the Oral Cavity and Oropharynx.* Springfield, IL: Charles Thomas; 1962.
17. Hopewell JW, Nyman J, Turesson I. Time factor for acute tissue reactions following fractionated irradiation: A balance between repopulation and enhanced radiosensitivity. *Int J Radiat Biol* 2003;79:513–524.
18. Horiot JC, Bontemps P, van den Bogaert W et al. Accelerated fractionation (AF) compared to conventional fractionation (CF) improves loco-regional control in the radiotherapy of advanced head and neck cancers: Results of the EORTC 22851 randomized trial. *Radiother Oncol* 1997;44:111–121.
19. Landuyt W, Fowler J, Ruifrok A, Stuben G, van der Kogel A, van der Schueren E. Kinetics of repair in the spinal cord of the rat. *Radiother Oncol* 1997;45:55–62.
20. Maciejewski B, Zajusz A, Pilecki B et al. Acute mucositis in the stimulated oral mucosa of patients during radiotherapy for head and neck cancer. *Radiother Oncol* 1991;22:7–11.
21. Moulder JE, Fischer JJ. Radiation reaction of rat skin. The role of the number of fractions and the overall treatment time. *Cancer* 1976;37:2762–2767.
22. Paulus U, Potten CS, Loeffler M. A model of the control of cellular regeneration in the intestinal crypt after perturbation based solely on local stem cell regulation. *Cell Prolif* 1992;25:559–578.

23. Rosenthal DI. Consequences of mucositis-induced treatment breaks and dose reductions on head and neck cancer treatment outcomes. *J Support Oncol* 2007;5:23–31.

24. Ruifrok AC, Kleiboer BJ, van der Kogel AJ. Reirradiation tolerance of the immature rat spinal cord. *Radiother Oncol* 1992;23:249–256.

25. Shirazi A, Liu K, Trott KR. Epidermal morphology, cell proliferation and repopulation in mouse skin during daily fractionated irradiation. *Int J Radiat Biol* 1995;68: 215–221.

26. van den Aardweg GJ, Hopewell JW, Simmonds RH. Repair and recovery in the epithelial and vascular connective tissues of pig skin after irradiation. *Radiother Oncol* 1988;11:73–82.

27. van Rongen E, Kal HB. Acute reactions in rat feet exposed to multiple fractions of X-rays per day. *Radiother Oncol* 1984;2:141–150.

28. Withers HR. Cellular kinetics of intestinal mucosa after irradiation. In: Burdette WJ, editor. *Carcinoma of the Colon and Antecedent Epithelium*. Springfield, IL: Charles Thomas; 1970, pp. 243–257.

29. Wygoda A, Rutkowski T, Hutnik M, Skladowski K, Golen M, Pilecki B. Acute mucosal reactions in patients with head and neck cancer. Three patterns of mucositis observed during radiotherapy. *Strahlenther Onkol* 2013;189:547–551.

## ■ FURTHER READING

30. Bentzen SM. Radiobiological considerations in the design of clinical trials. *Radiother Oncol* 1994;32:1–11.

31. Denekamp J. Changes in the rate of proliferation in normal tissues after irradiation. In: Nygaard OF, Adler HI and Sinclair WK, editors. *Radiation Research. Biomedical, Chemical and Physical Perspectives*. New York, NY: Academic Press; 1975, pp. 810–825.

32. Denham JW, Walker QJ, Lamb DS et al. Mucosal regeneration during radiotherapy. Trans Tasman Radiation Oncology Group (TROG). *Radiother Oncol* 1996;41:109–118.

33. Trott KR, Kummermehr J. The time factor and repopulation in tumors and normal tissues. *Semin Radiat Oncol* 1993;3:115–125.

# The dose-rate effect

## ALBERT J. VAN DER KOGEL AND MICHAEL C. JOINER

## 13.1 INTRODUCTION

Low dose-rate (LDR) irradiation is the ultimate form of fractionation, equivalent to multiple infinitely small fractions being given without radiation-free intervals, and thereby, damage induction and repair take place at the same time. In clinical radiotherapy, continuous low dose rate (CLDR) is used in brachytherapy either by permanent or temporary implantation of radioactive sources (e.g. I-125, Pd-103) into tumours. By utilising remote afterloading of medium or high dose-rate sources, notably Ir-192, various combinations of dose rate and fractionation can also be chosen, such as pulsed dose-rate (PDR) and high dose-rate (HDR) brachytherapy. With external beam treatments using intensity modulated radiotherapy (IMRT) or other techniques using interruptions like breathholding, the dose-rate effect may also have some impact as the longer treatment times per session which can be needed in more complex plans may lead to a reduction in effectiveness. Increasing dose rates by using flattening-filter-free linacs or other technologies also raises the possibility of a change in biological effectiveness for these treatments.

## 13.2 MECHANISMS UNDERLYING THE DOSE-RATE EFFECT

The dose rates used for most radiobiological studies on cells and tissues tend to be in the range of $1-5$ Gy min$^{-1}$, as are average dose rates used clinically for external beam radiotherapy. Exposure times for a dose of, for example, 2 Gy may be therefore no more than a few minutes. Within this short time, the initial *chemical* (i.e. free radical) processes that are generated by radiation can take place but such exposure times are not usually long enough for repair of DNA damage or for any other *biological* processes to occur significantly. As the dose rate is lowered, the time taken to deliver a particular radiation dose increases; it then becomes possible for a number of biological processes to take place *during* irradiation and to modify the observed radiation response. These processes have been described by the *4 R's of radiotherapy*: recovery (or repair), redistribution in the cell cycle, repopulation (proliferation) and reoxygenation (see Chapter 8).

Figure 13.1 illustrates the operation of these processes in producing the dose-rate effect. The range of dose rates over which each process has an effect depends upon its speed. Intracellular repair is the fastest of these processes (half-time $\sim$1 hour) and when the exposure duration is of the order of 1 hour considerable repair will take place. Calculations show that repair at this speed will modify radiation effects over the dose-rate range from around 1 Gy min$^{-1}$ down to $\sim$0.1 cGy min$^{-1}$ (Figures 13.2 and 13.3). Even in the range of clinical external beam dose rates, small effects on tolerance may arise from changes in dose rate. In contrast, repopulation is a much slower process. Doubling times for repopulation in human tumours (or normal tissues) cannot be less than 1 day; the range is probably very wide, from a few days to weeks (Tables 8.4 and 8.5). Therefore, only when the exposure duration exceeds about a day, will significant repopulation occur *during* a single radiation exposure. Repopulation, either in tumours or normal tissues, will therefore influence cellular response over a much lower range of dose rates, below say 2 cGy min$^{-1}$, depending upon the cell proliferation rate. Redistribution (i.e. cell-cycle progression) will modify response over an intermediate range of dose rates, as will reoxygenation in tumours. The kinetics of reoxygenation are variable among tumour types and may involve various mechanisms (see Chapter 17); this could, nevertheless, be a significant factor reducing the effectiveness of brachytherapy given over a short overall time.

## 13.3 EFFECT OF DOSE RATE ON CELL SURVIVAL

As the radiation dose rate is lowered in the range 1 Gy min$^{-1}$ down to 1 cGy min$^{-1}$, the effect per unit dose decreases and shouldered cell-survival curves which are observed at high dose rates gradually become straighter. This is illustrated in Figure 13.2. At 150 cGy min$^{-1}$, the survival curve has a marked curvature; at 1.6 cGy min$^{-1}$ it is almost straight (on the semi-log plot) and seems to extrapolate the initial slope of the HDR curve. The amount of sparing associated with the dose-rate reduction can be expressed by reading off the radiation doses that give a fixed surviving fraction, for example 0.01: these values are 7.7 Gy at 150 cGy min$^{-1}$ and 12.8 Gy at 1.6 cGy min$^{-1}$. The ratio of these doses $(12.8/7.7 = 1.6)$ is called the dose-recovery factor (DRF).

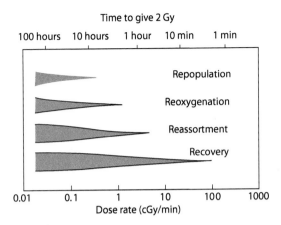

Time to give 2 Gy

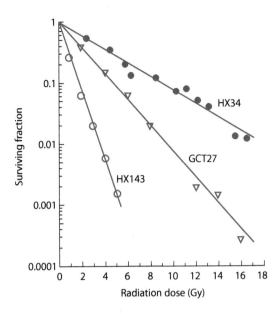

Figure 13.1 The range of dose rates over which repair, reassortment, and repopulation modify radiosensitivity depends upon the speed of these processes. (From (18), with permission.)

The data at all three dose rates in Figure 13.2 have been simultaneously fitted by Curtis' lethal, potentially lethal (LPL) model (see Chapter 4), a model that is useful for describing the dose-rate effect. This allows an estimate to be made of the half-time for cellular recovery (0.16 hours) and it also predicts cell survival under conditions of no repair (line A) or full repair (line B). Three further examples of LDR survival curves in human tumour cell lines are shown in Figure 13.3: they well illustrate the (near) linearity of LDR survival curves.

For four selected human tumour cell lines (Figure 13.4), cell-survival curves are shown at two dose rates (150 and 1.6 cGy min$^{-1}$). These four sets of data illustrate the dose-rate effect and the range of radiosensitivities seen among human tumour cells (17). At HDR there is a range of approximately

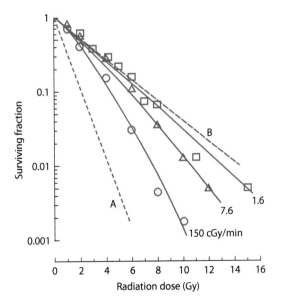

Figure 13.2 Cell-survival curves for a human melanoma cell line irradiated at dose rates of 150, 7.6 or 1.6 cGy min$^{-1}$. The data are fitted by the LPL model, from which the lines A and B are derived (see text). (From (17), with permission.)

Figure 13.3 Cell-survival curves for three human tumour cell lines irradiated at the LDR of 1.6 cGy min$^{-1}$. HX143: neuroblastoma, GCT27: germ-cell tumour of the testis, HX34: melanoma. (From (16), with permission.)

three in the radiation dose that gives a survival of 0.01, the $D_{0.01}$. At LDR the curves fan out and become straight or nearly so: the range of $D_{0.01}$ values is now roughly 7. This demonstrates an important characteristic of LDR irradiation: it can usually discriminate better than HDR irradiation, between cell lines of differing radiosensitivity.

## 13.4 DOSE-RATE EFFECT IN NORMAL TISSUES

Most normal tissues show considerable sparing as the dose rate is reduced. An example is shown in Figure 13.5. The thorax of conscious mice was irradiated with $^{60}$Co $\gamma$ rays and damage to the lung was measured using a breathing-rate assay (6). The radiation dose that produced early pneumonitis in 50% of the mice (i.e. the $ED_{50}$) was 13.3 Gy at 100 cGy min$^{-1}$ but it increased to 34.2 Gy at the lowest dose rate of 2 cGy min$^{-1}$ (DRF = 2.6). Note that a similar degree of sparing could be achieved (in studies of other investigators) by fractionated HDR irradiation using 2 Gy per fraction, and even more sparing at 1 Gy per fraction. Note also that at 2 cGy min$^{-1}$ the curve is still rising rapidly. It was not possible in these experiments to go down to dose rates below 2 cGy min$^{-1}$ because of the difficulty of immobilizing the mice for those very long periods of time.

The data in Figure 13.5 have been fitted by the incomplete repair model (20) as explained in Chapter 9. This model simulates the effect of recovery (repair) on tissue sensitivity; it does not account for *cell proliferation* during irradiation. The model fits the data well and it also allows extrapolation down to LDRs. It predicts, in this example, that dose-sparing due to recovery will continue to increase down to about 0.01 cGy min$^{-1}$ at which the $ED_{50}$ is 59 Gy and the recovery

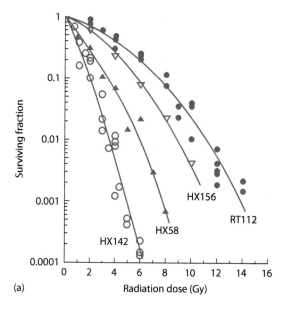

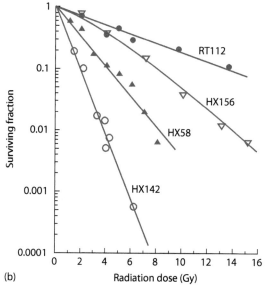

(a)

(b)

**Figure 13.4** Cell-survival curve for four representative human tumour cell lines irradiated (a) at HDR, 150 cGy min$^{-1}$ or (b) at LDR, 1.6 cGy min$^{-1}$. HX142, neuroblastoma; HX58, pancreas; HX156, cervix; RT112, bladder carcinoma. (From (16), with permission.)

factor (i.e. DRF value) is 4.4. Proliferation of putative stem cells in the lung may lead to even greater sparing at very low dose rates.

The comparison between a single LDR exposure (2 cGy min$^{-1}$) and fractionated HDR irradiation (2 Gy per fraction) allows an important conclusion to be drawn. If the fractions are delivered once per day then the overall time to deliver an ED$_{50}$ dose of 34 Gy is 17 days. The same effect is produced by a single LDR treatment in 28 hours. *Continuous LDR exposure is thus the most efficient way of allowing maximum tissue recovery in the shortest overall time.* It minimises the effects of cell proliferation, which is an advantage in terms of damage to tumour cells but a disadvantage for the tolerance of those early responding

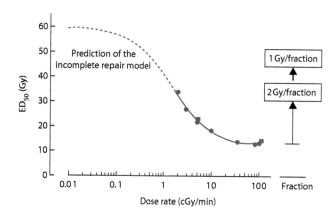

**Figure 13.5** The dose–rate effect for pneumonitis in mice. The full line fitted to the data was calculated on the basis of the incomplete repair model; the broken line shows its extrapolation to very low dose rates. The boxes on the right show the ED$_{50}$ values for fractionated irradiation. (From (6), with permission.)

normal tissues that rely more on proliferation than (intra) cellular recovery.

Figure 13.6 shows some examples of other studies of the dose-rate effect on normal tissues in rodents: lip mucosa, lung, spinal cord and bone marrow. When comparing two typical late-responding tissues (lung and spinal cord) with an early responding tissue (lip mucosa in the mouse) the patterns of recovery are similar, with the largest sparing in the spinal cord. This is to be expected for the central nervous system as this tissue shows the largest increase in tolerance when decreasing the fraction size (low $\alpha/\beta$ value). For early responding epithelial tissues like the lip mucosa the dose-rate effect is less pronounced, but for overall times longer than 1–2 days proliferation adds to a rapid increase in tolerance, in contrast to late-responding tissues.

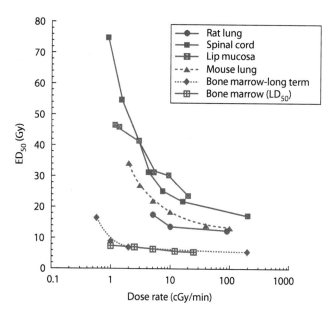

**Figure 13.6** The dose-rate effect in various rodent normal tissues: lung, spinal cord, lip mucosa and bone marrow.

The two bone-marrow endpoints, lethality due to bone-marrow syndrome and long-term repopulation of haemopoietic stem cells, show only a minimal recovery for dose rates as low as 1 cGy min$^{-1}$. This is predominantly due to the high sensitivity of the bone marrow, as a LD$_{50}$ dose in the range of 6–9 Gy is even at 1 cGy min$^{-1}$ delivered in a total time of only 10–15 hours. It is of interest to note that a slow proliferating haemopoietic stem cell population showed a significant recovery when lowering the dose rate to approximately 0.5 cGy min$^{-1}$, in agreement with a low $\alpha/\beta$ value (22).

## 13.5 ISOEFFECT RELATIONSHIPS BETWEEN FRACTIONATED AND CONTINUOUS LDR IRRADIATION

A variety of theoretical descriptions of the dose-rate effect have been made but for clinical application the most widely used is the incomplete repair model of Thames (20). The calculations of Dale and Deehan (5) make the same basic assumptions, although the formulation is slightly different. The basic equation of the incomplete repair model for continuous irradiation is

$$E = \alpha D + \beta D^2 g \tag{13.1}$$

where $E$ is the level of effect, $\alpha$ and $\beta$ are parameters of the linear-quadratic (LQ) equation, $D$ is the total dose, and $g$ is a function of the duration of continuous exposure. Note that the time-dependent recovery factor modifies only the quadratic term in the LQ equation, a feature that is supported by experimental data (17,23) (Figure 13.2). Note also that repopulation is ignored in these calculations.

The value of $g$ depends upon the half-time for recovery ($T_{1/2}$) and the duration of continuous exposure ($t$) according to the following relation:

$$g = \frac{2[\mu t - 1 + \exp(-\mu t)]}{(\mu t)^2} \tag{13.2}$$

where $\mu = 0.693/T_{1/2}$. Values of $g$ for a wide range of $T_{1/2}$ and $t$ are given in Tables 9.3 and 9.4.

This model allows isoeffect relationships to be calculated and as shown in Figure 13.5, it is successful in describing experimental data over a range of dose rates. Further examples of calculated curves are shown in Figure 13.7. On the left is the purely fractionated case, with HDR irradiation, described by the LQ model. The line in this chart corresponds to Equation 9.5 with $D_1 = 60$ Gy, $d_1 = 2$ Gy and $\alpha/\beta = 10$ Gy. The inter-fraction intervals have here been assumed to be long enough to allow complete recovery between fractions. The centre panel in Figure 13.7 shows isoeffect curves for a single continuous exposure at any dose rate, calculated using Equation 13.1 and with values of the half-time for recovery of 1.0, 1.5 or 2.0 hours. The three curves are slightly different, and this illustrates the dependence of the isoeffect curve for continuous exposure on the speed of recovery: the curve shifts laterally to lower dose rates as the half-time is prolonged. Running these calculations, we have to rely mostly on experimental data, as knowledge of recovery half-times for clinical endpoints is limited.

The curves in the panels of Figure 13.7 are *mutually isoeffective*. They are calculated for the same effect level and for the same $\alpha/\beta$ value of 10 Gy, chosen to give an extrapolated dose of 72 Gy at infinitely small doses per fraction or infinitely LDR, which corresponds to an EQD2 of 60 Gy. This example illustrates the equivalence that is predicted by the mathematical models between a particular continuous dose rate and a corresponding dose per fraction. For the parameters assumed here (as shown by the vertical arrows), a dose rate of around 1–2 cGy min$^{-1}$ (roughly 1 Gy per hour) is equivalent to fractionated treatment with approximately 2 Gy per fraction, for both of which the isoeffective dose is 60 Gy.

A further important conclusion can be drawn from calculations of the type shown in Figure 13.7. In Chapter 9 (see Figure 9.7) we have seen how the use of large fraction sizes leads to a therapeutic disadvantage in tumours with a high $\alpha/\beta$ value, relative to late normal tissue injury. The

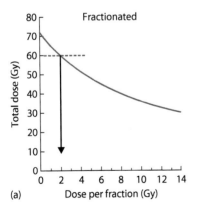
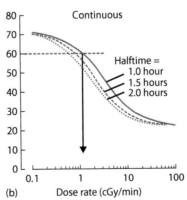
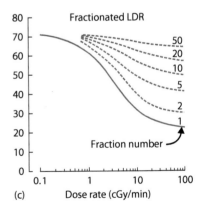

Figure 13.7 Isoeffect curves calculated with the incomplete repair model (20) for fractionated, continuous or fractionated LDR radiation exposure (the three panels are mutually isoeffective). Repopulation is ignored. The $\alpha/\beta$ value is 10 Gy and the EQD2 is 60 Gy. (Adapted from (16,19), with permission.)

same is true for high continuous dose-rate treatments. By drawing further horizontal lines between panels A and B in Figure 13.7, it can be seen that a dose rate of 5 cGy min⁻¹ is equivalent to around 6–8 Gy per fraction and 10 cGy min⁻¹ to over 10 Gy per fraction.

Figure 13.7c shows the results of calculations for *fractionated LDR irradiation*. Once again using the incomplete repair model, isoeffect curves were calculated for treatment with 2–50 fractions, each given at the dose rate shown on the abscissa and with full recovery between fractions. Again, repopulation is ignored. This diagram indicates the basic feature of fractionated LDR exposure: as we increase the number of fractions the dose-rate effect is reduced (i.e. the curves become flatter), and as we lower the dose rate the effect of fractionation is reduced (as seen by the vertical spread between the curves). This results from a simple principle. As we protract irradiation it is cellular recovery (DNA repair) that produces all these effects and there is a limit to how much recovery the cells can accomplish. If we allow recovery between fractions then there is less to be recovered *during* each fraction, and vice versa.

An alternative approach to the description of the dose-rate effect is the LPL model of Curtis (4). This is a mechanistic model that is described in Chapter 4. It has theoretical advantages for studies that seek to explore the cellular mechanisms of radiation cell killing but is less appropriate for clinical calculations than the empirical equations of Thames and Dale referred to previously.

## Effect of cell proliferation

The effect of proliferation at very low dose rates is graphically illustrated in Figure 13.8. These calculations are made for a hypothetical cell population with an $\alpha/\beta$ value of 3.7 Gy and a repair half-time of 0.85 hours. Cell proliferation is assumed to occur with the doubling times shown in the figure and no account has been taken of radiation effects on the rate of proliferation (if this occurred it would reduce the effect of proliferation at the higher dose rates). For these parameter values, there is no effect of proliferation at dose rates above 1 cGy min⁻¹ but as the dose rate is lowered to 0.1 cGy min⁻¹ the isoeffective dose rises steeply. The implication for brachytherapy is that above 1 cGy min⁻¹ repopulation effects can be ignored, but below this dose rate they will be substantial, both in tumours and in early responding normal tissues.

## The inverse dose-rate effect

Although in situations affecting clinical practice it is a general rule that cellular sensitivity decreases with decreasing dose rate, exceptions to this rule have been noted. Mitchell and Bedford in early studies of cell killing in mammalian cell lines occasionally found a slight inversion which they attributed to a lower dose rate allowing cells to progress through the

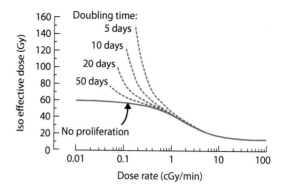

**Figure 13.8** The effect of cell proliferation as a function of dose rate. Isoeffect curves are shown for no proliferation or with the doubling times indicated. The calculations are based on a simple model of exponential growth, ignoring radiation effects on the rate of cell proliferation.

cell cycle into more sensitive phases, thus suffering greater damage. The mechanism of the inverse dose-rate effect has been elucidated further in more recent experimental work related to the 'low-dose hyper radiosensitivity' (HRS) process discovered by Joiner and colleagues (see Chapter 4). In cell lines showing a pronounced HRS response below doses of 0.4 Gy, also a reversal of the usual sparing at LDRs can be observed at dose rates below 1.5 cGy min⁻¹. An example of this HRS-driven inverse dose-rate effect is shown in Figure 13.9 (11). This phenomenon could be a factor promoting the effectiveness of LDR permanent I-125 implants, for example in the treatment of prostate cancer, where exposure rates over much of the target volume are generally less than 1 cGy min⁻¹.

## 13.6 RADIOBIOLOGICAL ASPECTS OF BRACHYTHERAPY

The principal reasons for choosing interstitial or intracavitary radiotherapy in preference to external beam treatment relate to dose delivery and dose distribution rather than to radiobiology. Irradiation from an implanted source within a tumour carries a distinct geometrical advantage for sparing the surrounding normal tissues that will inevitably tend to receive a lower radiation dose. Brachytherapy thus exploits the volume effect in normal tissues (see Chapters 16 and 26). Normal tissues will also often be exposed to a lower dose rate, which gives the additional advantage of 'negative double trouble', that is, 'double benefit' (see Chapter 10).

## Variation in cell killing around an implanted radioactive source

The non-uniformity of the radiation field around an implanted source has important radiobiological consequences. Close to the source the dose rate is high and the amount of cell killing will be close to that indicated by the acute-radiation survival curve. As we move away from the source, two

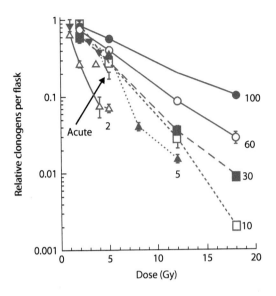

Figure 13.9 Survival curves obtained after exposure of asynchronously growing T98G glioblastoma cells to LDR ⁶⁰Co gamma radiation. Curve labels indicate the dose rate of radiation exposure in cGy h⁻¹. Relative clonogens per flask was calculated by multiplying the surviving fraction by the relative cell yield following irradiation. Each data point is plotted as the mean ± SEM. The acute dose rate was 33 Gy h⁻¹. This cell line is an example of those which demonstrate an inverse dose-rate effect on cell survival at dose rates below 100 cGy h⁻¹, whereby a decrease in dose rate results in an increase in cell killing per unit dose. Analysis of the cell cycle indicates that these inverse dose-rate effects are *not* due to accumulation of cells in G2/M phase or to other cell-cycle perturbations, but result from the process of low-dose HRS (see Chapter 4). (From (11), with permission.)

changes take place: cells will be less sensitive at the lower dose rates, and within a given period of implantation the accumulated dose will also be less. These two factors lead to a very rapid change in cell killing with distance from the source. Within tissues (tumour or normal) that are close to the source, the level of cell killing will be so high that cells of virtually any radiosensitivity will be killed. Further out, the effects will be so low that even the most radiosensitive cells will survive. Between these extremes there is a critical zone in which differential cell killing will occur. As shown by Steel et al. (19), for cells of any given level of radiosensitivity calculations imply that there will be cliff-like change from high to low local cure probability, taking place over a radial distance of a few millimetres (Figure 13.10). The distance of the cliff from the source is determined by the radiosensitivity of the cells at LDR, nearer for radioresistant cells and further away for radiosensitive cells (16).

## Is there a radiobiological advantage in LDR radiotherapy?

The question of whether LDR irradiation carries a therapeutic advantage is controversial. There is a considerable volume of

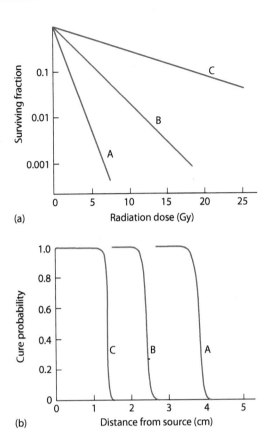

Figure 13.10 The likelihood of local tumour control varies steeply with distance from a point radiation source. The radius at which failure occurs depends upon the steepness of the survival curve at LDR (upper panel). (From (19), with permission.)

literature on the dose-rate effect, both in tumours and in normal tissues, on the basis of which it would be difficult to claim that under all circumstances LDR treatment would have the best therapeutic index. As shown in Figure 13.4, cells that are the least sensitive to radiation and have the largest shoulder on the cell-survival curve will show the greatest degree of dose sparing. These are not necessarily cell lines of low $\alpha/\beta$ value, for Peacock et al. (12) have shown that a range of human tumour cell lines, including those shown in Figure 13.4, have similar $\alpha/\beta$ values: radioresistant tumour cells tend to have both a lower $\alpha$ *and* a lower $\beta$ than more sensitive cells. In a particular therapeutic situation, we could make a calculation comparing the relative DRFs between tumour and critical normal tissues. This would tell us whether the normal tissues might be spared more or less than the tumour cells if we were to lower the dose rate. But this does not answer the therapeutic question, because to treat with one large HDR fraction has for a long time not been a clinical option. However, with the advances in functional imaging and combination of positron emission tomography/computed tomography/magnetic resonance imaging with high-precision IMRT, hypofractionation and even one to five large doses stereotactic body radiation therapy are now being used in modern radiation oncology. This is similar to comparing hypofractionation with the use of conventional or reduced dose per fraction. The appropriate clinical question is whether a single continuous LDR treatment is better than using a conventional fractionation schedule.

As illustrated in Figure 13.7, there is, on the basis of the incomplete repair model, an equivalence between *dose per fraction* in fractionated radiotherapy and *dose rate* for a single continuous exposure. Roughly speaking, for a given level of cell killing the total dose required at a continuous dose rate of 1 Gy h$^{-1}$ is similar to that required by acute fractionated treatment with 2 Gy per fraction. This equivalence depends upon the half-time for recovery but it is relatively independent of the $\alpha/\beta$ value (7). In radiobiological terms, these two treatments should be equally effective. Lowering the (fractionated) dose per fraction will spare late-responding normal tissues whose $\alpha/\beta$ value is low, as also will lowering the dose rate (continuous) below 1 Gy h$^{-1}$ – unless $T_{1/2}$ is very long. But tumours with lower $\alpha/\beta$ value, for example breast and prostate, might also be spared.

The success of intracavitary therapy may result from two factors: (1) the lower volume of normal tissue irradiated to a dose that discriminates between tissue sensitivities; and (2) the practical and radiobiological benefits of short treatment times. The clearest advantage for LDR irradiation is that for a given level of cell killing, and without hazarding late-responding normal tissues, this treatment will be complete within the *shortest overall time* (Section 13.4). Tumour cell repopulation will therefore be minimised. This could confer a therapeutic advantage for the treatment of rapidly repopulating tumours.

A potential *disadvantage* of LDR irradiation is that because of the short overall treatment time there may be inadequate time available for the reoxygenation of hypoxic tumour cells and therefore greater radioresistance due to hypoxia.

## Pulsed brachytherapy

The availability of computer-controlled HDR afterloading systems provides the opportunity to deliver interstitial or intracavitary radiotherapy in a series of pulses (PDR). The gaps between pulses allow greater freedom for the patient, increased safety for nursing staff, as well as technical advantages, for instance in allowing corrections for the decay of the radioactive source that minimise effects on the quality of treatment.

In principle, any move away from continuous exposure towards treatment with gaps carries a radiobiological *disadvantage*. This is because the dose rate *within* each pulse is higher and this allows less opportunity for repair of radiation damage. Slowly repairing tissues will therefore be disadvantaged and as argued in Chapter 11, there will be a loss of therapeutic index between tumour tissues that repair fast and those late-responding normal tissues that repair more slowly. The magnitude of this effect was considered by Brenner and Hall (3), who concluded that for gaps between pulses of up to 60 minutes the radiobiological

deficit may be an acceptable trade-off for the increase in dosimetric localisation to the target volume. There has since been much theoretical discussion of the guidelines for safe treatment with pulsed brachytherapy. Extensive laboratory studies comparing PDR and CLDR with cells *in vitro* have been carried out in Oslo by the group of Pettersen (9). They concluded that in some cell lines PDR had a greater than predicted effect. This could not be explained by the inverse dose-rate effect (see Section 13.5). Cell lines that showed an inverse dose-rate effect did so similarly under both CLDR and PDR conditions.

Theoretical studies have examined the effect of half-times for repair in normal and tumour tissues, including the evidence for multiple half-time components within each tissue (8). Brachytherapy studies on laboratory animals are technically difficult, not least because of the differences in scale between rats and humans, but detailed studies of effects in the rat spinal cord have been carried out (14).

Clinical pulsed brachytherapy equipment that allows a single high-intensity source to be 'stepped' through the treatment field are now widely used. These systems provide an important degree of control. The method does, however, need to be applied with care, for there can be penalties in terms of the quality of treatment when pulse sizes are allowed to be too large or when time between pulses is increased much above 1 hour. HDR afterloading systems create the temptation to shorten the overall time and, as indicated above, this could lead to increased early reactions to radiotherapy and greater tumour radioresistance due to inadequate reoxygenation. A prospective clinical trial comparing CLDR and PDR for cervix cancer was carried out in the Princess Margaret Hospital in Toronto, Canada (1). No statistical difference was observed in survival or late toxicity, and the authors concluded that PDR has the advantage of a better dose optimization. The use of PDR as a boost in combination with IMRT might yield the best options for dose escalation, as high doses are obtained within the target volume (13).

## 13.7 IMRT AND DOSE RATE

IMRT, a high-precision implementation of external beam radiotherapy, is generally accepted as the best tool to allow dose escalation with conventional photons in the target volume while sparing the surrounding normal tissues. Initially this higher precision was achieved by a more complex technology, including a high number of separate segments and thereby often longer delivery times of the complete dose fraction of more than 30 minutes. Thus, part of the escalated dose may be biologically lost by repair during the treatment. Various investigators have addressed this question by *in vitro* cell culture experiments. In such a series of experiments, along with a review of the literature, it was concluded that in general the effectiveness in terms of cell kill may decrease by up to 20% for treatment times of 20–30 minutes (2). It was shown that a similar loss of effectiveness did not occur if cells were irradiated with high linear energy transfer $d(48.5)$ + Be neutrons instead of megavoltage X-rays, thus confirming DNA repair as the mechanism (10). An important observation is that these figures differ for various cell lines, and are more dependent on the rate of repair than the $\alpha/\beta$ value, as also predicted by the LPL and incomplete repair models (see Chapters 4 and 9). Thus far, no indications of a reduced effectiveness of IMRT treatments were reported, and it should be realized that the outcome of therapy is not only determined by the intrinsic sensitivity of tumour cells. Of interest in this respect is an experimental study comparing *in vitro* radiosensitivity with *in vivo* tumour response in the same cell line (21), which showed that the loss of effect due to lower cell kill was compensated *in vivo* by rapid reoxygenation.

In contrast to early implementations of IMRT, volumetric modulated arc therapy (VMAT) is an IMRT technique that now allows delivery of dose fractions in typically less than 10 minutes. Many treatment units also now offer flattening-filter-free (FFF) beams which can result in higher average dose rates and hence also allow faster treatment delivery (see Chapter 7 for a full description of the processes and platforms that are available for the delivery of radiotherapy). With faster treatment delivery has come the question as to whether such higher dose rates, particularly the instantaneous dose rate in beam pulses, could lead to any change in effectiveness compared with average dose rates less than 5 Gy min$^{-1}$. In a study on two human cell lines irradiated *in vitro* from a clinical linear accelerator (15), no change in effect was found up to average dose rates of 30 Gy min$^{-1}$ corresponding to instantaneous dose rates of 338 Gy s$^{-1}$, up to doses of 10 Gy. However, analysis of the literature (24) has found that much higher X-ray and electron dose rates of around $10^9$ Gy s$^{-1}$, 5–10 Gy *can* deplete cellular oxygen, significantly changing the radiosensitivity of cells particularly that may already be in low oxygen tension of around 3 mm Hg or 0.4% which could occur in tumours. While it is unlikely that such HDRs could be achieved in linear accelerator–based X-ray radiotherapy, high-energy proton or carbon-ion beams might be able to produce such localised oxygen depletion and hence possible radioresistance.

---

### Key points

1. LDR irradiation is the ultimate form of fractionation which allows the maximal amount of recovery in the shortest overall treatment time.
2. The dose-rate effect is due primarily to repair of sublethal damage, while repopulation may play a role for treatment times longer than 1–2 days.
3. Cell-survival curves become straighter at LDRs and approach the initial slope of the survival curve.
4. An inverse dose-rate effect, the reversal of sparing at dose rates less than ~1 cGy min$^{-1}$, is observed in cell lines showing the phenomenon of low-dose HRS.

---

5. PDR provides the same radiobiological advantage as continuous LDR with the added benefit of optimized dose distributions and patient logistics.
6. IMRT given in 20–30 minutes per fraction may be intrinsically less effective due to lower cell kill, but this may be compensated in tumours by rapid reoxygenation.
7. HDRs of up to 30 Gy min$^{-1}$, as potentially given by FFF linac photon beams, have not shown a difference in biological effectiveness though possible *radioresistance* through localised depletion of oxygen cannot theoretically be ruled out for high-energy proton beams.

---

### ■ BIBLIOGRAPHY

1. Bachtiary B, Dewitt A, Pintilie M et al. Comparison of late toxicity between continuous low-dose-rate and pulsed-dose-rate brachytherapy in cervical cancer patients. *Int J Radiat Oncol Biol Phys* 2005;63:1077–1082.
2. Bewes JM, Suchowerska N, Jackson M, Zhang M, McKenzie DR. The radiobiological effect of intra-fraction dose-rate modulation in intensity modulated radiation therapy (IMRT). *Phys Med Biol* 2008;53:3567–3578.
3. Brenner DJ, Hall EJ. Fractionated high dose rate versus low dose rate regimens for intracavitary brachytherapy of the cervix. I. General considerations based on radiobiology. *Br J Radiol* 1991;64:133–141.
4. Curtis SB. Lethal and potentially lethal lesions induced by radiation – A unified repair model. *Radiat Res* 1986;106: 252–270.
5. Dale RG, Deehan C. Brachytherapy. In: Dale RG and Jones B, editors. *Radiobiological Modelling in Radiation Oncology*. London: The British Institute of Radiology; 2007. pp. 113–137.
6. Down JD, Easton DF, Steel GG. Repair in the mouse lung during low dose-rate irradiation. *Radiother Oncol* 1986;6: 29–42.
7. Fowler JF. Dose rate effects in normal tissues. In: Mould RF, editor. *Brachytherapy 2, Proceedings of the Fifth International Selectron Users' Meeting 1988. Leersum*, The Netherlands: Nucletron International BV; 1989. pp. 26–40.
8. Fowler JF, Van Limbergen EF. Biological effect of pulsed dose rate brachytherapy with stepping sources if short half-times of repair are present in tissues. *Int J Radiat Oncol Biol Phys* 1997;37:877–883.
9. Hanisch PH, Furre T, Olsen DR, Pettersen EO. Radiobiological responses for two cell lines following continuous low dose-rate (CLDR) and pulsed dose rate (PDR) brachytherapy. *Acta Oncol* 2007;46:602–611.
10. Joiner MC, Mogili N, Marples B, Burmeister J. Significant dose can be lost by extended delivery times in IMRT with x rays but not high-LET radiations. *Med Phys* 2010;37: 2457–2465.

11. Mitchell CR, Folkard M, Joiner MC. Effects of exposure to low-dose-rate (60)co gamma rays on human tumor cells *in vitro. Radiat Res* 2002;158:311–318.

12. Peacock JH, Eady JJ, Edwards SM, McMillan TJ, Steel GG. The intrinsic alpha/beta ratio for human tumour cells: Is it a constant? *Int J Radiat Biol* 1992;61:479–487.

13. Pieters BR, van de Kamer JB, van Herten YR et al. Comparison of biologically equivalent dose-volume parameters for the treatment of prostate cancer with concomitant boost IMRT versus IMRT combined with brachytherapy. *Radiother Oncol* 2008;88:46–52.

14. Pop LA, Millar WT, van der Plas M, van der Kogel AJ. Radiation tolerance of rat spinal cord to pulsed dose rate (PDR-) brachytherapy: The impact of differences in temporal dose distribution. *Radiother Oncol* 2000;55:301–315.

15. Sorensen BS, Vestergaard A, Overgaard J, Praestegaard LH. Dependence of cell survival on instantaneous dose rate of a linear accelerator. *Radiother Oncol* 2011;101:223–225.

16. Steel GG. The ESTRO Breur lecture. Cellular sensitivity to low dose-rate irradiation focuses the problem of tumour radioresistance. *Radiother Oncol* 1991;20:71–83.

17. Steel GG, Deacon JM, Duchesne GM, Horwich A, Kelland LR, Peacock JH. The dose-rate effect in human tumour cells. *Radiother Oncol* 1987;9:299–310.

18. Steel GG, Down JD, Peacock JH, Stephens TC. Dose-rate effects and the repair of radiation damage. *Radiother Oncol* 1986;5:321–331.

19. Steel GG, Kelland LR, Peacock JH. The radiobiological basis for low dose-rate radiotherapy. In: Mould RF, editor. *Brachytherapy 2, Proceedings of the Fifth International Selectron Users' Meeting 1988.* Leersum, The Netherlands: Nucletron International BV; 1989. pp. 15–25.

20. Thames HD. An 'incomplete-repair' model for survival after fractionated and continuous irradiations. *Int J Radiat Biol Relat Stud Phys Chem Med* 1985;47:319–339.

21. Tomita N, Shibamoto Y, Ito M et al. Biological effect of intermittent radiation exposure *in vivo*: Recovery from sublethal damage versus reoxygenation. *Radiother Oncol* 2008;86:369–374.

22. van Os R, Thames HD, Konings AW, Down JD. Radiation dose-fractionation and dose-rate relationships for long-term repopulating hemopoietic stem cells in a murine bone marrow transplant model. *Radiat Res* 1993;136:118–125.

23. Wells RL, Bedford JS. Dose-rate effects in mammalian cells. IV. Repairable and nonrepairable damage in noncycling C3H 10T 1/2 cells. *Radiat Res* 1983;94:105–134.

24. Wilson P, Jones B, Yokoi T, Hill M, Vojnovic B. Revisiting the ultra-high dose rate effect: Implications for charged particle radiotherapy using protons and light ions. *Br J Radiol* 2012;85:e933–e939.

## ■ FURTHER READING

25. Baker S, Pooler A, Hendry J, Davidson S. The implementation of the Gynaecological Groupe Europeen de Curietherapie – European Society for Therapeutic Radiology and Oncology radiobiology considerations in the conversion of low dose rate to pulsed dose rate treatment schedules for gynaecological brachytherapy. *Clin Oncol (R Coll Radiol)* 2013;25: 265–271.

26. Mitchell CR, Joiner MC. Effect of subsequent acute-dose irradiation on cell survival *in vitro* following low dose-rate exposures. *Int J Radiat Biol* 2002;78:981–990.

# Pathogenesis of normal tissue side effects

## WOLFGANG DÖRR

## 14.1 INTRODUCTION

The target volume in curative radiotherapy must unavoidably include a substantial amount of normal tissue, despite optimum conformation of the treatment fields to the tumour and precise treatment planning and application, for several reasons: First, malignant tumours infiltrate microscopically into normal structures, which need to be included in the high-dose volume as a tumour margin. Second, normal tissues within the tumour, e.g. soft tissue and blood vessels, are exposed to the full tumour dose. Third, normal structures in the entrance and exit channels of the radiation beam may also be exposed to clinically relevant doses. Therefore, effective curative radiotherapy is inevitably associated with an accepted risk for (severe) early and late radiation side effects ('adverse events') in order to achieve adequate tumour cure rates. The optimum radiation dose in curative radiotherapy is defined as the dose, which is associated with a certain, low – usually ≤5% – incidence of sequelae of a defined severity in cured patients ('complication-free healing'). The clinical manifestation of side effects therefore must be considered an indicator for optimum treatment and maximum tumour cure probability; side effects cannot *a priori* be considered as a consequence of incorrect treatment.

Early (acute) side effects are observed during or shortly after a course of radiotherapy. In contrast, late (chronic) side effects become clinically manifest after latent times of months to many years. The cut-off time to differentiate early from late effects has arbitrarily been set to 90 days after the onset of radiotherapy. It must be emphasized that this classification is exclusively based on the time course, i.e. the time of first diagnosis of the pathological changes. However, typical early and late responses to irradiation also have specific (radio)biological features which distinguish them.

*Early radiation side effects* are usually found in tissues with a high proliferative activity that counteracts a permanent physiological cell loss (turnover tissues), such as bone marrow, epidermis or mucosae of the upper and lower intestinal tract. The clinical symptoms of radiation effects in these tissues are predominantly based on radiation-induced impairment of cell production in the face of ongoing cell loss, as the latter is usually independent of the treatment. The consequence of this imbalance is progressive cell depletion (hypoplasia). This response is regularly accompanied by inflammatory changes, which can either be directly induced by the radiation exposure, or secondary to the changes in the turnover compartment of the tissue. Healing, which is usually complete for early radiation effects, is based on the proliferation of surviving tissue stem cells within the irradiated volume, or on migration of stem cells into the irradiated volume from unirradiated tissue sites.

*Late radiation side effects* are basically found in all organs. In contrast to the development of early side effects, which are characterized by cell depletion as a leading mechanism, the pathogenetic pathways of chronic side effects are more complex, and include changes in the parenchyma of the organs, i.e. in their tissue-specific compartments, but also in the connective and vascular tissue components. Moreover, the immune system (macrophages, mast cells, NK cells, etc.) is involved in the chronic tissue reactions. Late radiation effects hence represent a complex multifaceted, orchestrated response (2,11,38,45).

Late radiation sequelae, in contrast to early effects, with some exceptions, are irreversible and progressive, with increasing severity occurring with longer follow-up times. Therefore, with improving survival rates and prolongation of survival times of the patients, i.e. with the continuous improvement of radiation therapy, the number of cancer survivors that are at risk for late reactions is continually increasing. The risk for the manifestation of a chronic reaction in most instances remains throughout the life of the patient (20).

Early and late radiation effects are independent of each other with regard to their pathogenesis and – in general – conclusions from the severity of early reactions on the risk of late effects cannot be drawn. However, in particular situations, interactions between early and chronic reactions can occur *within one organ*, resulting in *consequential late effects* (CLEs). This is predominantly the case when the early responding tissue compartments (e.g. epithelia) have a protective function against mechanical and/or chemical exposure (9). This barrier function can be substantially impaired during the early radiation reaction due to cell depletion. In consequence, secondary mechanical and/or chemical traumata can impact on the target structures of the late sequelae (i.e. connective tissue, vasculature) in addition to the direct effects of radiation. This can then aggravate the late radiation response (9). These consequential late effects have been demonstrated for intestine, urinary tract, oral mucosa and skin localizations that are subject to particular mechanical or chemical stress, as well as for lung (8,9).

In this chapter, after a description of the general pathogenesis of typical early and late radiation effects, specific effects in clinically relevant organs and tissues at risk (organ at risk [OAR]) is described. This latter part also includes side effects that follow an atypical pathogenesis, such as (very) late cardiovascular changes or radiation cataract induction. This chapter, however, does not include systemic sequelae of radiation exposure, such as fatigue or nausea and emesis. Moreover, responses to high single doses or a few large fractions, as administered in stereotactic radiotherapy, may show a shift towards additional or alternative pathogenetic pathways, e.g. predominantly endothelial damage. These responses, which usually are restricted to very small volumes, are also largely excluded. Also, this chapter focuses on the tissue basis of radiation pathogenesis rather than on molecular pathways. Precise knowledge of the (molecular) pathogenesis and radiobiology of radiation effects forms the essential basis for the identification of early biomarkers of morbidity as well as for the development of selective, biology-based interventions. Molecular pathogenetic mechanisms are therefore summarized in the chapter on biological response modification in normal tissues (Chapter 24). Dörr et al. (12) also provide a concise review and summary of normal tissue tolerance.

## 14.2 EARLY RADIATION EFFECTS

Radiation effects in the epidermis were dose limiting in radiotherapy during the orthovoltage era, with peak doses occurring near the entrance sites of the beam. In contrast, with modern treatment techniques, distributions of even high doses inside the body can in general be achieved without severe epidermal toxicity.

However, early radiation effects are still relevant even in face of the progress in the physical application of radiotherapy. Early reactions significantly impact upon the general status and the health-related quality of life of the patients and thus can result in unintended treatment interruptions. Some early responses are *dose limiting*, such as oral mucositis in radiotherapy of advanced head and neck tumours, and hence reduce the chance for tumour cure. Moreover, early reactions can result in consequential late effects (9). In addition, the costs of supportive care are an important socio-economic factor. As these effects usually are observed over several days to weeks, they should be termed *early* rather than acute, as the latter in medicine in general refers to a time course of hours to a few days.

*Additional traumata* can significantly aggravate early radiation responses. Chemotherapy is one prominent example. Moreover, in epithelial tissues, mechanical stress can influence early complications, such as epidermal irritation by clothing or in skin folds, or oral mucosal trauma through dental prostheses or sharp-edged food components. Similarly, chemical exposure can intensify the response, like smoking, alcohol or spicy diet in oral mucosa, as well as additional physical factors, such as exposure of irradiated epidermis to ultraviolet irradiation. Such exacerbating factors should hence be avoided during radiotherapy.

## Phases of early radiation reactions

Different pathogenetic phases and components can be distinguished for early radiation responses in normal tissues (11,30), as illustrated schematically in Figure 14.1. Regularly a *humoral* response is initially observed, based on the release of paracrine active substances, e.g. by vascular endothelial cells and macrophages, but also by fibroblasts or parenchymal cells like epithelial keratinocytes. The associated changes in the *function* of the target cells are accompanied by inflammatory changes. This phase usually precedes the clinically dominating reaction, i.e. the reduction in the number of functional cells in the proliferating tissue compartment. This *hypoplasia* response is seen, for example, as epidermal or mucosal epitheliolysis or as leukopenia. Based on the breakdown of epithelial structures, which normally constitute a protective barrier function, *secondary infections* frequently develop, which can even progress into septicaemia. Eventually, with the exception of very severe reactions, *healing* occurs, based on surviving stem cells within the irradiated volume or migrating from unirradiated sites, for example bone marrow stem cells from the circulation or epidermal/mucosal stem cells invading from the outside into the high-dose volume.

*Changes in cellular function.* Early after the onset of radiotherapy, already after the first or the first few fractions, increased protein expression is observed (27), e.g. in endothelial cells, vascular smooth muscle cells or macrophages. These proteins are initially predominantly pro-inflammatory, such as interleukin-1α (IL-1α) and other interleukins, tumour necrosis factor-α (TNF-α) or cyclooxygenase-2 (COX-2). Similarly, the activity of inducible nitric oxide synthase (iNOS) is increased (26,30). These are only a few examples. The paracrine, intercellular communication is further modified by the

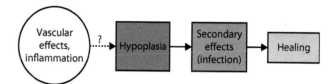

Figure 14.1 Components of early radiation effects. Early radiation effects usually start with vascular changes, clinically visible as erythema, accompanied by inflammatory changes. The depletion of functional cells, based on insufficient cellular supply in the face of ongoing differentiation and cell loss, is the dominating response to irradiation. The interaction of this phase with the vascular response is unclear. Progressive hypoplasia promotes secondary reactions, e.g. infections due to oral mucositis, moist skin desquamation or leukopenia. Eventually healing occurs, based on surviving stem cells within the irradiated volume or stem cells migrating in from outside the irradiated volume.

induction of cytokines, their receptors, adhesion molecules and components of the cell-matrix interaction, such as integrins (11). For example, keratinocytes of the epidermis and oral mucosa show an increased expression of epidermal growth factor (EGF), its receptor (EGFR) or the intercellular adhesion molecule-1 (ICAM-1). EGFR is subsequently internalized and translocated into the nucleus, and can act as a transcription factor and modulate DNA repair (6).

Initiation and regulation of these processes – because of their very early onset – cannot exclusively be attributed to the release of mediators during the disintegration of damaged cells or due to tissue hypoplasia. However, the signals underlying these changes in cellular function are unclear and are the focus of research. Their relevance for the pathophysiology of the early radiation effects is similarly indistinct. An impact on the clinical symptoms, like pain, is obvious, and modification of the tissue reaction, e.g. of the radiation-induced regeneration processes (repopulation, see Chapter 12), is very likely. The available data, however, do not allow us to clearly distinguish which of the intracellular, paracrine or humoral aspects are causally involved in the pathogenesis, and which are epiphenomena.

*Cellular depletion.* The cellular depletion phase, like leukopenia after bone marrow irradiation or hypoplasia in epidermis and mucosae, is – besides the inflammatory changes and the associated pain – the clinically most relevant component of early radiation responses. As mentioned above, these changes are found in the turnover compartment of the tissues, which physiologically display a precisely regulated equilibrium between permanent cell loss from the functional sub-compartment and cell production in the germinal sub-compartment. The hierarchical proliferative organisation of these tissues is illustrated in Figure 14.2.

The entire cell production per definition takes place in the germinal components of the tissue, e.g. basal and suprabasal

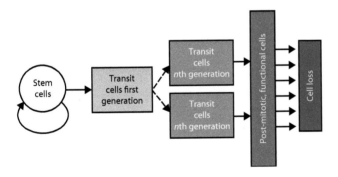

Figure 14.2 Proliferative organisation of turnover tissues. Typical early reactions occur in turnover tissues. The entire cell production is based on tissue stem cells, which generate on average one stem cell and one transit cell in asymmetrical divisions (see also Figure 14.3). Transit cells can undergo a limited number of divisions, which increase the cell yield per stem cell division. The cells undergo maturation and differentiation and are eventually lost. The turnover time from the initial stem cell division to cell loss is tissue specific.

layers of epithelia, intestinal crypts or bone marrow sinuses. The original basis of all cell production is the proliferation of *tissue-specific stem cells*. With very few exceptions, however, no cellular markers, such as surface antigens, have been identified that would allow for a differentiation between these stem cells and other proliferating (i.e. transit or post-irradiation doomed) cells. Therefore, the stem cell concept, also termed *target cell hypothesis*, although valid, must be regarded as strictly functional: the stem cell population consists of cells that can completely and correctly restore the integrity and structure of a tissue after an insult. Hence, the radiation tolerance of a tissue is defined by (1) the number and (2) the intrinsic radiosensitivity of these stem cells (7,33).

The equilibrium between cell production and cell loss is originally based on the division pattern of the stem cells. Physiologically, on average, each stem cell division results in one cell that remains in the stem cell pool, and one cell which eventually differentiates (7). This pattern, with two different daughter cells, is depicted as *asymmetrical division*. Those daughter cells which are not stem cells (transit or precursor cells) can undergo a limited number of transit divisions, which substantially increases the yield of cells per stem cell division. The regulation of these processes at present remains largely unclear. The number of functional cells seems to feed back on the general proliferative activity, i.e. both stem and transit cell divisions. However, the number of stem cells itself appears to modulate stem cell proliferation, indicating an (additional) autoregulation within this compartment (see also Chapter 12).

In most turnover tissues, transit cells by far dominate the proliferative cell population; the relationship between the numbers of transit and stem cells depends on the number of transit divisions. Therefore, any studies into the proliferative activity, such as S-phase labelling with BrdUrd, Ki67-labelling or mitotic counts, are mainly assessing transit cell proliferation and can by no means accurately characterize the proliferation parameters within the stem cell compartment.

The post-mitotic cells arising from the last transit division usually undergo several steps of maturation before they reach a terminal differentiation state and are eventually lost. Their lifespan is tissue specific, but can vary markedly between different tissues, from a few days in the epithelia of the upper and lower alimentary tract to many months in the urothelium of the urinary bladder. The overall *turnover time*, i.e. the time in which all cells are physiologically replaced once, defines the time course of the early radiation response (Figure 14.3).

The intrinsic radiosensitivity of the cells decreases during their differentiation process. Therefore, radiation doses administered in radiotherapy are predominantly lethal for stem cells, while transit cells are only minimally affected, and no effect (in terms of cell kill) is seen on post-mitotic cells. A number of studies in experimental *in vivo* models have investigated the progeny of surviving stem cells, e.g. with micro- or macro-colony-forming assays in intestinal epithelium and skin (43), or with the spleen colony assay for

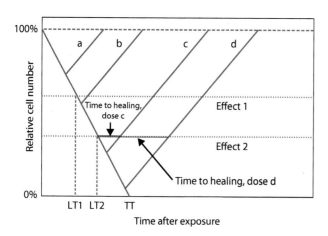

**Figure 14.3** Radiation-induced cell depletion and clinical manifestation of early radiation effects. Radiation exposure of turnover tissues results in an impairment of cell production, while cell loss continues independent of the treatment. The rate at which cells are lost is determined by the tissue turnover time (TT). If the residual proliferation of sterilised cells (abortive divisions) is not taken into consideration, then a complete loss of cells would be observed after one turnover time. A defined clinical effect 1, which is associated with a specific reduction of the cell number, can occur dependent on the dose (dose level b, c, d), and is not observed at lower radiation doses (dose level a). The latent time to clinical manifestation, however, is independent of dose. A more severe effect level 2 is based on a higher reduction in cell numbers, and hence is only observed at higher doses (c, d). Compared to effect 1, the latent time is longer, but is also independent of dose. In contrast, the time to clinical healing is longer with higher doses (d versus c).

surviving bone marrow stem cells (23). These investigations demonstrated that stem cell inactivation by radiation follows a dose-effect relationship, which corresponds to a typical cell survival curve *in vitro* (see Chapter 4). However, despite qualitative similarities in cell survival, there are significant quantitative differences between the *in vivo* and *in vitro* situations. Moreover, it must be emphasized that – in contrast to morphological endpoints such as oral mucosal ulceration – most functional clinical symptoms, like e.g. diarrhoea, may not be predominantly based on stem cell survival.

The radiation-induced impairment of proliferation in the stem-cell compartment results in a lack of cellular supply to the transit population(s), with the consequence of a decline in overall cell production. Furthermore, direct effects on transit proliferation are also possible at high to very high doses, which can further impact on the amplifying function of proliferation within the transit compartment. The latter may also apply to some chemotherapeutic drugs. Hence, increasing radiation doses result in a progressive decline in the number of precursor cells available for differentiation into post-mitotic cells. In contrast, despite the radiation exposure, differentiation and cell loss continue almost physiologically in qualitative and quantitative terms (7).

The radiation-induced imbalance between cell production and loss results in *progressive hypoplasia*, which becomes clinically manifest after a (tissue-specific) threshold cell depletion is reached (Figure 14.3). Different grades of severity of an early reaction, like dry and moist desquamation in skin, are based on different degrees of cell depletion, as also illustrated by different threshold levels in Figure 14.3. Because the cell loss rate depends on the turnover time of the tissue, and is independent of the treatment, the latent time until a clinical response is reached is tissue dependent but independent of dose, at least over a large dose range.

Usually, the turnover times are shorter than the latent time to complete cell depletion in the same tissue. For example, the turnover time in human and murine oral mucosa is in the range of 5 days (7), but it takes about 10 days for ulceration to develop in mouse mucosa after single-dose irradiation (13), and about 9 days after a cumulative (fractionated) dose of 20 Gy in human oral mucosa (41). This prolongation is due to the residual proliferative capacity (abortive divisions) of sterilized cells, which can occur even after high doses (see also Chapter 12).

Healing of early radiation effects is based on stem cells that survive within the irradiated volume or that migrate from outside into the lesion. The restoration of the *stem* cell population requires *symmetrical divisions*, with generation of two stem cell daughters (see also Chapter 12). It is likely that this process is regulated via the local environment, which does not provide the paracrine signals that allow the daughter cells of a stem cell division to differentiate. This is depicted as a *differentiation block*, which results in the recruitment of both daughter cells into the stem cell pool. The generation of transit cells through asymmetrical divisions, required to restore total in contrast to stem cell numbers, then re-occurs only when a sufficient number of stem cells have been produced.

The higher the dose, the lower is the number of stem cells that survive the treatment. Therefore, the clinically manifest response persists over a longer time with higher doses. This is illustrated, for example, by the EORTC 22851 study in head and neck tumours, where accelerated fractionation (and hence a biologically more effective treatment) resulted in clearly increased oral mucositis rates not only during but also at 6 weeks after the treatment (see Chapter 12). Also, complete restoration of cell numbers and tissue architecture takes longer with higher doses (Figure 14.3).

## 14.3 CHRONIC (LATE) RADIATION EFFECTS

Tissue organisation models have been developed that define late-responding tissues as flexible or *F-type tissues* (22). In these tissues, in contrast to early responding, hierarchical tissues (see Section 14.2), no clear differentiation can be made between proliferating and functional cells. Only on demand, proliferating cells are recruited into the functional population, and vice versa. It is assumed that the clinical manifestation of late radiation effects is based on a defined, critical depletion of functional cells (like for early reactions). The compensatory proliferation of the surviving parenchymal cells, which were originally functional cells, results in mitotic death and hence accelerates cell loss, and therefore shortens the time to the loss of organ function. The higher the initial cell depletion, i.e. the higher the dose, the more relevant becomes this mechanism. Hence, this model predicts a dose-dependent shortening of the latent time to the clinical manifestation of the effect, which is indeed a general clinical observation with regard to chronic radiation sequelae.

An alternative model (44) assumes that in late-responding tissues, structures with stem cell–like characteristics, *tissue-rescuing units* (TRUs) or *functional sub-units* (FSUs) exist. Their radiation-induced inactivation results in the observed clinical radiation responses. For some tissues or organs, relatively independent structures can be identified, like nephrons in the kidney, or alveoli in the lung, which may represent TRUs. In general, the functional organisation of the TRUs in a tissue – predominantly in a parallel, independent or in a serial, interdependent manner – impacts on the effect of dose distribution or inhomogeneities ('volume effect') in that tissue (see Chapter 16).

Undoubtedly, parenchymal cells in any organ are inactivated by radiation exposure. However, it is also accepted that – besides the parenchyma of the organs and the organ-specific cells – further tissue structures and cell populations are involved in the pathogenesis of late effects (Figure 14.4). These are in particular *vascular endothelial cells*, mainly in small blood vessels and capillaries, and connective tissue cells, i.e. fibroblasts. Endothelial cell death, by apoptosis or as delayed mitotic death, can be induced by exposure to ionising radiation. In contrast, mitotic *fibroblasts* are triggered into differentiation to post-mitotic fibrocytes, with the consequence of a drastically increased collagen synthesis

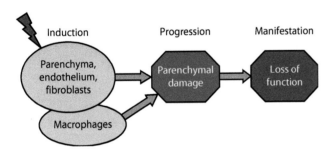

**Figure 14.4** Pathogenesis of late radiation effects. Chronic radiation effects are based on complex pathophysiological processes. These involve radiation-induced changes in organ-specific parenchymal cells (cell death), fibroblasts (differentiation) and vascular endothelial cells (loss of capillaries). All these cells, as well as macrophages, interact through a variety of cytokines and growth factors. This orchestrated response results in progressive parenchymal damage and eventually in loss of function within the irradiated volume. The clinical consequences depend on the architecture of the organ and the volume irradiated (see Chapter 16).

and deposition (25). Moreover, *macrophages*, irradiated or recruited into the tissue after irradiation, have been shown to significantly contribute to the signalling cascades involved in the pathogenesis of late radiation reactions in a number of tissues. Reactive oxygen and nitrogen species, chronically produced by various cell populations, in combination with chronic hypoxia, and a perpetual cascade of cytokines, seem to play an essential role in the pathogenesis of chronic radiation sequelae (2,10,26,27).

The interactive responses of these individual components of late radiation reactions result in progressive parenchymal damage and eventually in loss of function, within the volume exposed to a certain dose (Figure 14.4). The clinical consequences depend on the architecture of the organ, the radiation tolerance and at least partially on the localisation of the subvolume exposed within the entire organ (see Chapter 16).

Each of the participating cellular/tissue components of a late effect responds to radiation exposure with a specific dose dependence, and all these components then define the overall dose response for the different clinical endpoints in an orchestrated response. Hence, it is absolutely unlikely that the radiation sensitivity of one single cellular component can be used as a predictor of the sensitivity of the whole organ with regard to all potential or even only some clinical endpoints. For different organs, the relevance of the different pathogenetic components can differ (see Section 14.5). For example, in the liver the radiation response of the parenchymal cells (hepatocytes) is less important for the clinical symptoms, i.e. veno-occlusive disease (11). In the lung, type II pneumocytes (a slowly turning-over H-type tissue component), endothelial cells and fibroblasts seem to contribute similarly to radiation-induced fibrosis, in interaction with macrophages (10). In contrast, late fibrotic changes in the bladder are not primarily radiation induced, but rather secondary or even as a tertiary response to secondary functional and morphological impairment, which is predominantly based on urothelial and endothelial changes (11,19).

## Vasculature and endothelial cells

Irradiation causes changes in the function of the endothelial cells (11,29,36). Endothelial cell vacuolisation and foci of endothelial detachment are frequently seen, even at very early time points. Also, transudation of serum components into the vessel wall and subendothelial oedema have been observed, and formation of thrombi and occlusion of capillaries have been reported (14). Leukocyte adhesion and infiltration into the vessel wall is regularly found. Based on all these changes, irradiation eventually results in a progressive *loss of capillaries*, associated with a 'sausage-like' appearance of the arterioles, indicating a substantial impairment of perfusion. The detailed interrelation of the individual changes described above with the eventual capillary loss is unclear. Delayed mitotic death, based on the long turnover times of the endothelium, may contribute. The role of radiation-induced endothelial apoptosis, which occurs at early times after irradiation, is discussed controversially. As a result of the insufficient supply of oxygen and nutrients, atrophy of the downstream parenchyma develops. The morphological and functional consequences of this atrophy differ between the organs.

Telangiectasia, i.e. pathologically dilated capillaries, is observed in virtually all irradiated tissues and organs. The pathogenesis is unclear, but it is assumed that endothelial cell damage is involved. The loss of smooth muscle cells surrounding larger capillaries and veins may also contribute to the development of telangiectasia. In the intestine, the urinary system or also the central nervous system, telangiectasia can be clinically relevant because of the tendency for capillary haemorrhage. In the skin, telangiectasia are mainly a cosmetic problem; they also served, however, as a well-defined quantitative endpoint for radiobiological studies (see Section 14.5). Over longer time periods, the dilated, telangiectatic capillaries may collapse, thus resulting in a reversibility of their consequences, which has been demonstrated, e.g. after radiotherapy for uterine cervix or prostate cancer (15,16).

In arterioles, progressive *sclerosis* of the tunica media is observed, which also results in impaired supply of the downstream parenchyma. These changes presumably represent direct radiation effects on the cells in the media layer, in combination with endothelial changes.

Studies on the pathogenesis of late radiation effects have been performed in various experimental animal models, and predominantly with high single doses or few large fractions. Hence, no clear conclusions of such results on the correlation of the individual changes described above and their time course after (conventionally) fractionated radiotherapy can

be drawn, although it can be assumed that similar changes occur at low and intermediate doses per fraction, potentially with longer latent times.

## Fibroblasts

In mammals, a balance between mitotic fibroblasts and post-mitotic fibrocytes exists. Irradiation triggers the differentiation of fibroblasts into fibrocytes, with the consequence of substantially increased collagen synthesis and deposition (25), which significantly impacts on organ function. This process is predominantly modulated and regulated by the synthesis and release of transforming growth factor-$\beta$ (TGF-$\beta$) from various cell populations, which further triggers fibroblast differentiation (17). Increased expression of TGF-$\beta$ at the mRNA and protein level can be observed over long time intervals in various cell populations (2,45).

## Latent times

The latent times for chronic radiation effects, as well as the rate at which the severity of the clinical changes progresses, is inversely dependent on dose (Figure 14.5). This relationship results from several processes: with higher doses, more endothelial cells are damaged, and the progression rate of the loss of capillaries is higher. Therefore, less time is required until tissue function is lost. Similarly, higher doses trigger more fibroblasts into differentiation, which results in a higher synthesis rate of collagen, and the collagen level associated with loss of tissue function is reached earlier. Parenchymal radiation effects contribute to these processes in an organ-specific

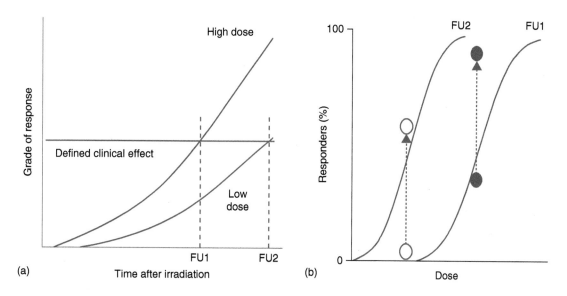

Figure 14.5 Time course and dose dependence of late radiation sequelae. Late radiation effects are progressive in nature. The latent time for a specific clinical effect as well as the progression rate are dependent on dose (a). In consequence, an increasing number of individuals presenting with the effect (responders) is found in the individual dose groups with prolongation of the follow-up time. Therefore, a shift of the dose effect curve to lower doses is found with increasing follow-up (b).

manner. As a consequence of the inverse dose dependence of latent time and progression rate, late normal tissue effects are increasingly observed also at lower dose levels with increasing follow-up time (Figure 14.5). Hence, the isoeffective doses for a defined clinical response decrease with increasing follow-up time. In consequence, the characterization of tolerance doses for late effects always requires information about the follow-up time on which the estimates are based.

## 14.4 ASSESSMENT AND DOCUMENTATION OF NORMAL TISSUE EFFECTS

Two aspects need to be considered with regard to the documentation and quantitation of normal tissue effects of radiation exposure: the frequency of assessment and the scoring system used. Early reactions can undergo considerable changes in their clinical manifestation in very short time periods. For example, oral mucositis can change from a slight erythema response to confluent epithelial denudation over just a few days, particularly if additional damage, e.g. by spicy food, etc., is inflicted. In contrast, chronic radiation sequelae develop slowly.

In conclusion, detailed assessment of early reactions requires scoring at least on a weekly basis during and for some weeks after radiotherapy. For studies on oral mucositis, even more frequent assessment is recommended. Late effects should be scored at intervals of several months after the end of radiotherapy, in order to assess the dynamics of their development, and may at later time points be documented at annual intervals. It must be emphasized that for some chronic reactions, such as in the heart or the urinary bladder (see Section 14.5), the time to clinical manifestation of the reaction, particularly after low radiation doses (see Section 14.3), can be in the range of decades. Hence, lifelong follow-up of patients is recommended.

For some late effects, it has been clearly demonstrated that they are not permanently observed over all follow-up visits, but rather are reversible or occur in waves. Prominent examples for this are chronic complications of radio(chemo)therapy in the urinary bladder and the rectum (15,28), but also xerostomia (35). In consequence, there is a clear discrepancy between the prevalence and the cumulative incidence of such late effects, and both parameters should be recorded and reported.

For documentation of normal tissue reactions – in order to be suitable for comparison between investigators, institutions and studies – standardised classification systems have been established. In general, complications are graded from 0 (no response) to 5 (lethal), as depicted in Table 14.1. Grade 1 reactions (mild) are reversible and in the case of early effects heal spontaneously without any specific therapeutic intervention or interruption of the oncological treatment. Grade 2 reactions (moderate/clear) can be treated on an outpatient basis and if occurring during treatment do not require a radiation dose reduction or treatment interruption. In contrast grade 3 effects (severe, pronounced) frequently require hospitalisation and intense supportive care and, if occurring early, may necessitate interruption of the treatment and/or dose modifications. Grade 4 reactions are life threatening, require immediate hospitalisation and require intense therapeutic interventions; early grade 4 reactions also result in cessation of the treatment.

The most widely used classification systems in radiation oncology (see references in 'Further Reading') are

- RTOG/EORTC classification, jointly developed by the Radiation Therapy and Oncology Group and the European Organisation for Research and Treatment of Cancer
- CTCAE, the Common Terminology Criteria for Adverse Events, developed by the National Cancer Institute (NCI)
- WHO classification (World Health Organisation)
- LENT/SOMA system (Late Effects of Normal Tissue/ Subjective Objective Management Analytic), developed specifically for scoring late sequelae resulting from oncological treatment

In principle, all these classification systems are comparable, and the scores from one system may be translated into the

Table 14.1 Systems for documentation of side effects, with examples for oral mucositis

| Grade | General | RTOG/EORTC | CTCAE (v3) | WHO |
|---|---|---|---|---|
| 0 | No change | No change | No change | No change |
| 1 | Mild | Erythema, mild soreness, painless erosions | Erythema; normal diet | Soreness, erythema |
| 2 | Moderate/clear | Painful erythema, oedema or ulcers; can eat | Patchy ulceration; can eat and swallow modified diet | Erythema, ulcers; can eat solids |
| 3 | Severe/significant | Painful erythema, enema or ulcers; cannot eat | Confluent ulcerations, bleeding with minor trauma; unable to adequately aliment or hydrate orally | Ulcers; requires liquid diet only |
| 4 | Life threatening | Requires parental or enteral support | Tissue necrosis; significant spontaneous bleeding | Alimentation not possible |
| 5 | Death due to side effects | Death due to side effects | Death due to side effects | Death due to side effects |

scores for another protocol (Table 14.1), but with certain exceptions. This translation is definitely precluded if sum scores are calculated, as has been suggested for LENT/SOMA, where the information on individual symptoms and endpoints is lost; this method hence cannot be recommended.

Besides these scores, more detailed protocols, or systems specifically designed for side effects in certain organs, e.g. OMAS (Oral Mucositis Assessment Scale), have been suggested. For clinical reports on side effects, the scoring protocol applied must be described in detail, particularly if modified versions of the original protocols are applied as has been described for the RTOG/EORTC oral mucositis score (24).

## 14.5 RADIATION EFFECTS IN SPECIFIC TISSUES AND ORGANS

In this section the response and tolerance of some clinically important dose-limiting normal tissues will be summarized. In general, an overview of clinical symptoms and consequences for the various radiation sequelae can be found in the classification protocols (see Section 14.4). More detailed descriptions are included in the reports of the QUANTEC initiative (Quantitative Analyses of Normal Tissue Effects in the Clinic) (21) as well as in the extensive review of the International Commission on Radiological Protection (5). Table 14.2 also provides estimated tolerance dose levels for various endpoints, and corresponding $\alpha/\beta$ values, as a guideline for clinical treatment planning. However, the numbers in this table should be used with considerable caution, as they are influenced by a number of factors, particularly the irradiated volume (see Chapter 16).

### Skin

The sequence of events in skin during radiotherapy is illustrated in Figure 14.6. Skin erythema is closely related to vascular radiation effects, with intermittent phases of vasodilation. In contrast, epidermal changes are based on the radiation-induced impairment of cell production, typical for early reactions (Section 14.2). The clinical manifestation is dry desquamation (radiodermatitis sicca), followed by moist desquamation. According to the turnover time of human epidermis of 20–45 days, this phase is usually seen at 2–3 weeks after the onset of radiotherapy. The skin reaction displays a significant area effect (see Chapter 16). Any variation in overall treatment time can have a large influence on epidermal tolerance: as an approximation, skin tolerance doses decrease by about 3–4 Gy/week when treatment duration is shortened from the standard 6–8 weeks.

Chronic subcutaneous fibrosis, clinically manifest as induration, is predominantly based on an increase in collagen fibres and a reduction of fatty tissue (see Section 14.3). The development of skin telangiectasia (Figure 14.7) illustrates

the progression of vascular injury in the dermis. The corresponding latent time distribution and the cumulative incidence for various grades of the response are shown in Figure 14.8. With high-energy X-rays, in contrast to orthovoltage radiotherapy, the maximum dose is deposited below the surface and late damage may therefore occur without any preceding early reactions.

*Skin appendices.* After a cumulative dose of 12 Gy, a loss in the function of *sebaceous glands* is observed, and at slightly higher doses the *perspiratory glands* also respond, both resulting in a typical dry skin. In *hair follicles*, single doses of 4 Gy or 10 Gy result in transient or permanent hair loss, respectively. In fractionated protocols, significantly higher doses up to 40 Gy still allow hair regrowth within 1 year, but is frequently associated with discolouration.

*Lymphoedema.* The occlusion of lymphatic vessels, as a direct radiation effect, but also significantly promoted by subcutaneous fibrosis, can result in chronic lymphoedema. This particularly applies to the limbs, if the entire circumference is included in the high-dose volume, as well as to the arms after breast cancer treatment, which does significantly impact on the patients' quality of life (e.g. [37]).

### Oral mucosa and oesophagus

Oral mucositis is the most severe and frequently dose-limiting early side effect of radio(chemo)therapy for head and neck tumours. Erythema, focal and confluent mucositis/ulceration are the lead symptoms (Table 14.1). Almost all patients with curative radiotherapy in this region develop some form of mucositis, with usually more than 50% confluent reactions (depending on the definition of 'confluency'). The latter typically develop during the third to fourth week of a conventionally fractionated protocol with 5 × 2 Gy/week. Oral mucosa is most sensitive to changes in dose intensity, i.e. weekly dose, and overall treatment time. Accelerated protocols regularly result in earlier onset, an aggravation of the response and/or an increase in the frequency of patients with severe reactions (Figure 14.9). Repopulation processes have been most intensely studied in this tissue (see Chapter 12).

Chronic effects of radiotherapy include mucosal atrophy and non-healing ulceration, and telangiectasia, which render the epithelium vulnerable; this is of particular importance for lip mucosa. Any additional trauma of the mucosa of the jaws may secondarily result in osteonecrosis. The early radiation response of the oesophagus mirrors that of the oral mucosa; in the chronic phase, strictures may develop.

### Teeth

Radiation caries, with a very fast manifestation, is a frequent complication of radiotherapy in adults. The response is based on both direct radiation effects at the dentin-enamel

Table 14.2  Tolerance doses and fractionation response (α/β value) for early and late organ damage in humans

| Organ | Endpoint[a] | Time to manifestation during/after irradiation[b] | $\alpha/\beta$ value (Gy)[c] | Tolerance dose for total volume (Gy)[d] | Comments |
|---|---|---|---|---|---|
| Cartilage, growing | Growth arrest | Next growth spurt | 6 | 20 | |
| Cartilage, adult | Necrosis | Months–years | | 70 | Associated with vascular damage |
| Bone, adult | Osteoradionecrosis | Years–decades | | 60 Mandible: 40–50 | Vascular damage and trauma |
| Connective tissue | Fibrosis | Months–years | 2 | 60 | Most frequent late reaction |
| Capillaries | Capillary changes/loss | Months–years | 3 | 60 | Contribute to a variety of (late) radiation effects |
| | | Years | | 70 | Resembles atherosclerotic changes |
| Large vessels | Wall changes, stenosis | | | 20 | Reversible |
| Heart | ECG-changes, arrhythmia | During RT | | | |
| | Cardiomyopathy (Pericarditis) | Months–years | 3 | 40 | Late myocardial infraction |
| Skin | Erythema | During RT | 9–10 | 40 | Varies with localisation (additional mechanical/chemical stress) |
| | Dry radiodermatitis | During RT | 10 | (100 cm²) | |
| | Moist radiodermatitis | During RT | 10 | 60 (100 cm²) | |
| | Gangrene, ulcer | | 3 | 55 (100 cm²) | Vasculature! |
| | | | | 40 | Discolouration! |
| Hair follicles | Hair loss | During RT (4th week) | 7 | | Transient loss of function |
| Sebaceous glands | Dry skin | During RT (2nd week) | | 12 | |
| Perspiratory glands | Dry skin, loss of transpiration | During RT (4th week) | | 30–40 | Long-lasting or permanent loss of function |
| Oral mucosa | Ulcerative mucositis | During RT (2nd–3rd weeks) | 10 | 20 | |
| Salivary glands | Atrophy/fibrosis | Months–years | | 60–70 | |
| | Transient loss of function – xerostomia | During RT (2nd week) | | 10–20 | |
| | Loss of function – xerostomia (partially reversible) | Continuous development from the early response | 3 | 25 | 1/3 capacity is sufficient for saliva production |
| Oesophagus | Dysphagia | During RT–months | | 40–45 | Early mucositis |
| | Ulcer–Fistula | During RT | | 55 | |
| Stomach | Atony | | | 20 | 'Radiation sickness' |
| | Ulcer | Months | 4 | 50 | |
| Small intestine | Malabsorption | During RT | 8 | 30 | |
| | Ulcer/obstruction | Months | 4 | 40 | Reduced tolerance due to fixation of intestinal loops, e.g. post-operative |

(Continued)

Table 14.2 (*Continued*) Tolerance doses and fractionation response ($\alpha/\beta$ value) for early and late organ damage in humans

| Organ | Endpoint[a] | Time to manifestation during/after irradiation[b] | $\alpha/\beta$ value (Gy)[c] | Tolerance dose for total volume (Gy)[d] | Comments |
|---|---|---|---|---|---|
| Large intestine | Diarrhoea, pain | During–post RT | | 10–20 | |
| Rectum | Ulcer/obstruction | Months–years | | 45 | Ileus–symptoms possible |
| | Proctitis | During RT | | 50 | |
| Liver | Chronic inflammation, ulcer | Months–years | 5 | 60 | Partial irradiation of the circumference increases tolerance |
| | Veno-occlusive disease (VOD) | 2–3 weeks | | 30 | Lethal after total organ irradiation; hence, late effects only after partial organ irradiation |
| Biliary tract | Fibrosis | Months–years | | | |
| Pancreas | Stenosis/stricture | Months–years | | | |
| | Fibrosis | Months–years | 1 | 50–60 | No early symptoms known, included in 'radiation sickness'? |
| Kidney | Nephropathy | 9 Months–years | 2 | 20 | |
| Ureter | Stricture | 2 years | | 60–70 | Vascular effects, potential interaction with surgery |
| Urinary bladder | Cystitis | During RT | 10 | 20–35 | Uncommon pathophysiology, no urothelial depletion |
| Urethra | Shrinkage, ulceration | Months–decades | 5–10 | 50 | Strong consecutive component |
| | Stricture | Months–years | | 60–70 | Reduced tolerance after transurethral resection of the prostate (TURP) |
| Larynx | Oedema | During RT | | 45 | |
| | Chronic enema, necrosis | Months | 2–4 | 70 | Permanent changes in voice quality, necrosis after decades |
| Lung | Pneumonitis | 2–6 weeks | 5 | 12–14 | Single-dose irradiation |
| | Pneumonitis | 4–6 weeks | 5 | 45 | |
| | Fibrosis | Months–years | 4 | | |
| Testis | Permanent sterility | Weeks–months | | 1.5 | Negative fractionation effect |
| Ovary | Permanent sterility | Weeks–months | | 2.5 | Strong inverse age dependence |
| Uterus | Atrophy | Months–years | | 100 | |
| Vagina | Mucositis | During RT | | 30 | |
| Breast, child | Ulcer, fibrosis | Months–years | | 50 | |
| | Growth arrest | At puberty | | 10 | |
| Breast, adult | Fibrosis/atrophy | Years | 2–3 | 60 | |
| Adrenal glands | Loss of function | Months–years | | 90 | |
| Pituitary gland/diencephalon (children) | Growth hormone deficit | Months–years | | 18–24 | Growth retardation |

*(Continued)*

**Table 14.2** (*Continued*) Tolerance doses and fractionation response ($\alpha/\beta$ value) for early and late organ damage in humans

| Organ | Endpoint[a] | Time to manifestation during/after irradiation[b] | $\alpha/\beta$ value (Gy)[c] | Tolerance dose for total volume (Gy)[d] | Comments |
|---|---|---|---|---|---|
| Cerebrum, child | Somnolence syndrome | During–post RT | | 24 | Specific response in children |
| Cerebrum, adult | Necrosis | Months–years | | 55 | |
| Spinal cord | Lhermitte syndrome | Weeks–months | | 35 | Reversible |
| • Cervical/thoracic | Radiation myelopathy | Months–years | 2 | 55 | |
| • Thoracic/lumbar | Radiation myelopathy | Months–years | 2 | 55 | |
| Peripheral nerves | Functional impairment | Months–years | | 60 | Frequently associated with connective tissue fibrosis |
| Eye lens[e] | Cataract | Months–years | 1–2[e] | <1[e] | Surgical management |
| Lacrimal system | Dry eye, ulceration | Weeks–months | 3 | 40 | Most critical radiation effect in the eye |
| Retina | Retinopathy | Weeks–months | | 45 | |
| Optic nerve | Neuropathy | Months–years | 2 | 55 | |
| Chiasma opticum | Loss of vision | Months–years | 2 | 55 | |
| Conjunctiva | Kerato–conjunctivitis | During–post RT | | 50 | Reversible |
| Ear | Serous otitis | During–post RT | | 30 | |
| | Inner ear injury | During RT + Months | | 30 | Slight hearing loss (15 dB) frequently not recognised by patients; overlap with age effects |
| Taste | Taste impairment, loss | During RT + months | | 30 | Reversible |
| Lymph nodes | Permanent atrophy | Months–years | | 70 | Frequently associated with connective tissue fibrosis |
| Lymphatic vessels | Sclerosis | Months–years | | 90 | |
| Bone marrow | Transient hypoplasia | During RT | 10 | 2 | Total-body irradiation |
| | Lethal aplasia (1 year) | | 5 | 4 | Total-body irradiation |
| | Permanent aplasia | During–post RT | | | Compensation by unirradiated parts; post-irradiation homing of circulating stem cells possible |

Adapted from (18).

*Note:* No shading: Early reaction. Shading: Late reaction.

a  Leading clinical symptom.

b  Relative to irradiation with 5 × 2 Gy per week. Times after the treatment relate to the last fraction.

c  See also Chapters 9 and 10. Missing values indicate that no valid estimates are possible.

d  Relates to irradiation of large volumes that include the entire organ or, for ubiquitous tissues (connective tissue, capillaries, etc.) to larger volumes. For partial organ irradiation, see Chapter 16.

e  Tolerance dose for the eye lens after single-dose exposure is clearly ≪1 Gy.

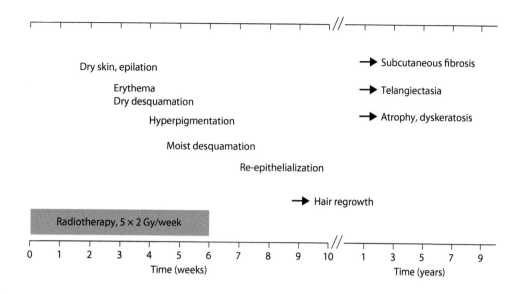

**Figure 14.6** Sequence of radiation effects in skin and appendices. The figure displays the time course of early and late skin reactions induced by conventional radiotherapy with 5 × 2 Gy per week over 6 weeks, if the same skin area is exposed to the maximum dose of 2 Gy at each dose fraction. The duration of radiotherapy is indicated on top of the abscissa.

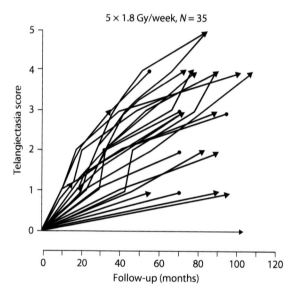

**Figure 14.7** Clinical manifestation of skin telangiectasia. Progression of skin telangiectasia in individual patients treated with five fractions of 1.8 Gy per week to a total of 35 fractions. Note the pronounced differences between patients and the continuous increase in severity even up to 8 years. (From (39), with permission.)

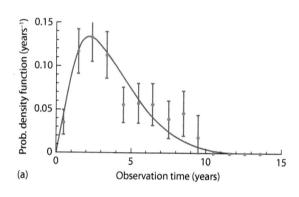

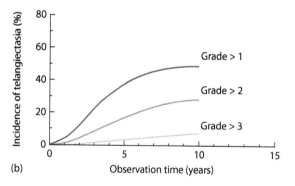

**Figure 14.8** Time course of telangiectasia. (a) The latent time distribution for any grade of telangiectasia as observed in 174 treatment fields with an intermediate probability of developing any response. The probability density function may be interpreted as the fraction of patients who developed the response within a specific year after irradiation. (b) The cumulative incidence of telangiectasia as a function of time for various grades, after radiotherapy with 44.4 Gy in 25 fractions. The model calculations are based on observations in 401 treatment fields. (From (4), with permission.)

border zone, and indirectly on radiation effects in the salivary glands (xerostomia, see below) and the associated changes in the oral micromilieu. Rigorous *pre*-treatment dental restoration or extractions are of major importance, because of the risk of osteoradionecrosis, if extractions are required after radiotherapy. In order to avoid dose peaks in the mucosa around metallic dental implants, mucosal retractors should be used to displace the mucosa by about 3 mm.

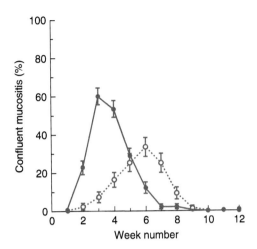

**Figure 14.9** Prevalence of confluent mucositis. The percentage of patients presenting with confluent mucositis within a given treatment week after onset of radiotherapy was plotted for accelerated radiotherapy, i.e. CHART (●), or conventional radiotherapy (○). (From (3), with permission.)

## Salivary glands

Salivary glands are sensitive to radiation exposure: already after the first week of therapy (accumulated dose of 10–15 Gy) saliva production is significantly reduced, frequently after a transient phase of hypersalivation. After total doses in excess of 40 Gy to both parotid glands, saliva production practically stops after about 4 weeks and does not recover at all after doses over 60 Gy. Volume effects are very pronounced, and sparing of partial volumes usually leads to recovery of function.

Chronic xerostomia has a major impact on the quality of life of the patients. It depends not only on reduced serous fluid production in the parotid glands, but also on the reduced mucin from the submandibular glands, and a reduced function of the small salivary glands. The submandibular glands produce most of the mucinous components of the saliva; by their water-binding capacity they keep the mucous membranes hydrated and also provide a barrier function.

## Stomach

Functional impairment, with a prolongation of the time for gastric emptying, and a reduction in HCl secretion are frequently seen. The symptoms are equivalent to those of gastritis. Ulceration, mainly based on vascular effects, can develop as a late effect at doses of 25–40 Gy.

## Intestine

Particularly at risk are 'fixed' intestinal loops, e.g. through postoperative adhesions, as these may be permanently located within a high-dose volume, in contrast to mobile loops. The same is true for the rectum.

The sequence of radiation-induced events in the intestine includes

- Initial increase in motility, followed by an atonic phase
- Loss of epithelium and villi due to proliferative impairment in the crypts, with the consequence of
  - Water electrolyte and protein loss into the lumen, resulting in diarrhoea
  - Changed resorption (including increased resorption of some substances, which must be considered if drugs are administered orally)
- Risk of sepsis

Late effects include chronic ulcers, based on an orchestrated response of all intestinal wall components, plus mechanical/chemical stress due to faeces, as well as infections. Fibrotic remodelling may result in stenosis and ileus. Frequently, telangiectasia are found, which may result in bleeding.

It has been demonstrated experimentally by inhibition of pancreatic secretion by somatostatin analogues that pancreatic enzymes contribute to the manifestation of the early effect. Interestingly, this treatment also reduces late fibrosis, underlining the consequential nature of chronic changes in the intestine.

## Liver

The liver is radiosensitive, with a tolerance dose of around 30 Gy in 2 Gy fractions. However, liver tolerance is only dose limiting when the whole organ is irradiated. An example is total-body irradiation preceding bone marrow transplantation. In this situation, the lung is well known as a dose-limiting organ, but also liver and kidney are at risk, especially after regimes equivalent to single doses of 10 Gy or higher.

Two phases of radiation hepatopathy are recognised, with early radiation hepatitis being the more dominant. This early phase develops approximately 2–6 weeks after irradiation, with signs of liver enlargement and ascites. Liver function tests during this period are abnormal. Early hepatitis usually presents as veno-occlusive disease (VOD), characterised by central vein thrombosis, whereby occlusion of the centrilobular veins causes atrophy and loss of the surrounding hepatocytes. Total liver VOD is usually lethal.

Chronic hepatopathy – which obviously can only develop after partial organ irradiation – has a variable latency ranging from 6 to more than 12 months post-irradiation, and shows progressive fibrotic changes in both centrilobular and periportal areas. These alterations are accompanied by blood-flow redistribution through recanalisation or newly formed veins, and regenerative proliferation of hepatocytes and bile ducts.

## Upper respiratory tract

The mucosae of the nose, paranasal sinuses and trachea respond to irradiation similarly to oral epithelium, but appear to be slightly more radioresistant. Early changes in the larynx are oedema and perichondritis. Doses above 50 Gy may result in a long-lasting impairment of the quality of the voice, which must be considered in patients depending on their voice in their professional life.

## Lung

In the lung, two separate radiation syndromes can be distinguished clinically: early pneumonitis, usually observed at 4–6 weeks after the end of radiotherapy, and fibrosis, which develops slowly over a period of several months to years. The lung is among the most sensitive late-responding organs, but with a pronounced volume effect (see Chapter 16). Besides a reduction in irradiated volume, reduced doses per fraction are most effective in avoiding severe (clinically manifest) lung reactions.

Clinical signs or symptoms of radiation pneumonitis are reduced pulmonary compliance, progressive dyspnoea, decreased gas exchange and dry cough. When there is insufficient functional reserve, cardiorespiratory failure may occur within a short time span. The development of chronic radiation pneumopathy, i.e. lung fibrosis, follows the general pathways described in Section 14.3. The complexity of the signalling cascades is illustrated in Figure 14.10. Local fibrotic responses must be expected in all patients with early reactions, indicating a strong consequential component of the late reaction (8). Higher age and tamoxifen treatment significantly increase the incidence of early pneumopathy.

## Kidney

The kidney is among the most sensitive of the late-responding critical organs. Radiation damage develops very slowly and may take many years to be recognised. Radiation nephropathy usually manifests as proteinuria, hypertension and impairment of the urine concentration function. Anaemia is usually present, and has been attributed both to haemolysis and to a decreased production of erythropoietin. A mild form of nephritis, presenting only as a sustained proteinuria, may be observed over a period of many years. Parts of one or both kidneys can receive much higher doses without affecting excretory function. However, after partial kidney irradiation, hypertension may develop after a latent period of up to or beyond 10 years.

The fractionation sensitivity of the kidney is high (i.e. the $\alpha/\beta$ value is low). The dose tolerated by the kidney does not increase with increasing time after radiotherapy, but even declines due to a continuous progression of damage, after doses well below the threshold for induction of functional deficit, which usually precludes reirradiation (see Chapter 23).

The pathogenesis of radiation nephropathy is complex. Most studies suggest glomerular endothelial injury as the start of a cascade leading to glomerular sclerosis and later tubulo-interstitial fibrosis. Several experimental studies have shown the importance of the renin-angiotensin system in the induction of glomerular sclerosis via upregulation of plasminogen activator inhibitor 1 (PAI-1) and enhanced fibrin deposition. Through loss of tubular epithelial cells, fibrin may then leak into the interstitium causing the onset of tubulo-interstitial fibrosis.

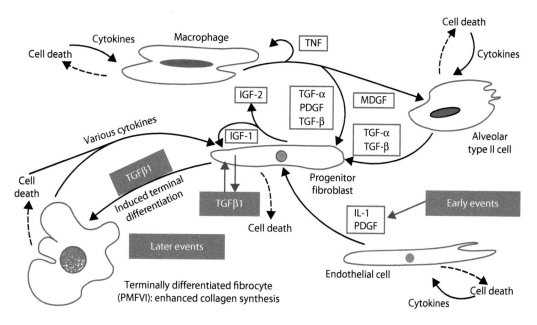

Figure 14.10 Possible cellular interactions and events after irradiation of lung tissue. (Modified from (25), with permission.)

## Urinary bladder

In patients, two phases of radiation-induced changes in the urinary bladder are observed, both with a reduction in bladder storage capacity and a consequential increase in micturition frequency. An early phase occurs 2–6 weeks after the start of radiotherapy, which is morphologically characterised by hyperaemia and mucosal oedema. Experimentally in mice, two waves of early injury have been observed. Mechanistically, the first phase seems to be related to direct radiation-induced changes of the prostaglandin metabolism (which regulates the tone of the bladder wall), as suggested by the beneficial effect of aspirin when administered during this phase. The second early phase is associated with changes in urothelial barrier function, but without epithelial cell depletion (which is not expected at this time due to the very long turnover time of the urothelium). Infection may complicate this early response, which then may progress to desquamation and ulceration.

A chronic phase develops with latent times that are inversely dose dependent and can range up to 10 years or longer. The morphological correlate in the initial late phase is a progressive mucosal breakdown, ranging from superficial denudation to ulceration and even the formation of fistulae. The urothelial changes are accompanied by urothelial areas of compensatory hyperproliferation. Vascular changes and signs of local ischaemia have been described. These processes progress into secondary fibrosis of the bladder wall. Telangiectasia can result in severe bleeding episodes.

The early changes clearly correlate with the chronic radiation sequelae, illustrating a strong consequential component. A schematic illustration of the sequence of events leading to late fibrosis, as concluded from animal studies, is given in Figure 14.11.

## Nervous system

The nervous system is less sensitive to radiation injury than some other late-responding tissues such as the lung or kidney. However, damage to this organ results in severe consequences such as paralysis: although tolerance doses are often quoted at the 5% complication level (TD5) the dose constraints for treatment planning generally are chosen to include a wide margin of safety.

A schematic outline of the development of various delayed lesions in the central nervous system as studied in animals is given in Figure 14.12.

### BRAIN

The most important radiation syndromes in the central nervous system develop a few months to several years after therapy. The often-used separation into early or late delayed injury is not very useful, as different types of lesions with overlapping time distributions occur. Some reactions occurring within the first six months comprise transient demyelination ('somnolence syndrome') or the much more severe leukoencephalopathy. The more typical radiation necrosis may also occur by 6 months, but even after as long as 2–3 years. Histopathologically, changes that occur within the first year are mostly restricted to the white matter. For times beyond 6–12 months, the grey matter usually also shows changes along with more pronounced vascular lesions (telangiectasia and focal haemorrhages). Radionecrosis of the brain with latent times between 1 and 2 years usually shows a mixture of histological characteristics.

The brain of children is more sensitive than in adults. Functional deficits, such as a reduction in IQ, can at least partly be attributed to radiotherapy after combined

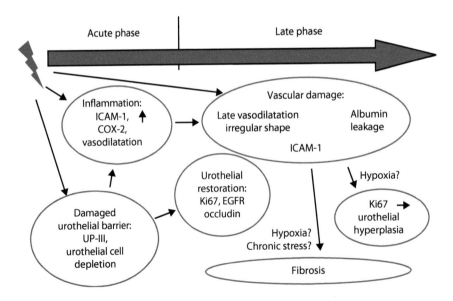

**Figure 14.11** Pathogenesis of radiation effects in the urinary bladder. The individual processes have been studied in mouse urinary bladder after single-dose irradiation. Morphological changes were related to functional impairment as assessed by transurethral cystometry. (Modified from (19), with permission.)

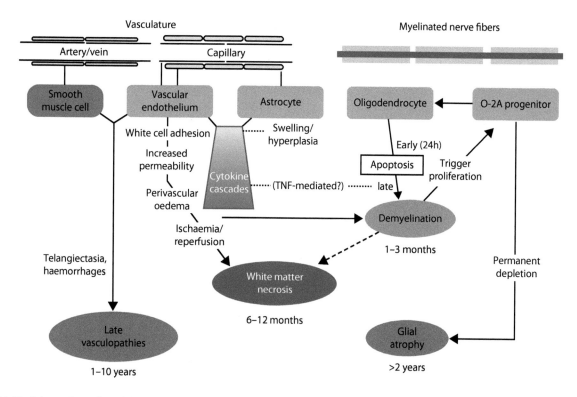

**Figure 14.12** Schematic outline of tissue components and cell types and their potential role in the pathophysiology of radiation-induced lesions in the central nervous system. (From (40), with permission.)

treatment protocols. Changes in the neurovascular unit may contribute to the impairments in learning and memory (42).

In the brain, neurogenesis persists into adulthood predominantly in two neurogenic centres: subventricular zone and subgranular zone. Neural stem cells are not only self-renewing and differentiating along multiple lineages in these regions, but also contribute to brain regeneration. Radiation exposure can sterilize these stem cells directly, or indirectly impact on neurogenesis by dose-dependent, inflammation-mediated mechanisms, even at doses <2 Gy (1).

### SPINAL CORD

Radiation-induced changes in the spinal cord are similar to those in the brain in terms of latent period, histopathology and radiation tolerance. Among the (relatively) early syndromes, the Lhermitte sign is a frequently occurring, usually reversible demyelinating reaction, which develops several months after completion of treatment and lasts for a few months to more than 1 year. It may occur at doses as low as 35 Gy in 2 Gy fractions, well below tolerance for permanent radiation myelopathy, when long segments of cord are irradiated, and does not predict for later development of permanent myelopathy.

As in the brain, the later types of myelopathy include two main syndromes. The first, occurring from about 6 to 18 months, is mostly limited to demyelination and necrosis of the white matter, whereas the second (with a latency of usually 1 to >4 years) is mostly based on vasculopathy. The tolerance dose of the spinal cord largely depends on the size

of the dose per fraction, while variations in overall treatment time up to 10–12 weeks have a negligible effect in conventional schedules using one fraction per day (see Chapter 12). For longer times or intervals, substantial recovery occurs which has important implications for retreatment (see Chapter 23).

### PERIPHERAL NERVES

Radiation effects in peripheral nerves, mainly plexuses and nerve roots, are probably more common than effects in the spinal cord but are less well documented. Peripheral nerves are often quoted as being more resistant to radiation than the cord or the brain, but this view is not supported by clinical data. As is the case for all nervous tissues, a dose of 60 Gy in 2 Gy fractions is associated with a less than 5% probability of injury, but this probability rises steeply with increasing radiation dose.

The brachial plexus is often included in treatments of the axillary and supraclavicular nodes in breast cancer patients. Clinically, plexopathy is characterized by mixed sensory and motor deficits, developing after a latent period ranging from 6 months to several years. The pathogenesis involves progressive vascular degeneration, fibrosis and demyelination with loss of nerve fibres.

## Heart and large vessels

With improvement of cancer therapies, the fraction of long-term cancer survivors in the population progressively increases. Cardiovascular disease, either as a consequence of the direct effects of cancer therapy or its adverse effects on traditional cardiac risk factors (e.g. obesity, hypertension, dyslipidemia and diabetes mellitus), hence gain increasing importance (e.g. [31]). The radiation effects can become manifest in various ways; the pathogenesis is complex, involving various inflammatory pathways (32).

In the heart, low doses can result in reversible functional changes in electrocardiogram, which are not predictive for late radiation sequelae. At higher doses, morphological changes can be observed. The most common type of radiation-induced heart effect is pericarditis with a variable degree of pericardial effusion. This complication has a relatively early onset (∼50% occurrence within the first 6 months, remainder within 2 years). It is asymptomatic and clears spontaneously in the majority of patients.

Radiation-induced cardiomyopathy is another form of complication that presents either as reduced ventricular ejection or conduction blocks and develops slowly over a period of 10–20 years. Current estimates of doses giving a 50% complication probability are approximately 50 Gy in 2 Gy fractions. With long-term follow-up of patients treated for Hodgkin disease or breast cancer, the enhanced risk of ischaemic heart disease after periods in excess of 10 years has increasingly been reported. The large variation in risk estimates reported in different studies suggests that volume effects are important, but also that sensitive substructures are present. In this respect the heart auricles and the proximal parts of the coronary arteries have been suggested to be particularly sensitive to radiation damage.

Histopathologically, late damage to the myocardium is characterised predominantly by diffuse interstitial and perivascular fibrosis, and loss of cardiomyocytes. Vascular radiation effects also contribute significantly to myocardial infarction after radiation exposure of the heart. However, the (molecular) pathophysiology of these effects remains unclear.

In large blood vessels, irradiation with doses over 8 Gy can initiate or promote atherosclerosis (32,34).

## Cartilage and bone

Growing cartilage (epiphyseal plate) is extremely radiosensitive; single doses of 4–7 Gy are sufficient to induce changes in chondrocytes within a few days, with a loss of the columnar structure and a reduction in cellular density. The reduced cell production translates into (bone) growth impairment, which is more pronounced at an earlier age. In contrast, adult cartilage, e.g. in joints, larynx or trachea, as well as adult bone is relatively radiation resistant. However, late effects in these structures, including osteoradionecrosis, must be considered as an interaction with vascular radiation effects.

## Sense organs

### EYE

Inclusion of the eye into the high-dose volume results in keratoconjunctivitis, which, however, resolves soon after the end of radiotherapy. In the eye lens, epithelial degeneration in the equator zone, where proliferation occurs physiologically, is observed after low radiation doses. The damaged fibres develop vacuolisation and partly retain their nuclei. Eventually, a usually posterior subcapsular radiation cataract develops in varying degrees. The latent times are inversely related to dose, and range from 6 months to several decades (hence, frequently preventing evaluation by the radiation oncologist). The tolerance doses usually reported are in the range of a few gray for fractionated irradiation, and clearly below 1 Gy for single-dose exposure. A fractionation effect seems to be pronounced for the eye lens. In contrast, no effect of overall exposure time is evident.

As cataracts can readily be treated with modern surgical techniques, late effects in the lacrimal glands (loss of function) and consequently in the cornea, depicted as 'dry eye', are more important and dose limiting. Already after moderate radiation doses, these can result in chronic corneal ulceration and eventually loss of the eye.

### EAR

The most frequent early radiation effect in the ear is a serous inflammation (otitis media), which impacts on hearing function. In addition, doses >30 Gy result in direct effects in the inner ear, with the consequence of permanent hearing impairment.

### TASTE

Radiation effects on taste acuity are a multifactorial process, including direct changes (cell loss) in taste buds, xerostomia with a reduced cleansing of the buds and changes in smelling ability. Taste impairment is usually observed after doses of around 30 Gy. Usually, the changes in the individual taste qualities resolve after radiotherapy, in intervals up to 1 year, but a general increase in threshold concentration may remain.

---

### Key points

1. Early radiation effects, developing in turnover tissues, are dominated by tissue hypoplasia.
2. The latent time of early effects is largely independent of dose, while severity and duration/time to healing are dose dependent.
3. Additional trauma aggravates early reactions.
4. Healing of early responses, based on surviving tissue stem cells, is usually complete.
5. Late radiation sequelae, observed after months to years after therapy, are progressive and often irreversible.
6. Late effects may occur in waves, thus leading to a clear discrepancy between cumulative incidence and prevalence. Hence, both parameters need to be documented.

7. Late effects are based on a complex and interactive response of parenchymal cells, vascular endothelium and fibroblasts, with a contribution of macrophages and other cell types.
8. The latent time of chronic reactions is inversely dependent on dose.

## ■ BIBLIOGRAPHY

1. Barani IJ, Benedict SH, Lin PS. Neural stem cells: Implications for the conventional radiotherapy of central nervous system malignancies. *Int J Radiat Oncol Biol Phys* 2007;68:324–333.

2. Bentzen SM. Preventing or reducing late side effects of radiation therapy: Radiobiology meets molecular pathology. *Nat Rev Cancer* 2006;6:702–713.

3. Bentzen SM, Saunders MI, Dische S, Bond SJ. Radiotherapy-related early morbidity in head and neck cancer: Quantitative clinical radiobiology as deduced from the CHART trial. *Radiother Oncol* 2001;60:123–135.

4. Bentzen SM, Turesson I, Thames HD. Fractionation sensitivity and latency of telangiectasia after postmastectomy radiotherapy: A graded-response analysis. *Radiother Oncol* 1990;18:95–106.

5. Clement CH, Stewart FA. International Commission on Radiological Protection (Eds). *ICRP Publ. 118: ICRP Statement on Tissue Reactions and Early and Late Effects of Radiation in Normal Tissues and Organs: Threshold Doses for Tissue Reactions in a Radiation Protection Context.* Vol 41 (1/2). Oxford: Published for the International Commission on Radiological Protection by Elsevier; 2012.

6. Dittmann K, Mayer C, Rodemann HP. Inhibition of radiation-induced EGFR nuclear import by C225 (Cetuximab) suppresses DNA-PK activity. *Radiother Oncol* 2005;76:157–161.

7. Dörr W. Three A's of repopulation during fractionated irradiation of squamous epithelia: Asymmetry loss, Acceleration of stem-cell divisions and Abortive divisions. *Int J Radiat Biol* 1997;72:635–643.

8. Dörr W, Bertmann S, Herrmann T. Radiation induced lung reactions in breast cancer therapy. Modulating factors and consequential effects. Strahlenther Onkol 2005;181:567–573.

9. Dörr W, Hendry JH. Consequential late effects in normal tissues. *Radiother Oncol* 2001;61:223–231.

10. Dörr W, Herrmann T. Pathogenetic mechanisms of lung fibrosis. In: Nieder C, Milas L and Ang KK (Eds). *Biological Modification of Radiation Response.* Berlin: Springer; 2003. pp. 29–36.

11. Dörr W, Herrmann T, Riesenbeck D (Eds). *Prävention und therapie von nebenwirkungen in der strahlentherapie.* Bremen: UNI-MED Science; 2005.

12. Dörr W, Herrmann T, Trott KR. Normal tissue tolerance. *Transl Cancer Res* 2017;6(Suppl 5):S840–S851.

13. Dörr W, Kummermehr J. Proliferation kinetics of mouse tongue epithelium under normal conditions and following single dose irradiation. *Virchows Arch B Cell Pathol Incl Mol Pathol* 1991;60:287–294.

14. Fajardo LF, Berthrong M, Anderson RE. *Radiation Pathology.* New York, NY: Oxford University Press; 2001.

15. Georg P, Boni A, Ghabuous A et al. Time course of late rectal- and urinary bladder side effects after MRI-guided adaptive brachytherapy for cervical cancer. *Strahlenther Onkol* 2013;189:535–540.

16. Goldner G, Pötter R, Kranz A, Bluhm A, Dörr W. Healing of late endoscopic changes in the rectum between 12 and 65 months after external beam radiotherapy. *Strahlenther Onkol* 2011;187:202–205.

17. Hakenjos L, Bamberg M, Rodemann HP. TGF-beta1-mediated alterations of rat lung fibroblast differentiation resulting in the radiation-induced fibrotic phenotype. *Int J Radiat Biol* 2000;76:503–509.

18. Herrmann T, Baumann M, Dörr W. *Klinische strahlenbiologie - kurz und bündig.* 4th ed. München: Elsevier; 2006.

19. Jaal J, Dörr W. Radiation induced late damage to the barrier function of small blood vessels in mouse bladder. *J Urol* 2006;176:2696–2700.

20. Jung H, Beck-Bornholdt HP, Svoboda V, Alberti W, Herrmann T. Quantification of late complications after radiation therapy. *Radiother Oncol* 2001;61:233–246.

21. Marks LB, Ten Haken RK, Martel MK. Guest editor's introduction to QUANTEC: A users guide. *Int J Radiat Oncol Biol Phys* 2010;76(3 Suppl):S1–S2.

22. Michalowski A. Effects of radiation on normal tissues: Hypothetical mechanisms and limitations of in situ assays of clonogenicity. *Radiat Environ Biophys* 1981;19:157–172.

23. Potten CS, Hendry JH (Eds). *Cytotoxic Insults to Tissues: Effects on Cell Lineages.* Edinburgh: Churchill-Livingstone; 1983.

24. Riesenbeck D, Dörr W. Documentation of radiation-induced oral mucositis. Scoring systems. *Strahlenther Onkol* 1998; 174(Suppl 3):44–46.

25. Rodemann HP, Bamberg M. Cellular basis of radiation-induced fibrosis. *Radiother Oncol* 1995;35:83–90.

26. Rubin P, Johnston CJ, Williams JP, McDonald S, Finkelstein JN. A perpetual cascade of cytokines postirradiation leads to pulmonary fibrosis. *Int J Radiat Oncol Biol Phys* 1995;33:99–109.

27. Schaue D, Kachikwu EL, McBride WH. Cytokines in radiobiological responses: A review. *Radiat Res* 2012;178:505–523.

28. Schmid MP, Pötter R, Bombosch V et al. Late gastrointestinal and urogenital side-effects after radiotherapy—Incidence and prevalence. Subgroup-analysis within the prospective Austrian-German phase II multicenter trial for localized prostate cancer. *Radiother Oncol* 2012;104:114–118.

29. Schultz-Hector S. Radiation-induced heart disease: Review of experimental data on dose response and pathogenesis. *Int J Radiat Biol* 1992;61:149–160.

30. Sonis ST. A biological approach to mucositis. *J Support Oncol* 2004;2:21–32; discussion 5–6.

31. Steingart RM, Yadav N, Manrique C, Carver JR, Liu J. Cancer survivorship: Cardiotoxic therapy in the adult cancer patient; cardiac outcomes with recommendations for patient management. *Semin Oncol* 2013;40:690–708.

32. Stewart FA. Mechanisms and dose-response relationships for radiation-induced cardiovascular disease. *Ann ICRP* 2012;41:72–79.

33. Stewart FA, Dörr W. Milestones in normal tissue radiation biology over the past 50 years: From clonogenic cell survival to cytokine networks and back to stem cell recovery. *Int J Radiat Biol* 2009;85:574–586.

34. Stewart FA, Hoving S, Russell NS. Vascular damage as an underlying mechanism of cardiac and cerebral toxicity in irradiated cancer patients. *Radiat Res* 2010;174:865–869.

35. Stock M, Dörr W, Stromberger C et al. Investigations on parotid gland recovery after IMRT in head and neck tumor patients. *Strahlenther Onkol* 2010;186:665–671.

36. Supiot S, Paris F. [Radiobiology dedicated to endothelium]. *Cancer Radiother* 2012;16:11–15.

37. Taghian NR, Miller CL, Jammallo LS, O'Toole J, Skolny MN. Lymphedema following breast cancer treatment and impact on quality of life: A review. *Crit Rev Oncol Hematol* 2014;92:227–234.

38. Trott KR, Dörr W, Facoetti A et al. Biological mechanisms of normal tissue damage: Importance for the design of NTCP models. *Radiother Oncol* 2012;105:79–85.

39. Turesson I. Individual variation and dose dependency in the progression rate of skin telangiectasia. *Int J Radiat Oncol Biol Phys* 1990;19:1569–1574.

40. van der Kogel AJ. Central nervous system radiation injury in small animal models. In: Gutin PH, Leibel SA and Sheline GE (Eds). *Radiation Injury to the Nervous System.* New York, NY: Raven Press; 1991. pp. 91–111.

41. Van der Schueren E, Van den Bogaert W, Vanuytsel L, Van Limbergen E. Radiotherapy by multiple fractions per day (MFD) in head and neck cancer: Acute reactions of skin and mucosa. *Int J Radiat Oncol Biol Phys* 1990;19:301–311.

42. Warrington JP, Ashpole N, Csiszar A, Lee YW, Ungvari Z, Sonntag WE. Whole brain radiation-induced vascular cognitive impairment: Mechanisms and implications. *J Vasc Res* 2013;50:445–457.

43. Withers HR, Elkind MM. Microcolony survival assay for cells of mouse intestinal mucosa exposed to radiation. *Int J Radiat Biol Relat Stud Phys Chem Med* 1970;17:261–267.

44. Withers HR, Taylor JM, Maciejewski B. Treatment volume and tissue tolerance. *Int J Radiat Oncol Biol Phys* 1988;14:751–759.

45. Yarnold J, Brotons MC. Pathogenetic mechanisms in radiation fibrosis. *Radiother Oncol* 2010;97:149–161.

## ■ FURTHER READING

46. Bentzen SM, Dörr W, Anscher MS et al. Normal tissue effects: Reporting and analysis. *Semin Radiat Oncol* 2003; 13:189–202.

47. Brown JM, Mehta MP, Nieder C (Eds). *Multimodal Concepts for Integration of Cytotoxic Drugs and Radiation Therapy.* Berlin: Springer; 2006.

48. Dörr W (Ed). *Growth Factors in the Pathogenesis of Radiation Effects in Normal Tissues.* Munich: Urban and Vogel; 2001.

49. Dörr W. Skin and other reactions to radiotherapy – Clinical presentation and radiobiology of skin reactions. *Front Radiat Ther Oncol* 2006;39:96–101.

50. Grötz KA, Riesenbeck D, Brahm R et al. Chronic radiation effects on dental hard tissue (radiation caries). Classification and therapeutic strategies. *Strahlenther Onkol* 2001;177:96–104.

51. National Cancer Institute. *Common Terminology Criteria for Adverse Events (CTCAE) v4.* Washington: https://evs.nci.nih.gov/ftp1/CTCAE/About.html; 2010.

52. Pavy JJ, Denekamp J, Letschert J et al. EORTC Late Effects Working Group. Late effects toxicity scoring: The SOMA scale. *Radiother Oncol* 1995;35:11–15.

53. Wong RK, Bensadoun RJ, Boers-Doets CB et al. Clinical practice guidelines for the prevention and treatment of acute and late radiation reactions from the MASCC Skin Toxicity Study Group. *Support Care Cancer* 2013;21:2933–2948.

54. Zhao W, Robbins ME. Inflammation and chronic oxidative stress in radiation-induced late normal tissue injury: Therapeutic implications. *Curr Med Chem* 2009;16:130–143.

# Stem cells in radiotherapy

ROBERT P. COPPES, MICHAEL BAUMANN, MECHTHILD KRAUSE AND RICHARD P. HILL

## 15.1 INTRODUCTION

The field of stem cell research has opened exciting new avenues for development of stem cell-based therapies for regeneration of tissues or treatment of cancers. Stem cells play a pivotal role in the response to radiotherapy since for the tumour these are the target cells that ultimately determine treatment outcome, while in normal tissues they play an important role in tissue repair. With the discovery and experimental handling of many different types of stem cells, the road has been paved for new therapeutic options. Stem cell-based therapies may in the near future be used to enhance the response of the tumour to radiation; inhibit post-treatment tumour regrowth; and protect, accelerate or enhance normal tissue regeneration. Stem cells are cells that are capable of self-renewal (produce more stem cells) and the production of more committed progenitor or functional cells in the tissues (differentiation), see Figure 15.1.

Three different types of stem cells exist; embryonic stem (ES) cells, induced pluripotent stem (iPS) cells and adult stem cells (ASCs). ES cells, derived from the inner cell mass of blastocysts, can be cultured for experimental purposes and can form all tissues of the body. In 2006, the 2012 Nobel-prizewinning team of Shinya Yamanaka at Kyoto University, Japan, managed to culture ES cell-like iPS cells from adult somatic cells, such as fibroblasts, by introduction of pluripotency genes like the transcription factors Oct-3/4, SOX2, c-Myc and Klf4 (43). Similar to ES cells, iPS cells can indefinitely self-renew, are pluripotent and are able to produce all cell types of the body after injection into blastocytes. As such, iPS cells hold high promise for fundamental and therapeutic applications. ASCs are a population of undifferentiated cells that are maintained through development and into adulthood. Such ASCs are believed to be present in every tissue or organ in the body and are committed to that specific tissue type and can proliferate and/or differentiate to repair damage. During life ASCs may accumulate DNA damage causing a reduction in number, in self-renewal and/or differentiation potential and may therefore be less capable of restoring damage (26). It has been postulated that stem cells are a critical target population for radiation carcinogenesis and there is increasing experimental evidence that stem cells, due to their longevity, may represent a major target for mutations leading to cancer (8,32).

Interestingly, tumours seem to harbour (cancer) stem cells, potentially derived from ASCs. Like normal stem cells, cancer stem cells (CSCs) can self-renew and form more differentiated cells within the tumour. Similar to normal tissue stem cells, CSCs are thought to be the cells that repopulate the tumour after therapies and are therefore also termed tumour-initiating cells (TICs) or cancer-initiating cells (CICs). Considerable overlap between normal stem cells and CSCs has been postulated and this can extend to the expression of specific proteins on the surface of the cells that can act as detectable surface markers of their status (see Table 15.1). Examples of specific surface markers of (cancer) stem cells include CD34 and CD38 for hematopoietic cells and leukaemias and CD133, CD44, and CD24 for different types of solid tumour cells. These markers have been used extensively to enrich tumour cell populations for stem cells by sorting techniques to allow analysis of the features of such cells (10,11,49), including measurements of radiosensitivity (see text that follows).

The characteristics of normal and cancer stem cells hold great potential for post-irradiation normal tissue regeneration and tumour treatment. Interfering with signalling pathways involved in self-renewal or differentiation of stem cells before, during or after irradiation may strongly affect treatment outcome both for the normal tissue and the tumour.

## 15.2 ADULT TISSUE STEM CELLS

Many tissues and organs contain ASCs that maintain tissue homeostasis during adult life and repair tissue after cell loss due to daily use, disease or injury. These cells have the capacity to self-renew and differentiate into the different cell types in the tissue. Rapid turnover tissues like gut, bone marrow and skin are thought to contain high numbers of stem cells, whereas slowly proliferating tissues are viewed as containing quiescent stem cells (28). ASCs may have various specific features (15), one or more for every tissue, and include multipotent stromal cells, also known as mesenchymal stem cells (MSCs), that can be derived from various tissues including bone marrow and adipose tissue. MSCs can easily be cultured for experimental purposes and are characterized as being able to differentiate into a range of cell types such as osteoblasts, chondrocytes and adipocytes. During development and repair, mesenchymal cells and

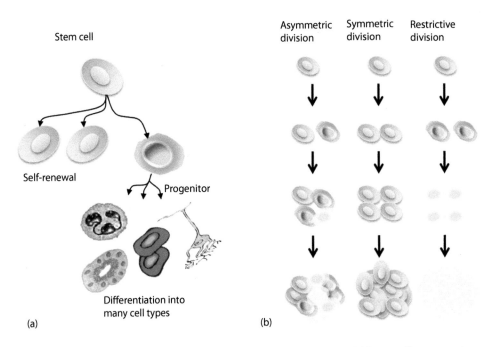

Figure 15.1 Stem cell fate. (a) Development of differentiated cells from stem cell with potential intermediate progenitor cell. (b) Stem cell division options. Asymmetric division commonly present in normal tissue and tumours, symmetric division results in expansion of stem cell pool and enhance regenerative capacity, whereas restrictive division results in exhaustion of stem cells pool and degeneration of tissue or tumour.

Table 15.1 Examples of surface markers of normal stem cells and cancer stem cells in different tissues

| Organ | Cancer type | Cancer stem cell markers | Normal stem cell markers |
|---|---|---|---|
| Bladder | Bladder cancer | CD44 | – |
| Breast | Mammary cancer | CD44+/ESA+/CD24−/CD90−, ALDH1+, Lin− | CD24med |
| Brain | Brain tumour | CD44+, CD133+, Nestin+ | CD133+, Lin− |
| Colon | Colorectal cancer | CD44+/ESA+, CD166+, CD133+, CD24+, EpCAM+, ALDH1+ | CD133+ |
| Oesophagus | Oesophageal cancer | CD44+, CD133+, CD24+, ABCG2+, CXCR4+, ALDH1+ | – |
| Hematopoietic | ALL, AML, MM | CD34+/−, CD38+/−, CD90+/−, CD123+, CD19+, CD45RA+, CD33+, CD13+, CD44+, CD96+, CD47+, CD32+, CD25+, CD138−, CD27+, CLL-1+, TIM3+ | CD34+, CD38−, CD90−, Lin− |
| Hemangioblastic | CML | Flk1+, CD31−, CD34− | Flk1+, CD31−, CD34− |
| Liver | Liver cancer | CD44+, CD133+, CD45−/CD90+, CD13+, EpCAM+ | CD133+, ESA+ |
| Lung | Lung cancer | CD44+, CD133+, Lin−/CD166+, ALDH1+ | CD133+ |
| Ovaries | Ovarian cancer | CD44+, CD133+, CD24+, CD117+, EpCAM+, ALDH1+ | CD117+ |
| Pancreas | Pancreatic cancer | CD44+/CD24+, CD133+, ESA+, ALDH1+ | CXCR4+, Nestin+ |
| Prostate | Prostate cancer | CD44+/CD24−, CD133+, $\alpha_2\beta_1$high, ALDH1+ | $\alpha_2\beta_1$high, CD133+ |
| Skin | Melanoma | CD20+, CD133+, CD271+, CD166+, Nestin+, ABCB5+ | K19+$\beta_1$+, CD133+, CD166+, Nestin+ |
| Stomach | Gastric cancer | CD44+, CD44V8-10+, CD133+, CD24+, CD54+, CD90+, CD49f+, CD71+, EpCAM+, ALDH1+ | – |
| Tongue, larynx, throat and sinus | Head and neck squamous cell carcinoma | CD44+, CD133+, Lin−, ALDH1+ | CD44+, Lin− |

Data from (1,2,49).

*Abbreviations:* ABCB5, ATP-binding cassette sub-family B member 5; ABCG2, ABC subfamily G member 2; ALDH1, aldehyde dehydrogenase 1; ALL, acute lympho-blastic leukemia; AML, acute myeloid leukemia; CLL-1, C-type lectin-like molecule-1; CML, chronic myelogenous leukemia; CXCR4, C-X-C chemokine receptor type 4; EpCAM, epithelial cellular adhesion molecule; ESA, epithelial surface antigen; Flk1, fetal liver kinase 1; Lin, lineage; MM, multiple myeloma; TIM3, T-cell immunoglobulin and mucin domain-containing-3; –, not known.

the tissue stem cells cross-talk through cytokine-receptor signalling to build a specific organ (40).

ASCs can divide to self-renew and to provide a continual population of more restricted progenitor cells. Depending on the tissue, several types of progenitor cells may exist, such as common myeloid progenitor and common lymphoid progenitor for haematopoiesis or none at all such as for neurogenesis (Figure 15.1a). These progenitor cells can further divide into many cell types that are necessary to perform the function of an organ or tissue. Progenitor cells are more restricted than stem cells in that they have no or a limited capacity to self-renew and differentiate into only a specific cell type in the tissue (oligopotent). However, it has become apparent that the stem cell–progenitor cell–differentiated cell pathway may not be a one-way route. Tissue damage to tissue or the tissue stem cells may induce progenitor cells to revert to stem cells and form an injury-inducible reserve stem cell population (12) through sensors of the structural and mechanical features of the cell microenvironment (35). Interestingly, cancer stem–progenitor cells also seem to behave as two-way traffic (48). This leads to concerns about the absolute validity of the use of cell surface markers to identify cancer stem cells, since cells not expressing such markers may have the capacity to revert to a stem cell phenotype at some time post-selection and thus the effective stem cell proportion in a tumour may be underestimated. This may be a particular concern if such plasticity of the stem cell phenotype can be induced by treatment.

Stem cells are capable of three types of divisions: (1) asymmetric division of a stem cell involving the generation of one stem cell and a more differentiated progenitor cell, (2) symmetric division in which a stem cell is able to maintain and multiply its own cell number and (3) restrictive division where two more differentiated daughter cells are produced. For normal homeostasis, asymmetric division would be preferred, whereas restrictive division would lead to tissue aging. After severe tissue damage the stem cells may first perform symmetric division to expand the number of stem cells where after asymmetric or restrictive division regenerates the tissue. When these processes are not properly controlled and in conjunction with stromal and vascular effects, it may result in tumour formation (4,26).

## 15.3 CANCER STEM CELLS

The current CSC hypothesis defines them as cancer cells that have the ability to self-renew, to differentiate into all subpopulations of tumour cells and to drive recurrence and metastasis (36). This is an attractive hypothesis since it implies that the CSCs are the cells that all need to be killed to cure a cancer. However, as noted above, the stem cell/progenitor cell phenotype may be quite plastic particularly in cancer cells, such that there can be two-way traffic between these states. Such capacities may be a constant feature of a defined cell or may be acquired through the

impact of microenvironmental conditions within tumours. Such plasticity may make it difficult to definitively identify CSC in a tumour cell population. For radiotherapy, the CSC definition translates into the fact that all CSCs need to be inactivated to reach permanent tumour cure, or, that a single surviving CSC has the potential to cause a tumour recurrence (6). It should be noted that the probability that a single putative CSC will regrow a tumour may not be unity, since it is possible that during early divisions it will transit to a completely differentiated cell population and extinguish (restrictive division, Figure 15.1b). Nevertheless, the evaluation of permanent local tumour control is an indirect or functional marker for the survival of CSCs, which includes the possibility that some CSCs may not die as a direct consequence of the treatment but might later be eliminated by the host, e.g. through the immune system.

Early studies on the ability to transplant tumours demonstrated that usually many cells were required to be injected to achieve a successful growth. Using limiting-dilution assays, similar to those used in current cancer stem cell studies, Hewitt and colleagues used unsorted populations of tumour cells from 26 spontaneously arising murine tumour models and found that for the different tumours the number of cells required to achieve tumour growth in 50% of injected sites ($TD_{50}$) varied from close to unity to greater than 10,000 cells (24). For a number of the tumours these authors also demonstrated that addition, to the viable tumour cell inoculum, of a large number ($10^5$–$10^6$) of lethally irradiated (to prevent their growth) cells from the same tumour significantly reduced the $TD_{50}$ value of the viable tumour cells. Current interpretation of these findings would be that stromal cell populations (vascular cell components, cancer-associated fibroblasts or various bone marrow-derived cell populations) known to be present in tumours may enhance the ability of the cancer stem cells to grow at the (new) injection site.

Using modern sorting techniques, it is today possible to select cell populations that are found to show a higher expression of putative stem cell surface markers from populations with lower expression, leading to an enrichment (but not purification) of putative cancer stem cells in the first population. The gold standard for validation of the stemness of tumour cells (e.g. sorted by using marker assays) is the limiting-dilution quantitative transplantation assay ($TD_{50}$ assay as described above), see Figure 15.2. Studies of single radiation treatments (given under clamped hypoxia) required to achieve local tumour control (tumour control dose 50%, $TCD_{50}$) were found to correlate with the $TD_{50}$ value, underlining the importance of the number of CSCs for radiocurability (6), see Figure 15.3. Functional assays like $TCD_{50}$ and $TD_{50}$, therefore, are essential to validate the results determined in marker-based biological experiments, which as noted previously may underestimate the true stem cell potential of a tumour cell population, particularly following treatment. They are also of high importance for the evaluation of the efficacy of new radio-oncological treatment

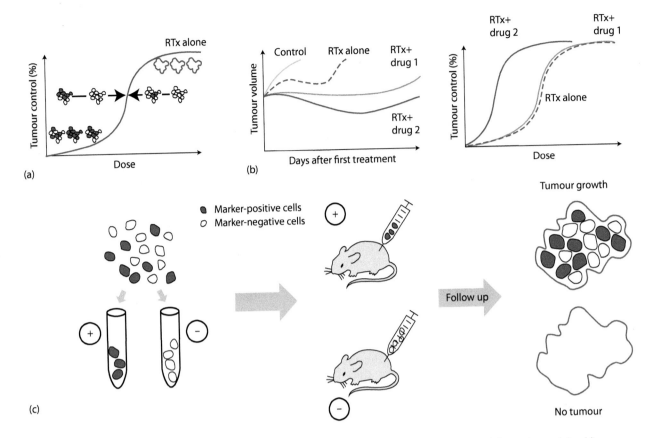

Figure 15.2 Local tumour control increases as a sigmoid function with increasing irradiation dose, which can be explained by exponential CSC kill and Poisson statistics (a). The combination of radiotherapy with drugs may significantly enhance tumour regression or growth delay without improving local tumour control (drug 1) or with enhanced local tumour control (drug 2). Currently only local tumour control assays functionally test the effect of irradiation or combined modality treatments on CSCs (b). In order to evaluate stem cell characteristics of marker-positive cells compared to marker-negative cells, *in vivo* transplantation assays are used (c). (From (10), with permission.)

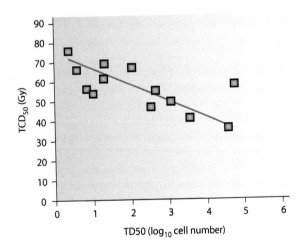

Figure 15.3 Correlation of transplantability and curability by irradiation of 13 different experimental tumour models. Transplantability has been evaluated as the number of vital tumour cells that needs to be injected to induce a growing tumour in 50% of the animals ($TD_{50}$). Curability has been assessed as the irradiation dose that needs to be applied to obtain permanent local control in 50% of the tumours ($TCD_{50}$). (From (6), with permission.)

approaches. Studies of the combination of radiotherapy and new molecular-targeted agents have observed a dissociation of the effects on curative ($TCD_{50}$) or palliative endpoints (tumour growth delay or tumour volume) with considerable overestimation of effects by the latter endpoints (27). A likely explanation is that many of those approaches inactivate the majority of non-CSCs, but are inefficient in enhancing the radiation effect on CSC inactivation, although it is possible that the treatments are also inducing surviving non-CSCs to revert to the stem cell state (6). Thus, the induced tumour shrinkage or prolongation of growth delay does not translate into improved local tumour control (Figure 15.2).

## 15.4 RADIOSENSITIVITY OF ADULT TISSUE STEM CELLS

For normal tissue homeostasis the lifespan of differentiated functional cells determines the underlying requirement for proliferation of the stem cells of that tissue (Figure 15.4). This, in turn, determines the response time of rapid proliferating tissues to radiation (see Chapter 12). After irradiation of a tissue, unrepaired DNA damage in stem

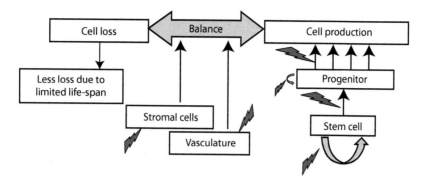

**Figure 15.4** Tissue homeostasis. Cell loss and cell production should be in balance for tissue homeostasis. Irradiation may affect all processes involved in the production of cells and potentially leading to premature aging of the tissue. Stromal cells and the vasculature potentially facilitate or inhibit cell production.

cells may prevent division or result in stem cell death when division is required to replace a differentiated functional cell to maintain homeostasis (Figure 15.4). Consequentially, the tissue function deteriorates with the speed of cell turnover. The long-term recovery of a tissue after radiation exposure, therefore, strongly depends on the number of surviving stem cells, which, in turn, depends on the radiation dose. Considerable evidence shows that in general DNA damage compromises ASC function (32). Moreover, function can also be influenced by other radiation-induced cytokine-driven processes, such as inflammation and fibrosis (see Chapter 14). These processes may affect stem cell maintenance that is a complex interaction between growth factor signalling pathways and extra cellular matrix interactions that can both be altered after irradiation (Figure 15.4).

The primary insult for any cell after irradiation is DNA damage. The ability to repair such damage is pivotal for the survival of the cell, in this case the stem cell. Although not well understood, ASCs may use different DNA repair pathways compared to more committed cells (32) and the DNA damage response (DDR) may differ between different types of ASCs. For example, whereas haematopoietic stem cells (HSCs) and hair-follicle-bulge stem cells (of the skin) trigger active repair and prevent cell death, gastrointestinal tract stem cells, such as those that reside in the ileum, do not. They rely on an active p53 transcription factor and apoptosis pathways to cause cell death.

Adult stem cells under normal circumstances are mostly quiescent residing in the G0 phase of the cell cycle, until cell loss requires them to proliferate. While this makes the study of DNA repair in stem cells in culture problematic, using *in vivo* long-term single-cell labelling and imaging techniques to track ASCs, but not their descendants, DNA repair in stem cells can be studied *in vivo*. Such studies have revealed several intriguing differences between ASCs and progenitor/differentiated cells. Quiescent stem cells have a low metabolic activity and often-high levels of anti-apoptotic proteins such as Bcl-2 and decreased production of reactive oxygen species (ROS) necessary for longevity. The use of glycolytic pathways for energy instead of mitochondrial respiration, the maintenance of a hypoxic niche, high levels of ABC transporters and the expression of BMI-1 in many ASCs may all contribute to a

more radioresistant phenotype. ASCs are also intrinsically more efficient in base and nucleotide excision repair and repair single- and double-strand breaks better. This may relate to the fact that DNA damage checkpoints and several repair pathways are cell-cycle dependent. However, if ASCs accumulate DNA damage and are then forced to enter the cell cycle, the higher levels of DNA-PKs in ASCs lead primarily to repair by error-prone non-homologous end joining. This potentially results in ASC exhaustion, premature differentiation and senescence and reduced regenerative response, acquisition of mutations and predisposition to cancer (8).

An important question is the extent to which the sensitivity of normal tissues to radiation is explained by the response of the ASCs? Next to the DDR of the stem cells and progenitor cells, the stem cell niche plays a pivotal role in the response of a tissue to irradiation. Irradiation may destroy the niche that is required to support repopulation of the tissue. Excessive inflammation and fibrosis occurring in many tissues after radiotherapy may destroy the stem cell niche and prevent stem cells-induced tissue regeneration. The radiation-induced secretion of inflammatory and pro-fibrotic cytokines such as TGF-ß not only promotes scar tissue formation but may also inhibit stem cell proliferation and differentiation. TGF-ß inhibitors are widely used in the culturing of stem cells. Studies of salivary glands and other tissue have shown that, after a dose of radiation that completely abrogates regeneration and secretory function, significant numbers of stem cells still survived and could be cultured *in vitro* (30). Moreover, administration of growth factors such as KGF induced the remaining stem cells to regenerate the tissue to some extent depending on the number of surviving stem cells. Next to this, tissue vascularization may play an important role in the tissue response to radiation (Figure 15.4). Hypoxia not only induces the constant production of toxic ROS but also seems to keep stem cells in a quiescence state reducing their regenerative capacity. Thus, a complex balance between surviving stem cells, the state of the stem-cell niche, inhibitory and stimulating signalling growth factors and cytokines and the response of the stromal elements of the tissue, ultimately determines the regenerative capacity of a tissue after irradiation.

## 15.5 RADIOSENSITIVITY OF CANCER STEM CELLS

Resulting from the importance of CSC inactivation for tumour cure, different CSC-related parameters and mechanisms affect radioresistance of tumours (14). First, radiocurability is known to correlate with the *number of CSCs* that need to be sterilized. This was shown already in the 1980s by proving a significant correlation between transplantability ($TD_{50}$) and tumour cure rate ($TCD_{50}$) after single-dose irradiation under homogeneous hypoxia in different animal tumour models (25). In line with these data, radiocurability of tumours inversely correlates with tumour volume (20) or with a combination of transplantability and intrinsic radiosensitivity *in vitro* (21). The importance of CSC density is shown by the fact that even curability after clinically relevant fractionated irradiation, which is influenced by several other factors, strongly correlates with the number and intrinsic radiosensitivity of CSCs (46). For expression of the putative CSC marker CD44, a correlation with local tumour control after radiotherapy in

patients with early laryngeal cancer has been shown (17). For other clinical tumours evidence is accumulating that markers related to CSC number or density correlate with outcome (10), see Table 15.2. For more heterogeneous patient groups, a high impact of other factors like differences in CSC radiosensitivity, tumour micromilieu or tumour cell repopulation is expected (see Chapters 8 and 18).

The potential of repopulation appears to be highest in squamous cell carcinomas, but is expected to be present in all malignant tumours. Repopulation of CSCs is one of the most important determinants of local tumour control after fractionated irradiation (5,23). With modern real-time imaging techniques and tracking of CSCs, using the absence of 26S proteasome activity as a marker, an increase of the percentage of CSCs 72 hours after irradiation with $5 \times 3$ Gy in a human glioma model could be shown to correlate with increased Ki-67 positive proliferating cells in marker-positive versus marker-negative cells (44). While proliferation appears to be the most important factor contributing to the fractionation effect, the possibility of a contribution from treatment-induced plasticity in the stem cell potential of

Table 15.2 Clinical studies investigating the correlation between CSC markers and the outcome of radiotherapy

| Entity | Marker | Outcome | Prognostic correlation | Author |
|---|---|---|---|---|
| **Glioblastoma** | | | | |
| $n = 88$ | CD133CD15 Nestin | Overall survival<br>Prognostic-free survival | − | Kim et al. (2011) (51) |
| $n = 80$ | CD133 | Overall survival | + | Murat et al. (2008) (52) |
| $n = 44$ | CD133 | Overall survival<br>Prognostic-free survival | + | Pallini et al. (2008) (53) |
| $n = 48$ | CD133 | Overall survival<br>Prognostic-free survival | + | Metellus et al. (2011) (54) |
| **HNSCC** | | | | |
| $n = 52$ | CD44 | Local tumour control | + | De Jong et al. (2010) (55) |
| $n = 74$ | CD44 Integrin-β1 | Local prognostic-free survival<br>Metastasis-free survival<br>Overall survival | + | Koukourakis et al. (2102) (56) |
| **Oesophageal cancer** | | | | |
| $n = 24$ | $CD44^+/CD24^-$ | Pathological tumour response | + | Smit et al. (2013) (57) |
| **Rectal cancer** | | | | |
| $n = 73$ | CD133 | Disease-free survival<br>Overall survival | + | Wang et al. (2009) (58) |
| $n = 210$ | CD44v6 | Disease-free survival<br>Disease-specific survival | + | Avoranta et al. (2012) (59) |
| $n = 99$ | CD133 | Disease-free survival<br>Cancer-specific overall survival | + | Sprenger et al. (2013) (60) |
| $n = 52$ | CD133CD44 | Disease-free survival | + | Kawamoto et al. (2012) (61) |
| **Cervical cancer** | | | | |
| $n = 73$ | CD24 | Metastasis-free survival<br>Loco-regional failure rate | +<br>− | Kwon et al. (2007) (62) |
| $n = 140$ | CD24 | Metastasis-free survival<br>Loco-regional failure-free survival<br>Overall survival | + | Sung et al. (2010) (63) |

Modified from (10).

the progenitor cell population in the tumours cannot yet be ruled out.

There are several data sets which support a higher *intrinsic radioresistance of CSCs* compared to non-CSCs. In extensive experiments, an increase of the *ex vivo* fraction of CD133 positive cells, confirmed as CSCs by transplantation assays, has been shown after *in vivo* irradiation of glioma xenografts. The more pronounced increase after fractionated irradiation (5 × 3 Gy) as compared to single-dose irradiation (9 Gy) may be explained by repopulation, repair of sublethal damage or induced plasticity of the CSC phenotype. Interestingly, DNA damage checkpoints were preferentially activated in marker-positive versus marker-negative cells (3). Another resistance mechanism may be related to ROS, a critical mediator of radiation damage in cells. Breast CSCs have been shown *in vitro* to contain a lower level of ROS versus progenitor cells and to have increased potential defence against ROS with higher expression of genes involved in ROS scavenging and a modulation of the initially higher post-irradiation clonogenic cell survival of CSC by pharmacological modulation of the ROS levels (18). However, a higher intrinsic radioresistance of CSCs cannot be regarded as a general phenomenon, since marked heterogeneity seems to exist between individual tumours of the same histology, the mechanisms of which are currently not understood (50).

Hypoxia, but also other *micromilieu factors* like lactate content, can increase radioresistance of tumour cells including stem cells, thereby reducing tumour control probability (41,42,47). A direct link between hypoxia and putative stem cells has been shown with the increase in the fraction of CD133 positive cells in brain tumour cells *in vitro* (9,37) and the preferential expression of hypoxia-inducible factor HIF2α and HIF-regulated genes in glioma stem cells compared to non-stem tumour cells and to normal neural stem cells (29). Expression of the HIF-induced gene CA-9 has also been linked with CSCs in breast cancers (16). Specific microenvironmental factors, but also cell-cell interactions and genetically regulated cellular signals, are important determinants for stem cell maintenance and survival. Currently, different kinds of *niches* have been described that contain a higher number of CSCs or maintain the stem-like phenotype of tumour cells, like the perivascular niche, the hypoxic niche and the niche at the invasion front of a tumour.

It should be noted that if CSCs are characterized by very different radiobiology compared to non-CSCs, prognostic and predictive tests would only be expected to reveal valid results if they measure parameters of CSCs. However, as outlined in Chapters 8 and 18, some parameters that are prognostic for the outcome of radiotherapy can today be derived from *in vitro* or bioimaging assays which measure all tumour cells and not specifically CSCs. This suggests that the radiobiological characteristics of CSCs and non-CSCs are not completely different in the clinical setting (10). Further research needs to address this very important question for biologically driven radiotherapy.

Overall, CSCs mediate radioresistance of tumours by tumour-specific factors like CSC number, repopulation and/or reoxygenation. The intrinsic radioresistance of CSCs appears to be higher compared to non-CSCs at least in some tumours. This could be especially important for the development of stem cell–specific predictive biomarkers of treatment outcome if this finding holds true.

## 15.6 TREATMENT OPTIONS

### Stem cell therapy to repair radiation-damaged normal tissues

Many factors play a role in the response of tissue to irradiation, but, ultimately, the (in)ability of stem cells to reconstitute functional cells determines the onset and the severity of the radiation effects. Stem cell therapy provides the potential for prevention or treatment of radiation-induced normal tissue damage. More than 50 years ago, radiobiologists showed that bone marrow transplantation could rescue the hematopoietic system in animals that were exposed to lethal doses of total-body radiation (45). These studies led to the first hematopoietic stem cell transplantations; treatments that are common clinical practice nowadays. A similar strategy may be able to rescue other organs from radiation damage. Currently, a wide variety of stem cell therapies are being investigated for their potential to treat radiation-induced normal tissue damage.

Interestingly, transplantation of cultured MSCs has been shown to elicit beneficial effects on skin, gut and salivary glands after irradiation (7). Although it was not shown that MSCs contribute to the regrowth of actual tissue, they are thought to suppress the inflammatory response and secrete growth factors, hereby potentially normalizing the stem cell niche (40). However, the success of such a therapy still depends on the number of (quiescent) surviving stem cells (30).

The identification of resident ASC populations in tissues and the capability to isolate and expand them *in vitro* for therapeutic purposes has enabled the investigation of the potential of regenerating radiation-injured tissue. An example of the possibilities of such a therapy is represented by studies on the salivary gland. Radiation-induced hyposalivation and consequent xerostomia (dry mouth syndrome, see Chapter 14) are currently untreatable and lead to a dramatic loss of quality of life of post-radiotherapy patients. Therapy with stem cells obtained from biopsies taken from the patient prior to treatment (autologous transplantation) may have great potential. Indeed, preclinical studies demonstrated the regenerative potential of cells cultured from rodent salivary glands. Cells obtained from salivary gland could be cultured as salispheres, resembling a cell population as shown in Figure 15.1, asymmetric division. From these salispheres cells could be isolated using stem cell markers, which were able to restore saliva production in irradiated mice. Murine cell therapy indicated that rescue of hyposalivation could be achieved with as few as 100 c-Kit+, or 10,000 CD24/CD29 or CD133 -expressing salisphere cells (34). Notably, the donor-derived cells integrated into the recipient tissue, even after

Table 15.3 Summary of salivary gland stem cell phenotypic studies presented in chronological order within species

| Species | Marker or markers of interest | Culture method | Tested for | | Author |
|---------|------------------------------|----------------|-------------|---------|--------|
| | | | *in vitro* differentiation | *in vivo* function | |
| Mouse | CD117 | Salispheres | Yes | Yes | Lombaert et al. (2008) (64) |
| | CD49f, CD117, CD29, CD24 | Salispheres | No | Yes | Nanduri et al. (2011, 2014) (65,76) |
| | CD117 and ALDH | Salispheres | Yes | No | Banh et al. (2011) (66) |
| | SP cells, Sca-1, clusterin | No culture | No | Yes | Mishima et al. (2012) (67) |
| | Ascl-3 | Salispheres | Yes* | No | Rugel-Stahl et al. (2012) (68) |
| Rat | No marker | Monolayer | Yes | No | Kishi et al. (2006) (69) |
| | CD49f, CD29 | Monolayer | No | No | David et al. (2008) (70) |
| | CD49f, CD29, CD117 | Monolayer | Yes | No | Neumann et al. (2012) (71) |
| Human | CD49f, CD90 | Monolayer | Yes** | No | Sato et al. (2007) (72) |
| | CD117 | Salispheres | Yes | No | Feng et al. (2009) (73) |
| | CD34, CD117, ALDH, CD90, CD44 | Salispheres | Yes | No | Banh et al. (2011) (66) |
| | CD44, CD166 | No culture | – | – | Maria et al. (2012) (74) |
| | CD49f, CD29 | Monolayer | No | No | Palmon et al. (2012) (75) |

Modified from (39).

*Note:* Dash indicates not applicable in study. *Lineage tracing data. **Pancreatic-like differentiation shown. ALDH, aldehyde dehydrogenase; SP, side population cells. Cluster of differentiation (CD) nomenclature are given where possible. Pseudonyms are CD24, heat stable antigen (HAS); CD29, integrin β1; CD49f, integrin α6; CD90, Thy-1; CD117, c-Kit; CD166, activated leukocyte cell adhesion molecule (ALCAM).

serial transplantation, and differentiated into several salivary gland lineages including acinar cells, the parenchymal cell type responsible for saliva production. Similar characteristics have been found in cells obtained from human salivary glands (39), see Table 15.3. Moreover, human salivary gland-derived salisphere cells can functionally restore irradiated murine salivary glands after xeno-transplantation (38), showing the great potential of such a therapy. Although so far only preclinically tested, progress has been made also with other options of stem cells therapy, such as embryonic stem cells and neuronal stem cells for brain damage, MSCs + osteoblasts for osteoradionecrosis, MSCs and adipose-derived stem cells to treat skin damage, liver sinusoidal endothelial cells and hepatocytes for radiation-induced liver disease and MSCs for gut damage (7). It can be anticipated that iPS cells may also become a source of cells for tissue repair following radiotherapy in the future. In addition to cell replacement, trophic support (such as that provided by MSC as discussed previously) or addition of endothelial progenitors may be beneficial or even necessary to improve regeneration of the tissue studied. Stem cell-based therapies have great potential and may provide a more durable cure for normal tissue damage after radiotherapy. It seems to be only a matter of time until the first therapies are tested in the clinic.

## Cancer stem cell-directed therapy combined with irradiation

Radiotherapy is a targeted treatment and it has high efficacy to inactivate CSCs, but it is not specific to CSCs.

Additional treatment options arise from the potential to develop drugs that specifically target CSCs. Currently, there is not a single drug treatment approved for clinical use that shows an anti-CSC efficacy in the curative range for solid tumours. However, if drugs are combined with irradiation, even inactivation of limited numbers of CSCs should significantly improve local tumour control (6). An example for such treatment approaches is the application of CD44(v6) directed antibodies, loaded with highly cytotoxic drugs (bivatuzumab mertansine). Combination of these antibodies with irradiation led to an improvement of permanent local tumour control, in experimental models of head and neck cancers (22). Other potential targets may be developmental pathways, receptor tyrosine kinases, ROS scavenging, DNA damage signalling, aldehyde metabolism, apoptosis, PI3K/AKT/mTor, hypoxia, CAF, ECM binding and immune responses (14). However, there are major limitations that need to be overcome for successful introduction of targeted drugs into the clinic. One is the specificity of the targeting. If the target is relevant not only in CSCs but also in normal tissue stem cells as may be the case for some of the current surface markers and for targeting of the developmental pathways, such as Hedgehog, Notch or Wnt, that may be aberrantly expressed in some tumours, increased toxicity is to be expected. Another limitation is the diversity of CSCs, not only between different patients, but also within one tumour and even within one CSC clone (reviewed in [10]). The possibility to directly target the CSC niches may also be a useful approach either by direct targeting (radiotherapy dose painting) or with specific drugs. However, it can presently not be judged whether this approach is realistic.

Although promising, the translation of cancer stem cell-based therapies to the clinic still has many hurdles before routine use.

## Organotypic cultures

Methods have been developed to culture patient-specific organ-stem-cell-containing 'organoids' (13). These organoids, which closely resemble organ tissues, contain tissue stem cells and differentiated cells of all tissue lineages, such as those of the salivary gland (31,38). Interestingly, three-dimensional organoid cultures have also been developed from transformed tissue resembling tumour architecture, multilineage differentiation and stem cells (19). This allows the modelling of cancer and determination of chemoradiation response of CSC-cultured organoids (33). Patient-derived normal and tumour organoids might therefore provide the functional assays needed to validate cancer-resistant signatures and predict patients' response to radiation, and to test cancer stem cell-based therapies.

---

### Key points

1. Three different types of stem cells exist: ES cells, iPS cells and ASCs.
2. ASCs exist in normal tissues and are potent cells capable of forming all parenchymal cell types within that tissue. They are usually quiescent.
3. ASCs have the ability to proliferate and repair normal tissues following damage caused by radiation but this ability can be compromised by the extent of inflammation and damage to stromal elements of the tissue.
4. ASCs may have increased ability to repair radiation-induced DNA damage relative to proliferating progenitor cells in the tissue but data are currently quite limited.
5. CSCs are a subpopulation (often <1%) of tumour cells that have the capacity to self-renew, generate progenitor cells and regrow a whole tumour and thus cause recurrences and metastasis following radiation treatment.
6. Cancer cell populations enriched in CSCs can be sorted from tumour cell populations using specific surface (molecular) markers.
7. The phenotype of CSCs (and early tumour progenitor cells) may be plastic and affected by the microenvironmental conditions in tumours, particularly hypoxia.
8. CSCs mediate radioresistance of tumours by tumour-specific factors like CSC number and repopulation.
9. The intrinsic radioresistance of CSCs may be higher compared to non-CSCs at least in some tumours.

---

## ■ BIBLIOGRAPHY

1. Abbaszadegan MR, Bagheri V, Razavi MS, Momtazi AA, Sahebkar A, Gholamin M. Isolation, identification, and characterization of cancer stem cells: A review. *J Cell Physiol* 2017;232:2008–2018.
2. Baccelli I, Trumpp A. The evolving concept of cancer and metastasis stem cells. *J Cell Biol* 2012;198:281–293.
3. Bao S, Wu Q, McLendon RE et al. Glioma stem cells promote radioresistance by preferential activation of the DNA damage response. *Nature* 2006;444:756–760.
4. Barcellos-Hoff MH, Nguyen DH. Radiation carcinogenesis in context: How do irradiated tissues become tumors? *Health Phys* 2009;97:446–457.
5. Baumann M, Dorr W, Petersen C, Krause M. Repopulation during fractionated radiotherapy: Much has been learned, even more is open. *Int J Radiat Biol* 2003;79:465–467.
6. Baumann M, Krause M, Hill R. Exploring the role of cancer stem cells in radioresistance. *Nat Rev Cancer* 2008;8:545–554.
7. Benderitter M, Caviggioli F, Chapel A et al. Stem cell therapies for the treatment of radiation-induced normal tissue side effects. *Antioxid Redox Signal* 2014;21:338–355.
8. Blanpain C. Tracing the cellular origin of cancer. *Nat Cell Biol* 2013;15:126–134.
9. Blazek ER, Foutch JL, Maki G. Daoy medulloblastoma cells that express CD133 are radioresistant relative to CD133– cells, and the CD133+ sector is enlarged by hypoxia. *Int J Radiat Oncol Biol Phys* 2007;67:1–5.
10. Butof R, Dubrovska A, Baumann M. Clinical perspectives of cancer stem cell research in radiation oncology. *Radiother Oncol* 2013;108:388–396.
11. Clarke MF, Dick JE, Dirks PB et al. Cancer stem cells – Perspectives on current status and future directions: AACR Workshop on cancer stem cells. *Cancer Res* 2006;66:9339–9344.
12. Clevers H. The intestinal crypt, a prototype stem cell compartment. *Cell* 2013;154:274–284.
13. Clevers H. Modeling development and disease with organoids. *Cell* 2016;165:1586–1597.
14. Coppes RP, Dubrovska A. Targeting stem cells in radiation oncology. *Clin Oncol (R Coll Radiol)* 2017;29:329–334.
15. Coppes RP, van der Goot A, Lombaert IM. Stem cell therapy to reduce radiation-induced normal tissue damage. *Semin Radiat Oncol* 2009;19:112–121.
16. Currie MJ, Beardsley BE, Harris GC et al. Immunohistochemical analysis of cancer stem cell markers in invasive breast carcinoma and associated ductal carcinoma in situ: Relationships with markers of tumor hypoxia and microvascularity. *Hum Pathol* 2013;44:402–411.
17. de Jong MC, Pramana J, van der Wal JE et al. CD44 expression predicts local recurrence after radiotherapy in larynx cancer. *Clin Cancer Res* 2010;16:5329–5338.
18. Diehn M, Cho RW, Lobo NA et al. Association of reactive oxygen species levels and radioresistance in cancer stem cells. *Nature* 2009;458:780–783.
19. Drost J, Clevers H. Translational applications of adult stem cell-derived organoids. *Development* 2017;144:968–975.

20. Dubben HH, Thames HD, Beck-Bornholdt HP. Tumor volume: A basic and specific response predictor in radiotherapy. *Radiother Oncol* 1998;47:167–174.

21. Gerweck LE, Zaidi ST, Zietman A. Multivariate determinants of radiocurability. I: Prediction of single fraction tumor control doses. *Int J Radiat Oncol Biol Phys* 1994;29:57–66.

22. Gurtner K, Hessel F, Eicheler W et al. Combined treatment of the immunoconjugate bivatuzumab mertansine and fractionated irradiation improves local tumour control in vivo. *Radiother Oncol* 2012;102:444–449.

23. Hessel F, Krause M, Petersen C et al. Repopulation of moderately well-differentiated and keratinizing GL human squamous cell carcinomas growing in nude mice. *Int J Radiat Oncol Biol Phys* 2004;58:510–518.

24. Hewitt HB, Blake ER, Walder AS. A critique of the evidence for active host defence against cancer, based on personal studies of 27 murine tumours of spontaneous origin. *Br J Cancer* 1976;33:241–259.

25. Hill RP, Milas L. The proportion of stem cells in murine tumors. *Int J Radiat Oncol Biol Phys* 1989;16:513–518.

26. Kenyon J, Gerson SL. The role of DNA damage repair in aging of adult stem cells. *Nucleic Acids Res* 2007;35:7557–7565.

27. Krause M, Zips D, Thames HD, Kummermehr J, Baumann M. Preclinical evaluation of molecular-targeted anticancer agents for radiotherapy. *Radiother Oncol* 2006;80:112–122.

28. Li L, Clevers H. Coexistence of quiescent and active adult stem cells in mammals. *Science* 2010;327:542–545.

29. Li Z, Bao S, Wu Q et al. Hypoxia-inducible factors regulate tumorigenic capacity of glioma stem cells. *Cancer Cell* 2009;15:501–513.

30. Lombaert IM, Brunsting JF, Wierenga PK, Kampinga HH, de Haan G, Coppes RP. Keratinocyte growth factor prevents radiation damage to salivary glands by expansion of the stem/progenitor pool. *Stem Cells* 2008;26:2595–2601.

31. Maimets M, Rocchi C, Bron R et al. Long-term in vitro expansion of salivary gland stem cells driven by Wnt signals. *Stem Cell Reports* 2016;6:150–162.

32. Mandal PK, Blanpain C, Rossi DJ. DNA damage response in adult stem cells: Pathways and consequences. *Nat Rev Mol Cell Biol* 2011;12:198–202.

33. Nagle PW, Hosper NA, Ploeg EM et al. The in vitro response of tissue stem cells to irradiation with different linear energy transfers. *Int J Radiat Oncol Biol Phys* 2016;95:103–111.

34. Nanduri LS, Lombaert IM, van der Zwaag M et al. Salisphere derived c-Kit+ cell transplantation restores tissue homeostasis in irradiated salivary gland. *Radiother Oncol* 2013;108:458–463.

35. Panciera T, Azzolin L, Fujimura A et al. Induction of expandable tissue-specific stem/progenitor cells through transient expression of YAP/TAZ. *Cell Stem Cell* 2016;19:725–737.

36. Peitzsch C, Tyutyunnykova A, Pantel K, Dubrovska A. Cancer stem cells: The root of tumor recurrence and metastases. *Semin Cancer Biol* 2017;44:10–24.

37. Platet N, Liu SY, Atifi ME et al. Influence of oxygen tension on CD133 phenotype in human glioma cell cultures. *Cancer Lett* 2007;258:286–290.

38. Pringle S, Maimets M, van der Zwaag M et al. Human salivary gland stem cells functionally restore radiation damaged salivary glands. *Stem Cells* 2016;34:640–652.

39. Pringle S, Van Os R, Coppes RP. Concise review: Adult salivary gland stem cells and a potential therapy for xerostomia. *Stem Cells* 2013;31:613–619.

40. Prockop DJ. Repair of tissues by adult stem/progenitor cells (MSCs): Controversies, myths, and changing paradigms. *Mol Ther* 2009;17:939–946.

41. Quennet V, Yaromina A, Zips D et al. Tumor lactate content predicts for response to fractionated irradiation of human squamous cell carcinomas in nude mice. *Radiother Oncol* 2006;81:130–135.

42. Sattler UG, Meyer SS, Quennet V et al. Glycolytic metabolism and tumour response to fractionated irradiation. *Radiother Oncol* 2010;94:102–109.

43. Takahashi K, Yamanaka S. Induction of pluripotent stem cells from mouse embryonic and adult fibroblast cultures by defined factors. *Cell* 2006;126:663–676.

44. Vlashi E, Kim K, Lagadec C et al. In vivo imaging, tracking, and targeting of cancer stem cells. *J Natl Cancer Inst* 2009;101:350–359.

45. Vos O, Davids JA, Weyzen WW, Van Bekkum DW. Evidence for the cellular hypothesis in radiation protection by bone marrow cells. *Acta Physiol Pharmacol Neerl* 1956;4:482–486.

46. Yaromina A, Krause M, Thames H et al. Pre-treatment number of clonogenic cells and their radiosensitivity are major determinants of local tumour control after fractionated irradiation. *Radiother Oncol* 2007;83:304–310.

47. Yaromina A, Kroeber T, Meinzer A et al. Exploratory study of the prognostic value of microenvironmental parameters during fractionated irradiation in human squamous cell carcinoma xenografts. *Int J Radiat Oncol Biol Phys* 2011;80:1205–1213.

48. Zanconato F, Cordenonsi M, Piccolo S. YAP/TAZ at the roots of cancer. *Cancer Cell* 2016;29:783–803.

49. Zhao RC, Zhu YS, Shi Y. New hope for cancer treatment: Exploring the distinction between normal adult stem cells and cancer stem cells. *Pharmacol Ther* 2008;119:74–82.

50. Zielske SP, Spalding AC, Wicha MS, Lawrence TS. Ablation of breast cancer stem cells with radiation. *Transl Oncol* 2011;4:227–233.

51. Kim KJ, Lee KH, Kim HS et al. The presence of stem cell marker-expressing cells is not prognostically significant in glioblastomas. *Neuropathology* 2011;31:494–502.

52. Murat A, Migliavacca E, Gorlia T et al. Stem cell-related "self-renewal" signature and high epidermal growth factor receptor expression associated with resistance to concomitant chemoradiotherapy in glioblastoma. *J Clin Oncol* 2008;26:3015–3024.

53. Pallini R, Ricci-Vitiani L, Banna GL et al. Cancer stem cell analysis and clinical outcome in patients with glioblastoma multiforme. *Clin Cancer Res* 2008;14:8205–8212.

54. Metellus P, Nanni-Metellus I, Delfino C et al. Prognostic impact of CD133 mRNA expression in 48 glioblastoma patients treated with concomitant radiochemotherapy: a prospective patient cohort at a single institution. *Ann Surg Oncol* 2011;18:2937–2945.

55. de Jong MC, Pramana J, van der Wal JE et al. CD44 expression predicts local recurrence after radiotherapy in larynx cancer. *Clin Cancer Res* 2010;16:5329–5338.

56. Koukourakis MI, Giatromanolaki A, Tsakmaki V, Danielidis V, Sivridis E. Cancer stem cell phenotype relates to radio-chemotherapy outcome in locally advanced squamous cell head-neck cancer. *Br J Cancer* 2012;106:846–853.

57. Smit JK, Faber H, Niemantsverdriet M et al. Prediction of response to radiotherapy in the treatment of esophageal cancer using stem cell markers. *Radiother Oncol* 2013;107:434–441.

58. Wang Q, Chen ZG, Du CZ, Wang HW, Yan LGuJ. Cancer stem cell marker CD133+ tumour cells and clinical outcome in rectal cancer. *Histopathology* 2009;55:284–293.

59. Avoranta ST, Korkeila EA, Syrjanen KJ, Pyrhonen SO, Sundstrom JT. Lack of CD44 variant 6 expression in rectal cancer invasive front associates with early recurrence. *World J Gastroenterol* 2012;18:4549–4556.

60. Sprenger T, Conradi LC, Beissbarth T et al. Enrichment of CD133-expressing cells in rectal cancers treated with preoperative radiochemotherapy is an independent marker for metastasis and survival. *Cancer* 2013;119:26–35.

61. Kawamoto A, Tanaka K, Saigusa S et al. Clinical significance of radiation-induced CD133 expression in residual rectal cancer cells after chemoradiotherapy. *Exp Ther Med* 2012;3:403–409.

62. Kwon GY, Ha H, Ahn G, Park SY, Huh SJ, Park W. Role of CD24 protein in predicting metastatic potential of uterine cervical squamous cell carcinoma in patients treated with radiotherapy. *Int J Radiat Oncol Biol Phys* 2007;69:1150–1156.

63. Sung CO, Park W, Choi YL et al. Prognostic significance of CD24 protein expression in patients treated with adjuvant radiotherapy after radical hysterectomy for cervical squamous cell carcinoma. *Radiother Oncol* 2010;95:359–364.

64. Lombaert IM, Brunsting JF, Wierenga PK et al. Rescue of salivary gland function after stem cell transplantation in irradiated glands. *PLoS One* 2008;3:e2063.

65. Nanduri LSY, Maimets M, Pringle SA et al. Regeneration of irradiated salivary glands with stem cell marker expressing cells. *Radiother Oncol* 2011;99:367–372.

66. Banh A, Xiao N, Cao H et al. A novel aldehyde dehydrogenase-3 activator leads to adult salivary stem cell enrichment in vivo. *Clin Cancer Res* 2011;17:7265–7272.

67. Mishima K, Inoue H, Nishiyama T et al. Transplantation of side population cells restores the function of damaged exocrine glands through clusterin. *Stem Cells* 2012;30:1925–1937.

68. Rugel-Stahl A, Elliott ME, Ovitt CE. Ascl3 marks adult progenitor cells of the mouse salivary gland. *Stem Cell Res* 2012;8:379–387.

69. Kishi T, Takao T, Fujita K et al. Clonal proliferation of multipotent stem/progenitor cells in the neonatal and adult salivary glands. *Biochem Biophys Res Commun* 2006;340:544–552.

70. David R, Shai E, Aframian DJ et al. Isolation and cultivation of integrin $\alpha6\beta1$-expressing salivary gland graft cells: A model for use with an artificial salivary gland. *Tissue Eng Part A* 2008;14:331–337.

71. Neumann Y, David R, Stiubea-Cohen R et al. Long-term cryopreservation model of rat salivary gland stem cells for future therapy in irradiated head and neck cancer patients. *Tissue Eng Part C* 2012;18:710–718.

72. Sato A, Okumura K, Matsumoto S et al. Isolation, tissue localization, and cellular characterization of progenitors derived from adult human salivary glands. *Cloning Stem Cells* 2007;9:191–205.

73. Feng J, van der Zwaag M, Stokman MA et al. Isolation and characterization of human salivary gland cells for stem cell transplantation to reduce radiation-induced hyposalivation. *Radiother Oncol* 2009;92:466–471.

74. Maria O, Maria A, Cai Y et al. Cell surface markers CD44 and CD166 localized specific populations of salivary acinar cells. *Oral Dis* 2012;18:162–168.

75. Palmon A, David R, Neumann Y et al. High-efficiency immunomagnetic isolation of solid tissue-originated integrin-expressing adult stem cells. *Methods* 2012;56:305–309.

76. Nanduri LSY, Baanstra M, Faber H, Rocchi C, Zwart E, de Haan G, van Os RP, Coppes RP. Purification and ex vivo expansion of fully functional salivary gland stem cells. *Stem Cell Reports* 2014;3:1–8.

## ■ FURTHER READING

77. Bartfeld S, Clevers H. Stem cell-derived organoids and their application for medical research and patient treatment. *J Mol Med (Berl)* 2017;95:729–738.

78. Krause M, Dubrovska A, Linge A, Baumann M. Cancer stem cells: Radioresistance, prediction of radiotherapy outcome and specific targets for combined treatments. *Adv Drug Deliv Rev* 2017;109:63–73.

79. Wang D, Plukker JTM, Coppes RP. Cancer stem cells with increased metastatic potential as a therapeutic target for esophageal cancer. *Semin Cancer Biol* 2017;44:60–66.

# Normal tissue tolerance and the effect of dose inhomogeneities

## WOLFGANG DÖRR AND ALBERT J. VAN DER KOGEL

## 16.1 INTRODUCTION

Volume specifications in radiotherapy (Figure 16.1) are defined in reports 50 and 62 of the International Commission on Radiation Units and Measurements (ICRU) (6,7). In 2013, ICRU Report 89 also focused on volume concepts in image-guided, adaptive radiotherapy including brachytherapy, mainly based on studies in cervix cancer (8). Even the smallest tumour volume defined, i.e. the gross tumour volume (GTV), contains normal tissue elements, e.g. blood vessels and connective tissue components. In addition, the clinical target volume (CTV) also encompasses a relevant number of normal parenchymal cells of the respective organ, with the suspected tumour cells intermingled. Moreover, the volume difference between the CTV and the treated volume (TV), i.e. the volume enclosed by a surface of a clinically effective isodose, is exclusively composed of normal tissue components. In all these normal cells and structures within the high-dose volume, radiation effects and hence adverse events of therapy may be induced. However, all the normal tissues within the TV are unavoidably exposed to the complete radiation dose applied to the tumour; the clinical consequences of this normal tissue exposure therefore may limit the TV dose, depending on the size of the TV.

The irradiated volume (IV) receives a dose that is considered significant with regard to the tolerance of the normal tissues, and is dependent on the physical parameters of the radiation delivery, for example the type of radiation (photons, electrons, ions) and its quality (energy), the mode of treatment planning (number of beam directions, etc.) and the radiotherapy technique (brachytherapy, three-dimensional-conformal teletherapy, intensity-modulated radiotherapy, volumetric modulated arc therapy [VMAT]). Technological improvements in the physical administration of radiotherapy over the last decades have led to increasing conformation of the TV with the planning target volume and of the IV with the TV. In this process, the volume of organs at risk (OARs) exposed to significant, i.e. clinically relevant, doses has significantly decreased, but has also resulted in substantial dose gradients within these organs. This has stimulated progressive interest in the identification of the consequences of inhomogeneities

in the dose distribution – the 'volume effect' – in normal tissues. The definition of the 'volume effect' is, however, not straightforward. In the present context, it relates to the relative or absolute volume of an OAR that is exposed to a certain, defined dose, or the dose within a defined volume of the OAR, but – importantly – also to the spatial localisation of the dose within the OAR. As a consequence of the above-mentioned modern radiotherapy techniques, the IV needs to be integrated into the list of R's (21) that define the radiation response of normal tissues.

The volume of normal tissues exposed to significant radiation doses is an important determinant of clinical tolerance, even without having any influence on tissue sensitivity per unit volume. An example of this is epidermal or mucosal ulceration. If this occurs over a large tissue area, the ulceration will lead to pain and will heal only slowly. A small area of ulceration, by contrast, may only lead to minor discomfort and will heal more rapidly. In this situation the *clinical tolerance* is strongly dependent on the IV, although *structural tolerance* is not. In fact, there is very little evidence for any increase in *cellular radiosensitivity* when the IV is increased, in clear contrast to the *clinical consequences*. However, the radiopathology underlying similar clinical changes and symptoms may change with dose, as has been demonstrated for the lung (16). Also, the (volume-dependent) interaction between radiation effects in different organs, e.g. heart-lung (2) needs to be considered.

## 16.2 THE QUANTEC INITIATIVE

The QUANTEC initiative (Quantitative Analyses of Normal Tissue Effects in the Clinic [14]) summarized then-current knowledge on radiation effects, with special emphasis on the impact of the exposed volume, in a panel of clinically important OARs. A number of subsequent studies and analyses on the same subject have continuously been published since.

Mathematical multi-parameter models of normal tissue complication probability (NTCP) have been developed, see Section 16.6 for overview and Chapters 7 and 26 for details. These models, however, typically have many limitations

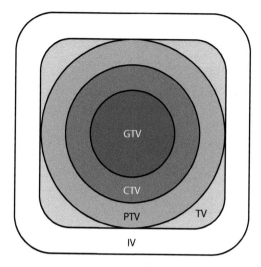

Figure 16.1 Volume definitions in radiotherapy according to ICRU report 62 (7). GTV: gross tumour volume (detectable tumour volume); CTV: clinical target volume (GTV plus volumes with expected subclinical spread); PTV: planning target volume (CTV plus safety margin for movements or deformations of CTV, technical uncertainties, etc.); TV: treatment volume (receiving the prescribed dose); IV: irradiated volume (i.e. exposed to significant doses with regard to normal tissue tolerance).

and uncertainties (20). The data obtained from newer clinical studies, combined with more precise knowledge of dose-distributions and dose-volume histograms, should in the future allow for the development of more realistic parameters for mathematical modelling and a validation and optimization of the existing mathematical models used for describing volume effects and consequences of inhomogeneous dose distributions. Because of this highly dynamic development and compilation of knowledge on individual organ 'volume effects', this chapter does not describe the consequences of dose inhomogeneities in individual human OARs in any detail but focuses on general aspects. If the reader of this chapter is searching for specific up-to-date information, particularly on specific clinical cases, then it is recommended to study the current literature. Description of important experimental data in animal models is given in Chapter 26.

## 16.3 THE CONCEPT OF ORGAN TOLERANCE DOSE

In general, the 'tolerance dose' of a tissue or organ is defined as the dose at which radiation exposure of the entire volume or a sub-volume of this organ in a specified irradiation protocol induces a (severe) pathological change or clinical symptom (an 'endpoint') within a defined follow-up period with a certain probability (i.e. a certain 'risk'). The latter is usually less than or equal to 5%. The concept of OAR tolerance doses therefore requires a series of definitions and specifications (4). These include the

- Organ/tissue under consideration
- Pathological change/symptom ('endpoint'), including the respective diagnostic procedures and the classification system applied
- Induction probability ('risk') under consideration
- Radiation type and quality
- Exposure protocol
- Follow-up period and procedures and – most importantly in the present context – also the
- Exposed volume and dose distribution

The specification of the tissue or OAR under consideration is obvious. The same applies for radiation type and quality, which effects are illustrated in Chapters 6 and 25. The appreciation of the exposure protocol, i.e. mainly fractionation as described, e.g. by the $\alpha/\beta$ value or even half-times for recovery of sublethal radiation damage, is accomplished by mathematical models of equieffective doses (1). It should be cautioned, however, that the fractionation parameters (see Chapters 9, 10, 11 and 12) are usually associated with broad confidence intervals, i.e. with a significant variability. These uncertainties should be considered in clinical treatment planning, particularly in critical cases.

The definition of endpoints, including aspects of diagnosis, classification and the impact of follow-up, and particularly dose distribution and dose inhomogeneities are also subject to significant uncertainties, which are discussed later in this chapter. These uncertainties also significantly impact on the quality of the estimation of the NTCP ('risk') for the induction of a certain radiation effect, i.e. endpoint or symptom.

It should be emphasized that the radiation tolerance of an OAR in general, or regarding individual endpoints, can be significantly affected by the functional status of the organ volume that is exposed to no or only small radiation doses. For example, lung function in heavy smokers can be substantially impaired, and the usually accepted tolerance limits must thus be significantly lowered compared to a 'standard' patient. Similar situations are met, e.g. with impaired liver function due to alcohol consumption, and many others. In general, any co-morbidity may have a potential to impact on OAR tolerance. This has to be considered for treatment planning and any NTCP estimation. Previous or additional, but also subsequent, chemotherapy also has a potential to impact on the function of the un-irradiated or less-exposed organ volume, depending on the type of chemotherapy. The same applies to surgery. Consideration of the impact of functional impairment of un-irradiated tissue on the tolerance limits for radiotherapy must therefore unconditionally and definitely be subject to the experience and expert knowledge of the responsible radiation oncologist. Similar to functionally inoperable patients, 'functionally un-irradiatable' patients may be identified.

In addition to the purely biological aspects of tissue tolerance, it should be noted that besides this 'biological' tolerance, based on evidence from various (pre-)clinical studies, there is also a judicial aspect, defining a 'legal' tolerance. For example, the radiation tolerance for spinal cord, using paralysis in <1% of the patients as a consequence of tissue necrosis as the endpoint, has been defined by QUANTEC at an equieffective dose of 2 Gy per fraction (EQD2) to 54 Gy (10). In clear contrast, in some countries, a maximum total dose of only 45 Gy is considered acceptable with regard to legal implications.

## 16.4 ORGAN TOLERANCE AND TISSUE ARCHITECTURE

Withers et al. (21) originally introduced the concept of tissue radiation tolerance based on functional sub-units (FSUs) present within the individual tissues. These FSUs may be considered as anatomical structures, e.g. bronchioli or nephrons, or simply as individual tissue-specific stem cells. Per their definition, a FSU is 'the largest tissue volume, or unit of cells, that can be regenerated from a single surviving clonogenic cell'. FSUs are sterilized by irradiation independently of each other, which results in structural damage within the exposed volume. In this concept, the number of FSUs that are sterilised by a certain irradiation protocol, and hence the consequent severity of the changes, depends on the intrinsic radiosensitivity of the FSU, and on dose and other radiobiological parameters, such as fractionation (see Chapters 9 and 10) or overall treatment time (see Chapter 12).

However, the *clinical* consequences of FSU sterilization are dependent on the *arrangement* of the FSUs within the exposed organ (Figure 16.2). Similar to the connection of elements in an electrical circuit, the FSUs in a biological tissue can be arranged either in a parallel or in a serial manner. In organs with a *parallel structure* (Figure 16.2a), FSUs function independently. Hence, a clinical radiation effect is only observed if the number of surviving FSUs is too low to sustain the physiological organ function. Hence, a threshold volume must be considered in treatment planning, which must not be exceeded, but within which large doses – sterilizing all FSUs relevant for the endpoint under consideration – may be administered. The risk of complications depends on the distribution of the total dose within the organ rather than on individual 'hot spots'. Typical examples of organs with a (predominantly) parallel architecture are lung, kidney and liver.

In contrast, in organs with a *serial* (or *tubular*) *architecture* (Figure 16.2b), the function of the entire organ depends on the function of each individual FSU. Inactivation of only one FSU may result in clinical side effects in the downstream part of the organ in a binary response pattern. In such organs, the risk of complications is highly dependent on 'hot spots', while the dose distribution within the entire organ is less relevant. Examples of (mainly) serially structured organs are spinal cord, oesophagus or intestine.

A purely parallel or serial organisation of any organ, however, only describes an extreme, hypothetical scenario.

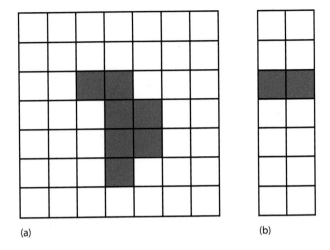

Figure 16.2 Parallel and serial organisation of functional sub-units (FSUs) in normal tissues. In parallel organised tissues (a), a critical number of functional sub-units must be damaged before a clinical response, i.e. loss of function, becomes manifest (threshold volume), although structural damage may be diagnosed in individual FSU. In contrast, in serial organs (b), failure of only one FSU results in a loss of function of the entire organ. (Adapted from (21), with permission.)

In reality, no organ is organized simply as a (serial) chain or a (parallel) conglomerate of FSUs. Importantly, as described in Chapter 14, one major component of late radiation effects in normal tissues is the response of the (micro)vasculature, and individual vessels must be considered as tubular structures, which introduces a serial factor into any tissue.

Many organs are per se better described by an intermediate type of organisation, which is neither serial/tubular nor parallel. One prominent example for this is the brain. Here, individual areas perform specific functions. The clinical tolerance of brain tissue is therefore much more dependent on the area of brain exposed to a certain dose rather than the total volume. Damage to even a small area may lead to permanent loss of the particular function controlled by that area, since the undamaged parts of the brain are not able to cover these specific functions, while other brain functions may be completely unaffected. Similarly, the eye is an organ with many very different tissues and structures, and hence displays specific volume characteristics.

The target structures for different endpoints within one OAR may be inhomogeneously distributed, and may also be organised in different ways. For example, in the urinary bladder, various clinical endpoints are observed, ranging from incontinence, with the target presumably located in the sphincter region (e.g. [18]), to decreased storage capacity/increased micturition frequency based on a complex response of the entire bladder wall (5), and haematuria with the vasculature within the bladder wall as the primary target. The same, for example applies for the rectum, with endpoints ranging from incontinence, frequency and bleeding to such complex consequences as the impact on quality of life (19), which is based on a specific combination of pathophysiological changes. In many organs, the target structures for individual endpoints still have to be identified, and their radiobiology (the 'R's') still has to be characterised.

## 16.5 EFFECT OF TISSUE STEM CELLS OUTSIDE THE TREATMENT VOLUME

An important factor impacting on the influence of the irradiated volume and dose inhomogeneities on tissue radiation effects is the potential of un-irradiated clonogenic/stem cells to migrate into the irradiated and thus damaged volume. The most prominent example is the bone marrow. After complete sterilisation of the stem and precursor cells in a fraction of active marrow, this volume – provided the supportive structures are either damaged only incompletely or regenerated – can be repopulated by haematopoietic stem cells that are already present in the circulation or recruited from un-irradiated active bone marrow. Further examples are epithelial tissues, which display a high cellular migratory capacity, like skin, oral mucosa or intestinal epithelium. They exhibit a steep increase in tolerance as the irradiated field size decreases to small areas.

This type of volume effect is also seen in some other tissues with a relatively linear or tubular structural organisation, e.g. spinal cord. Repopulation from neighbouring sub-units is much less likely in tissues with a parallel type of arrangement of the FSUs, with long migratory distances between FSUs, and has not been demonstrated in the kidney or lung. However, none of the existing NTCP models (see Section 16.8 and Chapter 26) incorporates such effects. Hence, these models are not capable of adequately describing the volume effect data for tissues and endpoints for which these phenomena are relevant.

## 16.6 ENDPOINTS AND SYMPTOMS

An endpoint in this context is defined as any potential pathological change or clinical symptomatology that is observed as the consequence of a therapeutic administration of ionizing radiation, and which can be detected with certain diagnostic procedures (4). In reporting the incidence, severity and time course of endpoints in clinical, but also in preclinical, studies the diagnostic procedures applied need to be specified in detail, as they may significantly impact on both the quality and the incidence/severity of the reported parameters. The same applies to the adverse event classification protocol used. If OAR events are only generally classified, i.e. when the endpoint with the highest severity defines the grading, then it remains completely unclear on which of the individual endpoints the classification is based.

Different endpoints related to one specific OAR may follow their own individual time course in their clinical manifestation. As a consequence, a similar severity of OAR morbidity at different intervals of follow-up may be related to the manifestation of different endpoints. Therefore, information on the time of diagnosis and the sequence and total duration of follow-up investigations is essential for the reporting of NTCP.

## 16.7 DOSE-VOLUME HISTOGRAMS AND THEIR LIMITATIONS

With the implementation of conformal three-dimensional radiotherapy and the associated treatment planning procedures, dose-volume histograms (DVHs) have proved useful as a tool for the evaluation and comparison – and thus optimisation – of treatment plans. However, it should be emphasised that there are significant subjective influences and inter-individual differences with regard to the delineation of OAR and critical substructures, as illustrated, e.g. by Damato et al. (3), and also different departmental delineation strategies. Moreover, despite ample clinical data for some organs, it remains unclear which of the DVH-derived parameters are optimal for the prediction of NTCP, as has been summarised for the lung by Marks et al. (13).

The use of DVH parameters for the estimation of NTCP is associated with a complete loss of the information on the spatial distribution of the dose within an OAR. This represents a serious constraint in determining the relationship between local tissue damage and the consequent overall incidence and severity of a certain endpoint. For example, a high-dose region in the histogram may represent a single, large high-dose volume or a number of smaller hot spots within completely different and independent regions of the OAR. These different patterns could have quite different implications for tissue tolerance.

Due to the loss of information on the *position* of the dose within an OAR, DVHs also cannot differentiate between functionally or anatomically different sub-regions or compartments within an organ. This becomes particularly relevant if variations in radiosensitivity with regard to a specific endpoint exist, like in the lung (17). Moreover, the clinical consequences of a certain endpoint may vary with different spatial localisations within the organ, like radiation mucositis occurring in the buccal mucosa versus its manifestation in the lips. As other examples, a high-dose volume in the periphery of the lung parenchyma or at a pole of a kidney may result in local, confined fibrosis and localised loss of function, while the same volume/dose distribution close to the mediastinum or at the renal hilum will significantly impact on the function of the entire or large parts of the respective organ. This represents a switch from a predominantly parallel to a more serial organisation scenario.

Information on the localisation of the dose is also highly relevant in OAR where different sub-volumes or sub-structures are associated with different endpoints, like in the brain and the eye, but also in the urinary bladder, rectum and others (see also Section 16.2).

## 16.8 MODELLING OF NORMAL TISSUE EFFECTS REGARDING DOSE INHOMOGENEITIES

Theoretical models have been developed to improve estimation of the NTCP for partial-volume irradiations and inhomogeneous dose distributions. Historically, power-law functions were the basis of the earliest models and were followed by models with some biophysical basis. The most important such models are described in detail in Chapter 7 and are summarised in the following text. Chapter 26 describes some of the further developments in this modelling.

The increasing importance of the OAR volume exposed and its relation to tissue architecture led to the concept of a variable *seriality* factor for different organs, which has been incorporated into some NTCP models. The modelling of volume effects on the basis of their serial or parallel organisation is useful and can explain the apparent paradox that relatively radiosensitive organs, like the kidney and lung, can sustain the loss of more than half their total mass without clinically significant loss of function, whereas relatively radioresistant tissues such as the spinal cord can be functionally inactivated by the irradiation of only a relatively small volume with a certain dose.

In the early model of *Lyman* (12), a power-law relationship was assumed between the tolerance dose for uniform whole-organ or partial-organ irradiation, where a parameter $n$ (the exponent of the partial volume) describes the volume dependence of the tolerance dose. When $n$ approaches 1, then the tolerance dose increases steeply with decreasing volume (described as a large volume effect); in contrast, when $n$ approaches 0, then the effect of a decrease in volume is small. The Lyman model has been extended to inhomogeneous irradiation by converting the original DVH into an equivalent DVH for uniform irradiation (see Section 16.7), usually by the effective-volume method (11). It should be stressed that this is associated with even more loss of information as in the original DVH. The resulting *Lyman Kutcher Burman* (LKB) model, however, is still one of the most commonly used models for predicting NTCP.

Intermediate between the purely empirical and more biophysically based models is the *relative seriality model* of Källman et al. (9). In this model, an extra parameter $s$ is introduced, i.e. the 'degree of seriality', to describe the functional organisation of a tissue (Section 16.2). A near-zero value of $s$ represents an almost exclusively parallel structure and an $s$ value close to unity represents an organ with a highly serial organisation.

The first model which assumed that an organ can be divided into physiologically discrete compartments, or FSUs, was *the integral response model* (21). This model allows for the spatial distribution of FSUs in the tissue to be non-uniform. The radiation response of each independent FSU is determined by Poisson statistics and the functional architecture of an FSU determines the organ's response to partial volume irradiation (see Section 16.4).

In the concept of the *equivalent uniform dose* (EUD), inhomogeneous dose distributions within one organ are also converted to a homogeneous organ dose, which would theoretically result in an identical survival of a hypothetical (stem) cell population (15). Hence, the concept is dependent on survival parameters of these hypothetical tissue stem cells, clonogenic cells or tissue rescuing units (FSUs). This may – if at all – to some extent be applicable for early radiation effects, although even their radiopathology is way more complex than solely based on cell kill (see Chapters 14 and 24). Moreover, late radiation effects are definitely based on a variety of target cell populations and largely on changes in cellular/tissue function rather than cell kill (see Chapter 14). Therefore, the NTCP estimates resulting from the EUD concept must be considered as purely empirical rather than in any way biology-based.

These present mathematical models used to estimate NTCP must therefore be considered phenomenological, i.e. consistent with current data collections, under certain conditions. Different models may be similarly applicable for the description of the same database, but may not be applicable to other data sets (20). All the available models, which are even being integrated into some treatment planning systems, should in the face of all these limitations and drawbacks only be used with great caution. They should be regarded as an aid to the evaluation and comparison of clinical data using different treatment setups, rather than giving accurate predictions of clinical outcome regarding NTCP.

---

### Key points

1. *Structural* tissue tolerance depends on cellular radiation sensitivity and is independent of volume irradiated. *Functional* tolerance depends on tissue organisation and functional reserve capacity.
2. Different individual endpoints related to one OAR may be based on exposure of specific target sub-volumes and follow different time course and radiobiological characteristics.
3. Tissues with a predominantly parallel organisation (e.g. lung) have a threshold volume below which functional damage does not occur. The risk of developing a complication depends on dose distribution throughout the whole organ rather than the maximum dose to a small area.
4. Tissues with a serial organisation (e.g. spinal cord) have little or no functional reserve and the risk of developing a complication is less dependent on volume irradiated than for tissues with a parallel organisation. The risk of complication is strongly influenced by high-dose regions and hot spots.
5. Migration of surviving clonogenic cells into the (margins of) irradiated volumes can lead to a steep increase in tissue tolerance for field diameters up to

20 mm in some tissues (e.g. spinal cord, intestine and skin).

6. Theoretical models have been developed to estimate NTCP for partial-volume irradiations and inhomogeneous dose distributions. Simple power-law and probability models have been expanded to incorporate parameters relating to tissue architecture and reserve capacity. These mainly phenomenological models always need to be validated against clinical data emerging from new conformal treatment schedules and new methods of delivery.

## ■ BIBLIOGRAPHY

1. Bentzen SM, Dorr W, Gahbauer R et al. Bioeffect modeling and equieffective dose concepts in radiation oncology – Terminology, quantities and units. *Radiother Oncol* 2012;105: 266–268.

2. Cella L, Palma G, Deasy JO et al. Complication probability models for radiation-induced heart valvular dysfunction: Do heart-lung interactions play a role? *PLOS ONE* 2014;9: e111753.

3. Damato AL, Townamchai K, Albert M et al. Dosimetric consequences of interobserver variability in delineating the organs at risk in gynecologic interstitial brachytherapy. *Int J Radiat Oncol Biol Phys* 2014;89:674–681.

4. Dörr W, Herrmann T, Baumann M. Application of organ tolerance dose-constraints in clinical studies in radiation oncology. *Strahlenther Onkol* 2014;190:621–627.

5. Dörr W, Jaal J, Zips D. Prostate cancer: Biological dose considerations and constraints in tele- and brachytherapy. *Strahlenther Onkol* 2007;183 Spec No 2:14–15.

6. International Commission on Radiation Units and Measurements (ICRU). Prescribing, recording and reporting photon beam therapy. ICRU Report 50. *J ICRU* 1993;os26:1–72.

7. International Commission on Radiation Units and Measurements (ICRU). Prescribing, recording and reporting photon beam therapy (supplement to ICRU report 50). ICRU Report 62. *J ICRU* 1999;os32:1–52.

8. International Commission on Radiation Units and Measurements (ICRU). Prescribing, recording, and reporting brachytherapy for cancer of the cervix. ICRU Report 89. *J ICRU* 2013;13:1–258.

9. Källman P, Agren A, Brahme A. Tumour and normal tissue responses to fractionated non-uniform dose delivery. *Int J Radiat Biol* 1992;62:249–262.

10. Kirkpatrick JP, van der Kogel AJ, Schultheiss TE. Radiation dose-volume effects in the spinal cord. *Int J Radiat Oncol Biol Phys* 2010;76:S42–S49.

11. Kutcher GJ, Burman C. Calculation of complication probability factors for non-uniform normal tissue irradiation: The effective volume method. *Int J Radiat Oncol Biol Phys* 1989;16:1623–1630.

12. Lyman JT. Complication probability as assessed from dose-volume histograms. *Radiat Res Suppl* 1985;8:S13–S19.

13. Marks LB, Bentzen SM, Deasy JO et al. Radiation dose-volume effects in the lung. *Int J Radiat Oncol Biol Phys* 2010;76:S70–S76.

14. Marks LB, Ten Haken RK, Martel MK. Guest editor's introduction to QUANTEC: A users guide. *Int J Radiat Oncol Biol Phys* 2010;76(3 Suppl):S1–S2.

15. Niemierko A. Reporting and analyzing dose distributions: A concept of equivalent uniform dose. *Med Phys* 1997;24:103–110.

16. Novakova-Jiresova A, van Luijk P, van Goor H, Kampinga HH, Coppes RP. Changes in expression of injury after irradiation of increasing volumes in rat lung. *Int J Radiat Oncol Biol Phys* 2007;67:1510–1518.

17. Seppenwoolde Y, De Jaeger K, Boersma LJ, Belderbos JS, Lebesque JV. Regional differences in lung radiosensitivity after radiotherapy for non-small-cell lung cancer. *Int J Radiat Oncol Biol Phys* 2004;60:748–758.

18. Steggerda MJ, Witteveen T, van den Boom F, Moonen LM. Is there a relation between the radiation dose to the different sub-segments of the lower urinary tract and urinary morbidity after brachytherapy of the prostate with I-125 seeds? *Radiother Oncol* 2013;109:251–255.

19. Stenmark MH, Conlon AS, Johnson S et al. Dose to the inferior rectum is strongly associated with patient reported bowel quality of life after radiation therapy for prostate cancer. *Radiother Oncol* 2014;110:291–297.

20. van der Schaaf A, Langendijk JA, Fiorino C, Rancati T. Embracing phenomenological approaches to normal tissue complication probability modeling: A question of method. *Int J Radiat Oncol Biol Phys* 2015;91:468–471.

21. Withers HR, Taylor JM, Maciejewski B. Treatment volume and tissue tolerance. *Int J Radiat Oncol Biol Phys* 1988;14:751–759.

## ■ FURTHER READING

22. Marks LB, Ten Haken RK, Martel MK. Guest editor's introduction to QUANTEC: A users guide. *Int J Radiat Oncol Biol Phys* 2010;76(3 Suppl):S1–S2.

23. Withers HR. The four R's of radiotherapy. In: Lett JT and Adler H, editors. *Advances in Radiation Biology*. Vol 5. New York, NY: Academic Press; 1975. pp. 241–271.

# The oxygen effect and therapeutic approaches to tumour hypoxia

MICHAEL R. HORSMAN, J. MARTIN BROWN, ALBERT J. VAN DER KOGEL, BRADLY G. WOUTERS AND JENS OVERGAARD

## 17.1 OXYGEN AND THE TUMOUR MICROENVIRONMENT

The response of cells to ionizing radiation is strongly dependent upon oxygen (11). This is illustrated in Figure 17.1a for mammalian cells irradiated in culture. Cell surviving fraction is shown as a function of radiation dose administered either under normal aerated conditions or under hypoxia. The enhancement of radiation damage by oxygen is approximately dose modifying (i.e. the radiation dose that gives a particular level of survival is reduced by the same factor at all levels of survival). This allows us to calculate an oxygen enhancement ratio (OER):

$$OER = \frac{\text{Radiation dose in hypoxia}}{\text{Radiation dose in air}}$$

for the same level of biological effect. For most cells the maximum OER in culture (comparing doses under 21% air and under anoxia) for X-rays is around 2.5–3. However, some studies suggest that at radiation doses of 3 Gy or less the OER is somewhat reduced (35). This is an important finding because this is the dose range for clinical fractionation treatments.

It has been demonstrated from rapid-mix studies that the oxygen effect only occurs if oxygen is present either during irradiation or within a few milliseconds thereafter (22). The dependence of the degree of sensitization on oxygen tension is shown in Figure 17.1b. As the oxygen concentration increases from zero (anoxia), there is a relatively steep increase in radiosensitivity. The greatest change occurs from about 0.5 to 20 mm Hg (equivalent to about 0.05%–2.5% $O_2$). A further increase in oxygen concentration, up to that seen in air (21% or 159 mm Hg) or even to 100% oxygen (760 mm Hg), produces a much smaller though definite increase in radiosensitivity. Oxygen tension typically found in arterial blood is between 75 and 100 mmHg and in venous blood between 30 and 40 mm Hg. Thus, from a radiobiological standpoint most normal tissues can be considered to be well oxygenated, although it is now recognized that moderate hypoxia is a feature of some normal tissues such as cartilage and skin.

The average oxygen concentration in tumours, however, is typically much lower with many cells at intermediate oxygen concentrations between 0.5 and 20 mm Hg where there is the maximum change of radiosensitivity.

The mechanism responsible for the enhancement of radiation damage by oxygen is generally referred to as the oxygen-fixation hypothesis and is illustrated in Figure 17.2. This explanation is based on radiation chemistry, and is independent of other effects of oxygen on cell biology (Chapter 18). When radiation is absorbed in a biological material, free radicals are produced. These radicals are highly reactive molecules and it is these that break chemical bonds, produce chemical changes, and initiate the chain of events that result in initial biological damage. They can be produced either directly in the target molecule (usually DNA) or indirectly in other cellular molecules and diffuse far enough to reach and damage critical targets. Most of the indirect effects occur by the OH$^\bullet$ free radicals produced in water, since this makes up 70%–80% of mammalian cells. It is the fate of the free radicals ultimately produced in the critical target, designated as R$^\bullet$ in Figure 17.2 that is important. If oxygen is present then it can react with R$^\bullet$ to produce RO$_2^\bullet$, which then undergoes further reaction ultimately to yield ROOH in the target molecule. This produces a change in the chemical composition of the target and the damage is then referred to as chemically 'fixed'. Subsequently, this damage is recognized by biological pathways that participate in the DNA damage response to invoke enzymatic processing of the lesions and subsequent repair (see Chapter 2). In the absence of oxygen, or in the presence of reducing species (e.g. sulfhydryls), the unstable R$^\bullet$ molecule can react with H$^+$, thus chemically restoring its original form.

Oxygen plays an important role in the radiation response of tumours. The growth of solid tumours requires the induction of a blood supply, a process that is referred to as angiogenesis. This new blood supply is primitive and chaotic in nature and may be inadequate for meeting all the needs of the growing tumour mass. As a result, nutrient-deprived, acidic and oxygen-deficient regions develop, yet the hypoxic cells existing in these areas may still be viable, at least for a limited time. The first clear indication that hypoxia could

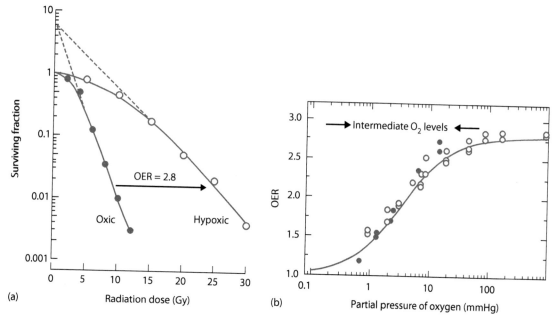

**Figure 17.1** (a) Survival curves for mammalian cells exposed to X-rays under oxic or hypoxic conditions, illustrating the dose-modifying effect of oxygen. (b) Variation of this OER with oxygen partial pressure with the oxygen concentrations found in venous (V) and arterial (A) blood indicated. (From (47), with permission.)

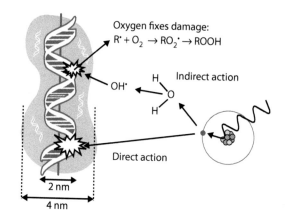

**Figure 17.2** The oxygen fixation hypothesis. Free radicals produced in DNA by either a direct or indirect action of radiation can be restored to their original state under hypoxia but fixed in the presence of oxygen. (Adapted from (12).)

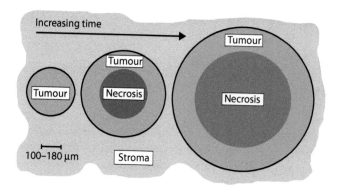

**Figure 17.3** Simplified description of the development of microscopic regions of necrosis in tumours. Conclusions by Thomlinson and Gray from studies on histological sections of human bronchial carcinoma showing the development of necrosis beyond a limiting distance from the vascular stroma. (Adapted from (12).)

exist in human tumours was made in 1955 by Thomlinson and Gray (43) from their observations on histological sections of fresh specimens from human carcinoma of the bronchus (Figure 17.3). They observed viable tumour regions surrounded by vascular stroma from which the tumour cells obtained their nutrient and oxygen requirements. As these regions expanded, areas of necrosis appeared at the centre. The thickness of the resulting shell of viable tissue (100–180 μm) was found to be similar to the calculated diffusion distance of oxygen in respiring tissues from the blood vessels; it was thus suggested that as oxygen diffused from the stroma it was consumed by the cells and, while those cells beyond the diffusion distance were unable to

survive, cells immediately bordering onto necrosis might still be viable yet hypoxic.

Tannock (42) made similar observations in mouse mammary tumours. The extent of necrosis in these tumours was much greater and each patent blood vessel was surrounded by a cord of viable tumour cells beyond which were necrotic cells. This 'corded' structure is also seen in other solid tumours and is illustrated in Figure 17.4. Cells at the edge of the cords are thought to be hypoxic and are often called 'chronically' hypoxic cells. Tannock showed, however, that since the cell population of the cord is in a dynamic state of cell turnover these hypoxic cells may have a short lifespan, being continually replaced as other cells are displaced away

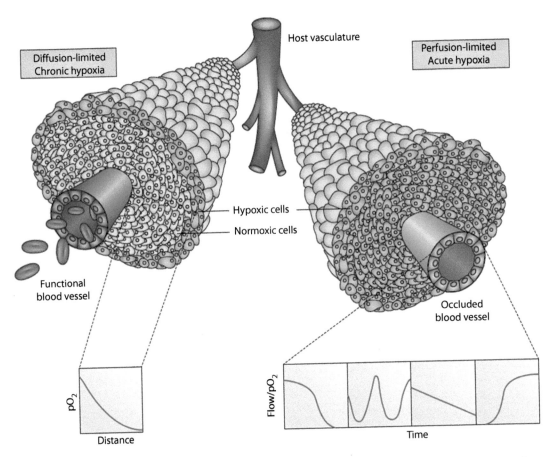

Figure 17.4 Representation of diffusion-limited chronic hypoxia and perfusion limited acute hypoxia within tumour cords. (From (18), with permission.)

from the blood vessel and in turn become hypoxic. Later it was shown that some tumour blood vessels may periodically open and wholly or partially close, leading to transient or acute hypoxia (Figure 17.4). The mechanisms responsible for intermittent blood flow in tumours are not entirely clear. They might include the plugging of vessels by blood cells or by circulating tumour cells; collapse of vessels in regions of high tumour interstitial pressure; or spontaneous vasomotion in incorporated host arterioles affecting blood flow in downstream capillaries.

## 17.2 SIGNIFICANCE FOR RADIATION THERAPY

The presence of hypoxic cells in tumours likely plays a significant role in influencing the response of that tumour to conventional cancer therapy. This has been shown for various types of chemotherapy, including bleomycin, 5-fluorouracil, methotrexate and cis-platinum, all of which are less effective at killing tumour cells when they are hypoxic than when they are well oxygenated (9). In most, though not all, circumstances, this is not a consequence of hypoxia per se, but rather because hypoxic cells are normally distant from blood vessels, thus creating problems for drug delivery, or because such cells are typically non-cycling and

exist in areas of low (acid) pH, both of which can influence drug activity.

The degree of tumour hypoxia impacts radiation response, especially with large doses of radiation. This is illustrated in Figure 17.5a for SCCVII mouse carcinomas that were irradiated *in situ* either in air-breathing mice or in mice in which the tumours were made fully hypoxic (anoxic) by clamping off the blood flow to the tumour. Cell survival was estimated 24 hours after irradiation using an *ex vivo* clonogenic survival assay following tumour excision. The survival curve for the clamped tumours resembles the *in vitro* anoxic survival curve shown previously in Figure 17.1a, confirming that at the time of irradiation all the tumour cells were completely anoxic. For tumours irradiated in air-breathing mice the response is biphasic. At low radiation doses the response is dominated by the aerobic cells and the curves are similar to the oxic curve in Figure 17.1a. But, at higher radiation doses the presence of hypoxic cells begins to influence the response and the survival curve eventually parallels the hypoxic curve. The proportion of maximally resistant hypoxic cells (the hypoxic fraction) can be calculated from the vertical separation between the clamped and air-breathing survival curves in the region where they are parallel. In this mouse model the hypoxic fraction was calculated to be around 1%. Note that the hypoxic fraction

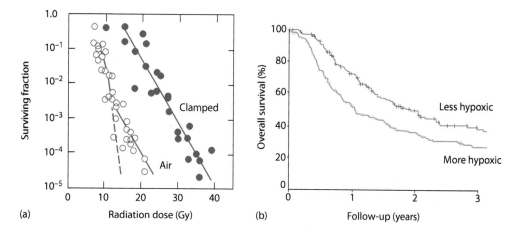

**Figure 17.5** (a) Survival curves for SCCVII tumours irradiated *in situ* and then excised and clonogenic survival measured *in vitro*. Points represent individual tumours from mice irradiated under normal air breathing conditions (open symbols) or when tumours were clamped (closed symbols) for 5 minutes before and during irradiation. (b) Survival for 397 head and neck cancer patients that had their oxygenation status assessed with the Eppendorf oxygen electrode prior to the start of conventional radiation therapy. More or less hypoxia was determined by whether the percentage of oxygen partial pressure values <2.5 mm Hg were above (more hypoxic) or below (less hypoxic) the median value of 19%. ([a] Unpublished observations from C. Grau. [b] From (30), with permission.)

calculated in this way refers to the fraction of viable, maximally resistant hypoxic cells in the tumour. In addition there are also viable cells at a range of oxygenation (and radiosensitivity) between those adjacent to blood vessels and the maximally hypoxic cells. These 'intermediate' hypoxic cells are probably the most important hypoxic cells for standard fractionated radiotherapy (47). There may also be additional non-viable hypoxic cells.

Figure 17.5b includes clinical data that not only illustrate the presence of hypoxia in human tumours, but that such hypoxia can significantly influence outcome. Here patients diagnosed with head and neck cancer had the oxygenation status of their tumours measured using the Eppendorf oxygen electrode prior to their receiving conventional radiation treatment. Patients were then divided into two groups depending on whether the tumours were less or more hypoxic based on the median number of values ≤2.5 mm Hg. Those patients who had tumours with more hypoxia had significantly lower overall survival.

The hypoxic fraction (as defined above) in a tumour is not necessarily constant and can change both before and after irradiation. This is illustrated in Figure 17.6a. Tumours less than 1 mm in diameter have been found to be fully oxygenated (41), but as they increase in size they usually develop hypoxic regions. If tumours are irradiated with a large single dose of radiation, most of the radiosensitive aerobic cells in the tumour will eventually die. The viable cells that survive are predominantly those that were hypoxic at the time of irradiation, and therefore the hypoxic fraction of the viable cells immediately after irradiation will be close to 100%. Subsequently, the hypoxic fraction falls and approaches its starting value. This is the phenomenon of reoxygenation, and it has been reported to occur in a variety of tumour systems, although the speed of this reoxygenation varies widely, occurring within a few hours in some tumours

and taking several days in others. Furthermore, the final viable hypoxic fraction after reoxygenation can also be higher or lower than its value prior to irradiation. Note that this phenomenon of reoxygenation does not necessarily involve a change in overall tumour oxygenation – it is a reflection of the changing oxygenation of the cells surviving a dose of irradiation consistent with a change in oxygen distribution within a tumour.

The mechanisms underlying reoxygenation in tumours are not fully understood. If reoxygenation occurs rapidly then it is likely the result of recirculation of blood through vessels that were temporarily closed at the time of irradiation. Reoxygenation occurring at longer time intervals is probably the result of cell death leading to tumour shrinkage and a reduction in intercapillary distances, thus allowing oxygen to reach hypoxic cells.

Reoxygenation has important implications in clinical radiotherapy. Figure 17.6b illustrates the hypothetical situation in a tumour following fractionated radiation treatments. In this example, 90% of the viable tumour cells are considered well oxygenated (OER = 2.8) and 10% are hypoxic. The responses of the oxic and hypoxic cells to repeated dose fractions of 2 Gy are illustrated. In this example a surviving fraction at 2 Gy (SF2) of 0.47 for the oxic cells has been assumed. If no reoxygenation occurs, then each successive dose of radiation would be expected to kill fewer and fewer cells with increasing total dose because the surviving cell population becomes dominated by the 10% originally hypoxic cells after only about six fractions. At the end of a 60 Gy treatment, cell survival is more than 6 logs (one million fold) higher compared with a tumour with no hypoxia. However, if reoxygenation occurs between fractions then the radiation killing of initially hypoxic cells will be greater and the hypoxic cells then have less impact on response. In the example shown in Figure 17.6b, 'full'

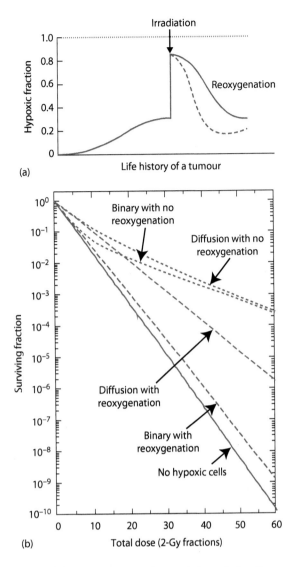

**Figure 17.6** (a) The time-course changes in hypoxic fraction during the life history of a tumour. Hypoxia increases as the tumour grows, but when treated with a single dose of radiation the hypoxic fraction increases as a result of the oxic cells being killed. The subsequent decrease is termed *reoxygenation*. (b) Calculated cell survival curves following repeated 2 Gy fractions in tumours containing originally 90% well-oxygenated and 10% hypoxic cells. Two models are shown, one in which there is a binary distribution of oxygenated and hypoxic cells, and a more physiologically realistic one in which oxygen diffusion defines the distribution of oxygenation in tumours. A surviving fraction at 2 Gy of 0.47 for oxic cells has been assumed with an OER of 2.8. (From (47), with permission.)

rexoygenation has been estimated, meaning that the hypoxic fraction returns to the same starting value of 10% before each 2 Gy fraction. In this case, the overall effect of hypoxia is much smaller with about only a 1 log (10-fold) difference. The existence of such extensive reoxygenation is supported by the fact that local control can be achieved in a variety of tumours given fractionated radiotherapy with 30–35 fractions of 2 Gy. However, assuming a binary distribution of oxygenated

and hypoxic cells is not biologically realistic. The study of Wouters and Brown (47) showed that cells at intermediate levels of oxygenation (i.e. those with an intermediate radiosensitivity) can cause significant radioresistance during fractionated radiotherapy despite extensive reoxygenation. This is shown in Figure 17.6b, demonstrating that even with full reoxygenation hypoxia can make a large difference to the tumour cell survival following low-dose (2 Gy) fractionated irradiation. However, these cells do not influence response to large single doses, which is determined solely by the most resistant fraction of hypoxic cells. As noted above, however, they do contribute to the response to clinically relevant doses and therefore may play an important role in determining the outcome of fractionated treatment.

## 17.3 IDENTIFYING TUMOUR HYPOXIA

The significance of hypoxia on response to radiotherapy means that we need to be able to identify those tumours in which it exists. For animal models three well-tested assay techniques are routinely used that not only allow us to show the presence of hypoxia, but also put a value on the percentage of viable cells at very low levels of oxygen (29). These are the clamped clonogenic assay (as shown in Figure 17.5a); the clamped tumour growth delay assay, which involves measuring the time taken for tumours to grow to a specific size after irradiation; and the clamped tumour control assay, in which the percentage of animals showing local tumour control at a certain time after treatment is recorded. For each technique it is necessary to produce full radiation dose-response curves under normal and totally hypoxic (anoxic) conditions (hence, the use of clamping, although other methods to induce full hypoxia can also be used), and the hypoxic fractions can then be calculated from the displacement of the dose-response curves. It is important to recognize that these techniques assay the fraction of viable radiation-resistant hypoxic cells. This is commonly referred to as the 'radiobiological' hypoxic fraction, but can be very different from the overall fraction of hypoxic cells measured using other methods (see the following discussion). The radiobiological hypoxic fraction is a relevant value for radiotherapy (at least for large dose fractions) since it directly measures cells that can contribute to treatment failure. Using these classical assays, it has been reported that the radiobiological hypoxic fraction of experimental solid tumours can range from below 1% to well over 50% of the total viable cell population.

Attempts to estimate the level of hypoxia in human tumours have proven more difficult. A major reason is that the direct procedures that have been used in animal tumours are not applicable to the human situation. Instead, clinical estimates of tumour hypoxia need to rely on more indirect approaches, as listed in Table 17.1 (18). Some of the earliest attempts to determine hypoxia in human tumours focused on the vascular supply, since it is only via the tumour vasculature that oxygen can be delivered. The endpoints included

**Table 17.1** Methods used for monitoring hypoxia in human tumours

**Vascular–based methods**
　Biopsy/immunohistochemistry
　　Intercapillary distance
　　Vascular density
　　Cell to nearest vessel distance
　　$HbO_2$ saturation (oxyhaemoglobin)
　Imaging approaches
　　CT perfusion (computed tomography)
　　$HbO_2$ saturation (NIRS, BOLD-MRI)
　　DCE-MRI
　　PET ($^{15}$Oxygen labelled water)

**Direct oxygen measurements**
　Electrodes (glass/Eppendorf)
　EPR (electron paramagnetic resonance) imaging

**Exogenous markers**
　Biopsy/immunohistochemistry
　　Nitroimidazole markers
　Imaging approaches
　　PET (nitroimidazoles)
　　CuATSM – copper(II) (diacetyl-bis
　　[N4-methylthiosemicarbazone])
　　MRI (nitroimidazoles)
　　SPECT (nitroimidazoles/technetium)

**Endogenous markers**
　Individual genes/proteins
　　Biopsy studies
　　Serum/plasma
　Gene signatures

**Surrogate markers**
　Metabolism
　　Biopsy/bioluminescence (lactate/ATP/glucose)
　　Imaging (FDG/MRS)
　DNA damage
　　Comet assay
　　H2AX phosphorylation
　Interstitial fluid pressure
　　Probes
　　DCE-MRI

*Abbreviations:* BOLD, blood oxygen level dependent; DCE, dynamic contrast enhanced; FDG, fluorodeoxyglucose; MRI, magnetic resonance imaging; MRS, magnetic resonance spectroscopy; NIRS, near-infrared spectroscopy; PET, positron emission tomography; SPECT, single-photon emission computed tomography.

histological measurements of intercapillary distance, vascular density and the distance from tumour cells to the nearest blood vessels; estimates of the oxygen-carrying capacity of the blood by monitoring oxyhaemoglobin ($HbO_2$) saturation either invasively using a cryophotometric technique on tumour biopsies or non-invasively with near infrared spectroscopy (NIRS) or blood oxygen level dependent (BOLD) contrast magnetic resonance imaging (MRI); or non-invasive assessment of tumour perfusion estimated with positron emission tomography (PET) using [$^{15}$O]-labelled water,

computed tomography (CT) and dynamic contrast-enhanced (DCE) MRI. While many of these studies reported positive correlations between the various vascular parameters and outcome to radiation therapy it was not always the case. This is perhaps not surprising because each method only focused on one aspect that could contribute to hypoxia.

A more direct method for identifying hypoxia involves determining oxygen partial pressure (pO$_2$) distributions using electrodes. Early attempts to do this used 'home-made' glass electrodes, which were cumbersome, fragile and could obtain a few pO$_2$ values 3–4 mm below the tumour surface. However, clinical data obtained in cervix and head and neck cancer clearly demonstrated a relationship between such oxygenation measurements and outcome to radiation therapy. This whole area was revolutionized with the development of the Eppendorf electrode, which had the oxygen sensor inside a metal needle that was attached to a stepping motor and so could make multiple measurements along a needle track through the tumour. Using this machine hypoxia was found to exist in virtually all human tumours investigated, although the degree varied. Unfortunately, it was impossible to state whether the values obtained were from viable tissue or whether the cells in viable hypoxic regions were clonogenic. Furthermore, the tumours had generally to be easily accessible and the technique was invasive. These limitations have made this approach obsolete. Nevertheless, studies in head and neck, cervix, prostate and soft tissue sarcomas were able to clearly demonstrate that pre-treatment measurements of hypoxia could influence outcome to radiation therapy, with less well-oxygenated tumours showing the poorest response (see Figure 17.5b). An alternative non-invasive approach to directly measure oxygenation status involves electron paramagnetic resonance (EPR) imaging, but while this can provide quantitative and repeated three-dimensional estimates of oxygenation and has been used extensively in pre-clinical studies and even in patients with a range of different clinical problems, its clinical application in cancer has been limited.

One of the more widely studied methods for detecting hypoxia involves the administration of exogenous compounds that under hypoxia undergo a chemical change to a product that can then be detected, usually as a result of binding to tumour macromolecules. The most popular agents used in this context have been 2-nitroimidazole-based markers of which the lead compound is pimonidazole. This agent can be detected immunohistochemically and its degree of binding has been correlated with radiobiological hypoxia in pre-clinical studies and local tumour control after radiation therapy in head and neck cancer, although not in cervix. Similar positive clinical findings between hypoxia levels and outcome in head and neck cancer were found for another nitroimidazole marker EF5, a fluorinated derivative of etanidazole. Labelling such compounds with a radioactive tracer allows for their non-invasive detection using PET, MRI or single photon emission computed tomography (SPECT). Although non-invasive imaging is clearly the future, the current use of these approaches is still far from ideal. The tumour cells need to be hypoxic for significant time periods to be detected, which means that such markers are far more sensitive to chronic hypoxia than acute; the time at which measurements are typically made may be too short and thus detect unbound non-hypoxic material; and the resolution of the images is such that voxel sizes identified are often larger than most hypoxic structures. Despite these limitations a variety of clinical studies using $^{18}$F-labelled fluoromisonidazole (FMISO), fluoroerythronitroimidazole (FETNIM) and fluorazomycin arabinoside (FAZA) have shown outcome to radiation therapy to be correlated with hypoxia imaging. Copper(II) diacetyl-bis (N4-methylthiosemicarbazone) (Cu-ATSM) belongs to a chemically different group of PET agents that has been suggested of being able to identify hypoxia, but the results so far obtained are somewhat inconsistent so its role in this context is unclear.

Hypoxia is also well known to increase the cellular expression of a wide variety of genes and proteins (Chapter 18) which has led to the suggestion that measurements of these elevated expression patterns could be indicative of hypoxia and thus prognostic for outcome (13). The principal endogenous agents investigated as potential hypoxia markers include the hypoxia inducible factor 1 (HIF-1), carbonic anhydrase IX (CAIX), the glucose transporters GLUT-1 and GLUT-3 and osteopontin (OPN). Attempts to relate expression levels with more established assays for hypoxia has reported mixed results, which is perhaps not entirely unexpected since the expression of many endogenous agents can be regulated by factors other than hypoxia. Furthermore, the oxygen dependency of these endogenous proteins may be significantly different than the oxygen dependency for labelling by the nitroimidazole exogenous markers. Regardless of these issues, several studies were able to correlate increased expression with outcome, especially when a hypoxic gene signature was applied.

Table 17.1 also includes a number of surrogate markers. These are factors like metabolism, DNA damage and interstitial fluid pressure that are known to be altered by/associated with hypoxia. However, their potential to categorically relate hypoxia to radiotherapy outcome remains unclear.

## 17.4 MODIFYING OXYGEN DELIVERY

Substantial effort has been made to find methods that can effectively overcome tumour radioresistance resulting from hypoxia. One of the earliest clinical attempts to achieve this involved patients breathing high-oxygen-content gas under hyperbaric conditions (7). An increase in barometric pressure of the gas breathed by the patient during radiotherapy is termed *hyperbaric oxygen (HBO) therapy* with pressures up to around 3 atmospheres of pure oxygen having been used. Most trials were small in size and suffered from the use of unconventional fractionation schedules but the results demonstrated that HBO therapy was superior to radiotherapy given in air, especially when a few large fractions were applied (31). This was clearly seen in the largest multicentre clinical trials of HBO, by

the British Medical Research Council, in which the results both from advanced head and neck cancer and carcinoma of the cervix cancers showed a significant benefit in local tumour control and subsequent survival (Figure 17.7a and 17.7b). No benefit was observed in bladder cancer, and these results were not confirmed by a number of smaller studies (31). In retrospect, the use of HBO therapy was discontinued somewhat prematurely. This was partly due to the introduction of chemical radiosensitizers (see later) and because of problems with patient compliance. It has been claimed that hyperbaric treatment caused significant suffering, but the discomfort associated with such a treatment must be considered minor compared with the life-threatening complications associated with chemotherapy that is used with a less restrictive indication.

High-oxygen gas breathing, either as 100% oxygen or carbogen (95% oxygen + 5% carbon dioxide) under normobaric conditions has also been tried clinically to radiosensitize tumours, but failed to show significant therapeutic gain. One reason for this may have been the failure to achieve the optimum pre-irradiation gas breathing time; a number of experimental studies have shown this to be critical for the enhancement of radiation damage and that results can vary from tumour to tumour. The failure of this approach may also have been related to the fact that normobaric oxygen would only be expected to deal with diffusion-limited chronic hypoxia and not with perfusion-limited acute hypoxia. Experimental studies demonstrated that nicotinamide, a vitamin-B3 analogue, could preferentially enhance radiation damage in a variety of murine tumours using both single-dose and fractionated schedules (16), and additional studies suggested the mechanism for this enhanced radiation response to be due to nicotinamide preventing the transient fluctuations in tumour blood flow that lead to the development of acute hypoxia. This led to the suggestion that the optimal approach would be to combine nicotinamide with treatments that specifically target chronic hypoxia. Benefit has been seen when nicotinamide was combined with hyperthermia, perfluorochemical emulsions, pentoxifylline and high oxygen-content gas breathing. Clinical testing involved combining nicotinamide with carbogen in two European randomized trials: the BCON (bladder, carbogen and nicotinamide) trial in bladder (21) and the ARCON (accelerated radiation, carbogen and nicotinamide) trial in the head and neck (25). Local control in the ARCON laryngeal cancer trial was approximately 80%, equal in both treatment arms, which was to be expected since the control rates were already very high, while the experimental arm did receive two fractions of 2 Gy less to the primary target. However, a significant improvement was observed in patients with more hypoxic tumours (Figure 17.8).

It is well established that haemoglobin concentration is an important prognostic factor for the response to radiotherapy in certain tumour types, especially squamous cell carcinomas (15). Generally, patients with low haemoglobin levels have a reduced local-regional tumour control and survival probability.

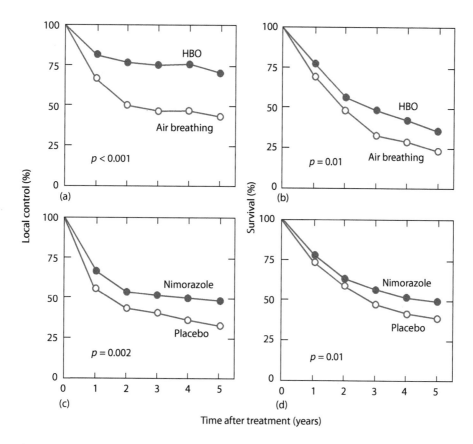

**Figure 17.7** Influence of hypoxic modification on local tumour control and survival in cancer patients. Results are from the Medical Research Council (MRC) hyperbaric oxygen (HBO) trial in patients with stage III carcinoma of the cervix (a + b) or the DAHANCA 5 nimorazole study in patients with carcinoma of the pharynx and supraglottic larynx (c + d). For the MRC study the patients were given conventional radiation treatments under either air breathing conditions (open symbols; 124 patients) or while breathing HBO (closed symbols; 119 patients). In the DAHANCA study patients received placebo (open symbols; 195 patients) or nimorazole (closed symbols; 219 patients) in conjunction with conventional radiotherapy. (Modified from (34,45).)

While several mechanisms can be proposed to explain this relationship, tumour hypoxia is clearly one of the major factors.

Although there is no clear relationship between the 'steady-state' haemoglobin concentration and the extent of tumour hypoxia, experimental and clinical studies have both indicated that a rapid, albeit transient, increase of the haemoglobin concentration by transfusion can result in an increase in tumour oxygenation (14). Furthermore, studies have shown that the amount of oxygen delivered to tumours by the blood is especially important for a curative result. This is clearly illustrated in Figure 17.9, in which head and neck cancer patients who smoked were found to have a significantly lower loco-regional control than those who did not. Smoking can lead to a loss of more than 30% of the oxygen-unloading capacity of the blood and this would be expected to significantly reduce tumour oxygenation and subsequently decrease tumour control (10).

The importance of haemoglobin led to two randomized trials of the effect of transfusion in patients with low haemoglobin values (8,34). Despite an initial positive report from the Canadian trial in uterine cervix carcinoma, both studies concluded that the use of such transfusions did not significantly improve treatment outcome. In the

DAHANCA 5 study, transfusion was given several days prior to radiotherapy and adaptation may have occurred. Using preclinical data, Hirst (14) hypothesised that any increase in tumour hypoxic fraction induced by anaemia will be only transient, with tumours adapting to the lowered oxygen delivery. Transfusing anaemic animals decreased tumour hypoxia, but this effect also was only transient and the tumours were able to adapt to the increased oxygen level within 24 hours. This suggests that when correcting for anaemia it may not necessarily be the final haemoglobin concentration by itself that is important. Rather, an increasing haemoglobin concentration occurring at the time when the tumours are regressing during radiotherapy may be more likely to result in an increased oxygen supply to tumours and a subsequent improvement in response to radiotherapy.

Although a well-documented causal relationship between haemoglobin concentration, tumour oxygenation and response to radiotherapy has not been shown, it is likely that such a relationship does exist and there is thus still a rationale for investigating the possibility of improving the outcome of radiotherapy in relevant tumour sites in patients with low haemoglobin concentration given curative radiotherapy. One approach where this was tried

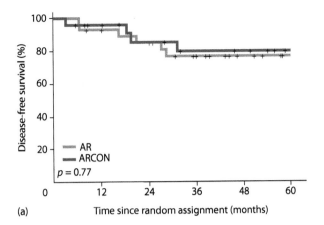

(a)

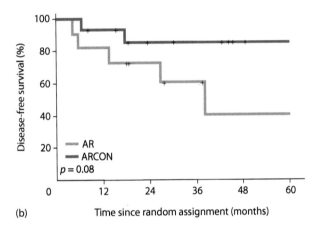

(b)

Figure 17.8 The effect of hypoxia on the response of laryngeal cancer to treatment with accelerated radiotherapy (AR) alone or when combined with nicotinamide and carbogen (ARCON). Results show disease-free survival for patients with either low (a) or high (b) hypoxic fraction, estimated with the hypoxic marker pimonidazole following immunohistochemical analysis of biopsies using a cut-off value of 2.6%, prior to irradiation with AR or ARCON. (From (25), with permission.)

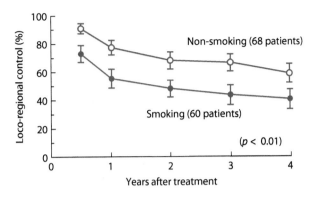

Figure 17.9 Influence of smoking during treatment on outcome of radiotherapy in patients with advanced head and neck carcinoma. Results are for local control from a prospective study in patients treated with curative radiotherapy alone. (Modified from (10).)

involved using erythropoietin (EPO), a hormone normally secreted from the kidney in response to tissue hypoxia and low serum EPO levels are often seen in anaemic cancer patients (15). Several studies demonstrated that administration of recombinant human EPO was capable of producing a gradual increase in haemoglobin concentration in patients and thus a number of multicentre phase III studies were initiated to evaluate the importance of EPO in radiotherapy. However, although patients showed the expected increase in haemoglobin levels, those treated with EPO had a poorer outcome than the non-EPO-treated control arms (15). This has been attributed to the finding that EPO receptors have been found on tumour cells (26), but the fact that the tumour could adapt to the gradually rising higher haemoglobin levels is also likely to be a factor. Nonetheless, this result does not make the concept of increasing the haemoglobin concentration immediately prior to irradiation an irrelevant issue.

Another approach focuses on changing oxygen delivery not through vascular-mediated effects, but rather by decreasing the oxygen consumption of cells close to blood vessels and thereby increasing the oxygen diffusion distance, making more oxygen available to the hypoxic cells. This may be achieved using the drug metformin which has undergone extensive clinical evaluation for the treatment of diabetes and has been linked to decreased rates of certain types of cancer, especially prostate (40), and pre-clinically shown to enhance radiation response. While this may be attributed to an interaction with a number of signalling cascades, it may also be the result of metformin decreasing hypoxia through a reduction of cellular oxygen consumption (48) but this has not yet been proven and is an area where more research is needed.

## 17.5 HYPOXIC CELL RADIOSENSITIZERS

The concept of chemical radiosensitization of hypoxic cells was introduced by Adams and Cooke (2) when they showed that certain compounds were able to mimic oxygen and thus enhance radiation damage. They also demonstrated that the efficiency of sensitization was directly related to the electron affinity of the compounds. It was postulated that such agents would diffuse out of the tumour blood supply and unlike oxygen, which is rapidly metabolized by tumour cells, these compounds would be able to diffuse further, reach the more distant hypoxic cells and thus sensitize them. Since these drugs mimic the sensitizing effect of oxygen, they would not be expected to increase the radiation response of well-oxygenated cells in surrounding normal tissues; radiation tolerance should therefore not be compromised.

The first electron-affinic compounds to show hypoxic radiosensitization were the nitrobenzenes. These were followed by the nitrofurans and finally nitroimidazoles, the most potent of which was found to be the 2-nitroimidazole, misonidazole. Its *in vitro* activity is illustrated in

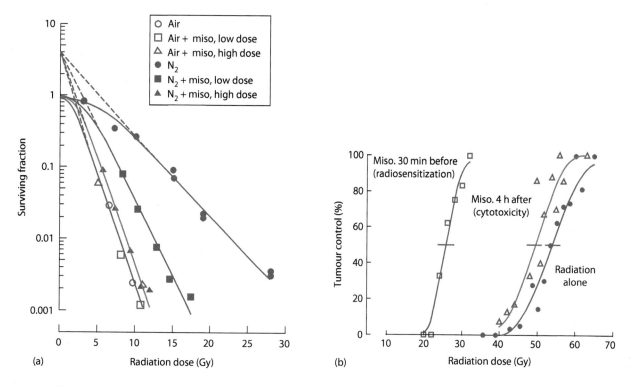

**Figure 17.10** (a) Survival of Chinese hamster cells irradiated under aerobic or hypoxic conditions in the presence or absence of low (1 mM) or high (10 mM) doses of misonidazole. (b) Control of a C3H mammary carcinoma measured 120 days after receiving local radiation alone, or when mice were given an intraperitoneal injection of misonidazole (1 g/kg) either 30 minutes before or 4 hours after irradiating. ([a] From (1), with permission. [b] J. Overgaard, Unpublished observations.)

Figure 17.10a. Note that in these experiments misonidazole is radiation dose modifying: the survival curves have the same extrapolation number (i.e. 4). The radiation response of hypoxic cells can thus be enhanced substantially by irradiating the cells in the presence of misonidazole; in fact, at a drug concentration of 10 mM the radiosensitivity of hypoxic cells approaches that of aerated cells. The response of the aerated cells is unaffected, as expected for an oxygen-mimetic agent.

Radiosensitizers such as misonidazole can also enhance radiation damage in experimental tumours *in vivo*, as shown in Figure 17.10b. The magnitude of the sensitizing effect is usually expressed by the sensitizer enhancement ratio (SER):

$$ \text{SER} = \frac{\text{Radiation dose without sensitizer}}{\text{Radiation dose with sensitizer}} $$

for the same level of biological effect. Large enhancement ratios (>2) have been found in a variety of animal tumours when the sensitizer was administered prior to single-dose irradiation – owing to the importance of hypoxic cells in single treatments. However, when misonidazole was combined with fractionated radiation, the SER values were lower. This probably results from both reoxygenation between radiation fractions reducing the therapeutic impact of hypoxia, and from the fact that these hypoxic radiosensitizers are less effective at intermediate oxygen concentrations which become important with fractionated

irradiation. Also shown in Figure 17.10b is the effect of giving misonidazole after irradiation, where a small but significant enhancement was still seen. This obviously cannot be due to hypoxic cell radiosensitization, but probably results from the well-demonstrated observation that misonidazole is also directly toxic to hypoxic cells; the level of cell killing increases considerably with the duration of exposure to the sensitizer.

The first clinical studies of radiosensitizers were with metronidazole in brain tumours and together with encouraging laboratory studies of misonidazole they were followed by a boom in the late 1970s of trials exploring the potential of this latter agent as a radiosensitizer (31). Most of the trials with misonidazole were unable to demonstrate a significant improvement in radiation response, although benefit was seen in some trials in certain subgroups of treated patients. This was certainly true for the Danish head and neck cancer trial (DAHANCA 2), which found a highly significant improvement in pharynx tumours but not in the prognostically better glottic carcinomas (33). The generally disappointing clinical results with misonidazole may partly be because it was evaluated in unpromising tumour sites and with too few patients. However, the most likely explanation is the fact that the misonidazole doses were too low for adequate sensitization, being limited by the risk of neurotoxicity (3).

The difficulty of achieving sufficiently large clinical doses of misonidazole led to a search for better radiosensitizing drugs. Of the many compounds synthesized and tested, two of the most promising were etanidazole and pimonidazole. Etanidazole was selected as being superior to misonidazole for two reasons. First, although it has a sensitizing efficiency equivalent to that of misonidazole, it has a shorter half-life *in vivo*, which should lead to reduced toxicity. Second, it also has a reduced lipophilicity (a lower octanol/water partition coefficient) and therefore is less readily taken up in neural tissue, leading to less neurotoxicity (6). Etanidazole was tested in two large head and neck cancer trials, one in the United States and the other in Europe. In neither case was there a significant therapeutic benefit although in a later subgroup analysis a positive benefit was reported. Pimonidazole contained a side chain with a weakly basic piperidine group. This compound is more electron affinic than misonidazole and thus is more effective as a radiosensitizer; it is also uncharged at acid pH, thus promoting its accumulation in ischaemic regions of tumours. A pimonidazole trial was started in uterine cervix, but was stopped when it became evident that those patients who received pimonidazole showed a poorer response.

In Denmark, an alternative strategy was taken that involved searching for a less toxic drug and thus nimorazole was chosen. Although its sensitizing ability was less than could theoretically be achieved by misonidazole or etanidazole, nimorazole was far less toxic and thus could be given in much higher doses. At a clinically relevant dose the SER was approximately 1.3. Furthermore, the drug could be given in association with a conventional radiation therapy schedule and was therefore amenable to clinical use. When given to patients with supraglottic and pharyngeal carcinomas (DAHANCA 5) a highly significant benefit in terms of improved locoregional tumour control and disease-free survival were obtained (34). These results are shown in Figure 17.7c and d and are consistent with the earlier DAHANCA 2 study for misonidazole. As a consequence, nimorazole has now become part of the standard treatment schedule for head and neck tumours in Denmark.

Additional studies are still ongoing in an attempt to find other drugs that have low systemic toxicity but superior hypoxic radiosensitization. In that context, one such drug looks clinically promising: the nitroimidazole doranidazole, in which promising preliminary results were obtained in a phase III study with intraoperative radiotherapy in advanced pancreatic cancer. However, it is unlikely to be useful when added to standard fractionated radiotherapy for previously discussed reasons, but like other hypoxic radiosensitizers might be extremely effective if added to high-dose/fraction stereotactic body radiation therapy (5).

One of the most effective radiation sensitizers is hyperthermia (19). Numerous pre-clinical studies have shown that irradiating tumours and heating with temperatures up to 43°C at around the same time substantially enhanced radiation response. The benefit seen is dependent on the temperature applied and the time of heating, but the effect becomes reduced as the time interval between the heat and radiation increases, so eventually no sensitization is seen, yet the response to radiation is still enhanced as a result of the heat killing some of the radioresistant hypoxic cell population. As a result of the extensive pre-clinical studies, a number of clinical trials have been undertaken and a meta-analysis of those trials in which patients were randomized to radiation or radiation and heat demonstrated significant improvements in local tumour control (Table 17.2). Some of the studies listed in Table 17.2 also reported improvements in overall survival (19).

## 17.6 HYPOXIC CYTOTOXINS

Another approach to the hypoxia problem is the use of agents specifically toxic to hypoxic cells – 'hypoxic cytotoxins' (Figure 17.11). These should be relatively tumour specific and since it is the hypoxic cells that are the ones resistant to standard therapy, they should be able to overcome the resistance to standard therapy of the tumour as a whole.

Table 17.2 Meta-analysis of 23 randomised clinical trials of radiation (RT) ± hyperthermia (HT) including 1919 patients

| Tumour site | Number of trials | Number of patients | RT + HT[a] (%) | RT alone[a] (%) | Odds ratio (95%CL[b]) |
|---|---|---|---|---|---|
| Advanced breast | 2 | 143 | 68 | 67 | 1.06 (0.52–2.14) |
| Chest wall | 4 | 276 | 59 | 38 | 2.37 (1.46–3.86) |
| Cervix | 4 | 248 | 77 | 52 | 3.05 (1.77–5.27) |
| Rectum | 2 | 258 | 19 | 9 | 2.27 (1.08–4.76) |
| Bladder | 1 | 101 | 73 | 51 | 2.61 (1.14–5.98) |
| Prostate | 1 | 49 | 81 | 79 | 1.16 (0.28–4.77) |
| Melanoma | 1 | 128 | 56 | 31 | 2.81 (1.36–5.80) |
| Head and neck | 5 | 274 | 51 | 33 | 2.08 (1.28–3.39) |
| Mixed | 3 | 442 | 39 | 34 | 1.24 (0.84–1.82) |
| All trials | 23 | 1919 | 52 | 38 | 1.80 (1.50–2.16) |

Modified from (19), with permission.

[a] All results are for locoregional control.
[b] Errors are 95% confidence limits (CL).

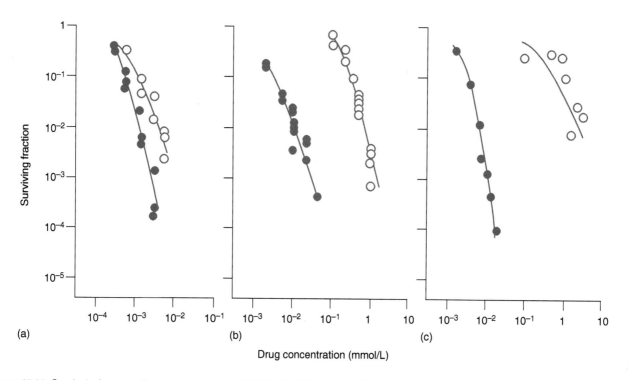

**Figure 17.11** Survival of mammalian cells exposed to (a) MMC, (b) RSU-1069 or (c) tirapazamine under aerobic (open symbols) or hypoxic (closed symbols) conditions. (Redrawn from (17), with permission.)

Mitomycin C, a quinone antibiotic that requires reductive metabolism for activity, is the prototype anticancer drug of this class. Introduced into clinical use in 1958, mitomycin C has demonstrated activity against a number of different tumours in combination with other chemotherapeutic drugs and radiation. Sartorelli and Rockwell (39) were able to show that this drug preferentially kills hypoxic compared to aerobic cells *in vitro*. However, the differential toxicity is modest: the ratio of drug concentrations under aerobic to hypoxic conditions for the same level of cell kill (hypoxic cytotoxicity ratio [HCR]) is in the range of 1 (no differential) to 5. Nonetheless, clinical trials have reported higher cure rates for head and neck cancers by adding mitomycin C to radiotherapy compared with radiotherapy alone. However, as mitomycin C is a standard chemotherapy drug with toxicity also towards well-oxygenated cells, it is not clear whether the improved cure rates over radiotherapy alone were the result of selective killing of hypoxic cells.

Tirapazamine (TPZ), a drug discovered by Brown and Lee, is the first purely hypoxic cytotoxin for which antitumour activity has been demonstrated to enter clinical trials. TPZ was a significant advance over the previously known classes of hypoxic cytotoxins, including quinone antibiotics and nitroimidazoles, because its differential toxicity towards hypoxic cells was much larger, in the range of 50- to 300-fold (Figure 17.11), and combination studies with fractionated radiation demonstrated its ability to kill hypoxic cells in transplanted tumours. TPZ potentiates the antitumour effect of radiation by selectively killing the hypoxic cells in the tumours. As these are the most radiation-resistant cells in tumours, TPZ and radiation act as complementary cytotoxins, each one killing the cells resistant to the other, thereby potentiating the efficacy of radiation on the tumour (Figure 17.12).

Following promising early phase I and II studies Rischin and Peters led a large Phase III multicentre trial of TPZ added to chemoradiotherapy of head and neck cancer. The outcome of the trial was disappointing: There was no benefit to adding TPZ to the standard regime. However, the authors noted that many patients were found to have major deviations in the radiotherapy plan and for patients without major radiotherapy deviations the TPZ arm was superior in loco-regional control compared to the radiation-only arm (37). So TPZ may have failed this trial because of poor radiotherapy in some centres. But that is not the only problem. It is clear from many studies that no benefit could be expected for patients who do not have hypoxic tumours and the inclusion of such patients in a trial such as this will clearly dilute the effect. This is most clearly seen in data obtained at the Peter MacCallum Cancer Centre in Melbourne by Rischin and Peters and colleagues which shows the TPZ is very effective when given to patients with hypoxic tumours as assessed by PET scanning using the hypoxia-specific radiotracers [18]F-MISO or [18]F-FAZA, but not at all for patients with non-hypoxic tumours (Figure 17.13). So this leads to the clear conclusion that, for TPZ, as for any hypoxia-targeted agent, one should only select those patients for treatment who have hypoxic tumours.

Tirapazamine has also been studied in the clinic with platinum-based chemotherapy, though the mechanism of the potentiation is not through killing hypoxic cells (as

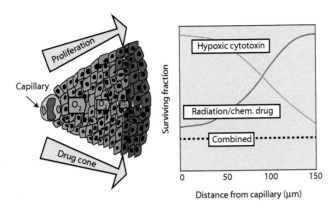

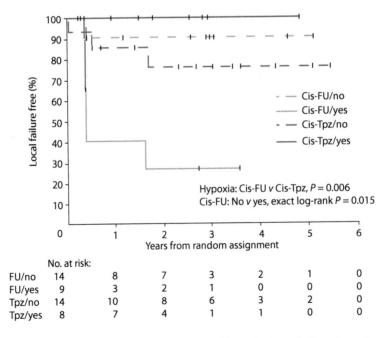

**Figure 17.12** *Left*: Cartoon of part of a tumour cord showing decreasing oxygen concentration as well as decreasing cellular proliferation and drug concentration as a function of distance from the capillary. *Right*: The profiles on the left lead to the prediction that cell killing by radiation and most anticancer drugs will be reduced as a function of distance from the capillary. However, a hypoxic cytotoxin will show the opposite profile. The combination of standard treatment with such a hypoxic cytotoxin would be expected to overcome the problem of hypoxic cells by producing a relatively uniform cell profile of cell killing as a function of distance from the capillary (combined). Such profiles have been demonstrated experimentally for human tumours transplanted into mice. (Reprinted from (4), with permission.)

time and response rates without increasing cisplatin toxicity to normal organs. However, when TPZ was tested either to substitute for etoposide (cisplatin + etoposide versus cisplatin + TPZ), or was added to carboplatin + paclitaxel there was no benefit.

In addition, other classes of hypoxia-activated agents have been developed and tested including PR-104, TH-302 (evofosfamide), E09 (apaziquone), AQ4N (banoxantrone) and many more that have been developed and tested preclinically (46). PR-104, a 2-nitroimidazole hypoxia-activated mustard developed by Denny and Wilson in Auckland, has several features that are different from TPZ. One is that the hypoxia-produced active metabolite can diffuse from the hypoxic area to kill the surrounding oxygenated cells. This means that, unlike TPZ, PR-104 can show antitumour activity alone (36). PR-104 is a bifunctional mustard that is inactivated by nitro groups that because of their strong electron-withdrawing capacity pull reactivity away from the mustard groups that will cross-link DNA. But under hypoxic conditions cellular reductases reduce one of the nitro groups to an amine and activate the mustard moiety to become a cytotoxin, which not only kills the cells in which it is produced but also diffuses to kill both aerobic and hypoxic cells.

TH-302 (evofosfamide), a 2-nitroimidazole hypoxia-activated prodrug of the DNA alkylator, bromo-isophosphoramide mustard, developed by Threshold Pharmaceuticals, has a mechanism of action similar to PR-104. After promising phase II data, two randomized phase III studies combining evofosfamide with gemcitabine in pancreatic cancer (MAESTRO), and with doxorubicin in soft tissue sarcoma (TH-CR-406/SARC021) were

with radiation), but is the result of inhibiting the repair of cisplatin-induced DNA interstrand cross links. A phase III study with non-small cell lung cancer showed that the addition of TPZ to cisplatin significantly increased survival

| No. at risk: | | | | | | |
|---|---|---|---|---|---|---|
| FU/no | 14 | 8 | 7 | 3 | 2 | 1 | 0 |
| FU/yes | 9 | 3 | 2 | 1 | 0 | 0 | 0 |
| Tpz/no | 14 | 10 | 8 | 6 | 3 | 2 | 0 |
| Tpz/yes | 8 | 7 | 4 | 1 | 1 | 0 | 0 |

**Figure 17.13** Kaplan-Meier plot of time to local failure by treatment arm and hypoxia status in the primary tumour (determined by FMISO-PET) demonstrates the importance of tumour hypoxia for the response to TPZ. Cis, cisplatin; FU, fluorouracil; TPZ, tirapazamine; yes/no refers to hypoxic or not. (From (38), with permission.)

initiated. Disappointingly, both failed to meet their primary endpoints. The company will continue two phase II trials with another hypoxia-activated drug, tarloxotinib bromide, which releases an irreversible epidermal growth factor receptor tyrosine kinase inhibitor under severe hypoxia.

AQ4N (banoxantrone) is a prodrug of AQ4 designed to prevent its binding to DNA until metabolized in hypoxic cells to give AQ4, a stable, $O_2$ insensitive metabolite that inhibits topoisomerase II. AQ4N has antitumour activity in mice when combined with radiation or anticancer drugs and was evaluated in a phase I/II trial with radiotherapy and temozolomide in subjects with newly diagnosed glioblastoma multiforme but did not meet its target.

It is worth noting that N-oxide-based hypoxic cytotoxins (such as TPZ) and nitro-based hypoxic cytotoxins (such as evofosfamide), though both activated by hypoxia, are quite different. TPZ and analogues can be metabolized to toxic species at both moderate and severe levels of hypoxia, whereas nitro-based drugs require stringent hypoxia for bioreduction. Also, TPZ kills only the cells in which it is metabolized, whereas evofosfamide (and PR-104 and tarloxotinib bromide) when metabolized release a toxic product that can diffuse to well-oxygenated regions. Thus, evofosfamide has single agent activity, whereas TPZ has not. It is unclear which of the two classes of drugs will be superior; it is likely that the tumour type, the companion therapy (e.g. chemotherapy or radiation) and the level of hypoxia will determine this. Figure 17.14 shows the structures of these hypoxic cytotoxins.

## 17.7 VASCULAR-BASED APPROACHES

The inadequate vascular supply to tumours is one of the major factors responsible for the development of hypoxia.

The tumour vasculature develops from normal tissue vessels by the process of angiogenesis. This is an essential aspect of tumour growth, but this tumour neo-vasculature is primitive and chaotic in nature and is often unable to meet the oxygen demands of rapidly expanding tumour regions, thus causing hypoxia to develop. The importance of the tumour neo-vasculature in determining growth and the environmental conditions within a tumour therefore makes it an attractive target for therapy (20). The first and most popular is the use of drugs to prevent angiogenesis from occurring (angiogenesis inhibitors [AIs]), while the second involves the use of therapies that can specifically damage an already established vasculature (vascular disrupting agents [VDAs]). Examples of AIs clinically tested include inhibitors of vascular endothelial growth factor such as bevacizumab; tyrosine kinase inhibitors including sorafenib (Bay 43-9006/nexavar), sunitinib (SU11248/sutent), vanatanib (PTK787/ZX 222584) and vandetanib (ZD6474/zactima); and thalidomide and related analogues (lenalidomide, pomalidomide). Clinically relevant VDAs include tubulin binding agents like combretastatin A-1 phosphate, OXi4503, ombrabulin (AVE8062) and plinabulin (NPI-2358); the flavonoid compound vadimezan (ASA404); and chemotherapeutic drugs such as the vinca alkaloids and arsenic trioxides.

Although both types of vascular targeting agents have anti-tumour activity when used alone, significant improvements in tumour response have been observed when they are combined with radiation. With AIs one proposed mechanism of action is that this improvement is the consequence of normalisation of the tumour vasculature resulting in a decrease in tumour hypoxia (24). While there are certainly preclinical studies showing an improved tumour oxygenation status with AI treatment, there are also many studies showing no change and even a decrease in tumour

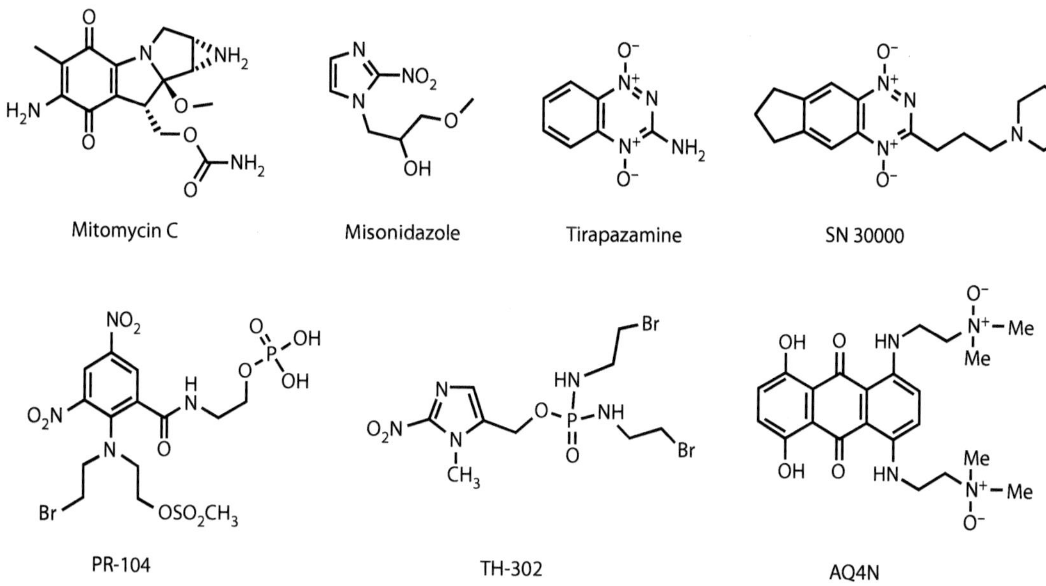

Figure 17.14 Chemical structures of the hypoxic cytotoxins discussed in the text.

oxygenation. These findings not only make it unclear as to the role of hypoxia in influencing the combination of AIs with radiation, they also suggest that timing and sequencing of the two modalities may be critical for the optimal benefit.

The ability of VDAs to enhance radiation response is shown in Figure 17.15. In these experiments tumour-bearing mice were injected with OXi4503, a combretastatin analogue in clinical testing, within a few hours after locally irradiating the tumours. Although the drug alone had no effect on tumour control, it significantly enhanced the response to radiation when given after irradiation. VDAs damage tumour blood vessels leading to a reduced blood flow to the affected tumour region. This gives rise to local hypoxia and ischaemia, and ultimately cell death. Since hypoxic cells are already under stress as a result of oxygen and nutrient deprivation, it is likely that these cells will be the first to die after this additional insult from vascular shutdown and it is probably this effect that explains the enhancement of the radiation response. Additional studies have shown that these effects are tumour specific. However, the tumour response may depend on timing and sequencing since with some VDAs administering them prior to irradiation can have a reduced effect on radiation response, presumably because although the VDAs kill some cells as a result of the vascular occlusion, there are other cells that become hypoxic yet survive and are then a source of radiation resistance. This has implications when VDAs are combined with radiation in a fractionated schedule. However, when appropriate schedules designed to minimize the hypoxia inducing effect of VDAs are used (as shown in Figure 17.15), a significant enhanced response can be observed with a fractionated radiation schedule. As a result, the combination of VDAs with radiation is currently under clinical evaluation.

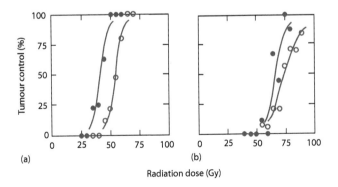

Figure 17.15 Effect of intraperitoneal injection of OXi4503 (50 mg/kg) on local control of a C3H mammary carcinoma measured 90 days after treatment with either single radiation doses (a) or a limited fractionated schedule of 10 fractions in 12 days (b). Results are for radiation alone (open symbols), or radiation + OXi4503 (closed symbols), with the OXi4503 given 2 hours after irradiating in the single-dose study or 1 hour after fractions 5 and 10 in the fractionated study. (Redrawn from (23), with permission.)

## 17.8 DOSE PAINTING

An idea to overcome the resistance of hypoxic cells that has garnered interest among some physicists and radiation oncologists is to use the precision in conforming treatment fields offered by image-guided radiotherapy to boost the radiation dose to regions of the tumour identified as hypoxic by PET imaging. This concept, commonly referred to as 'dose painting', was first suggested by Ling et al. (28), and has been followed by numerous clinical studies demonstrating the feasibility of boosting the dose to regions of tumour hypoxia identified by FMISO or FAZA PET imaging (e.g. [27]). However, there are several theoretical problems with this approach including the heterogeneity in time of tumour hypoxia (Chapter 18), and the inevitable lack of resolution of PET imaging. Indeed the regions of hypoxia identified by PET imaging bear little or no relationship to the microscopic and complex patterns of tumour hypoxia seen with immunohistochemistry (Figures 18.2, 18.4 and 18.10). It is likely that the positive PET regions identify the highest concentrations of hypoxic areas in the tumour, but could not be expected to show all the hypoxic regions. Thus, it seems unlikely that hypoxia dose painting can actually improve tumour response and a rigorous multicentre trial confirmed this prediction (44). Despite this, numerous studies, including this multicentre study, have shown that the identification of hypoxic regions by PET imaging is nevertheless prognostic for poor response to radiotherapy.

## 17.9 META-ANALYSIS OF CONTROLLED CLINICAL TRIALS MODIFYING HYPOXIA

The clinical role of hypoxia is one of the most thoroughly addressed issues in radiotherapy. However, of the numerous clinical trials that have been conducted during the last four decades, most have been inconclusive, which has raised serious concerns about the real importance of tumour hypoxia for cancer treatment. This question was addressed in a meta-analysis of all randomised clinical trials in which some form of hypoxic modification was performed in solid tumours undergoing radiotherapy with curative intent. The survey of published and unpublished data identified more than 10,000 patients treated in 86 randomised clinical trials, and the results are given in Table 17.3. The most relevant endpoint was considered to be local tumour control in view of the local nature of the radiation treatment, and this showed a significant improvement. This improvement persisted when the trials were evaluated separately for radiosensitizer or HBO treatment. When analysed according to site, significant improvements were only found for uterine cervix and head and neck. Overall survival was also significantly improved, again dominated by the head and neck patients, but no difference was found for distant metastases or radiation complications. From this meta-analysis it appears that the hypoxic problem in radiotherapy may be marginal in most

Table 17.3 Meta-analysis of 86 randomised clinical trials of hypoxic modifiers with radiotherapy including 10,108 patients

| Endpoint | Events/total | | Odds ratio and 95% confidence interval | P-value |
|---|---|---|---|---|
| | Modification | Control | | |
| Loco-regional control | 2144/4416 | 2465/4473 | 0.77 (0.71–0.84) | <0.001 |
| Survival | 3237/4921 | 3405/4952 | 0.87 (0.80–0.95) | <0.01 |
| Distant metastasis | 452/2332 | 480/2339 | 0.93 (0.81–1.07) | 0.24 |
| Complications | 374/2424 | 310/2305 | 1.17 (1.00–1.38) | 0.06 |
| **Tumour site (Loco-regional control)** | | | | |
| Bladder | 185/402 | 206/403 | 0.82 (0.62–1.08) | 0.15 |
| Head and neck | 1179/2261 | 1336/2225 | 0.73 (0.64–0.82) | <0.001 |
| Lung | 196/309 | 212/315 | 0.84 (0.61–1.17) | 0.23 |
| Uterine cervix | 499/1308 | 601/1383 | 0.80 (0.69–0.94) | <0.01 |
| Other | 88/132 | 104/141 | 0.71 (0.42–1.20) | 0.18 |
| **All sites** | **2147/4412** | **2459/4467** | **0.76 (0.70–0.83)** | **<0.001** |
| **Hypoxic modification (Loco-regional control)** | | | | |
| Normobaric oxygen | 107/307 | 135/335 | 0.79 (0.58–1.09) | 0.14 |
| Hyperbaric oxygen | 414/1038 | 550/1107 | 0.67 (0.57–0.80) | <0.001 |
| Hypoxic sensitizer | 1608/3022 | 1760/2998 | 0.80 (0.72–0.89) | <0.001 |

Modified from (32), with permission.

adenocarcinomas. Future efforts should, therefore, be focused on squamous cell carcinoma, especially of the head and neck, at least when radiotherapy is given in conventional treatment schedules. These positive results were obtained despite the fact that there was probably considerable heterogeneity among tumours with the same localization and histology, thus the trials likely included patients in which hypoxia was not an issue and so unlikely to benefit from the application of a hypoxic modifier. This suggests that future clinical studies with hypoxic modification should include some form of estimate of tumour hypoxia for patient selection.

## Key points

1. Hypoxic regions caused both by inadequate diffusion (chronic hypoxia) and inadequate perfusion (acute hypoxia) is a common feature of human and experimental tumours.
2. Radiation primarily kills the better-oxygenated cells in tumours, so the cells destined to survive are mostly hypoxic. This changes over the following hours or days, a process known as 'reoxygenation'.
3. Reoxygenation is the primary reason for the superiority of fractionated radiotherapy versus single doses comparing tumour control for equal levels of normal tissue toxicity.
4. Despite reoxygenation clinical studies have shown that better-oxygenated tumours respond to fractionated radiotherapy better than less well-oxygenated tumours.
5. There are numerous ways to assess the degree of hypoxia in human tumours with the most clinically available being PET imaging with one of the hypoxia imaging agents such as F-MISO or FAZA.
6. Many strategies to overcome tumour hypoxia have been investigated, broadly categorized as oxygenating the cells, radiosensitizing the cells and killing the hypoxic cells.
7. Meta-analysis of randomized clinical trials has shown a benefit for local tumour control of hypoxia modification in head and neck and cervix tumours.
8. Selection of hypoxic tumours is essential in future trials of hypoxia modifying agents.

## ■ BIBLIOGRAPHY

1. Adams GE. Hypoxic cell sensitizers for radiotherapy. In: Becker FF, editor. *Cancer: A Comprehensive Treatise.* Vol 6. New York, NY: Plenum Press; 1977. pp. 181–223.
2. Adams GE, Cooke MS. Electron-affinic sensitization. I. A structural basis for chemical radiosensitizers in bacteria. *Int J Radiat Biol Relat Stud Phys Chem Med* 1969;15:457–471.
3. Brown JM. Clinical trials of radiosensitizers: What should we expect? *Int J Radiat Oncol Biol Phys* 1984;10:425–429.
4. Brown JM. The hypoxic cell: A target for selective cancer therapy – Eighteenth Bruce F. Cain Memorial Award lecture. *Cancer Res* 1999;59:5863–5870.
5. Brown JM, Diehn M, Loo BW, Jr. Stereotactic ablative radiotherapy should be combined with a hypoxic cell radiosensitizer. *Int J Radiat Oncol Biol Phys* 2010;78:323–327.
6. Brown JM, Yu NY, Brown DM, Lee WW. SR-2508: A 2-nitroimidazole amide which should be superior to misonidazole as a radiosensitizer for clinical use. *Int J Radiat Oncol Biol Phys* 1981;7:695–703.
7. Churchill-Davidson I. The oxygen effect in radiotherapy: Historical review. *Front Radiat Ther Oncol* 1968;1:1–15.
8. Fyles AW, Milosevic M, Pintilie M, Syed A, Hill RP. Anemia, hypoxia and transfusion in patients with cervix cancer: A review. *Radiother Oncol* 2000;57:13–19.
9. Grau C, Overgaard J. Effect of etoposide, carmustine, vincristine, 5-fluorouracil, or methotrexate on radiobiologically oxic and hypoxic cells in a C3H mouse mammary carcinoma *in situ. Cancer Chemother Pharmacol* 1992;30:277–280.
10. Grau C, Overgaard J. Significance of hemoglobin concentration for treatment outcome. In: Molls M and Vaupel P, editors. *Medical Radiology: Blood Perfusion and Microenvironment of Human Tumours.* Heidelberg: Springer-Verlag; 1997. pp. 101–112.
11. Gray LH, Conger AD, Ebert M, Hornsey S, Scott OC. The concentration of oxygen dissolved in tissues at the time of irradiation as a factor in radiotherapy. *Br J Radiol* 1953;26:638–648.
12. Hall EJ. *Radiobiology for the Radiologist.* 3rd ed. Philadelphia, PA: Lippincott; 1988.
13. Harris AL. Hypoxia – A key regulatory factor in tumour growth. *Nat Rev Cancer* 2002;2:38–47.
14. Hirst DG. Anemia: A problem or an opportunity in radiotherapy? *Int J Radiat Oncol Biol Phys* 1986;12:2009–2017.
15. Hoff CM. Importance of hemoglobin concentration and its modification for the outcome of head and neck cancer patients treated with radiotherapy. *Acta Oncol* 2012;51:419–432.
16. Horsman MR. Nicotinamide and other benzamide analogs as agents for overcoming hypoxic cell radiation resistance in tumours. A review. *Acta Oncol* 1995;34:571–587.
17. Horsman MR, Lindegaard JC, Grau C, Nordsmark M, Overgaard J. Dose-response modifiers in radiation therapy. In: Gunderson LL and Tepper JE, editors. *Clinical Radiation Oncology.* 2nd ed. Philadelphia, PA: Churchill Livingstone; 2007. pp. 59–73.
18. Horsman MR, Mortensen LS, Petersen JB, Busk M, Overgaard J. Imaging hypoxia to improve radiotherapy outcome. *Nat Rev Clin Oncol* 2012;9:674–687.
19. Horsman MR, Overgaard J. Hyperthermia: A potent enhancer of radiotherapy. *Clin Oncol (R Coll Radiol)* 2007;19:418–426.
20. Horsman MR, Siemann DW. Pathophysiologic effects of vascular-targeting agents and the implications for combination with conventional therapies. *Cancer Res* 2006;66:11520–11539.
21. Hoskin PJ, Rojas AM, Bentzen SM, Saunders MI. Radiotherapy with concurrent carbogen and nicotinamide in bladder carcinoma. *J Clin Oncol* 2010;28:4912–4918.

22. Howard-Flanders P, Moore D. The time interval after pulsed irradiation within which injury to bacteria can be modified by dissolved oxygen. I. A search for an effect of oxygen 0.02 second after pulsed irradiation. *Radiat Res* 1958;9:422–437.

23. Iversen AB, Busk M, Horsman MR. Induction of hypoxia by vascular disrupting agents and the significance for their combination with radiation therapy. *Acta Oncol* 2013;52:1320–1326.

24. Jain RK. Normalization of tumor vasculature: An emerging concept in antiangiogenic therapy. *Science* 2005;307:58–62.

25. Janssens GO, Rademakers SE, Terhaard CH et al. Accelerated radiotherapy with carbogen and nicotinamide for laryngeal cancer: Results of a phase III randomized trial. *J Clin Oncol* 2012;30:1777–1783.

26. Lai SY, Grandis JR. Understanding the presence and function of erythropoietin receptors on cancer cells. *J Clin Oncol* 2006;24:4675–4676.

27. Lee NY, Mechalakos JG, Nehmeh S et al. Fluorine-18-labeled fluoromisonidazole positron emission and computed tomography-guided intensity-modulated radiotherapy for head and neck cancer: A feasibility study. *Int J Radiat Oncol Biol Phys* 2008;70:2–13.

28. Ling CC, Humm J, Larson S et al. Towards multidimensional radiotherapy MD-CRT: Biological imaging and biological conformality. *Int J Radiat Oncol Biol Phys* 2000;47:551–560.

29. Moulder JE, Rockwell S. Hypoxic fractions of solid tumors: Experimental techniques, methods of analysis, and a survey of existing data. *Int J Radiat Oncol Biol Phys* 1984;10:695–712.

30. Nordsmark M, Bentzen SM, Rudat V et al. Prognostic value of tumor oxygenation in 397 head and neck tumors after primary radiation therapy. An international multi-center study. *Radiother Oncol* 2005;77:18–24.

31. Overgaard J. Sensitization of hypoxic tumour cells – Clinical experience. *Int J Radiat Biol* 1989;56:801–811.

32. Overgaard J. Hypoxic radiosensitization: Adored and ignored. *J Clin Oncol* 2007;25:4066–4074.

33. Overgaard J, Hansen HS, Andersen AP et al. Misonidazole combined with split-course radiotherapy in the treatment of invasive carcinoma of larynx and pharynx: Report from the DAHANCA 2 study. *Int J Radiat Oncol Biol Phys* 1989;16:1065–1068.

34. Overgaard J, Hansen HS, Overgaard M et al. A randomized double-blind phase III study of nimorazole as a hypoxic radiosensitizer of primary radiotherapy in supraglottic larynx and pharynx carcinoma. Results of the Danish Head and Neck Cancer Study DAHANCA Protocol 5-85. *Radiother Oncol* 1998;46:135–146.

35. Palcic B, Skarsgard LD. Reduced oxygen enhancement ratio at low doses of ionizing radiation. *Radiat Res* 1984;100:328–339.

36. Patterson AV, Ferry DM, Edmunds SJ et al. Mechanism of action and preclinical antitumor activity of the novel hypoxia-activated DNA cross-linking agent PR-104. *Clin Cancer Res* 2007;13:3922–3932.

37. Peters LJ, O'Sullivan B, Giralt J et al. Critical impact of radiotherapy protocol compliance and quality in the treatment of advanced head and neck cancer: Results from TROG 02.02. *J Clin Oncol* 2010;28:2996–3001.

38. Rischin D, Hicks RJ, Fisher R et al. Trans-Tasman Radiation Oncology Study Group. Prognostic significance of [18F]-misonidazole positron emission tomography-detected tumor hypoxia in patients with advanced head and neck cancer randomly assigned to chemoradiation with or without tirapazamine: A substudy of Trans-Tasman Radiation Oncology Group Study 98.02. *J Clin Oncol* 2006;24:2098–2104.

39. Sartorelli AC, Hodnick WF, Belcourt MF et al. Mitomycin C: A prototype bioreductive agent. *Oncol Res* 1994;6:501–508.

40. Spratt DE, Zhang C, Zumsteg ZS, Pei X, Zhang Z, Zelefsky MJ. Metformin and prostate cancer: Reduced development of castration-resistant disease and prostate cancer mortality. *Eur Urol* 2013;63:709–716.

41. Stanley JA, Shipley WU, Steel GG. Influence of tumour size on hypoxic fraction and therapeutic sensitivity of Lewis lung tumour. *Br J Cancer* 1977;36:105–113.

42. Tannock IF. The relation between cell proliferation and the vascular system in a transplanted mouse mammary tumour. *Br J Cancer* 1968;22:258–273.

43. Thomlinson RH, Gray LH. The histological structure of some human lung cancers and the possible implications for radiotherapy. *Br J Cancer* 1955;9:539–549.

44. Vera P, Thureau S, Chaumet-Riffaud P et al. Phase II study of a radiotherapy total dose increase in hypoxic lesions identified by 18F-Misonidazole PET/CT in patients with non-small cell lung carcinoma RTEP5 study. *J Nucl Med* 2017;58:1045–1053.

45. Watson ER, Halnan KE, Dische S et al. Hyperbaric oxygen and radiotherapy: A Medical Research Council trial in carcinoma of the cervix. *Br J Radiol* 1978;51:879–887.

46. Wilson WR, Hay MP. Targeting hypoxia in cancer therapy. *Nat Rev Cancer* 2011;11:393–410.

47. Wouters BG, Brown JM. Cells at intermediate oxygen levels can be more important than the 'hypoxic fraction' in determining tumor response to fractionated radiotherapy. *Radiat Res* 1997;147:541–550.

48. Zannella VE, Dal Pra A, Muaddi H et al. Reprogramming metabolism with metformin improves tumor oxygenation and radiotherapy response. *Clin Cancer Res* 2013;19:6741–6750.

## ▪ FURTHER READING

49. Brown JM, Giaccia AJ. The unique physiology of solid tumors: Opportunities (and problems) for cancer therapy. *Cancer Res* 1998;58:1408–1418.

50. Vaupel P, Kallinowski F, Okunieff P. Blood flow, oxygen and nutrient supply, and metabolic micro-environment of human tumors: A review. *Cancer Res* 1989;49:6449–6465.

# The tumour microenvironment and cellular hypoxia responses

BRADLY G. WOUTERS, MARIANNE KORITZINSKY, J. MARTIN BROWN AND ALBERT J. VAN DER KOGEL

## 18.1 OXYGENATION PATTERNS OF TUMOURS

The steady-state oxygen concentration in tissues is determined by the balance between oxygen supply and demand. Oxygen is supplied from the blood, mainly in a form that is bound to haemoglobin in red blood cells and is consumed by cells primarily through the process of oxidative respiration in the mitochondria. In this process, mitochondria use oxygen as the terminal electron acceptor in a cascade of reactions collectively termed the electron transport chain. Here, nutrients are oxidized to produce the cellular energy currency ATP (adenosine triphosphate). Respiration plays a very important role in energy production by extracting the maximum amount of energy from cellular nutrients. For example, 1 molecule of glucose produces 36 molecules of ATP under conditions where oxygen is present but only 2 molecules of ATP when oxygen is absent (anaerobic glycolysis). The consumption of oxygen in this process gives rise to a limited ability of oxygen to diffuse through unvascularised tissues. Estimates of the oxygen diffusion distance range from 75 to 200 microns depending on the actual respiration rate (oxygen consumption rate) of the tissue/cells in question.

The oxygen concentration of most normal tissues is stably maintained at an equivalent atmospheric concentration of 5%–7%. When oxygen concentrations drop to 3% or below, the tissue is considered hypoxic. Below this value, oxygen deprivation leads to the activation of biological pathways which serve to alter the behaviour or 'phenotype' of the cell. Many of these pathways are activated to allow adaptation of the cell or the tissue to the stress associated with oxygen deprivation. For example, these pathways can increase the capacity for anaerobic glycolysis (to maintain energy production), mediate changes in blood flow and stimulate angiogenesis (new blood vessel growth) to increase the oxygen supply to the tissue. For the most part, these pathways operate in both normal tissues and in tumours.

## Two distinct mechanisms cause tumour hypoxia

The rapid and uncontrolled proliferation of tumour cells often results in a demand for oxygen that exceeds the capacity of the vascular network. Although the resulting hypoxia may stimulate tumour angiogenesis (through mechanisms described in the following text), the developing vessels are often still unable to provide adequate oxygenation for the rapidly proliferating tumour. Thus, although angiogenesis becomes a 'hallmark' of cancer, hypoxic tumour areas remain a common feature throughout the lifetime of the tumour. The lack of sufficient numbers of tumour blood vessels gives rise to one of the two main causes of hypoxia in human tumours known as 'chronic' or 'diffusion-limited' hypoxia. It is important to recognize that although this term has become ubiquitous, hypoxia arises because of oxygen consumption and not from the 'diffusion' properties of oxygen itself. In this type of hypoxia, individual perfused vessels are characterized by a gradient of oxygenation surrounding them. Diffusion-limited hypoxia in tumours was first documented in 1955 (21) (see Chapter 17) and its presence indicates the existence of cells at all possible oxygen concentrations ranging from anoxia at distal locations to normal values next to the vessels.

In some situations, hypoxic cells can also be found much closer to blood vessels than would be expected from oxygen consumption limitations. This observation reflects the poor functionality of tumour vasculature which is characterized by being highly tortuous and poorly organized (Figure 18.1) (19). Tumour vessels are often immature, leaky, lack smooth muscle cells, and have structural abnormalities including blind ends and arterial-venous shunts that together result in unstable blood flow, the cause of what is termed *acute* or *perfusion-limited* hypoxia. Perfusion-limited hypoxia is characterized by rapidly changing oxygen concentrations in areas where blood flow through the vessel is unstable (10). As a result, cells may be exposed to oxygen

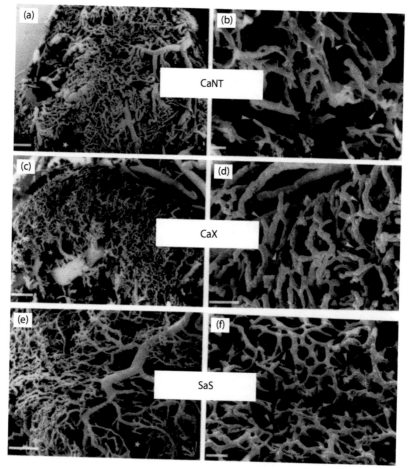

Figure 18.1 Scanning electron micrographs of vascular corrosion casts of murine carcinomas (CaX and CaNT) and sarcoma (SaS) grown subcutaneously in mice. Left-hand panels represent low magnifications (bars = 500 μm) and right-hand panels represent high magnifications (bars = 100 μm). (From (8), with permission.)

concentrations that vary transiently between normal (well perfused) to anoxia (complete vessel blockage) and anywhere in between. Examples of perfusion (acute) and diffusion (chronic) hypoxia observed in experimental tumour models are shown in Figure 18.2.

## 18.2 THE HETEROGENEITY OF TUMOUR HYPOXIA

### Heterogeneity in severity (oxygen concentration)

Both limitations in diffusion and perfusion give rise to tumour cells at widely different oxygen levels. As cells are pushed away from blood vessels by the proliferation of cells close to the vessel, they experience a steady decline in oxygen availability. Eventually these cells may reach distances where the oxygen concentration drops to zero and they can then die and contribute to the necrotic areas in the tumour. Diffusion-limited hypoxia therefore is characterized by an oxygen gradient where cells exist at all possible oxygen concentrations from normoxic to anoxic. Likewise, the

limitations in perfusion that give rise to acute hypoxia can be complete or partial, resulting in surrounding tumour cells at varying oxygen tensions. As a result, both mechanisms of tumour hypoxia are expected to produce cells at a wide range of oxygen concentrations. Consistent with this prediction, direct measurements made in patients using polarographic oxygen electrodes have demonstrated the presence of a large range of oxygen concentrations. Vaupel and Höckel were among the first to use this technique in the clinic and an example of their data from a series of breast cancers and normal tissues is shown in Figure 18.3. Immunohistological staining of tumour sections also reveals variable degrees of staining intensities that reflect the presence of cells at a wide range of oxygen concentrations (see Figures 18.2, 18.4 and 18.10).

The fact that tumours contain cells at many different oxygen concentrations is an important factor to consider when assessing the consequences of tumour hypoxia. In fact, the term *hypoxia* is rather ill-defined and can refer to different cell populations in different contexts. As discussed in Chapter 17, hypoxia-associated radioresistance is due to the participation of oxygen in *radiochemical* events that take place immediately after irradiation. Thus, we can think of

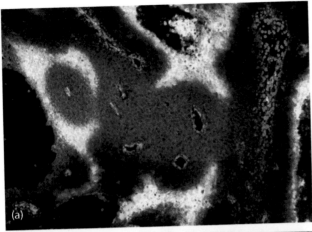

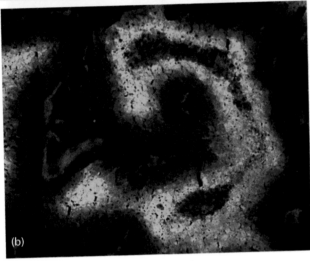

Figure 18.2 (a) Multimarker image of human mucoepidermoid carcinoma MEC82 grown as xenograft, with vasculature (white), Hoechst 33342 (blue) staining nuclei of cells adjacent to perfused vessel, first hypoxia marker (pimonidazole, green) and second hypoxia marker (CCI-103F, red). Spatial co-localization of both markers (red and green) appears as yellow. At an injection interval of 2 hours, most of the hypoxic cells were labelled by both the first and second hypoxia marker. Acute (or transient) hypoxia is illustrated as an area that was not hypoxic at the time of the injection of the first marker but had become hypoxic at the time of the second hypoxia marker injection (red only). (b) Gray-scale image of C38 murine colon carcinoma, showing vessels (red) and hypoxia stained by pimonidazole (green). (From (11), with permission.)

'radiobiological hypoxia' as oxygen concentrations below those causing maximum resistance to radiation, e.g. 0.05%. However, oxygen also influences a number of *biological* responses that are governed by several distinct molecular pathways. The sensitivity of these molecular pathways to oxygen deprivation can be very different from the relationship between oxygen concentration and radiosensitivity. For example, activation of some molecular pathways reaches a maximum at much more moderate hypoxia (~1%–2% $O_2$). These biological responses may in turn affect many tumour

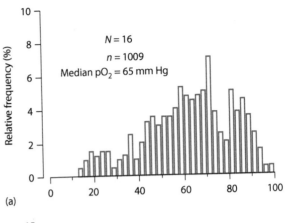

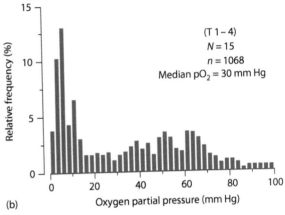

Figure 18.3 Frequency distributions of oxygen partial pressures for normal breast tissue (a) and breast cancers (b). Measurements were performed with a polarographic $O_2$-sensitive needle electrode with multiple recordings along three tracks for each patient. N: number of patients; n: number of measurements. (From (23), with permission.)

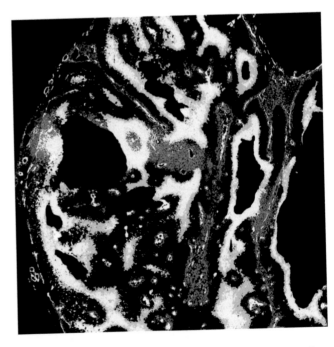

Figure 18.4 Composite binary image of a larger tumour area of the same tumour shown in Figure 18.2a.

properties that are important for treatment outcome, including the response to radiation. Therefore, the relevant fraction of hypoxic cells may be considerably different from the radiobiological hypoxic fraction (6).

Despite this confusion about the definition of hypoxia, it has become commonplace in clinical situations to try to define the level of tumour hypoxia by a single number, the 'hypoxic fraction'. In Chapter 17, we emphasized the importance of considering cell viability and we defined the radiobiological hypoxic fraction as the fraction of *viable/clonogenic* radiation-resistant hypoxic cells. For assessments made by oxygen electrodes, the hypoxic fraction is usually defined as the fraction of measurements below some arbitrary low value of oxygen partial pressure, often 5 or 10 mm Hg. For immunohistochemical detection with hypoxic markers (e.g. the nitroimidazoles), the hypoxic fraction is typically calculated as the fraction of cells that reach a certain threshold of staining intensity. In either case, the values arrived at are typically interpreted as a surrogate for the radiobiological hypoxic fraction. It is important to realize that because these thresholds are arbitrary and do not distinguish clonogenic from non-clonogenic cells, these two techniques will not necessarily give similar results and may not even correlate with each other. Furthermore, when used in this way, both of these methods ignore potentially important hypoxic cells that lie *above* the threshold and perhaps even more importantly, the variation in oxygen concentrations found within the tumour.

## Heterogeneity in space

Hypoxia arising from either diffusion or perfusion limitations also gives rise to substantial intra-tumour heterogeneity in space. This spatial heterogeneity exists at the cellular level and is beautifully illustrated in immunologically stained tumour sections that cover a large area of the tumour (see Figures 18.2, 18.4 and 18.10). This staining demonstrates the existence of steep oxygen gradients over distances of only a few cell diameters, contrasting with a common misconception that hypoxia is found mainly in the 'cores' of large tumours. In reality, hypoxia has the potential to exist around every blood vessel in the tumour and thus has no strong association with tumour size. The misconception of 'central tumour hypoxia' may stem from the common observation of central *necrotic* regions in human tumour xenografts grown in mice. However, in human tumours, hypoxia typically exists throughout the tumour volume, albeit at greater levels in certain regions.

The extent of spatial oxygen heterogeneity also has implications for the way in which tumour hypoxia is evaluated in the clinic. It is important to obtain a sufficient number of measurements in different parts of the tumour in order to get a picture of the overall level of hypoxia and its variation, a task that is difficult with immunohistochemical techniques that are often limited to small biopsies. In

this situation, one is forced to assume that the biopsy is representative of the overall tumour. This may often not be the case, as demonstrated by non-invasive imaging of positron emission tomography (PET) labelled hypoxia probes (e.g. misonidazole) that are able to assess the entire tumour volume. These PET images often show macroscopic 'hot spots' where hypoxia is more common.

Measurements in the clinic using oxygen probes are performed along more than one track in the tumour, with several samplings along each track. This gives rise to a frequency histogram that should reasonably reflect the overall distribution of oxygen values. However, a word of caution is appropriate here since not only does this technique lose all spatial information, but each measurement made by the oxygen electrode represents an average concentration over a volume that contains several hundred cells. It is likely that oxygen gradients exist even within these small volumes. Consequently, the actual cellular oxygen concentration will not be the same as that measured by the electrode. This 'averaging' problem is even greater with non-invasive techniques to image hypoxia. In this case, each imaging voxel can contain thousands or millions of cells. The limitations of all methods to reflect the true spatial heterogeneity (microscopic or macroscopic) need to be considered in the ongoing efforts to target radiotherapy specifically to hypoxic areas in tumours. Although areas with a larger proportion of hypoxic cells can receive higher doses, it will never be possible to specifically target *all* hypoxic tumour cells.

## Heterogeneity in time

The biological consequences of hypoxia are influenced not only by the severity of oxygen deprivation, but also by the length of time that cells are exposed to this stress. If we consider diffusion-limited hypoxia, the oxygen concentration is expected to decrease as a function of distance away from the blood vessel. Due to cellular proliferation in well-oxygenated areas close to the vessel, individual cells within a diffusion-limited gradient experience a slow decline in oxygen concentration over time as they are gradually pushed away from the vessel. The rate at which cells move through this gradient, and thus the length of exposure to various oxygen concentrations, is determined by the rate of cell proliferation. This can vary dramatically from one tumour to another, and even within different regions of the same tumour. Consequently, the lifetime of hypoxic tumour cells ranges from hours to days.

Much more rapid and dramatic oxygen fluctuations can occur as a result of limited perfusion as a vessel shuts down or reopens. Transient hypoxia has been convincingly demonstrated using several different methods in experimental tumours. For example, serial administration of two different hypoxia-specific markers analysed by immunohistochemistry identifies cells that stain for only one of the two markers (Figures 18.2 and 18.4). This indicates

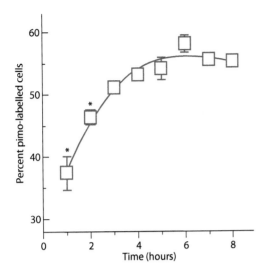

Figure 18.5 Percentage of SiHa tumour cells (human cervical squamous carcinoma) labelled with pimonidazole (pimo) as a function of labelling time. Tumours were grown subcutaneously in mice which were administered pimo by i.p. injection hourly before tumour excision. Tumours were processed to a single-cell suspension and the pimonidazole signal detected by flow cytometry. (From (1), with permission.)

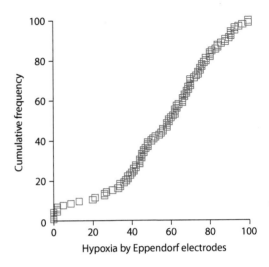

Figure 18.6 Cumulative frequency of tumour oxygenation in 105 patients with primary uterine cervix cancer. Measurements were performed with a polarographic $O_2$-sensitive needle electrode with multiple recordings along three tracks for each patient. The percentage of measurements $\leq 5$ mm Hg ($HP_5$) was used as a parameter for tumour oxygenation status. (From (14), with permission.)

that these cells were sufficiently hypoxic at one of the times to stain for hypoxia, but not at the other. Similarly, if a hypoxia marker is administered in a short pulse (1 hour), a much smaller number of cells are labelled, compared to when it is given for a longer period of time (Figure 18.5). This is due to the fact that many cells are only transiently hypoxic during this period. Continuous recordings from spatially fixed oxygen probes have also directly demonstrated temporal fluctuations in oxygenation (10). The results from these studies indicate that a substantial proportion of tumour cells can experience transient periods of hypoxia lasting less than 1 hour.

The potentially rapid changes in oxygenation associated with perfusion-limited hypoxia present an additional problem associated with attempts to measure oxygenation in tumours. Such measurements are typically made only once, and it is unclear how representative they are of the actual oxygenation *during* treatment.

### Heterogeneity among patients

Although there is large intra-tumour spatial and temporal heterogeneity, the variability in oxygenation between different tumours is even greater. Tumours with similar clinical characteristics can display very different patterns and overall levels of hypoxia at any given time. Figure 18.6 illustrates this fact using data obtained from a group of tumours whose oxygenation status was determined using an oxygen electrode (14). In these cases, the hypoxic fraction within a tumour was defined as the percentage of oxygen readings which were less than 5 mm Hg. Defined in this way,

the hypoxic fraction of individual tumours shows a dramatic level of variation and in this study ranged from 0% to 100% across 105 cervical cancers. About half of these tumours had hypoxic fractions above 50%.

The heterogeneity in oxygenation among different patients is one of the features of tumour hypoxia that makes it so interesting to study. Because oxygenation differs markedly among patients, it can be used as a factor to categorize otherwise similarly presenting patients into different prognostic subgroups that may receive different treatments (6). Indeed, a multi-centre meta-analysis identified the hypoxic fraction measured by oxygen electrodes as a significant negative prognostic factor in radiotherapy-treated head and neck cancer (Figure 18.7).

## 18.3 HYPOXIA AND ITS ASSOCIATION WITH THE MALIGNANT PHENOTYPE

The long-standing interest in tumour hypoxia within the radiation oncology community stems primarily from its association with radioresistance (see Chapter 17) and this aspect certainly remains an important contributor to patient response in the clinic (20). However, clinical studies also support a role for hypoxia that is unrelated to treatment sensitivity. For example, in a study of uterine cervix cancers treated with surgery alone, patients with more hypoxic tumours had poorer disease-free and overall survival and more frequent parametrial spread as well as lymph-vascular space involvement (Figure 18.8). This study, albeit small, indicated that hypoxic tumours are somehow biologically different from well-oxygenated tumours.

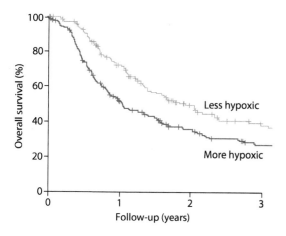

Figure 18.7 Overall survival rate for 397 patients with primary head and neck cancers. Measurements were performed with polarographic $O_2$-sensitive needle electrodes with multiple recordings along ±5 tracks for each patient. Thin and bold lines represent patients with less or more hypoxic tumours, respectively. More hypoxia was defined as a patient having more than 19% of measurements yielding less than 2.5 mm Hg $O_2$. (From (13), with permission.)

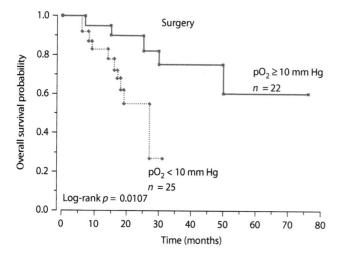

Figure 18.8 Overall survival probability for 47 patients with uterine cervix cancer treated with primary surgery. Measurements were performed with polarographic $O_2$-sensitive needle electrodes with multiple recordings along two tracks for each patient. Full or broken lines represent patients with median $pO_2$ higher or lower than 10 mm Hg, respectively. (From (7), with permission.)

Similarly, several clinical studies have demonstrated that hypoxia is a strong predictor for the presence of distant metastasis (e.g. [3]).

Although a correlation between hypoxia and tumour progression, infiltration and metastasis has been established, these correlative studies alone cannot address whether this is a cause-and-effect relationship. In other words, is the increased malignancy a result of tumour hypoxia or is tumour hypoxia a consequence of a more malignant tumour? These possibilities are not mutually exclusive, and

there is evidence supporting both. On one hand, hypoxia would be expected to be a reflection of aggressive growth because high proliferation rates will cause cells to become rapidly 'pushed away' from vessels, and angiogenesis would have a hard time keeping up. Furthermore, proliferation must also be supported by energy production which consumes oxygen and limits diffusion. On the other hand, data from the laboratory and experimental tumour models indicate that hypoxia functionally influences malignancy through the activation of physiological responses that facilitate adaptation to low oxygen.

## 18.4 HYPOXIA-DRIVEN BIOLOGICAL ADAPTATION

During evolution, organisms have developed a number of different pathways whose function is to allow adaptation to low oxygen availability (5). Adaptation occurs at the cellular, tissue and whole animal levels. For example, hypoxia associated with high altitude causes increased production of erythropoietin (EPO) which stimulates oxygen delivery by promoting the differentiation and proliferation of red blood cells and synthesis of the oxygen carrier haemoglobin. Similarly, during intense exercise, oxygen consumption may exceed supply in muscles and cause hypoxia. The muscle cells respond to hypoxia by increasing their capacity to carry out anaerobic metabolism in order to produce sufficient ATP. The by-product of anaerobic metabolism is lactate which causes pain in the athlete's muscles, a signal that exercise should be reduced. Hypoxia is also a powerful regulator of angiogenesis in both tumours and normal tissues. In fact, cellular responses to hypoxia play a fundamental role in controlling normal development of our vascular system.

Increased red blood cell and haemoglobin production, anaerobic metabolism and angiogenesis are adaptive processes that act to improve cellular oxygen supply and maintain energy homeostasis. Cancer cells utilize these same physiological response pathways to support the growth and spread of tumours. They switch to glycolysis for energy production and stimulate angiogenesis to improve oxygenation. In many cases, cancer cells have even undergone genetic alterations that allow them to hijack physiological responses to hypoxia, and they exhibit high rates of anaerobic metabolism and angiogenesis even during well-oxygenated conditions. This can occur through mutations in genes that regulate the hypoxic molecular response pathways to render them constitutively 'on' even during aerobic conditions. As noted above, however, tumour hypoxia persists in spite of high tumour vascularization, due to poor organization and functionality of these vessels.

Since hypoxia response pathways contribute both to hypoxia tolerance and overall malignancy, there is great interest in understanding these responses at the molecular level. Ultimately, this knowledge should lead to the development of hypoxia-specific biomarkers and new molecular targeting agents that can be tested in the clinic. Biological changes that occur during hypoxia result from the oxygen dependency of specific cellular enzymes that ultimately results in changes in protein abundance or activity. This concept is perfectly exemplified by the oxygen-dependent regulation of the hypoxia inducible factor (HIF) family of transcription factors.

## HIF – The master transcriptional regulator of hypoxic responses

Many of the known changes in biology that occur during hypoxia in humans and other organisms are controlled by the activation of HIF (18). This is summarized in Figure 18.9. The most widely expressed family member is HIF-1, although HIF-2 also functions in various cell types. HIF-1 and HIF-2 have similar functions and they regulate the transcriptional induction of more than 100 different known genes during hypoxia. These HIF targets regulate several important processes including erythropoiesis, metabolism, angiogenesis, invasion, proliferation and cell survival.

The HIF transcription factors consist of a constitutively expressed HIF-1β subunit, and an oxygen-sensitive HIF-1α or HIF-2α subunit. When oxygen is present, HIF-1α and HIF-2α are synthesized normally, but are unstable and degraded with a half-life of only about 5 minutes. Their degradation occurs because during aerobic conditions two proline amino acids are hydroxylated by enzymes known as the HIF PHDs (prolyl hydroxylases) that use molecular oxygen as a co-factor. When they are hydroxylated, HIF-1α

and HIF-2α are recognized by the von Hippel-Lindau (VHL) protein and targeted for ubiquitination and degradation. Under hypoxic conditions, HIF-1α and HIF-2α cannot be hydroxylated and thus are not recognized by VHL. This leads to their stabilization, allowing them to bind the HIF-1β subunit and activate gene transcription. The direct oxygen dependence of the PHD enzymes hence result in increased abundance of numerous proteins that are transcriptional targets of HIF, and that profoundly influence cell phenotype.

## HIF activity as a hypoxia biomarker and therapeutic target

The reduction in oxygen concentration required to stabilize and activate HIF is much less than that necessary to induce radioresistance. The dependency of HIF on oxygen concentration is determined by the enzymes that hydroxylate HIF-1α and HIF-2α. The HIF PHDs have a comparatively high Km for oxygen. Thus, HIF becomes active when oxygen concentrations drop to only 1% or 2% oxygen, a level that would cause virtually no increase in radioresistance. Consequently, the fraction of cells expressing HIF or HIF-dependent genes in a tumour can be significantly greater than the fraction of radiation-resistant cells. This is an important consideration in clinical studies that have investigated 'endogenous' hypoxia markers. Several HIF target genes, including carbonic anhydrase 9 (CA9), glucose transporter 1 or 3 (GLUT-1, GLUT-3) and vascular endothelial growth factor (VEGF) have been used in studies to assess hypoxia. These markers are

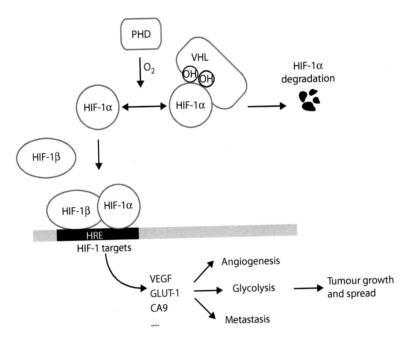

Figure 18.9 Cartoon illustrating the regulation of hypoxia-inducible factor-1 (HIF-1). During normoxia, HIF-1α is hydroxylated by the PHD enzymes. This makes it a substrate for VHL-mediated proteasomal degradation. In the absence of oxygen, HIF-1α is stabilized and can dimerize with its partner HIF-1β to form the transcription factor HIF-1. HIF-1 binds hypoxia responsive elements (HRE) in the promoter of its target genes, resulting in increased transcription. These target genes regulate angiogenesis, metabolism and metastasis.

assessing HIF activity and thus reflect the type of hypoxia necessary to activate it. One should not expect that this will necessarily also reflect the radiobiological hypoxic fraction or the hypoxic fraction measured through other methods (Figure 18.10).

Although HIF is controlled primarily through oxygen, several common genetic alterations in cancer result in hypoxia-independent regulation of HIF-1α. VHL is a classic tumour suppressor gene, and its loss prevents degradation of HIF-1α and HIF-2α. Consequently, VHL-deficient tumours show constitutive HIF activity, and greatly enhanced angiogenesis. Oncogenic activation of the PI3-kinase and Ras pathways has also been reported to influence HIF-1α protein levels. This regulation also needs to be taken into account when using HIF targets as biomarkers of hypoxia. In some cases, HIF activation may occur in ways that are largely independent of hypoxia.

The activation of HIF and its target genes may be highly clinically relevant in spite of not always reflecting tumour hypoxia. The malignant cancer phenotype is highly linked

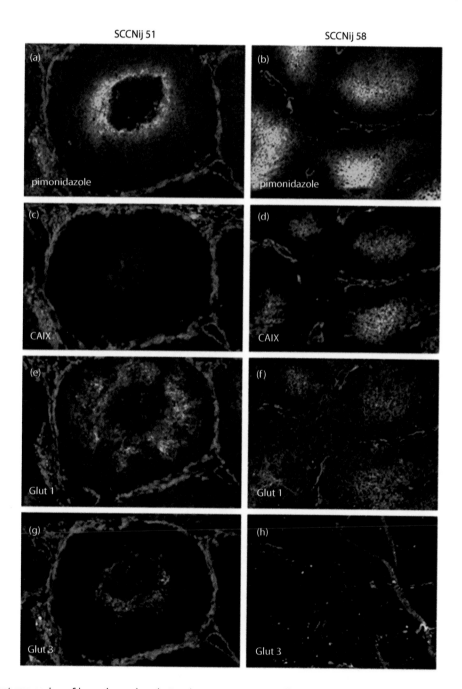

**Figure 18.10** Different expression of hypoxia markers in two human squamous-cell carcinoma xenograft models (SCCNij51 and SCCNij58). The images show the differences in localisation of the exogenous marker pimonidazole (a and b) compared to three endogenous hypoxic markers: CAIX (c and d), GLUT-1 (e and f) and GLUT-3 (g and h) (all in green), relative to the vasculature (in red). (From (15), with permission from Elsevier.)

to processes like angiogenesis, metastasis and glycolysis which can all be stimulated by activation of HIF (16,24). Genetic alterations that cause constitutive activation of the HIF pathway can therefore be envisaged to both promote and reflect malignancy. On the basis of this, there is great interest in evaluating HIF and its transcriptional targets as prognostic factors, even in the absence of a direct correlation with hypoxia (17). Furthermore, the central role that HIF plays in regulating gene expression has caused widespread interest in its potential as a molecular target in cancer therapy. HIF-mediated gene expression presumably helps cells to survive better during low oxygen availability, so disrupting this signalling in tumours is expected to promote hypoxia-induced death. In this way, targeting HIF in cancer therapy can be seen as an attractive approach to complement radiotherapy which kills well-oxygenated cells. The current efforts to target HIF have been spurred on by a detailed understanding of how HIF is regulated at the molecular level. This knowledge provides a basis for the targeting approach and makes the rational design of specific small-molecule inhibitors feasible. Experiments *in vitro* and *in vivo* have also provided some proof-of-principle supporting this approach. These studies have shown that cells which have been genetically engineered to lack functional HIF-1 die more rapidly from hypoxic stress and form fewer and slower growing tumours in animal models. A somewhat improved response to radiation has also been achieved experimentally when HIF has been targeted in established tumours using genetic approaches. It remains to be seen whether these encouraging results can be repeated and further improved with drugs that can be administered in the clinic.

## HIF-independent biological adaptation to hypoxia

There are numerous other cellular enzymes that, like the PHDs, require oxygen for their function and hence cause altered phenotypes in hypoxia. Oxygen availability can thereby affect regulation of protein abundance and function on multiple levels, including chromatin organization, DNA transcription, mRNA stability, mRNA translation, protein folding, protein stability and activity. The oxygen-sensitive HIF PHD proteins are part of a large family of enzymes that include the Jumonji-family of histone demethylases that influence chromatin organization and hence gene-specific transcriptional activity. The most famous example of an oxygen-dependent enzyme is probably the mitochondrial cytochrome c oxidase that uses oxygen as a terminal electron acceptor in the final step of the electron transport chain. Oxygen is also used as an electron acceptor in other oxidative processes such as disulphide bond formation that determines three-dimensional conformation and activity of secreted proteins. It is the changes in these and many other cellular pathways that in concert determine biological response, adaptation and phenotype in hypoxia (9,12).

## Hypoxia and genetic instability

One specific result of signalling in hypoxia of particular relevance to both tumour development and treatment is the effect of hypoxia on DNA repair capacity and genomic instability. Hypoxia has been shown to influence multiple DNA repair pathways, and thus promote the acquisition of genetic changes and development of cancer (2). Reporter gene and genomic minisatellite assays have shown that cells have increased mutation frequency and genetic instability when grown in the microenvironment of tumours compared to growth *in vitro*. Hypoxia and reoxygenation also cause aberrant DNA synthesis, leading to over-replication and gene amplification which are other frequent alterations observed in cancer cells. Cycling oxygenation has particularly been linked to DNA damage through the production of reactive oxygen species (ROS) upon reoxygenation. This is accompanied by reduced expression of DNA repair genes under subsequent hypoxic conditions and functional decreases in the nucleotide excision repair (NER), mismatch repair (MMR) and homologous recombination (HR) pathways. Both increased damage and response to damage are ultimately a result of altered activity of oxygen-dependent enzymes. Decreased expression of DNA repair genes is a consequence of regulation of transcription and translation in hypoxia. However, it may also be possible to exploit hypoxia-induced loss of DNA repair capacity therapeutically in other ways, and this represents a current research focus.

## 18.5 GENETIC DETERMINANTS OF TUMOUR HYPOXIA

Increased understanding of biological responses and adaptation to hypoxia has provided insight into why the patterns and severity of hypoxia can be so different between patients. Ultimately, these differences must be a consequence of the biology of the cell of origin and the numerous genetic alterations that the cell has acquired during carcinogenesis. The variation in steady-state levels of hypoxia across patients are influenced by three major factors: variations in oxygen *supply*, oxygen *demand* and hypoxia tolerance.

Oxygen supply is a consequence of the distribution and functionality of blood vessels. This is determined by the abundance and balance of angiogenic factors, which are regulated by signalling pathways such as HIF as well as by other oncogenic pathways. Genetic alterations in these pathways can therefore influence vascular development, function and ultimately oxygen delivery to the tumour. Oxygen demand is determined by cell number and by oxygen consumption. If consumption rates are high, the gradients will be steep and hypoxia will arise closer to vessels than if consumption is low. Consumption is driven by overall metabolic activity as well as the cells' preference for aerobic versus anaerobic metabolism. Genetic alterations that stimulate rapid proliferation therefore produce cells

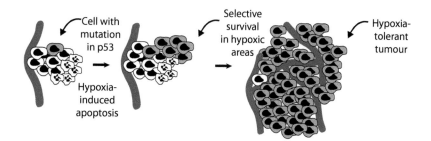

**Figure 18.11** Cartoon illustrating selection of apoptosis resistant cells in a hypoxic microenvironment. Early in tumour genesis, apoptosis susceptible cells die rapidly if they experience hypoxia. In the genetically unstable tumour, a clonal mutation in an apoptosis gene (e.g. p53) arises that makes a cell resistant to hypoxia-induced death. Due to its extended lifespan, this clone expands relative to the wild-type cells and eventually its progeny dominate the tumour mass.

with a higher oxygen demand to support their biosynthetic and energy needs, while mutations in metabolic enzymes can shunt nutrients and metabolites through alternative pathways that affect the demand. Finally, steady-state levels of tumour hypoxia are influenced by hypoxia tolerance mechanisms. This is because the longer a cell can survive in a hypoxic micro-milieu, the longer it can contribute to the (viable) hypoxic fraction. In spite of adaptive mechanisms, oxygen deficiency ultimately becomes toxic and results in cell death if it is severe and long lasting. Cancer cells are in general more tolerant to hypoxia than normal cells, but there is a large range which is a function of the cell's ability to launch biological adaptation programs, such as those governed by HIF, and its propensity to die which can be influenced by mutations in tumour suppressors or oncogenes (see the next section). Given that angiogenesis and deregulated proliferation, metabolism and cell death all are processes known to represent 'Hallmarks of Cancer' which are arrived upon by the unique genetic alterations in individual tumours, it is not surprising that these present with highly heterogeneous patterns and levels of hypoxia.

## 18.6 HYPOXIA-DRIVEN SELECTION OF MALIGNANT CELLS

The fact that hypoxia can cause cell death in a manner influenced by mutational patterns suggests that the hypoxic environment may also create a selection pressure for the outgrowth of cells that have increased tolerance to hypoxia. Furthermore, the 'selection' of such hypoxia-tolerant cells may also contribute to the known association of hypoxia with more aggressive disease. This principle of hypoxia-mediated selection has been elegantly illustrated in an experiment where rare cells that lack the tumour suppressor gene p53 (p53 knockout cells) are mixed with identical cells where p53 is functional and then exposed to periods of hypoxia (4). The p53 is required for the induction of apoptosis in response to many stimuli, including hypoxia, and the knockout cells are therefore resistant to apoptosis. In the mixing experiment, the cells with functional p53 die during hypoxia, while the p53 knockout cells survive. The p53 knockout cells thus

rapidly outgrow their counterparts and eventually dominate the cell population (Figure 18.11). One can easily envisage this selection process occurring in a genetically unstable tumour. Single cells with random mutations that cause tolerance to hypoxia will have a growth advantage and expand relative to the other cells. Thus, hypoxia can act as a strong selective force during tumour development.

The selection of cells with increased hypoxia tolerance can occur through a number of different ways affecting various molecular pathways. Importantly, the genetic alterations selected for by hypoxia may also render the cells resistant to other forms of stress. Consequently, a high level of tumour hypoxia may indicate not only that the tumour cells have a unique ability to survive against hypoxic exposure, but also an increased ability to survive during radiotherapy or other forms of cancer treatment. In other words, hypoxia can co-select highly resistant or highly malignant cells.

---

### Key points

1. Tumour oxygenation is heterogeneous with respect to severity, time and space.
2. Most tumours have some hypoxic cells.
3. High levels of hypoxia are associated with poor treatment outcome.
4. Hypoxia can select for outgrowth of cells with mutations.
5. Cellular responses to hypoxia influence malignancy.

---

### ■ BIBLIOGRAPHY

1. Bennewith KL, Durand RE. Quantifying transient hypoxia in human tumor xenografts by flow cytometry. *Cancer Res* 2004;64:6183–6189.
2. Bristow RG, Hill RP. Hypoxia and metabolism. Hypoxia, DNA repair and genetic instability. *Nat Rev Cancer* 2008;8:180–192.
3. Brizel DM, Scully SP, Harrelson JM et al. Tumor oxygenation predicts for the likelihood of distant metastases in human soft tissue sarcoma. *Cancer Res* 1996;56:941–943.

4. Graeber TG, Osmanian C, Jacks T et al. Hypoxia-mediated selection of cells with diminished apoptotic potential in solid tumours. *Nature* 1996;379:88–91.

5. Harris AL. Hypoxia – A key regulatory factor in tumour growth. *Nat Rev Cancer* 2002;2:38–47.

6. Hill RP, Bristow RG, Fyles A, Koritzinsky M, Milosevic M, Wouters BG. Hypoxia and predicting radiation response. *Semin Radiat Oncol* 2015;25:260–272.

7. Höckel M, Schlenger K, Aral B, Mitze M, Schaffer U, Vaupel P. Association between tumor hypoxia and malignant progression in advanced cancer of the uterine cervix. *Cancer Res* 1996;56:4509–4515.

8. Konerding MA, Malkusch W, Klapthor B et al. Evidence for characteristic vascular patterns in solid tumours: Quantitative studies using corrosion casts. *Br J Cancer* 1999;80:724–732.

9. Koritzinsky M, Wouters BG. The roles of reactive oxygen species and autophagy in mediating the tolerance of tumor cells to cycling hypoxia. *Semin Radiat Oncol* 2013;23:252–261.

10. Lanzen J, Braun RD, Klitzman B, Brizel D, Secomb TW, Dewhirst MW. Direct demonstration of instabilities in oxygen concentrations within the extravascular compartment of an experimental tumor. *Cancer Res* 2006;66:2219–2223.

11. Ljungkvist AS, Bussink J, Kaanders JH, van der Kogel AJ. Dynamics of tumor hypoxia measured with bioreductive hypoxic cell markers. *Radiat Res* 2007;167:127–145.

12. Nakazawa MS, Keith B, Simon MC. Oxygen availability and metabolic adaptations. *Nat Rev Cancer* 2016;16:663–673.

13. Nordsmark M, Bentzen SM, Rudat V et al. Prognostic value of tumor oxygenation in 397 head and neck tumors after primary radiation therapy. An international multi-center study. *Radiother Oncol* 2005;77:18–24.

14. Nordsmark M, Loncaster J, Aquino-Parsons C et al. The prognostic value of pimonidazole and tumour pO2 in human cervix carcinomas after radiation therapy: A prospective international multi-center study. *Radiother Oncol* 2006;80:123–131.

15. Rademakers SE, Span PN, Kaanders JH, Sweep FC, van der Kogel AJ, Bussink J. Molecular aspects of tumour hypoxia. *Mol Oncol* 2008;2:41–53.

16. Rankin EB, Nam JM, Giaccia AJ. Hypoxia: Signaling the metastatic cascade. *Trends Cancer* 2016;2:295–304.

17. Semenza GL. Evaluation of HIF-1 inhibitors as anticancer agents. *Drug Discov Today* 2007;12:853–859.

18. Semenza GL. Hypoxia-inducible factor 1 (HIF-1) pathway. *Sci STKE* 2007;2007:cm8.

19. Siemann DW, Horsman MR. Modulation of the tumor vasculature and oxygenation to improve therapy. *Pharmacol Ther* 2015;153:107–124.

20. Tatum JL, Kelloff GJ, Gillies RJa et al. Hypoxia: Importance in tumor biology, noninvasive measurement by imaging, and value of its measurement in the management of cancer therapy. *Int J Radiat Biol* 2006;82:699–757.

21. Thomlinson RH, Gray LH. The histological structure of some human lung cancers and the possible implications for radio-therapy. *Br J Cancer* 1955;9:539–549.

22. van Laarhoven HW, Bussink J, Lok J, Punt CJ, Heerschap A, van Der Kogel AJ. Effects of nicotinamide and carbogen in different murine colon carcinomas: Immunohistochemical analysis of vascular architecture and microenvironmental parameters. *Int J Radiat Oncol Biol Phys* 2004;60:310–321.

23. Vaupel P, Schlenger K, Knoop C, Höckel M. Oxygenation of human tumors: Evaluation of tissue oxygen distribution in breast cancers by computerized O2 tension measurements. *Cancer Res* 1991;51:3316–3322.

24. Xie H, Simon MC. Oxygen availability and metabolic reprogramming in cancer. *J Biol Chem* 2017;292:16825–16832.

## ■ FURTHER READING

25. Fang JS, Gillies RD, Gatenby RA. Adaptation to hypoxia and acidosis in carcinogenesis and tumor progression. *Semin Cancer Biol* 2008;18:330–337.

26. Koumenis C, Wouters BG. 'Translating' tumor hypoxia: Unfolded protein response (UPR)-dependent and UPR-independent pathways. *Mol Cancer Res* 2006;4:423–436.

27. Magagnin MG, Koritzinsky M, Wouters BG. Patterns of tumor oxygenation and their influence on the cellular hypoxic response and hypoxia-directed therapies. *Drug Resist Updat* 2006;9:185–197.

28. Vaupel P. Hypoxia and aggressive tumor phenotype: Implications for therapy and prognosis. *Oncologist* 2008;13(Suppl 3):21–26.

29. Wouters BG, van den Beucken T, Magagnin MG, Koritzinsky M, Fels D, Koumenis C. Control of the hypoxic response through regulation of mRNA translation. *Semin Cell Dev Biol* 2005;16:487–501.

# Combined radiotherapy and chemotherapy

## VINCENT GRÉGOIRE, JEAN-PASCAL MACHIELS AND MICHAEL BAUMANN

## 19.1 INTRODUCTION: CLINICAL OVERVIEW OF COMBINED RADIOTHERAPY AND CHEMOTHERAPY

In solid adult tumours, owing to its limited clinical efficacy, chemotherapy is very seldom used as a sole curative treatment modality. It is, however, more and more used in combination with curative treatments such as surgery and radiotherapy, at least for locally advanced diseases. Chemotherapy can be delivered before a local treatment in an induction or neo-adjuvant setting, it can be delivered during a local treatment (i.e. during the course of radiotherapy) in a concomitant setting, and it can be delivered after a local treatment in an adjuvant setting. The rationale for these various schedules of administration is discussed in Section 19.3. Table 19.1 summarizes the evidence-based data supporting the combined use of chemotherapy and radiotherapy in the most common adult tumours.

In brain high-grade glioblastoma, *Cochrane Reviews* recently published a report on all the randomised controlled trials performed on the use of temozolomide and radiotherapy (26). In summary, in primary glioblastoma, temozolomide significantly increased overall survival (OS) (hazard ratio 0.60, *p*-value 0.0003) and progression-free survival (hazard ratio 0.63, *p*-value 0.02) without modification of the quality of life; the benefit was mainly observed when temozolomide was given both concomitantly and in an adjuvant setting. The risks of haematological complications, fatigue and infections were increased with temozolomide. The benefit of temozolomide was particularly striking in patients expressing silencing of the MGMT (O6-methyl-guanine-DNA methyltransferase) DNA repair gene by promoter methylation (27). In recurrent glioblastoma, the use of concomitant temozolomide and radiotherapy also significantly increased the progression-free survival in a subgroup of patients with grade IV glioblastoma (*p*-value 0.008) without increase in toxicity.

In head and neck squamous cell carcinoma (SCC), meta-analyses have been conducted to ascertain the benefit and optimal scheduling of chemotherapy administration in relation to primary radiotherapy (8,45,46). A significant benefit in survival was observed only when chemotherapy was associated *concomitantly* with radiotherapy. The benefit was higher in patients receiving platinum-based chemotherapy and was observed in all tumour locations (7). In patients with laryngeal or hypopharyngeal SCC, the use of induction chemotherapy with platinum and 5FU is an alternative to total laryngectomy followed by post-operative radiotherapy (14,35). But platinum-5FU induction chemotherapy followed by radiotherapy translated into significantly worse loco-regional control when compared to concomitant platinum radiotherapy; this advantage, however, did not translate into an improvement in OS, likely due to increased late morbidity of concomitant chemo-radiotherapy (16,17). Also, induction chemotherapy has not been shown to add any significant advantage over concomitant chemo-radiotherapy (25,28). In patients with a high risk of loco-regional recurrence after primary surgery (R1 or R2 resection, extra-capsular tumour extension), post-operative concomitant chemo-radiotherapy with 3-weekly cisplatin (100 mg m$^{-2}$) was also associated with a significant benefit in survival (6,10,11). In all of the above-mentioned studies, an increased risk of acute and late toxicity was however seen with the use of concomitant chemo-radiotherapy (36). In nasopharyngeal carcinoma, the superiority of concomitant chemo-radiotherapy over radiotherapy alone has also been demonstrated, whereas the use of induction or adjuvant chemotherapy is still debated (4).

Meta-analyses based on individual patient data have been conducted to determine the effectiveness and toxicity of concomitant chemo-radiotherapy regimens compared to radiotherapy alone or sequential chemo-radiotherapy for non-small cell lung carcinoma. Based on nine trials including a total of 1764 patients and a median follow-up of 7.2 years, it was shown that the use of chemotherapy (cisplatin or carboplatin based) translated into an absolute benefit in OS of 4% at 2 years (1). This meta-analysis could not define the optimal schedule of chemotherapy administration in relation to radiotherapy. In a subsequent meta-analysis comparing concomitant and sequential chemo-radiotherapy, the same group demonstrated that with a median follow-up of 6 years, concomitant chemo-radiotherapy improved OS over sequential treatment with an absolute benefit of 5.7% and 4.5% at 3 and 5 years, respectively (hazard ratio 0.84, *p*-value 0.004) (2). Concomitant radiochemotherapy increased acute oesophageal toxicity (grade 3–4) from 4% to 18% with a relative risk of 4.9. There was no significant difference regarding acute pulmonary toxicity.

In limited stage small-cell lung cancer, a meta-analysis has also demonstrated the benefit of combining chemotherapy with thoracic radiotherapy, indicating

Table 19.1 Evidence-based data supporting combined chemotherapy and radiotherapy

| Disease site | Induction CH | Concomitant CH | Adjuvant CH | References |
|---|---|---|---|---|
| Brain glioblastoma | n.a. | + (level 1) | + (level 1) | 26 |
| Head and neck squamous cell carcinoma | ± (level 1) | +++ (level 1) | − (level 2) | 6,8,10,11,16,17,25,28,45,46 |
| Non-small cell lung cancer | − (level 1) | +++ (level 1) | n.a. | 1,2 |
| Small-cell lung cancer | +++ (level 1) | +++ (level 1) | +++ (level 1) | 44,47 |
| Cancer of uterine cervix | ± (level 1) | +++ (level 1) | n.a. | 9,19,42 |
| Oesophageal carcinoma | n.a. | +++ (level 1) | n.a. | 50 |
| Rectal carcinoma | n.a. | +++ (level 1) | n.a. | 13,49 |
| Anal carcinoma | − (level 2) | +++ (level 1) | − (level 2) | 3,24,31,43 |

*Note:* 'n.a.': no information; '+++' many data in favour of; '−' data not in favour of; '±' conflicting data not allowing a definite conclusion.

*Level of evidence:* level 1: multiple randomised studies/meta-analysis; level 2: one or two randomised studies, requiring further confirmation.

an improved absolute overall survival of $5.4 \pm 1.4\%$ at 3 years (44). For platinum-based concomitant chemotherapy, it was also shown that the benefit was higher when early chest radiotherapy was used (47).

In cancer of the uterine cervix, several meta-analyses have been performed to evaluate the benefit of combining radiotherapy with chemotherapy. A review including 24 trials totalling 4921 patients (from which data were available for 61% to 75% of patients) has shown that concomitant chemo-radiotherapy improved absolute survival by 10% (95% confidence interval: 8%–16%) over radiotherapy alone (19). Cisplatin was the most commonly used chemotherapy. The benefit was observed for both loco-regional control (odds ratio of 0.61, $p < 0.0001$) and distant recurrence (odds ratio 0.57, $p$-value $< 0.0001$) (20). However, this improvement was associated with an increased risk of haematological and gastrointestinal early toxicities. A similar analysis was performed to evaluate the benefit of induction chemotherapy (42). The results are much more heterogeneous and no definite conclusion can be drawn. There was a trend towards improved survival for regimens with cisplatin dose intensities greater than 25 mg m$^{-2}$ per week or cycle lengths shorter than 14 days. Conversely, in all other settings, a detrimental effect of induction chemotherapy on survival was found. In a more recent meta-analysis on individual patient data, the Chemotherapy for Cervical Cancer Meta-Analysis Collaboration (CCCMAC) group confirmed previously published data on the benefit of concomitant chemo-radiotherapy on both the loco-regional control and the distant metastasis rates, with a 5-year OS benefit of 6% (hazard ratio 0.81, $p$-value $< 0.001$) (9). This benefit was observed at the price of a higher rate of haematological and gastro-intestinal toxicity. The advantage of adjuvant chemotherapy requires further testing.

In localized oesophageal carcinoma, a meta-analysis of 19 randomised trials comparing radiotherapy and concomitant chemotherapy to radiotherapy alone has shown an absolute survival benefit of 9% (95% confidence interval: 5%–12%) and 4% (95% confidence interval: 3%–6%) at 1 and 2 years, respectively (50). However, this benefit was associated with a significant increase in severe and life-threatening toxicities.

The results from sequential radiotherapy-chemotherapy (RT-CT) studies showed no significant benefit in survival or local control but significant toxicities.

For patients with Dukes' B and C carcinoma of the rectum, a randomised study conducted by the National Surgical Adjuvant Breast and Bowel Project (NSABP) demonstrated that post-operative concomitant chemo-radiotherapy reduced the incidence of locoregional relapse compared to post-operative chemotherapy alone (13% versus 8% at 5 years, $p = 0.02$) (49). However, post-operative chemo-radiotherapy did not have any influence on disease-free survival or overall survival. In patients with resectable stage II and III carcinoma of the rectum, a meta-analysis of five randomised studies has showed that pre-operative 5FU-based chemo-radiotherapy significantly increased the rate of pathological complete response ($p < 0.00001$) and decreased the rate of 5-year local recurrence ($p < 0.001$) compared to radiotherapy alone (13). No difference was observed between pre-operative radiotherapy or concomitant chemo-radiotherapy regarding disease free survival (DFS) or overall survival (OS) at 5 years. The rate of grade III and IV acute toxicity was significantly increased ($p < 0.002$) as was the rate of post-operative overall morbidity ($p < 0.05$) in the group of patients treated with concomitant chemo-radiotherapy, but no difference in post-operative mortality or anastomotic leak rate was observed.

In patients with locally advanced squamous cell carcinoma of the anal canal, concomitant 5-fluorouracil, mitomycin and radiotherapy (45 Gy plus a boost of 15–20 Gy) resulted in an 18% increase in 5-year loco-regional control and a 32% increase in colostomy-free survival in comparison with radiotherapy alone (3). No significant difference in early and late side effects was observed between the two arms. More recent trials have failed to show a benefit of induction or adjuvant chemotherapy in addition to concomitant chemo-radiotherapy (24,31,43).

In summary, the combined use of chemotherapy with radiotherapy has typically translated into a significant benefit in loco-regional control probability and in overall survival in sites where radiotherapy plays a definitive role. With the exception of cervix carcinoma where concomitant chemo-radiotherapy also decreased the risk of distant metastasis, this benefit is mainly a consequence of an improvement in loco-regional control. In all the reported studies, the therapeutic ratio (defined as the advantage in efficacy over the disadvantage in toxicity) was, however, less clearly assessed and/or reported. In general, an increase in early toxicity was observed in all the trials. For late toxicity, systematic reporting of data is lacking, but the few available reports also indicate an increase in late radiation effects. Even if the benefits of combined modality chemoradiotherapy appear irrefutable, the reported clinical trials generally do not allow any information to be derived on the actual underlying mechanisms of interaction between chemotherapeutic drugs and ionizing radiation. Have the benefits and side effects resulted from a simple additivity of two effective therapeutic interventions, or from a more complex molecular interplay between the two modalities? If the latter is the case, was the combination of treatments appropriately designed based on the known mechanisms of interaction and the biodistribution and pharmacokinetics of the drugs? These issues remain largely unaddressed.

## 19.2 CLASSES OF CHEMOTHERAPEUTIC AGENTS AND THEIR MECHANISMS OF ACTION

Classically, cytotoxic anti-neoplastic drugs are divided into different classes based on their mechanisms of action, i.e. anti-metabolites, alkylating agents, topoisomerase inhibitors, anti-microtubule agents and antibiotics. Compared to radiotherapy or surgery, chemotherapy is a systemic treatment administered mainly intravenously or orally. Chemotherapy agents are used alone (monochemotherapy) or in combination (polychemotherapy). Typically, chemotherapeutic agents are biologically active by killing dividing cells, thus exerting both their efficacy and their toxicity (Table 19.2). The main side effects typically observed with chemotherapy, but with important variations in intensity from one drug to another, include nausea, vomiting, alopecia, mucositis, fatigue, anaemia, thrombopenia and neutropenia. In addition, some specific toxicities can be observed with specific agents (e.g. cardiac dysfunction with anthracyclines, bladder toxicity with ifosfamide). Table 19.2 describes the main cytotoxic agents with their biological activity and specific toxicities.

### Anti-metabolites

Anti-metabolites interfere with DNA and/or RNA synthesis (15). The majority have a chemical structure similar to the nucleotides with modifications in one or several chemical groups. They can block enzymes required for DNA synthesis with interference with DNA duplication and/or can be misincorporated into DNA and RNA with consequent induction of apoptosis. Anti-metabolites are cell-cycle dependent drugs, acting mainly in S-phase. The main different subgroups are the anti-folates (e.g. methotrexate

and pemetrexed), the fluoropyrimidines (e.g. 5-fluorouracil and capecitabine), the deoxynucleoside analogues (e.g. gemcitabine, cytarabine and fludarabine) and the thiopurines (e.g. ioguanine and mercaptopurine).

### Alkylating agents

Alkylating agents bind covalently to DNA and RNA through their alkyl groups, thus causing DNA intra- and/or inter-strand cross-linking, and more generally interfere with replication and transcription processes (48). Alkylating agents include the platinum compounds (e.g. cisplatin, carboplatin and oxaliplatin), the nitrogen mustards (e.g. cyclophosphamide, ifosfamide, melphalan and busulfan), the nitrosoureas (e.g. carmustine, lomustine and fotemustine), the tetrazines (e.g. temozolomide and dacarbazine), the aziridines (e.g. mitomycin and thiotepa) and procarbazine.

### Topoisomerase inhibitors

Topoisomerase inhibitors are agents that inhibit the topoisomerase I or II enzymes which allow DNA unwinding during replication and transcription (32). The camptothecins inhibit topoisomerase 1 and include irinotecan and topotecan. Doxorubicin, mitoxantrone, etoposide and teniposide are topoisomerase II inhibitors. Doxorubicin acts as an intercalating drug leading to topoisomerase II inhibition, as do all the anthracyclines. Mitoxantrone is an anthracenedione that blocks topoisomerase II. Etoposide forms a ternary complex with DNA and the topoisomerase II enzyme.

### Anti-microtubule agents

Anti-microtubule agents were derived originally from plants and interfere with microtubule function, thus blocking cell division. The two main groups are the vinca alkaloids and the taxanes. The vinca alkaloids interfere with the microtubule formation and the taxanes block microtubule disassembly. Mitosis is therefore impossible leading to cell-cycle arrest and subsequent cell death. The vinca alkaloids include vincristine, vinblastine, Navelbine and vinflunine and the taxanes include docetaxel, paclitaxel and cabazitaxel. These compounds are cell-cycle dependent.

### Antibiotics

This group includes a variety of drugs with different mechanisms of action. We have already discussed the anthracyclines, mitoxantrone and mitomycin. In addition, bleomycin can also act as an intercalating agent but causes also DNA strand breaks. Actinomycin can block transcription by complexing with DNA.

Table 19.2 Main classes of cytotoxic agents with their biological activity and specific toxicities[a]

| | Main mechanism of action | Specific toxicities if relevant |
|---|---|---|
| **Anti-metabolites** | | |
| Methotrexate | Inhibition of dihydrofolate reductase | Kidney dysfunction |
| Pemetrexed | Inhibition of thymidylate synthase | |
| 5-Fluorouracil | Nucleotide analogue and inhibition of thymidylate synthase | |
| Capecitabine | 5-Fluorouracil pro-drug | Hand-foot syndrome |
| Gemcitabine | Nucleotide analogue | |
| Fludarabine | Nucleotide analogue | |
| **Alkylating agents** | | |
| Cyclophosphamide | Binds to guanine | Haemorrhagic cystitis |
| Ifosfamide | Binds to guanine | Haemorrhagic cystitis |
| Cisplatin | Binds to bases | Kidney dysfunction |
| Carboplatin | Binds to bases | Myelosuppression |
| Oxaliplatin | Binds to bases | Polyneuritis |
| Carmustine | Binds to bases | |
| Lomustine | Binds to bases | |
| Fotemustine | Binds to bases | |
| Temozolomide | Binds to bases | |
| Dacarbazine | Binds to bases | |
| Mitomycin | Binds to bases | |
| Procarbazine | Not fully understood | |
| **Topoisomerase inhibitors** | | |
| Doxorubicin | Intercalant, topoisomerase II inhibitor | Cardiac dysfunction |
| Liposomal doxorubicin | Intercalant, topoisomerase II inhibitor | Hand-foot syndrome |
| Mitoxantrone | Topoisomerase II inhibitor | Cardiac dysfunction |
| Etoposide | Topoisomerase II inhibitor | |
| Irinotecan | Topoisomerase I inhibitor | Diarrhoea |
| Topotecan | Topoisomerase I inhibitor | |
| **Anti-microtubule agents** | | |
| Vinblastine | Inhibition of microtubule assembly | Polyneuritis |
| Vincristine | Inhibition of microtubule assembly | Polyneuritis |
| Navelbine | Inhibition of microtubule assembly | Polyneuritis |
| Docetaxel | Inhibition of microtubule disassembly | Polyneuritis, capillary leak syndrome |
| Paclitaxel | Inhibition of microtubule disassembly | Polyneuritis, capillary leak syndrome |
| Cabazitaxel | Inhibition of microtubule disassembly | |
| **Antibiotics** | | |
| Actinomycin | Blocks transcription | |
| Bleomycin | Causes DNA strand breaks | Interstitial lung disease |
| Trabectedin | Targets transcription-coupled nucleotide excision repair system to induce lethal DNA strand breaks | |

[a] Besides alopecia, gastrointestinal disorders, mucositis, fatigue, neutropenia and thrombocytopenia.

## 19.3 INTERACTION BETWEEN CHEMOTHERAPY AND RADIOTHERAPY

### Spatial cooperation

Spatial cooperation is the term used to describe the use of radiotherapy and chemotherapy to target disease in different anatomical sites. The most common situation is where radiation is used to treat the primary tumour and chemotherapy is added to deal with systemic spread. There is an analogous situation in small cell lung cancer where chemotherapy is the main systemic treatment and radiotherapy is used to deal with disease in a 'seclusion site' such as the brain. Another example is the treatment of breast cancer where surgery and post-operative radiotherapy deal with the loco-regional disease and adjuvant chemotherapy deals with the micro-metastatic disease.

If spatial co-operation is effective, this should result in a reduction of distant failures after the combined therapy. The successful exploitation of spatial co-operation depends critically on the effectiveness of the chemotherapy used. In the common solid tumours, chemotherapy alone seldom achieves a surviving fraction lower than $10^{-6}$. Even small metastatic deposits of $< 0.1$ g may contain $10^7$–$10^8$ tumour cells and, if the majority of these are also clonogenic, standard chemotherapy may fail to control even a small amount of disseminated disease. For spatial co-operation to succeed more widely, we need more effective drugs or methods of specifically targeting existing drugs to the tumour cells, thus allowing dose escalation.

If the rationale underlying spatial co-operation between radiotherapy and chemotherapy is indeed to target different anatomical sites, the optimal way of combining these modalities is sequentially in order to avoid the likely increase in side effects if given concomitantly. The choice of the sequence between the two modalities may depend on the evaluation of the respective risk of relapse at the loco-regional and distant site. For example, in locally advanced breast carcinoma, chest wall radiotherapy may precede systemic treatment, while the reverse may be proposed for patients with higher risk of distant metastasis.

## Independent cell kill and 'shared' toxicity

This term describes the simple concept that if two effective therapeutic modalities can both be given at full dose then, even in the absence of interactive processes, the tumour response (total cell kill) should be greater than that achieved with either agent alone. To exploit this mechanism, the radiotherapy and chemotherapy should have non-overlapping toxicities and the chemotherapy should not enhance normal tissue damage within the radiation field. Such a situation may be obtained by temporal separation of the two modalities but, even if this can be achieved without a negative influence on tumour control, the patient will probably have to tolerate a wider range of toxic reactions.

This needs to be taken into account when assessing the overall benefit. If independent cell killing can be successfully exploited, it could potentially lead to both improved local control and reduced distant failure, without any interactions between the modalities.

The treatment of early stage Hodgkin disease is a good illustration of this concept. Both radiation (mantle field irradiation up to a total dose of 40 Gy) and chemotherapy (including alkylating agents) are highly effective in providing long-term cure for these patients (Table 19.3). However, the use of both these modalities alone is associated with a relatively high incidence of late complications, e.g. mainly induction of secondary solid tumours and cardiopathy for radiotherapy, and induction of lymphoma and leukaemia for chemotherapy. Hence, modern treatment of early stage Hodgkin disease combines different chemotherapy regimens (fewer courses and different drugs) with radiotherapy delivered on the involved fields only and to a lower dose (e.g. 30 Gy or lower) (34). Long-term efficacy is similar. Data are not yet mature enough to inform conclusively about any reduced incidence of late toxicity, but preliminary results have already shown both a significant reduction in cardiopathy and in radiation-induced second primary tumours.

When independent cell kill is the mechanism of interaction between radiotherapy and chemotherapy, obviously the optimal way of combining these modalities is sequentially to avoid the likely increase in side effects when given concomitantly.

## Cellular and molecular interaction

This term describes the situation in which radiation and chemotherapy interact with each other at the cellular or molecular level such that the net effect is greater than the simple addition of the individual effects of the two modalities. As illustrated in Figure 19.1, this interaction is likely to translate into a modification of the shape of the cell survival curves, i.e. a steeper slope of the tangent to the initial part of the curve (increase in the $\alpha$ parameter of the linear-quadratic model) for the combined treatment. A classical way

Table 19.3 Comparative efficacy and toxicity between several treatment options for early stage Hodgkin disease

|  | Radiotherapy (extended field, 40 Gy) | Chemotherapy (MOPP-ABVD) | Chemotherapy-radiotherapy (involved field, ≈30 Gy) |
|---|---|---|---|
| 10-year overall survival | 80%–90% | 80%–90% | ≈90% |
| **Complications (RR)** | | | |
| Leukaemia induction | 11.0 | 70.0 | Significantly reduced[a] |
| Lymphoma induction | 21.0 | 22.0 | Significantly reduced[a] |
| Solid tumour induction | 2.8 | 1.1 | Significantly reduced[a] |
| Cardiopathy | 2.2–3.1 | ≈1.0 | Significantly reduced[a] |

*Abbreviation:* RR: relative risk.

[a] Awaiting longer follow-up analysis.

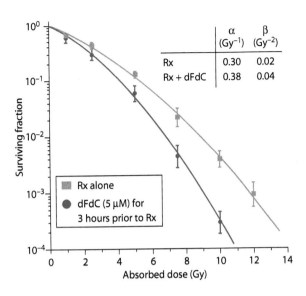

| | α (Gy⁻¹) | β (Gy⁻²) |
|---|---|---|
| Rx | 0.30 | 0.02 |
| Rx + dFdC | 0.38 | 0.04 |

Rx alone

dFdC (5 µM) for 3 hours prior to Rx

Figure 19.1 Head and neck SQD-9 cell survival curves with or without pre-incubation with gemcitabine (dFdC) at a dose of 5 µM for 3 hours. In the presence of the drug, the initial slope of the cell survival curve became steeper reflecting an interaction with ionizing radiation.

of expressing the benefit of a combined treatment is through the use of a dose modifying factor (DMF), which is defined as the ratio of isoeffective radiation doses in the absence and presence of the radiosensitizer. The concept of DMF can be used in describing tumour effect or normal tissue toxicity.

A good clinical illustration of this type of interaction between chemotherapy and radiotherapy is in the treatment of locally advanced head and neck squamous cell carcinoma, in the meta-analysis of over 17,000 individual patients (46). Patients were categorized according to whether chemotherapy had been given before (induction chemotherapy), during (concomitant chemotherapy) or after radiotherapy (adjuvant chemotherapy). A significant absolute 5-year benefit of 6.5 ± 1% was found only when *concomitant* chemotherapy was given. For induction or adjuvant chemotherapy, the 5-year survival was only improved by 2.4 ± 1.4% and by −1 ± 2.2%, respectively. This example illustrates that the two modalities needed to be given within a narrow window of temporal proximity to translate into a clinical benefit. This mechanism of interaction is likely to play a substantial role in achieving a benefit of combined chemo-radiotherapy in the majority of solid tumours in adults.

## 19.4 MOLECULAR MECHANISMS OF INTERACTION BETWEEN CHEMOTHERAPY AND RADIOTHERAPY

### Enhanced DNA/chromosome damage and repair

Little is known about the capacity of chemotherapeutic agents to increase the efficiency with which ionizing radiation induces DNA damage. Compounds such as iododeoxyuridine (IdUrd) and bromodeoxyuridine (BrdUrd) when incorporated into DNA have been shown to enhance radiation-induced DNA damage, likely through the production of reactive uracilyl radicals and halide ions, which in turn induce DNA single-strand breaks (SSBs) in the neighbouring DNA (29). Several commonly used chemotherapy agents have been shown to inhibit the repair of radiation damage, i.e. DNA and/or chromosome damage. Examples are nucleoside analogues, cisplatin, bleomycin, Adriamycin and hydroxyurea. Some of these drugs inhibit repair processes by interfering with the enzymatic machinery involved in the restoration of the DNA/chromosome integrity. Fludarabine, for example, is a nucleoside analogue, which is incorporated into DNA and blocks DNA primase, DNA polymerases δ and ε and DNA ligase I, and which has been shown to inhibit the repair of chromosome breaks (Figure 19.2) (22).

Some of these drugs, like radiation, can directly produce DNA damage such as DNA breaks, adducts and intercalation. Cisplatin for example, induces DNA adducts with guanine, thus leading to intra- or inter-stand cross links. These adducts are normally removed through base excision repair mechanisms followed by homologous recombination. When occurring in close proximity to radiation-induced SSBs, especially those located on the opposite stand, an easily repairable DNA adduct lesion is converted into a double-strand break (DSB) (5). Inhibition of repair, or the conversion of SSB to DSB, has the effect of increasing the slope of the radiation survival curve and leads to an enhanced radioresponse. Another example is the plant derivative etoposide, a topoisomerase-II inhibitor, which creates by itself DNA DSB. When in close vicinity to radiation-induced DNA damage, such lesions become

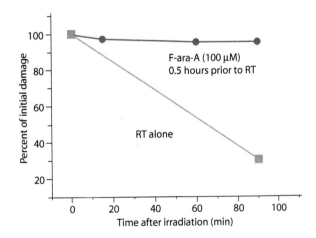

F-ara-A (100 µM) 0.5 hours prior to RT

RT alone

Figure 19.2 Repair inhibition of chromosome breaks by the nucleoside analogue F-ara-A. Human lymphocytes were irradiated with a single X-ray dose of 2 Gy and incubated at 37°C in presence or absence of F-ara-A. At 90 minutes post-irradiation 70% of the chromosome breaks have repaired in the control sample; in the sample incubated with F-ara-A, only 5% of breaks have repaired.

non-repairable leading to a supra-additive interaction with radiation (18).

Enhancement, which occurs as a result of DNA repair inhibition, will be more pronounced in fractionated radiation schedules than for single doses. A major problem with DNA repair inhibition as an exploitable mechanism for obtaining a therapeutic gain is the lack of evidence for a selective antitumour effect. For this strategy to be effective, some sort of tumour drug targeting may be required.

## Cell-cycle synchronization

The vast majority of chemotherapeutic agents are inhibitors of cell division and are thus mainly active on proliferating cells. Agents such as gemcitabine, fludarabine, methotrexate and 5-fluorouracil inhibit various enzymes involved in DNA synthesis and repair in S-phase cells; agents such as etoposide, Adriamycin, doxorubicin, alkylating agents and platinum compounds induce DNA strand breaks and DNA strand cross links in any phase of the cell cycle, but will only become potentially lethal in replicating cells; agents like Taxol, Taxotere and vinca-alkaloids inhibit mitotic spindle formation or disassembly and thus are mainly active during mitosis.

As a consequence of this cell-cycle phase selective cytotoxicity of chemotherapeutic agents, the remaining surviving cells could in principle be synchronized. If radiation could be delivered when these 'synchronized' cells have reached a more radiosensitive phase of the cell cycle (e.g. G2–mitosis), a tremendous potentiation of the radiation effect could be observed. Such a mechanism of interaction between drugs and ionizing radiation has often been reported in pre-clinical experimental models (e.g. [23]). However, in the clinic, due to much greater intra-tumour heterogeneity and also the difficulty in assessing the appropriate timing between drug administration and radiotherapy delivery, it is unlikely that cell synchronization can be successfully exploited. Furthermore, considering that radiotherapy is typically delivered on a fractionated basis, it is also likely that this effect would be lost after a few fractions.

## Enhanced apoptosis

Apoptosis (or interphase cell death) is a common mechanism of cell death induced by chemotherapeutic agents (33). These drugs can trigger one or more of the pathways leading to apoptosis. For the anti-metabolites, DNA incorporation is a necessary event to ensure a robust apoptotic response, hence the specific sensitivity of S-phase cells to these agents. Within this framework, it has been hypothesized that combining these drugs with ionizing radiation, which is very effective in inducing DNA SSBs or DSBs in every phase of the cell cycle, could facilitate their DNA incorporation and thus trigger an enhanced apoptotic reaction. This hypothesis was investigated in tumour models *in vivo*, using single doses of X-rays combined with gemcitabine (39). An increased apoptotic response was indeed observed when the two modalities were combined, but comprehensive analysis of the data did not demonstrate any synergistic enhancement, only an additive effect. Overall, it is fair to say that increased apoptosis as a general mechanism to account for enhanced response to combined drug and radiation treatment is not firmly established and requires further investigation.

## Reoxygenation and vascular disrupting agents

As discussed in Chapters 17 and 18, hypoxia, a common feature of the majority of human solid tumours, is associated with a poorer response to radiotherapy. One reason for this is that the functionally insufficient tumour vascular network does not permit an adequate diffusion of oxygen throughout the whole tumour mass. It has therefore been proposed that chemotherapy, by inducing some degree of tumour shrinkage, might facilitate a more even diffusion of oxygen and increase overall tumour oxygenation, which in turn would increase tumour radiosensitivity. In the murine mammary carcinoma MCA-4, it was indeed shown that intra-tumoural $pO_2$ increased progressively in the few hours following Taxol administration, from 6.2 mm Hg in untreated tumours to 10 mm Hg in treated tumours (40). This progressive tumour reoxygenation was associated with a significant parallel increase in the tumour radioresponse compared with control animals that did not get Taxol. Similar observations have been reported following gemcitabine treatment (37). This mechanism, which could likely play a role with any chemotherapeutic drug, has however never been tested with other agents.

As an opposite paradigm, angiogenesis being an essential component of tumour growth, the use of vascular disrupting agent, which would further enhance hypoxia leading to anoxia and cell death, has been widely tested with radiation. Combretastatin A4 phosphate (CA4P) is the lead compound of this class of agents and has been shown to increase tumour hypoxia and induce rapid necrosis in the centre of the tumour leaving a rim of viable cells at the periphery. When combined with radiation, providing an appropriate timing and schedule of administration was used, an enhanced effect could be observed after both single and fractionated doses of radiation (30).

## Inhibition of cell proliferation

Table 19.4 summarizes information from pre-clinical experiments on the mechanisms of interaction between chemotherapeutic agents and ionizing radiation. For the majority of these agents, the exact cellular and molecular mechanisms of interaction are not precisely known. Nevertheless, these agents are routinely used in the clinic and have been shown to be effective in combination with

Table 19.4 Summary of the pre-clinical data regarding the mechanisms of interaction between ionizing radiation and chemotherapeutic agents

| | DNA damage induction | repair | Chromosome aberrations | Cell cycle | Apoptosis | Reoxygenation |
|---|---|---|---|---|---|---|
| **Anti-metabolites** | | | | | | |
| 5-Fluorouracil | − | ± | − | + | ? | ? |
| Methotrexate | ? | ? | ? | ? | ? | ? |
| Hydroxyurea | ? | ± | + | + | ? | ? |
| Gemcitabine | − | − | + | + | − | + |
| Fludarabine | − | − | + | + | − | ? |
| **Alkylating agents** | | | | | | |
| Cisplatin | +? | + | ? | − | ? | ? |
| BCNU | ? | + | − | ? | ? | ? |
| Cyclophosphamide | ? | ? | − | ? | ? | ? |
| **Topoisomerase inhibitors** | | | | | | |
| Etoposide | ? | + | − | + | + | ? |
| Camptothecin | ? | ? | − | ± | ± | ± |
| Adriamycin | − | ± | ± | + | ? | ? |
| **Anti-microtubule agents** | | | | | | |
| Vinca-alkaloids | ? | − | ? | + | ? | ? |
| Taxanes | ? | − | + | + | + | + |
| **Antibiotics** | | | | | | |
| Mitomycin-C | ? | ? | − | ? | ? | ? |
| Bleomycin | ? | − | ± | + | ? | ? |
| Actinomycin-D | ? | +? | ? | ? | − | − |

*Note:* '−': not demonstrated; '+': demonstrated; '±': conflicting data; '?': unknown.

*Abbreviation:* BCNU: β-chloro-nitrosourea.

radiotherapy. Furthermore, even for those agents for which mechanisms of interaction with radiation have been elucidated in experimental models, it is unlikely that the clinical regimen has been designed to fully benefit from these interactions. Indeed, in the clinic, logistical considerations may come into play to explain ways in which drugs and radiotherapy are combined, and such considerations may not be entirely compatible with a full exploitation of the molecular and cellular interactions between drugs and ionizing radiation.

It is therefore reasonable to propose that a prominent mechanism of interaction between drugs and radiotherapy would be a simple inhibition of the cellular proliferation that takes place during the radiation inter-fraction interval. Such a mechanism is illustrated in Figure 19.3 (22). This interaction would be much less sensitive to the exact timing between drug and radiation dose delivery, so long as the drug is delivered at some point during the radiotherapy schedule. This being the case, it may be best to administer the drug towards the end of the radiation treatment course, when tumour cell repopulation had been triggered (see Chapter 11). This was the rationale of a phase II trial conducted on head and neck squamous cell carcinoma, where two courses of cisplatin/5FU were given over the last 2 weeks of radiotherapy as a 'chemoboost' (12). Results were encouraging but have not yet been tested in a randomised phase III trial.

## 19.5 TOXICITY RESULTING FROM CONCOMITANT USE OF CHEMOTHERAPY AND RADIOTHERAPY

### Early toxicity

As discussed in Chapter 14, early toxicity after radiotherapy (e.g. oral mucositis, skin reaction, oesophagitis, proctitis and bone marrow depletion) typically results from an imbalance between physiologic loss of mature cells and renewal from the stem cells or the precursor cells. As mentioned previously, all chemotherapeutic agents are active on proliferative cells, and thus on their own also produce an imbalance between precursors and mature cells. It is thus anticipated that concomitant association between drugs and radiation will

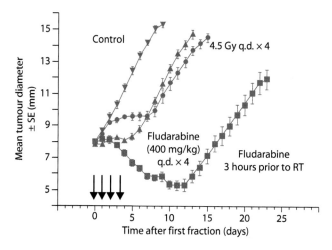

Figure 19.3 Regrowth delay experiment in a mouse sarcoma (SA-NH). Eight mm diameter tumours were treated with 4 daily i.p. injections of fludarabine (arrows), irradiated with 4 daily fractions of 4.5 Gy, or injected with 4 daily doses of fludarabine 3 hours prior to 4 daily fractions of 4.5 Gy. Control mice were injected with saline. Each data point represents the mean of 9–10 mice. When treated with radiation alone, tumours kept growing and only a 5.3 ± 0.5 (sem) day regrowth delay was observed compared to control animals. During fludarabine treatment alone, tumour proliferation was inhibited, but tumours started growing again as soon as the injection stopped; overall a regrowth delay of 5.5 ± 0.7 (sem) days was observed. When both modalities were combined, a decrease in tumour size was already observed during treatment and the regrowth delay of 14.3 ± 0.9 (sem) days was much larger than the additive effect of the two modalities alone.

Table 19.5 Summary of the pre-clinical data regarding the toxicity of concomitant chemo-radiation

| | Acute effects | Late effects |
|---|---|---|
| **Anti-metabolites** | | |
| 5-Fluorouracil | + (GI, skin) | ? |
| Methotrexate | + (GI) | ? |
| Hydroxyurea | + (GI) | ? |
| Gemcitabine | + (GI) | ± (lung) |
| Fludarabine | + (GI) | ± (CNS) |
| **Alkylating agents** | | |
| Cisplatin | + (GI) | + (kidney) |
| BCNU | + (GI) | + (lung) |
| Cyclophosphamide | + (GI, skin) | + (lung, bladder, CNS) |
| **Topoisomerase inhibitors** | | |
| Adriamycin | + (GI, skin) | + (heart, lung) |
| Etoposide | ? | ? |
| **Anti-microtubule agents** | | |
| Vinca-alkaloids | − (GI, BM) | ? |
| Taxanes | + (GI) | ? |
| **Antibiotics** | | |
| Mitomycin-C | + (GI, BM) | + (lung) |
| Bleomycin | + (GI, skin) | + (skin, lung) |
| Actinomycin-D | + (GI, BM, skin) | + (lung) |

*Note:* '−': not demonstrated; '+': demonstrated; '±': conflicting data; '?': unknown.

*Abbreviations:* GI: gastrointestinal; BM: bone marrow; CNS: central nervous system; BCNU: β-chloro-nitrosourea.

result in an increased early toxicity. Table 19.5 summarizes experimental data on early toxicity observed during concomitant association between drugs and radiation. It shows that for all classes of drugs, an increase in radiation-induced early toxicity has been reported. These findings are in agreement with the clinical trials that compared radiotherapy alone versus concomitant chemo-radiation, which systematically indicated a significant increase in early toxicity in the combined modality arm.

There is a considerable body of experimental data which demonstrates that normal tissue damage after combined modality treatment is strongly influenced by the sequence and timing of the modalities. Many commonly used drugs cause a substantial increase in normal tissue radiation injury when the modalities are given in close sequence but not when they are separated in time (Figure 19.4) (21). However, this finding conflicts with the requirement to use concomitant chemo-radiation (thus with a narrow window of association) for improving loco-regional tumour control. Thus, unless pharmacokinetic studies show different patterns of drug biodistribution between tumour cells and normal cells, it is likely that the optimal sequence of drug administration for tumour radiosensitization is unfortunately the one that will also produce the largest increase in early radiation toxicity.

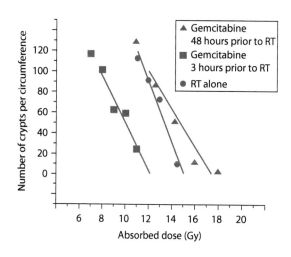

Figure 19.4 Radioenhancement of acute jejunal damage after single-dose irradiation in mice. Mice were total-body irradiated with single doses of 250 kV X-rays with or without prior injection (3 hours or 48 hours) of a single dose (150 mg kg$^{-1}$) of gemcitabine. The crypt cell regeneration assay was used. When injected 3 hours prior to irradiation, gemcitabine induced a marked radiosensitization (DMF of 1.3). When injected 24 hours prior to irradiation a small radioprotection was observed (DMF of 0.9).

## Late toxicity

In contrast with early radiation effects, which typically occur during treatment and in rapidly renewing tissues, late effects can affect all types of tissues after a latent period, which typically is expressed in months to years. Also late damage tends more to be irreversible and a radiation dose-dependency has been well documented in a large number of tissues. The pathophysiology of late radiation effects is discussed at length in Chapter 14. Although it may involve various cell types, any therapeutic intervention that may affect the repair of radiation (DNA) damage in the tumour is likely to also increase late normal tissue radiation damage (Table 19.5). Furthermore, the risk of late effects after combined chemo-radiotherapy can be further increased when the drugs have a specific toxicity for tissues within the irradiated volume, e.g. bleomycin for lung toxicity, Adriamycin for cardiac toxicity and cisplatin for renal toxicity. In the clinic, the design of protocols and the choice of the various drugs to combine with radiotherapy need to integrate this knowledge. For example, bleomycin should be avoided together with radiotherapy for tumours of the mediastinum. For post-operative irradiation of the left breast or chest wall in women receiving Adriamycin, adequate planning should be made to avoid irradiation of the myocardium.

## 19.6 THE THERAPEUTIC RATIO

The therapeutic ratio (TR), or therapeutic gain, is the relative expected benefit of a combined modality treatment, integrating both the tumour and the normal tissue effects. It is defined as the ratio of DMFs for tumour over normal tissues. A therapeutic ratio above unity indicates that overall, the combined modality treatment is relatively more effective for tumour control than for normal tissue toxicity; conversely, a therapeutic ratio below unity indicates that the combined treatment is relatively more toxic than beneficial. The therapeutic ratio needs to be determined for both early and late normal tissue toxicity. Table 19.6 presents an example of a concomitant association of cisplatin and 5-fluorouracil with radiotherapy for the treatment of locally advanced squamous cell carcinoma of the cervix (41). It shows that when early toxicity is taken into account, the therapeutic ratio is far below unity. However, although very distressful, early side effects are usually manageable with extensive supportive care during treatment, and in this clinical example they fully resolved within a few weeks after the end of treatment. When late effects are considered, the therapeutic ratio is well above unity, illustrating the potential net benefit of the combined treatment strategy in this particular clinical setting.

When designing a new clinical trial or a new clinical strategy with concomitant chemotherapy and radiotherapy, one may need to slightly decrease the dose intensity of the standard treatment (i.e. radiotherapy) to get a therapeutic ratio above unity, but still have a beneficial effect at the tumour level. An example was the trial comparing radiotherapy alone (70 Gy in 7 weeks) for locally advanced head and neck squamous cell carcinoma, to intercalated chemotherapy-radiotherapy (three cycles of 20 Gy in 2 weeks alternating with four cycles of cisplatin-5FU) (38). At 3 years, the overall survival was increased from 23% to 41% without any increase in early toxicity. The choice between an 'equal toxicity' design or an 'equal dose' design therefore must be considered on a site-by-site basis depending on the objective of the trial or clinical strategy.

---

### Key points

1. Proper design combining drug and radiotherapy treatment depends on the objective desired. Sequential association (induction or adjuvant) is preferred when target cell populations are different and/or when the objective is to optimize the dose intensity of chemotherapy and radiotherapy in both chemo- and radiosensitive disease. Concomitant association is preferred when cellular or molecular interactions are used to improve loco-regional control of the disease.

---

Table 19.6 Comparison of efficacy and side effects after concomitant chemo-radiotherapy for locally advanced squamous cell carcinoma of the cervix

| | Radiotherapy alone[a] (n = 193) | Chemo[b]-radiotherapy (n = 195) | Therapeutic ratio |
|---|---|---|---|
| Recurrence rate at 5 years | 35% | 19% | — |
| Acute effects (G3–5) | 5% | 45% | 0.2 |
| Acute effects (excluding haematological toxicity) (G3–5) | 2% | 10% | 0.4 |
| Late effects (G3–5) | 11% | 12% | 1.7 |

Data from (41).

[a]  External pelvic radiotherapy up to 45 Gy in 4.5 weeks followed by a brachytherapy implant with a total dose equal or superior to 85 Gy.

[b]  Cisplatin (75 mg m$^{-2}$, d1) + 5-fluorouracil (1 g m$^{-2}$ d$^{-1}$, d1–d4) × 3 every 3 weeks.

2. Although several mechanisms of interaction between drugs and radiation have been identified (modulation of DNA and chromosome damage and repair, cell-cycle synchronization, enhanced induction of apoptosis and reoxygenation), in a clinical setting it is most likely that a key benefit is the inhibition of tumour cell proliferation by drugs during the radiation inter-fraction interval.

3. Concomitant administration of chemotherapy and radiation gives increased early normal tissue toxicity due to inhibition of stem cell or precursor cell proliferation. Late normal tissue damage is likely to be enhanced through inhibition of DNA repair, and by a specific mechanism of drug toxicity in sensitive tissues (e.g. Adriamycin in the heart and bleomycin in the lung).

4. The TR expresses the relative benefit of a combined modality treatment, integrating both the tumour and the normal tissue effects. For 'equal dose' trials, TR is typically below unity for early toxicity and above unity for late radiation damage.

5. Several randomised trials with concomitant chemo-radiotherapy have been conducted in brain, head and neck, lung, oesophagus, cervix and colo-rectal cancers. A significant increase in loco-regional control has been found in some disease sites (e.g. brain, head and neck and cervix) with a consequent improvement in patient survival.

## ■ BIBLIOGRAPHY

1. Auperin A, Le Pechoux C, Pignon JP et al. Meta-Analysis of Cisplatin/Carboplatin Based Concomitant Chemotherapy in Non-Small Cell Lung Cancer Group. Concomitant radio-chemotherapy based on platin compounds in patients with locally advanced non-small cell lung cancer (NSCLC): A meta-analysis of individual data from 1764 patients. *Ann Oncol* 2006;17:473–483.

2. Auperin A, Le Pechoux C, Rolland E et al. Meta-analysis of concomitant versus sequential radiochemotherapy in locally advanced non-small-cell lung cancer. *J Clin Oncol* 2010;28:2181–2190.

3. Bartelink H, Roelofsen F, Eschwege F et al. Concomitant radiotherapy and chemotherapy is superior to radiotherapy alone in the treatment of locally advanced anal cancer: Results of a phase III randomized trial of the European Organization for Research and Treatment of Cancer Radiotherapy and Gastrointestinal Cooperative Groups. *J Clin Oncol* 1997;15:2040–2049.

4. Baujat B, Audry H, Bourhis J et al. MAC-NPC Collaborative Group. *Cochrane Database Syst Rev* 2006;4:CD004329.

5. Begg AC. Cisplatin and radiation: Interaction probabilities and therapeutic possibilities. *Int J Radiat Oncol Biol Phys* 1990;19:1183–1189.

6. Bernier J, Domenge C, Ozsahin M et al. Postoperative irradiation with or without concomitant chemotherapy for locally advanced head and neck cancer. *N Engl J Med* 2004;350:1945–1952.

7. Blanchard P, Baujat B, Holostenco V et al. MACH-CH Collaborative Group. Meta-analysis of chemotherapy in head and neck cancer (MACH-NC): A comprehensive analysis by tumour site. *Radiother Oncol* 2011;100:33–40.

8. Budach W, Hehr T, Budach V, Belka C, Dietz K. A meta-analysis of hyperfractionated and accelerated radio-therapy and combined chemotherapy and radiotherapy regimens in unresected locally advanced squamous cell carcinoma of the head and neck. *BMC Cancer* 2006; 6:28.

9. Chemoradiotherapy for Cervical Cancer Meta-Analysis Collaboration. Reducing uncertainties about the effects of chemoradiotherapy for cervical cancer: A systematic review and meta-analysis of individual patient data from 18 randomized trials. *J Clin Oncol* 2008;26: 5802–5812.

10. Cooper JS, Pajak TF, Forastiere AA et al. Postoperative concurrent radiotherapy and chemotherapy for high-risk squamous-cell carcinoma of the head and neck. *N Engl J Med* 2004;350:1937–1944.

11. Cooper JS, Zhang Q, Pajak TF et al. Long-term follow-up of the RTOG 9501/intergroup phase III trial: Postoperative concurrent radiation therapy and chemotherapy in high-risk squamous cell carcinoma of the head and neck. *Int J Radiat Oncol Biol Phys* 2012;84:1198–1205.

12. Corry J, Rischin D, Smith JG et al. Radiation with concurrent late chemotherapy intensification ('chemoboost') for locally advanced head and neck cancer. *Radiother Oncol* 2000;54:123–127.

13. De Caluwe L, Van Nieuwenhove Y, Ceelen WP. Preoperative chemoradiation versus radiation alone for stage II and III resectable rectal cancer. *Cochrane Database Syst Rev* 2013;2:CD006041.

14. Department of Veterans Affairs Laryngeal Cancer Study Group. Induction chemotherapy plus radiation compared with surgery plus radiation in patients with advanced laryngeal cancer. *N Engl J Med* 1991;324:1685–1690.

15. Elion GB. The purine path to chemotherapy. *Science* 1989;244:41–47.

16. Forastiere AA, Goepfert H, Maor M et al. Concurrent chemotherapy and radiotherapy for organ preservation in advanced laryngeal cancer. *N Engl J Med* 2003;349:2091–2098.

17. Forastiere AA, Zhang Q, Weber RS et al. Long-term results of RTOG 91-11: A comparison of three nonsurgical treatment strategies to preserve the larynx in patients with locally advanced larynx cancer. *J Clin Oncol* 2013;31:845–852.

18. Giocanti N, Hennequin C, Balosso J, Mahler M, Favaudon V. DNA repair and cell cycle interactions in radiation sensitization by the topoisomerase II poison etoposide. *Cancer Res* 1993;53:2105–2111.

19. Green J, Kirwan J, Tierney J et al. Concomitant chemotherapy and radiation therapy for cancer of the uterine cervix. *Cochrane Database Syst Rev* 2005;20(3):CD002225.

20. Green JA, Kirwan JM, Tierney JF et al. Survival and recurrence after concomitant chemotherapy and radiotherapy for cancer of the uterine cervix: A systematic review and meta-analysis. *Lancet* 2001;358:781–786.

21. Gregoire V, Beauduin M, Rosier JF et al. Kinetics of mouse jejunum radiosensitization by 2',2'-difluorodeoxycytidine (gemcitabine) and its relationship with pharmacodynamics of DNA synthesis inhibition and cell cycle redistribution in crypt cells. *Br J Cancer* 1997;76:1315–1321.

22. Gregoire V, Hittelman WN, Rosier JF, Milas L. Chemo-radiotherapy: Radiosensitizing nucleoside analogues (review). *Oncol Rep* 1999;6:949–957.

23. Gregoire V, Van NT, Stephens LC et al. The role of fludarabine-induced apoptosis and cell cycle synchronization in enhanced murine tumor radiation response *in vivo*. *Cancer Res* 1994;54:6201–6209.

24. Gunderson LL, Winter KA, Ajani JA et al. Long-term update of US GI intergroup RTOG 98–11 phase III trial for anal carcinoma: Survival, relapse, and colostomy failure with concurrent chemoradiation involving fluorouracil/mitomycin versus fluorouracil/cisplatin. *J Clin Oncol* 2012;30:4344–4351.

25. Haddad R, O'Neill A, Rabinowits G et al. Induction chemotherapy followed by concurrent chemoradiotherapy (sequential chemoradiotherapy) versus concurrent chemoradiotherapy alone in locally advanced head and neck cancer (PARADIGM): A randomised phase 3 trial. *Lancet Oncol* 2013;14:257–264.

26. Hart MG, Garside R, Rogers G, Stein K, Grant R. Temozolomide for high grade glioma. *Cochrane Database Syst Rev* 2013;4:CD007415.

27. Hegi ME, Diserens AC, Gorlia T et al. MGMT gene silencing and benefit from temozolomide in glioblastoma. *N Engl J Med* 2005;352:997–1003.

28. Hitt R, Grau JJ, Lopez-Pousa A et al. Spanish Head and Neck Cancer Cooperative Group (TTCC). A randomized phase III trial comparing induction chemotherapy followed by chemoradiotherapy versus chemoradiotherapy alone as treatment of unresectable head and neck cancer. *Ann Oncol* 2014;25:216–225.

29. Iliakis G, Pantelias G, Kurtzman S. Mechanism of radiosensitization by halogenated pyrimidines: Effect of BrdU on cell killing and interphase chromosome breakage in radiation-sensitive cells. *Radiat Res* 1991;125:56–64.

30. Iversen AB, Busk M, Horsman MR. Induction of hypoxia by vascular disrupting agents and the significance for their combination with radiation therapy. *Acta Oncol* 2013;52:1320–1326.

31. James RD, Glynne-Jones R, Meadows HM et al. Mitomycin or cisplatin chemoradiation with or without maintenance chemotherapy for treatment of squamous-cell carcinoma of the anus (ACT II): A randomised, phase 3, open-label, 2 × 2 factorial trial. *Lancet Oncol* 2013;14:516–524.

32. Johnson IS, Armstrong JG, Gorman M, Burnett JP, Jr. The vinca alkaloids: A new class of oncolytic agents. *Cancer Res* 1963;23:1390–1427.

33. Kaufmann SH, Earnshaw WC. Induction of apoptosis by cancer chemotherapy. *Exp Cell Res* 2000;256:42–49.

34. Kelsey CR, Beaven AW, Diehl LF, Prosnitz LR. Combined-modality therapy for early-stage Hodgkin lymphoma: Maintaining high cure rates while minimizing risks. *Oncology (Williston Park)* 2012;26:1182–1189, 1193.

35. Lefebvre JL, Andry G, Chevalier D et al. Group EHaNC. Laryngeal preservation with induction chemotherapy for hypopharyngeal squamous cell carcinoma: 10-year results of EORTC trial 24891. *Ann Oncol* 2012;23:2708–2714.

36. Machtay M, Moughan J, Trotti A et al. Factors associated with severe late toxicity after concurrent chemoradiation for locally advanced head and neck cancer: An RTOG analysis. *J Clin Oncol* 2008;26:3582–3589.

37. Mason KA, Milas L, Hunter NR et al. Maximizing therapeutic gain with gemcitabine and fractionated radiation. *Int J Radiat Oncol Biol Phys* 1999;44:1125–1135.

38. Merlano M, Vitale V, Rosso R et al. Treatment of advanced squamous-cell carcinoma of the head and neck with alternating chemotherapy and radiotherapy. *N Engl J Med* 1992;327:1115–1121.

39. Milas L, Fujii T, Hunter N et al. Enhancement of tumor radioresponse *in vivo* by gemcitabine. *Cancer Res* 1999;59:107–114.

40. Milas L, Hunter N, Mason KA, Milross C, Peters LJ. Tumor reoxygenation as a mechanism of Taxol-induced enhancement of tumor radioresponse. *Acta Oncol* 1995;34:409–412.

41. Morris M, Eifel PJ, Lu J et al. Pelvic radiation with concurrent chemotherapy compared with pelvic and para-aortic radiation for high-risk cervical cancer. *N Engl J Med* 1999;340:1137–1143.

42. NACCCMA (Neoadjuvant Chemotherapy for Cervical Cancer Meta-Analysis) Collaboration. Neoadjuvant chemotherapy for locally advanced cervix cancer. *Cochrane Database Syst Rev* 2004:CD001774.

43. Peiffert D, Tournier-Rangeard L, Gerard JP et al. Induction chemotherapy and dose intensification of the radiation boost in locally advanced anal canal carcinoma: Final analysis of the randomized UNICANCER ACCORD 03 trial. *J Clin Oncol* 2012;30:1941–1948.

44. Pignon JP, Arriagada R, Ihde DC et al. A meta-analysis of thoracic radiotherapy for small-cell lung cancer. *N Engl J Med* 1992;327:1618–1624.

45. Pignon JP, Bourhis J, Domenge C, Designe L. Chemotherapy added to locoregional treatment for head and neck squamous-cell carcinoma: Three meta-analyses of updated individual data. MACH-NC Collaborative Group. Meta-Analysis of Chemotherapy on Head and Neck Cancer. *Lancet* 2000;355:949–955.

46. Pignon JP, le Maître A, Maillard E, Bourhis J. MACH-NC Collaborative Group Meta-analysis of chemotherapy in head and neck cancer (MACH-NC): An update on 93 randomised trials and 17,346 patients. *Radiother Oncol* 2009;92:4–14.

47. Pijls-Johannesma M, De Ruysscher D, Vansteenkiste J, Kester A, Rutten I, Lambin P. Timing of chest radiotherapy in patients with limited stage small cell lung cancer: A systematic review and meta-analysis of randomised controlled trials. *Cancer Treat Rev* 2007;33:461–473.

48. Rosenberg B, VanCamp L, Trosko JE, Mansour VH. Platinum compounds: A new class of potent antitumour agents. *Nature* 1969;222:385–386.
49. Wolmark N, Wieand HS, Hyams DM et al. Randomized trial of postoperative adjuvant chemotherapy with or without radiotherapy for carcinoma of the rectum: National Surgical Adjuvant Breast and Bowel Project Protocol R-02. *J Natl Cancer Inst* 2000;92:388–396.
50. Wong R, Malthaner R. Combined chemotherapy and radiotherapy (without surgery) compared with radiotherapy alone in localized carcinoma of the esophagus. *Cochrane Database Syst Rev* 2006, 2010:CD002092.

### ■ FURTHER READING

51. Hennequin C, Favaudon V. Biological basis for chemo-radiotherapy interactions. *Eur J Cancer* 2002;38:223–230.
52. Seiwert TY, Salama JK, Vokes EE. The concurrent chemoradiation paradigm – General principles. *Nat Clin Pract Oncol* 2007;4:86–100.
53. Steel GG. The search for therapeutic gain in the combination of radiotherapy and chemotherapy. *Radiother Oncol* 1988;11:31–53.
54. Steel GG, Peckham MJ. Exploitable mechanisms in combined radiotherapy-chemotherapy: The concept of additivity. *Int J Radiat Oncol Biol Phys* 1979;5:85–91.

# Molecular targeted agents for enhancing tumour response

## MICHAEL BAUMANN, MECHTHILD KRAUSE AND VINCENT GRÉGOIRE

## 20.1 INTRODUCTION

Today, combined radiochemotherapy is firmly established in clinical practice for a wide spectrum of tumours. Randomized trials have shown that in many cases, this strategy may lead to better local control and survival than radiotherapy alone. The radiobiological basis for radiochemotherapy and its current results are reviewed in Chapter 19. In this chapter we emphasise that, despite their proven benefit, currently available chemotherapeutic drugs are far from being perfect for combining with radiotherapy (44). Tumour cell kill by chemotherapy at clinically achievable doses is minor compared to that caused by radiation. Only in a relatively small proportion of patients is chemotherapy sufficiently effective to destroy subclinical metastatic deposits. Normal tissue toxicity is frequently increased after combined radiochemotherapy, which may limit doses of drugs or radiation. For these reasons it is obvious that more effective and less toxic substances are needed to further improve the results of systemic therapies combined with radiation.

Substantial research is ongoing in the design of targeted anticancer drugs. These drugs, also called molecular-targeted drugs, more or less specifically interfere with those molecular pathways which keep cells alive, and which allow cells to communicate with their environment and with other cells, or which govern the response of cells against stressors including radiation. Important examples of such molecular processes are outlined in Chapter 21. Recent advances in the field of biotechnology and cell biology have made it possible to unravel the details of this molecular signalling, and new pathways of molecular crosstalk are being detected at a rapid pace. As many of these pathways may be specifically inhibited or modified, the number of novel biology driven drugs, whose potential for radiotherapy warrants evaluation, is increasing rapidly.

### Rationale for combining molecular-targeted drugs with radiotherapy

Several reasons make the combination of molecular-targeted agents with irradiation a promising avenue for pre-clinical and clinical cancer research (44):

- The radiobiological basis of the response of tumours and normal tissues has been extensively studied and can in many cases be described not only qualitatively but also quantitatively (see Chapter 5).
- The molecular mechanisms underlying the radiobiology are being increasingly well understood and may be specifically targeted (see Chapters 2, 3 and 21).
- Molecular targets are often differentially expressed in tumours and normal tissues, offering a possible therapeutic gain (see Chapter 24).
- Molecular-targeted agents are in themselves not curative in solid tumours, whereas radiotherapy is highly efficient in eradicating cancer stem cells. As discussed in Chapter 5, it can be estimated from Poisson statistics that on average only 0.1–2.3 cancer stem cells per tumour survive at local tumour control probabilities between 10% and 90%, i.e. in the 'curative' dose range. This means that recurrences after high-dose radiotherapy may be caused by only one or a few cancer stem cells. This is illustrated in Figure 20.1, where histological sections of irradiated AT17 mouse mammary carcinomas are compared with the dose-response curve for local control in the same tumour model. A unique feature of the AT17 tumour is that regrowth of surviving cancer stem cells after irradiation can be directly visualized and measured as colony formation *in vivo* (44,45). Figure 20.1a–c shows that with increasing dose, the number of colonies per section decreases, and that after 54 Gy a single surviving colony was found (close-up in Figure 20.1d). Figure 20.1e shows the number of surviving clonogenic cells per tumour for groups of tumours treated with increasing doses. The number of colonies per tumour decreases and the proportion of tumours without any surviving cancer stem cell increases with increasing radiation dose. The histological data correspond well with the observed rate of permanent local tumour control after irradiation in the same tumour model. Those tumours which are not completely sterilized after irradiation with doses in the curative range (in this experiment >50 Gy) typically contain only 1 to a maximum of 100 surviving cancer stem cells. Thus, even if a novel molecular targeted agent has the potential to kill only a few cancer stem cells, or if

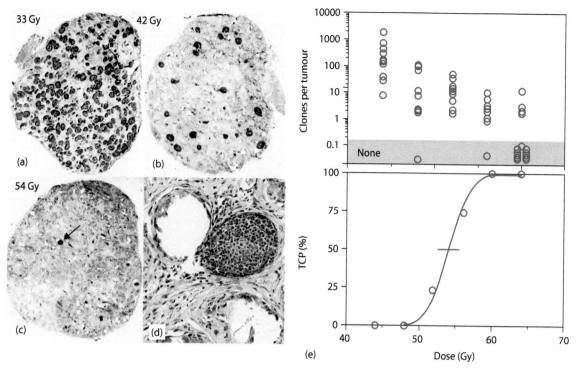

**Figure 20.1** Pattern of clonal regeneration of stem cells in the AT17 mouse mammary carcinoma after irradiation with single doses of 33 Gy (a), 42 Gy (b) and 54 Gy (c) under clamp hypoxic conditions. With increasing irradiation dose, the number of colonies per section decreases, after 54 Gy only one surviving colony was found (arrow, close-up in d). Panel (e) (upper) shows the number of surviving stem cells for individual AT17 tumours measured at day 19 after single-dose irradiation under clamp hypoxia. Panel (e) (lower) shows local tumour control (symbols) at 18 months follow-up and the calculated tumour control probabilities (line) for AT17 tumours irradiated with the same single doses under clamp hypoxia. The increase in local tumour control corresponds closely with the proportion of tumours without surviving stem cells. (From (44), with permission.)

it interferes in mechanisms of radioresistance of tumours, its combination with radiotherapy may still lead to an improvement in local tumour control.

## Research strategies to evaluate targeted drugs for radiotherapy

The large number of potential cellular target molecules and the rapid emergence of new drugs to interact with these targets requires a rational, radiobiology-driven approach for target selection. Attractive targets for drugs to be used specifically within the context of radiotherapy would be (over)expressed in a high proportion of tumours frequently treated by radiation, would be not expressed by normal tissues surrounding the tumour, would be linked to poor loco-regional tumour control after radiotherapy alone and would ideally be associated with known radiobiological mechanisms of tumour radioresistance (44). Identification of such targets requires specific research on pre-clinical model tumours and on tumour material of patients treated by radiotherapy. The biological data obtained from the tumours should be compared with high-quality clinical outcome data which incorporate comprehensive information on dose, fractionation and known prognostic factors.

Appropriate multivariate methods should be applied, not only in determining prognostic factors but also in assessing the results of biomarker studies. A good example of rational target identification in the context of radiotherapy is the epidermal growth factor receptor (EGFR), which is discussed in the next section.

In developing new molecular-targeted agents for use with radiation, the initial evaluation is typically performed on cells in culture. Endpoints include inhibition of cell proliferation and colony formation after irradiation with and without drug. However, it should be kept in mind that effects *in vitro* do not necessarily translate into the same effect *in vivo*. Typical problems are that higher drug concentrations can be achieved *in vitro* than *in vivo*, that the expression of target molecules may be different *in vitro* and *in vivo*, that cell culture conditions may significantly influence cell survival, and that many microenvironmental factors which are present in tumours (e.g. hypoxia, low pH and cell-cell interactions) are usually not reflected in cell culture (reviewed in [44]). However, because of the high number of potential targets, there is currently no practical alternative to initially screening molecular-targeted drugs combined with radiation using *in vitro* models, which can in a second step be complemented by more dedicated three-dimensional *in vitro* models. Experiments on cells in culture are also very important for unravelling the mechanisms of action of effects observed in animals or clinical studies.

The final step in the pre-clinical investigation of new targeted drugs for radiotherapy should include experiments on tumour models *in vivo*. The design and experimental endpoints of such studies are discussed in Chapter 8. For the discussion here, it is important to discriminate volume-dependent endpoints such as tumour regression or tumour growth delay from local tumour control. Those cells which may form a recurrence after therapy, i.e. cancer stem cells, constitute only a small proportion of all cancer cells, whereas the bulk of tumour cells are non-tumourigenic (17,35). Thus, changes in tumour volume after therapy are governed by the changes in the mass of tumour cells, that is primarily by the non-stem cells. By contrast, local tumour control is dependent on the complete inactivation of the subpopulation of cancer stem cells (8). The majority of current pre-clinical studies in cancer research use volume-dependent endpoints. This carries a substantial risk that new treatments may be optimized for their effect on the bulk of non-stem cancer cells, with no improvement in the curative potential. The existence of differential effects of molecular-targeted agents combined with radiation on non-stem cells versus cancer stem cells is supported by several recent studies that have shown a dissociation of tumour volume-dependent endpoints and tumour control (reviewed in [8,44]). An example is shown in Figure 20.2 where inhibition of the EGFR led to pronounced regression and growth delay of the tumour without improving local tumour control. Overall, these experiments support the principle that radiotherapy-specific pre-clinical research strategies need to be applied to test the efficacy of molecular-targeted drugs combined with radiation and that cancer stem cell specific endpoints such as local tumour control should be used whenever possible (see Chapter 8).

Some specific aspects need also to be mentioned with regard to testing molecular-targeted drugs for radiotherapy in clinical trials (5). First, pre-clinical data should be available from combining the drug with radiation, and there should be a valid radiobiological rationale to combine exactly the selected drug in the selected tumour entity. As outlined previously, pre-clinical data on tumour volume-dependent endpoints may not be sufficient, as these not always reflect survival of cancer stem cells which determine the outcome of curative radiotherapy. Furthermore, biomarkers which are established for use of the drug alone or combined with chemotherapy do not necessarily also work for the combination with radiation. Therefore, extensive biological co-investigations should be part of all clinical trials on combined modality treatments to establish radiotherapy-specific prognostic and predictive tests (see the following text). Last, the effects of molecular-targeted drugs on cancer stem cells are weak compared to the effects of radiation, where clear and often very steep dose-response relationships exist for tumours as well as for normal tissues. If the (biologically effective) radiation dose and the dose distribution are not standardized and of high quality, an effect of a new drug may be easily missed or normal tissue reactions might be increased.

Unfortunately, this pre-clinical and clinical research strategy has so far not been fully established in research laboratories and industry, leading to inadequate access to new drugs with specific activity when combined with radiotherapy (5). Today's laboratory mass screening of candidate anticancer drugs is usually done in the absence of radiotherapy. Thus, candidate compounds that are not effective alone, but could be promising for radiosensitizing tumour cells, will not be selected. Furthermore, pre-clinical studies usually apply new compounds as monotherapy or in combination with other chemotherapeutic agents, but not combined with radiotherapy. New drugs that are eventually included in clinical trials are usually tested only in combination with radiotherapy after they have shown promise alone or in combination with chemotherapy. Again, this selection could miss important opportunities (5).

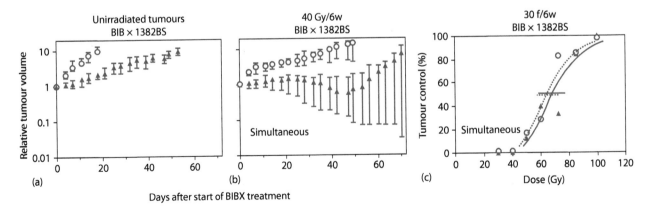

**Figure 20.2** Effect of EGFR TK inhibition on the tumour volume of unirradiated (a) and irradiated (b) FaDu HNSCC xenografts (40 Gy, 30 fractions, 6 weeks) and on local tumour control after 30 fractions within 6 weeks (c). Open symbols represent control tumours, closed symbols represent tumours treated with the TKI simultaneously with irradiation. Error bars show 95% C.I. (From (6), with permission.)

## Targeted drugs and distant metastases

A 'perfect' targeted drug for radiotherapy may have no impact on the survival of cancer cells when given without irradiation, but effectively decreases mechanisms of radiation resistance, thereby improving local tumour control. However, subclinical distant metastases might be already present outside the irradiated volume. The drug, because of its ineffectiveness without irradiation, will not eradicate these subclinical metastases, and the patient may succumb from distant metastases despite the fact that the primary tumour is controlled. This is a fundamental difference between a (pure) targeted radiation modifier compared to chemotherapeutic drugs which may kill tumour cells by themselves, and therefore, when combined with radiotherapy, may help to eradicate both the primary tumour and distant metastases. Therefore, most researchers aim to develop targeted drugs which also have efficacy against cancer cells by themselves and which therefore can eradicate subclinical metastases. Alternatively, pure radiation modifiers may be combined with radiation plus chemotherapy. In such trimodality treatments, systemic chemotherapy (potentially enhanced by the targeted drug) would be directed against the metastatic deposits, whereas radiotherapy, enhanced in its effect by the targeted drug and possibly by the chemotherapeutic agent, would eradicate the primary tumour. It should be noted that such novel strategies would not necessarily have to utilize *concurrent* radiochemotherapy which for most cancers is today's standard of care.

## 20.2 EGFR INHIBITORS

### Pre-clinical data in model tumours

In murine tumour models, a significant correlation between EGFR expression and radiation dose needed to achieve 50% local tumour control (TCD50) after single-dose exposure was demonstrated (1). These results may be explained by a higher number, an increased cellular radioresistance or greater hypoxia of cancer stem cells in EGFR-overexpressing tumours. A correlation has also been observed between accelerated repopulation of cancer stem cells and the expression kinetics of EGFR in one of several human squamous cell carcinoma models, suggesting that the EGFR might also be involved in specific radiobiological mechanisms of resistance in *fractionated* radiotherapy (7,25,55). It is important to note that not only EGFR expression but also the ligand-independent activation of the receptor by radiation may be involved in radioresistance (60).

A promising approach therefore is to combine radiotherapy with drugs which target the EGFR. Such drugs can either be monoclonal antibodies against the EGFR or small molecules which specifically inhibit phosphorylation of the EGFR (tyrosine kinase inhibitors [TKIs]). Figure 20.3 shows the downstream molecular pathways that may be altered by these two approaches. For a large number of tumour cell lines *in vitro* it has been demonstrated that EGFR inhibition with or without irradiation results in reduced cell proliferation. For some but not all of these cell lines, a radiosensitizing effect could also be shown which at least in part seems to be related to inhibition of repair of DNA damage (reviewed in [7]). Also, for many tumour models *in vivo*, prolonged growth delay was demonstrated for different EGFR inhibitors combined with radiotherapy ([32], and reviewed in [6]). Experiments demonstrated improved local tumour control when the monoclonal anti-EGFR antibody C225 was given with single-dose or fractionated irradiation (32,43,50,53), however, this effect is heterogeneous between different tumours of the same histology (32).

Several radiobiological mechanisms may explain the observed effects: direct inactivation of cancer stem cells by the drug, cellular radiosensitization, reduced repopulation and improved reoxygenation are all possible (7,42). The fact that the range of response in different head and neck cancer (head and neck squamous cell carcinoma [HNSCC]) models reaches from substantial improvement of local tumour control in some models to non-response in other models is so far not well understood. A candidate biomarker for the combined effect may be the genetic EGFR expression, i.e. the EGFR gene amplification status (32). It is interesting to note that so far, improved local tumour control in pre-clinical studies has only been shown for anti-EGFR antibodies but not for EGFR TKIs, even when tested in the same tumour models. This suggests that immune-response reactions or other EGFR-independent mechanisms might be important.

### Clinical data

The most clinical experience so far has been reported for head and neck cancer. The EGFR is highly expressed in HNSCC. In a retrospective Radiation Therapy and Oncology Group (RTOG) study on patients with locally advanced tumours treated by radiotherapy alone, EGFR expression has been shown to be an independent prognostic factor for both overall survival and disease-free survival (2); patients whose tumours overexpressed the EGFR did significantly worse than patients who did not. These clinical observations support the concept that EGFR inhibition might counteract mechanisms of intrinsic radioresistance. It was also shown in retrospective analyses from the Danish Head and Neck Cancer Study Group (DAHANCA) and the continuous hyperfractionated accelerated radiotherapy (CHART) trials that only patients with high EGFR expression benefited from accelerated radiotherapy (9,26). In line with pre-clinical results discussed above, these data suggest that the EGFR may be involved in accelerated repopulation of cancer stem cells.

Cetuximab (C225 or Erbitux) is so far the leading monoclonal antibody against EGFR that has been tested clinically. A randomized phase III trial comparing radiotherapy alone to the same radiotherapy with a loading

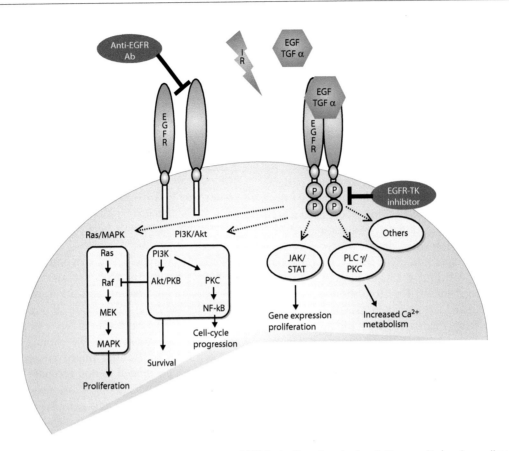

**Figure 20.3** EGFR-mediated signal transduction. Activation of the EGFR by its ligands or by irradiation results in a homodimerisation of two EGFR or a heterodimerisation with another member of the EGF receptor family, followed by internalisation and autophosphorylation of the intracellular tyrosine kinase domain. Different cascades can be activated, leading to proliferation, enhanced cell survival and cell-cycle progression. The EGFR can be inhibited by monoclonal antibodies, which block extracellular dimerisation and lead to internalisation of the EGFR-mAb complex, degradation and downmodulation of the EGFR. TK inhibitors pass the cellular membrane and block phosphorylation of the tyrosine kinase. (From (6), with permission.)

dose (400 mg m$^{-2}$) followed by weekly doses (250 mg m$^{-2}$) of C225 was undertaken in 424 patients with stage III–IV SCC of the oropharynx, hypopharynx and larynx (12,13). Patients were stratified according to the radiotherapy regimen (70 Gy in 35 fractions in 7 weeks or 72–76.8 Gy in 60–64 fractions in 7 weeks, or 72 Gy in 42 fractions over 6 weeks), the performance status, the nodal involvement (N0 versus N+) and the T-stage (T1–T3 versus T4). With a median follow-up of 54 months, patients in the combined treatment arm did significantly better than patients treated by radiotherapy alone in term of loco-regional control, progression-free survival and overall survival (Table 20.1). The rate of distant metastasis was not different between the two arms and although some differences were observed when subgroup analysis was performed, the study was not powered to detect any significant difference between them. An interesting observation of this trial was that with the exception of acneiform rash, no difference was observed between the two groups regarding toxicity and in particular, radiation-induced acute side effects (Table 20.1). It is important to note that, consistent with the above-mentioned inter-tumoural heterogeneity, the overall effect of the combined treatment was not higher as compared to the effect observed for

combined cisplatinum-based radiochemotherapy (15), so that combined radiotherapy with cetuximab is an alternative, but not generally preferable to cisplatinum-based radiochemotherapy (10). The toxicity profile is different with more skin reactions in the cetuximab regimens, but more kidney and haematological toxicity in the cisplatinum-based regimens. Triple combinations of radiochemotherapy and cetuximab have so far revealed negative results in randomised phase III trials. Addition of cetuximab to definitive radiochemotherapy with cisplatinum led to no improvement of loco-regional tumour control and survival in HNSCC (3) or even impaired survival together with higher toxicity in oesophageal cancer (21). These data are in line with low pathological complete response rates observed after simultaneous neoadjuvant radiochemotherapy and cetuximab in patients with rectal carcinoma in different phase II studies (11,48,59). The underlying reasons for this lower efficacy are not known. Biological explanations include counteractive effects between the treatment components that may either be caused by the cetuximab-induced increase of G0/G1 fraction of the cell cycle and its pro-inflammatory effects that could cause chemotherapy resistance as well as modulations of the cellular redox state by cetuximab (22,30).

Table 20.1 Comparison between radiotherapy alone and radiotherapy plus cetuximab in patients with locally advanced head and neck squamous cell carcinoma

| | Radiotherapy alone ($n = 213$) (%) | Radiotherapy + cetuximab ($n = 211$) (%) | p-Value |
|---|---|---|---|
| **Antitumour efficacy** | | | |
| 3-year loco-regional control | 34 | 47 | <0.01 |
| 3-year progression-free survival | 31 | 42 | 0.04 |
| 3-year overall survival | 45 | 55 | 0.05 |
| **Adverse effects (grades 3–5)** | | | |
| Mucositis | 52 | 56 | 0.44 |
| Dysphagia | 30 | 26 | 0.45 |
| Radiation dermatitis | 18 | 23 | 0.27 |
| Acneiform rash | 1 | 17 | <0.001 |

Data from (12).

However, for palliative treatment of HNSCC, addition of cetuximab to cisplatin has been shown in a phase III trial to be superior to cisplatin alone (14).

Other monoclonal antibodies directed against the EGFR have been developed and are being tested in various clinical phases. Nimotuzumab (H-R3) is a humanized antibody that has been tested in a phase I trial in combination with radiotherapy in patients with locally advanced disease (20). A phase II trial is ongoing in HNSCC. In anaplastic astrocytoma and glioblastoma, combination of radiotherapy with Nimotuzumab led to longer patient survival compared to radiotherapy alone in a randomised phase II trial that unfortunately did not include standard radiochemotherapy as a control arm (61). The safety profile of Zalutumumab (HuMax-EGFr), a fully humanized monoclonal antibody, has been evaluated in patients with metastatic or recurrent HNSCC (4). This antibody is undergoing testing in concomitant association with radiotherapy for locally advanced HNSCC. Panitumumab (ABX-EGF) and matuzumab (EMD 72000) are also fully humanized antibodies against EGFR (28,38) and have been tested in various human tumours. Combination of Panitumumab with neoadjuvant radiochemotherapy in locally advanced rectal cancer leads to high gastrointestinal toxicity and pathological complete response rates of 21% and 18%, which appear higher as compared to similar trials on cetuximab; however, long-term survival has not been evaluated yet (34,56).

For EGFR TKIs, several phase III trials are reported without radiotherapy (reviewed in [41]). In non-small cell lung cancer (NSCLC) the results were only positive when the TKI were given alone, whereas no improvement in tumour response or survival was observed when the TKIs were combined with chemotherapy. This is in contrast to pancreatic cancer where addition of erlotinib to gemcitabine improved survival. For combination with radiotherapy, one phase III trial has been reported on sequential, but none for simultaneous treatment. The trial investigating the administration of gefitinib after the end of radiochemotherapy compared to radiochemotherapy alone was stopped early because survival was significantly better after radiochemotherapy alone (37).

Applied simultaneously to primary radiochemotherapy or as maintenance therapy, the addition of Gefitinib did not improve local tumour control or survival in a phase II trial (31). This is in line with various other early clinical trials showing no or minor responses but in some cases higher toxicity compared to the standard treatment (e.g. [54,57,62]). For Erlotinib, several phase I and phase II studies have shown feasibility for combination with radio(chemo)therapy in different tumour entities, but no direct comparisons of response rates have been performed so far to standard treatments.

Overall, the data reported so far indicate that addition of targeted drugs to established anticancer treatments will not always improve the results even if the drug is effective when given alone. This calls for careful pre-clinical and clinical research into exactly the setting intended for use before introduction of novel drugs into multimodality treatments and for focusing research strategies already in the pre-clinical phase on the development of biomarkers for patient selection.

## 20.3 ANTI-ANGIOGENIC DRUGS

Very early tumour foci can be fed by diffusion alone; however, at a diameter larger than 1–2 millimetres, tumours need perfused blood vessels for further growth. For this neo-angiogenesis, the vascular endothelial growth factor (VEGF) plays an important role. A potential advantage of targeting VEGF signalling is that there is almost no physiological neo-angiogenesis in adults, thus making this target relatively tumour specific. The VEGF receptor (VEGFR) is expressed preferentially on endothelial cells and its activation is known to induce endothelial cell proliferation, migration and survival. High levels of VEGF are associated with poor prognoses in patients. In pre-clinical experiments, VEGFR inhibitors have been shown to radiosensitize endothelial cells, to inhibit proliferation and survival of endothelial and, secondarily, of tumour cells. Application of an anti-VEGFR antibody in combination with short-term fractionated irradiation led to improved local control in two different tumour models *in vivo* (40). With a VEGFR tyrosine kinase inhibitor, prolonged tumour growth delay could be shown after combination with fractionated irradiation in different tumour models; however, this effect did not translate into improved local tumour control (67,68). Interpreting these data, potential radiobiological effects on tumour hypoxia need to be considered. In theory, anti-angiogenic drugs could increase hypoxia by reduction of the vessel density. However, also improvement of tumour cell oxygenation by reduction of the interstitial fluid pressure and oxygen consumption and by normalisation of the chaotic tumour vasculature is possible (36). Pre-clinical data on the impact of transient normalisation of the tumour vasculature for tumour response after irradiation are contradictory.

Anti-angiogenic substances are also being tested clinically in combination with radiotherapy. A randomized trial has been performed in stage III NSCLC in which induction chemotherapy was followed by concomitant radiochemotherapy. The patients were randomized to receive AE-941 (Neovastat), a shark cartilage extract with anti-angiogenic properties, or placebo at the start of induction chemotherapy and continuing after radiochemotherapy as maintenance therapy. This trial was closed early because of insufficient accrual after 384 patients and showed no effect on overall survival (47). Early clinical experience is also available for the monoclonal anti-VEGF antibody bevacizumab (Avastin) in rectal cancer. A proof-of-concept study was performed with bevacizumab and radiotherapy in six patients with locally advanced adenocarcinoma of the rectum (65). Patients received bevacizumab 2 weeks before neoadjuvant 5FU-based radiochemotherapy. Twelve days after the first infusion of bevacizumab, overall improvement in the efficiency of blood vessels was observed as measured by various endpoints such as blood flow, blood volume, microvascular density and fluorodeoxyglucose (FDG) uptake and this supports the concept of transient normalization of tumour perfusion with anti-angiogenic drugs, allowing a more effective delivery of oxygen and chemotherapeutic agents (36). After phase II trials on simultaneous administration to neoadjuvant radiochemotherapy with capecitabine, contradictory results on pathological complete response rates have been reported (39,63). However, some in-field intestinal toxicity has occurred, underlining the need for further investigations to clarify the therapeutic potential of bevacizumab to improve the results of radiochemotherapy in gastrointestinal cancer (19,58,66). Also in other tumour entities like glioblastoma or pancreatic cancer, phase II trials are published and some phase III trials are ongoing.

## 20.4 INHIBITORS OF THE PI3K/AKT PATHWAY

PI3K/AKT signal transduction is an important downstream pathway of the receptor tyrosine kinases. Its activation results in increased cell survival and contributes to radioresistance. The mammalian target of rapamycin (mTOR) is a key signal transduction molecule of the PI3K/AKT pathway and constitutive mTOR activation contributes to radioresistance. However, using clonogenic endpoints *in vitro*, mTOR inhibition by rapamycin could not be shown to radiosensitize U87 glioma cells. When given combined with irradiation (4 × 4 Gy over 18 days) in the same tumour model, tumour growth delay was significantly prolonged compared to irradiation alone (27) and a significant effect on growth delay of U87 tumours could be shown in another *in vivo* experiment in the same tumour model. However, using a fractionated irradiation schedule with daily irradiation over 5 days and daily application of rapamycin, neither tumour growth delay nor local tumour control (TCD50) were influenced by addition of the drug (64). Except for a few feasibility studies, there are so far no published data on combined approaches with radiotherapy.

## 20.5 INHIBITORS OF THE RAS PATHWAY

Ras is a downstream molecule of several growth factor receptors, among others the EGFR. Its signal transduction leads to proliferation of tumour cells. Many human tumours overexpress activated H- or K-Ras isoforms, which may increase tumour radioresistance by promoting aberrant survival signals. Inhibition of the enzyme farnesyl transferase prevents Ras activation (reviewed in [16]). Farnesyl transferase inhibitors (FTIs) have been shown to radiosensitize tumour cells *in vitro* and to reduce tumour growth when combined with single-dose irradiation *in vivo*. Using an *ex vivo* clonogenic assay, a reduced survival of clonogenic tumour cells has been demonstrated after single-dose irradiation combined with a FTI in two different tumour models. This effect was considerably higher in H-RAS mutated compared to H-RAS wild-type tumour cells (18,23). Studies with tumour-control endpoints have not yet been performed. In clinical phase I trials, FTI combined with radiotherapy in NSCLC, HNSCC, glioma and pancreatic cancer has shown acceptable toxicity (24,33,49).

## 20.6 HDAC INHIBITORS

The main mechanisms underlying the effects of histone deacetylase (HDAC) inhibitors are physical modifications of the chromatin structure and hyper-acetylation of histone proteins, which leads to relaxation of the chromatin and possibly to radiosensitization of tumour cells. Indeed, HDAC inhibitors like valproic acid have been shown in pre-clinical experiments to radiosensitize tumour cells *in vitro* and to inhibit tumour growth when combined with single-dose irradiation *in vivo* (reviewed in [16]). So far there are no data from studies using local tumour control endpoints. Different HDAC inhibitors are currently being tested in combination with radio(chemo)therapy in early clinical trials.

## 20.7 CYCLOOXYGENASE-2 INHIBITORS

Cyclooxygenase-2 (COX-2), an enzyme involved in pro-staglandin synthesis, is overexpressed in a variety of human cancers and has been associated with poor prognosis after radiotherapy. Selective COX-2 inhibitors have been shown to increase the radiosensitivity of human glioma and lung cancer cells *in vitro*. In human tumour xenografts, COX-2 inhibitors have prolonged tumour growth delay and improved local tumour control after irradiation (46). Early clinical trials combining COX-2 inhibitors with radiotherapy have not shown unexpected toxicity (29). However, because of cardiovascular problems observed in patients receiving long-term treatment with COX-2 inhibitors for inflammation and pain, several clinical trials were terminated and not reported. Though, in light of the promising pre-clinical data, short-term use of COX-2 inhibitors combined with radiotherapy still appears to be a highly attractive avenue for further research. Indeed, the above described toxicity did not occur in a phase II trial on combined radiochemotherapy and the COX-2 inhibitor celecoxib; however, low tumour response rates led to early termination of the trial (52). Promising results have been reported from a small randomised trial for radiochemotherapy or radiochemotherapy with celecoxib in patients with nasopharyngeal cancer, where the 2-year local tumour control rate was improved from 80% to 100% (51).

## 20.8 OTHER TARGETED DRUGS

The combination of radiation with a variety of other targeted drugs including tumour necrosis factor–related apoptosis-inducing ligand (TRAIL), DNA repair inhibitors, broad-spectrum tyrosine kinase inhibitors, proteasome inhibitors and inhibitors of cell adhesion molecules, have shown promising effects when combined with radiation *in vitro* or *in vivo*, some of them have been evaluated in clinical feasibility trials. Conclusions on clinical efficacy cannot yet be drawn.

## 20.9 CONCLUSIONS

Tumour response and duration of patient survival, after treatment with molecular-targeted agents in combination with radiotherapy, vary considerably between different classes of drugs, different substances within one class of drugs, different combination schedules, and also between individual patients. So far, this heterogeneity has been best studied for the combination of radiotherapy with EGFR inhibitors. To rationally prescribe the many emerging molecular-targeted drugs within the context of radiotherapy, development and introduction of biomarkers is of high importance. Due to specific interactions of molecular-targeted drugs with the biological effects of irradiation, biomarkers are expected to differ for radiation oncology compared to application of the drugs alone or within

chemotherapy treatment schedules and therefore need to be established and tested separately. An example of this principle are the activating K-RAS mutations that have been shown to be negatively correlated with the effect of EGFR-TK inhibitors given alone or combined with chemotherapy in NSCLC, whereas pre-clinical data show radiosensitizing effects for EGFR-TK inhibitors. Currently there are still more open than answered questions in the field of biomarkers for combined radiotherapy and molecular-targeted agents (41). Further research into the mechanisms of action of these novel combined approaches will eventually contribute to the development of valid biomarkers enabling clinicians to take full advantage of the potential of molecular-targeted drugs for improving radiotherapy.

---

### Key points

1. Molecular-targeted drugs specifically modify intra- or intercellular signal transduction and may thereby radiosensitize tumours.
2. Molecular targets are often differentially expressed in tumours and normal tissues, offering the possibility of a therapeutic gain.
3. Radiotherapy offers a particularly promising scenario for utilizing targeted anticancer agents. These drugs by themselves kill only few cancer stem cells and are not curative in solid tumours, whereas radiotherapy is highly efficient in eradicating cancer stem cells. When combined with radiation, the additional cell kill by the targeted drug may enhance the curative potential of radiotherapy.
4. Identification and testing of molecular-targeted drugs for radiotherapy requires a radiotherapy-specific research strategy. The addition of targeted drugs to radiation may promote tumour regression and prolong tumour growth delay without improving local tumour control. As tumour control reflects the survival of cancer stem cells, this endpoint should be used whenever possible.
5. Considerable inter-tumoural and inter-substance heterogeneity exists for the efficacy of targeting the same pathway. This calls for better understanding of the mechanisms of action of molecular-targeted drugs in combination with radiation, and for the development of predictive assays.

---

■ BIBLIOGRAPHY

1. Akimoto T, Hunter NR, Buchmiller L, Mason K, Ang KK, Milas L. Inverse relationship between epidermal growth factor receptor expression and radiocurability of murine carcinomas. *Clin Cancer Res* 1999;5:2884–2890.
2. Ang K, Berkey BA, Tu X et al. Impact of epidermal growth factor receptor expression on survival and pattern of relapse

in patients with advanced head and neck carcinoma. *Cancer Res* 2002;62:7350–7356.

3. Ang KK, Zhang QE, Rosenthal DI et al. ASCO annual meeting. (*Journal of Clinical Oncology*) 2011, abstract 5500.

4. Bastholt L, Specht L, Jensen K et al. A novel fully human monoclonal antibody against epidermal growth factor receptor (EGFR). First clinical and FDG-PET imaging results from a phase I/II trial conducted by the Danish Head and Neck Cancer Study Group (DAHANCA) in patients with squamous cell carcinoma of the head and neck (SCCHN). *J Clin Oncol* 2005;23:507S.

5. Baumann M. Keynote comment: Radiotherapy in the age of molecular oncology. *Lancet Oncol* 2006;7:786–787.

6. Baumann M, Krause M. Targeting the epidermal growth factor receptor in radiotherapy: Radiobiological mechanisms, preclinical and clinical results. *Radiother Oncol* 2004;72: 257–266.

7. Baumann M, Krause M, Dikomey E et al. EGFR-targeted anti-cancer drugs in radiotherapy: Preclinical evaluation of mechanisms. *Radiother Oncol* 2007;83:238–248.

8. Baumann M, Krause M, Hill R. Exploring the role of cancer stem cells in radioresistance. *Nat Rev Cancer* 2008;8: 545–554.

9. Bentzen SM, Atasoy BM, Daley FM et al. Epidermal growth factor receptor expression in pretreatment biopsies from head and neck squamous cell carcinoma as a predictive factor for a benefit from accelerated radiation therapy in a randomized controlled/trial. *J Clin Oncol* 2005;23: 5560–5567.

10. Bernier J, Schneider D. Cetuximab combined with radiotherapy: An alternative to chemoradiotherapy for patients with locally advanced squamous cell carcinomas of the head and neck? *Eur J Cancer* 2007;43:35–45.

11. Bertolini F, Chiara S, Bengala C et al. Neoadjuvant treatment with single-agent cetuximab followed by 5-FU, cetuximab, and pelvic radiotherapy: A phase II study in locally advanced rectal cancer. *Int J Radiat Oncol Biol Phys* 2009;73:466–472.

12. Bonner JA, Harari PM, Giralt J et al. Radiotherapy plus cetuximab for squamous-cell carcinoma of the head and neck. *N Engl J Med* 2006;354:567–578.

13. Bonner JA, Harari PM, Giralt J et al. Radiotherapy plus cetuximab for locoregionally advanced head and neck cancer: 5-year survival data from a phase 3 randomised trial, and relation between cetuximab-induced rash and survival. *Lancet Oncol* 2010;11:21–28.

14. Burtness B, Goldwasser MA, Flood W, Mattar B, Forastiere AA. Phase III randomized trial of cisplatin plus placebo compared with cisplatin plus cetuximab in metastatic/recurrent head and neck cancer: An Eastern Cooperative Oncology Group study. *J Clin Oncol* 2005;23:8646–8654.

15. Caudell JJ, Sawrie SM, Spencer SA et al. Locoregionally advanced head and neck cancer treated with primary radiotherapy: A comparison of the addition of cetuximab or chemotherapy and the impact of protocol treatment. *Int J Radiat Oncol Biol Phys* 2008;71:676–681.

16. Chinnaiyan P, Allen GW, Harari PM. Radiation and new molecular agents, part II: Targeting HDAC, HSP90, IGF-1R, PI3K, and Ras. *Semin Radiat Oncol* 2006;16:59–64.

17. Clarke MF, Dick JE, Dirks PB et al. Cancer stem cells – Perspectives on current status and future directions: AACR Workshop on Cancer Stem Cells. *Cancer Res* 2006;66: 9339–9344.

18. Cohen-Jonathan E, Muschel RJ, Gillies McKenna W et al. Farnesyltransferase inhibitors potentiate the antitumor effect of radiation on a human tumor xenograft expressing activated HRAS. *Radiat Res* 2000;154:125–132.

19. Crane CH, Ellis LM, Abbruzzese JL et al. Phase I trial evaluating the safety of bevacizumab with concurrent radiotherapy and capecitabine in locally advanced pancreatic cancer. *J Clin Oncol* 2006;24:1145–1151.

20. Crombet T, Osorio M, Cruz T et al. Use of the humanized anti-epidermal growth factor receptor monoclonal antibody h-R3 in combination with radiotherapy in the treatment of locally advanced head and neck cancer patients. *J Clin Oncol* 2004;22:1646–1654.

21. Crosby T, Hurt CN, Falk S et al. Chemoradiotherapy with or without cetuximab in patients with oesophageal cancer (SCOPE1): A multicentre, phase 2/3 randomised trial. *Lancet Oncol* 2013;14:627–637.

22. Dahan L, Sadok A, Formento JL, Seitz JF, Kovacic H. Modulation of cellular redox state underlies antagonism between oxaliplatin and cetuximab in human colorectal cancer cell lines. *Br J Pharmacol* 2009;158:610–620.

23. Delmas C, Heliez C, Cohen-Jonathan E et al. Farnesyl-transferase inhibitor, R115777, reverses the resistance of human glioma cell lines to ionizing radiation. *Int J Cancer* 2002;100:43–48.

24. Desjardins A, Reardon DA, Peters KB et al. A phase I trial of the farnesyl transferase inhibitor, SCH 66336, with temozolomide for patients with malignant glioma. *J Neurooncol* 2011;105: 601–606.

25. Eicheler W, Krause M, Hessel F, Zips D, Baumann M. Kinetics of EGFR expression during fractionated irradiation varies between different human squamous cell carcinoma lines in nude mice. *Radiother Oncol* 2005;76:151–156.

26. Eriksen JG, Steiniche T, Overgaard J. The influence of epidermal growth factor receptor and tumor differentiation on the response to accelerated radiotherapy of squamous cell carcinomas of the head and neck in the randomized DAHANCA 6 and 7 study. *Radiother Oncol* 2005;74:93–100.

27. Eshleman JS, Carlson BL, Mladek AC, Kastner BD, Shide KL, Sarkaria JN. Inhibition of the mammalian target of rapamycin sensitizes U87 xenografts to fractionated radiation therapy. *Cancer Res* 2002;62:7291–7297.

28. Foon KA, Yang XD, Weiner LM et al. Preclinical and clinical evaluations of ABX-EGF, a fully human anti-epidermal growth factor receptor antibody. *Int J Radiat Oncol Biol Phys* 2004;58:984–990.

29. Ganswindt U, Budach W, Jendrossek V, Becker G, Bamberg M, Belka C. Combination of celecoxib with percutaneous radiotherapy in patients with localised prostate cancer – A phase I study. *Radiat Oncol* 2006;1:9.

30. Glynne-Jones R, Mawdsley S, Harrison M. Cetuximab and chemoradiation for rectal cancer – Is the water getting muddy? *Acta Oncol* 2010;49:278–286.

31. Gregoire V, Hamoir M, Chen C et al. Gefitinib plus cisplatin and radiotherapy in previously untreated head and neck squamous cell carcinoma: A phase II, randomized, double-blind, placebo-controlled study. *Radiother Oncol* 2011;100:62–69.

32. Gurtner K, Deuse Y, Butof R et al. Diverse effects of combined radiotherapy and EGFR inhibition with antibodies or TK inhibitors on local tumour control and correlation with EGFR gene expression. *Radiother Oncol* 2011;99:323–330.

33. Hahn SM, Bernhard EJ, Regine W et al. A Phase I trial of the farnesyltransferase inhibitor L-778,123 and radiotherapy for locally advanced lung and head and neck cancer. *Clin Cancer Res* 2002;8:1065–1072.

34. Helbling D, Bodoky G, Gautschi O et al. Neoadjuvant chemoradiotherapy with or without panitumumab in patients with wild-type KRAS, locally advanced rectal cancer (LARC): A randomized, multicenter, phase II trial SAKK 41/07. *Ann Oncol* 2013;24:718–725.

35. Hill RP, Milas L. The proportion of stem cells in murine tumors. *Int J Radiat Oncol Biol Phys* 1989;16:513–518.

36. Jain RK. Normalization of tumor vasculature: An emerging concept in antiangiogenic therapy. *Science* 2005;307:58–62.

37. Kelly K, Chansky K, Gaspar LE et al. Updated analysis of SWOG 0023: A randomized phase III trial of gefitinib versus placebo maintenance after definitive chemoradiation followed by docetaxel in patients with locally advanced stage III non-small cell lung cancer. *J Clin Oncol* 2007;25:18S, abstract 7513.

38. Kim T. Technology evaluation: Matuzumab, Merck KGaA. *Curr Opin Mol Ther* 2004;6:96–103.

39. Koukourakis MI, Giatromanolaki A, Tsoutsou P et al. Bevacizumab, capecitabine, amifostine, and preoperative hypofractionated accelerated radiotherapy (HypoArc) for rectal cancer: A Phase II study. *Int J Radiat Oncol Biol Phys* 2011;80:492–498.

40. Kozin SV, Boucher Y, Hicklin DJ, Bohlen P, Jain RK, Suit HD. Vascular endothelial growth factor receptor-2-blocking antibody potentiates radiation-induced long-term control of human tumor xenografts. *Cancer Res* 2001;61:39–44.

41. Krause M, Baumann M. Clinical biomarkers of kinase activity: Examples from EGFR inhibition trials. *Cancer Metastasis Rev* 2008;epub.

42. Krause M, Ostermann G, Petersen C et al. Decreased repopulation as well as increased reoxygenation contribute to the improvement in local control after targeting of the EGFR by C225 during fractionated irradiation. *Radiother Oncol* 2005;76:162–167.

43. Krause M, Schutze C, Petersen C et al. Different classes of EGFR inhibitors may have different potential to improve local tumour control after fractionated irradiation: A study on C225 in FaDu hSCC. *Radiother Oncol* 2005;74:109–115.

44. Krause M, Zips D, Thames HD, Kummermehr J, Baumann M. Preclinical evaluation of molecular-targeted anticancer agents for radiotherapy. *Radiother Oncol* 2006;80:112–122.

45. Kummermehr J, Trott KR. Tumour stem cells. In: Potten CS, editor. *Stem cells*. London: Academic Press; 1997. pp. 363–400.

46. Liao Z, Mason KA, Milas L. Cyclo-oxygenase-2 and its inhibition in cancer: Is there a role? *Drugs* 2007;67:821–845.

47. Lu C, Lee JJ, Komaki R et al. A phase III study of Æ-941 with induction chemotherapy (IC) and concomitant chemoradiotherapy (CRT) for stage III non-small cell lung cancer (NSCLC) (NCI T99-0046, RTOG 02-70, MDA 99-303). *J Clin Oncol* 2007;25:18S, abstract 7527.

48. Machiels JP, Sempoux C, Scalliet P et al. Phase I/II study of preoperative cetuximab, capecitabine, and external beam radiotherapy in patients with rectal cancer. *Ann Oncol* 2007;18:738–744.

49. Martin NE, Brunner TB, Kiel KD et al. A phase I trial of the dual farnesyltransferase and geranylgeranyltransferase inhibitor L-778,123 and radiotherapy for locally advanced pancreatic cancer. *Clin Cancer Res* 2004;10:5447–5454.

50. Milas L, Fang FM, Mason KA et al. Importance of maintenance therapy in C225-induced enhancement of tumor control by fractionated radiation. *Int J Radiat Oncol Biol Phys* 2007;67:568–572.

51. Mohammadianpanah M, Razmjou-Ghalaei S, Shafizad A et al. Efficacy and safety of concurrent chemoradiation with weekly cisplatin +/- low-dose celecoxib in locally advanced undifferentiated nasopharyngeal carcinoma: A phase II–III clinical trial. *J Cancer Res Ther* 2011;7:442–447.

52. Mutter R, Lu B, Carbone DP et al. A phase II study of celecoxib in combination with paclitaxel, carboplatin, and radiotherapy for patients with inoperable stage IIIA/B non-small cell lung cancer. *Clin Cancer Res* 2009;15:2158–2165.

53. Nasu S, Ang KK, Fan Z, Milas L. C225 antiepidermal growth factor receptor antibody enhances tumor radiocurability. *Int J Radiat Oncol Biol Phys* 2001;51:474–477.

54. Okamoto I, Takahashi T, Okamoto H et al. Single-agent gefitinib with concurrent radiotherapy for locally advanced non-small cell lung cancer harboring mutations of the epidermal growth factor receptor. *Lung Cancer* 2011;72:199–204.

55. Petersen C, Eicheler W, Frömmel A et al. Proliferation and micromilieu during fractionated irradiation of human FaDu squamous cell carcinoma in nude mice. *Int J Radiat Biol* 2003;79:469–477.

56. Pinto C, Di Fabio F, Maiello E et al. Phase II study of panitumumab, oxaliplatin, 5-fluorouracil, and concurrent radiotherapy as preoperative treatment in high-risk locally advanced rectal cancer patients (StarPan/STAR-02 Study). *Ann Oncol* 2011;22:2424–2430.

57. Ready N, Janne PA, Bogart J et al. Cancer LGBCIL. Chemoradiotherapy and gefitinib in stage III non-small cell lung cancer with epidermal growth factor receptor and KRAS mutation analysis: Cancer and leukemia group B (CALEB) 30106, a CALGB-stratified phase II trial. *J Thorac Oncol* 2010;5:1382–1390.

58. Resch G, De Vries A, Ofner D et al. Colorectal Cancer Study G. Preoperative treatment with capecitabine, bevacizumab and radiotherapy for primary locally advanced rectal cancer – A two stage phase II clinical trial. *Radiother Oncol* 2012;102:10–13.

59. Rodel C, Arnold D, Hipp M et al. Phase I-II trial of cetuximab, capecitabine, oxaliplatin, and radiotherapy as preoperative treatment in rectal cancer. *Int J Radiat Oncol Biol Phys* 2008;70:1081–1086.

60. Schmidt-Ullrich RK, Contessa JN, Dent P et al. Molecular mechanisms of radiation-induced accelerated repopulation. *Radiat Oncol Investig* 1999;7:321–330.

61. Solomon MT, Selva JC, Figueredo J et al. Radiotherapy plus nimotuzumab or placebo in the treatment of high grade glioma patients: Results from a randomized, double blind trial. *BMC Cancer* 2013;13:299.

62. Uhm JH, Ballman KV, Wu W et al. Phase II evaluation of gefitinib in patients with newly diagnosed Grade 4 astrocytoma: Mayo/North Central Cancer Treatment Group Study N0074. *Int J Radiat Oncol Biol Phys* 2011;80:347–353.

63. Velenik V, Ocvirk J, Music M et al. Neoadjuvant capecitabine, radiotherapy, and bevacizumab (CRAB) in locally advanced rectal cancer: Results of an open-label phase II study. *Radiat Oncol* 2011;6:105.

64. Weppler SA, Krause M, Zyromska A, Lambin P, Baumann M, Wouters BG. Response of U87 glioma xenografts treated with concurrent rapamycin and fractionated radiotherapy: Possible role for thrombosis. *Radiother Oncol* 2007;82:96–104.

65. Willett CG, Boucher Y, di Tomaso E et al. Direct evidence that the VEGF-specific antibody bevacizumab has antivascular effects in human rectal cancer. *Nat Med* 2004;10:145–147.

66. Willett CG, Boucher Y, Duda DG et al. Surrogate markers for antiangiogenic therapy and dose-limiting toxicities for bevacizumab with radiation and chemotherapy: Continued experience of a phase I trial in rectal cancer patients. *J Clin Oncol* 2005;23:8136–8139.

67. Zips D, Hessel F, Krause M et al. Impact of adjuvant inhibition of vascular endothelial growth factor receptor tyrosine kinases on tumor growth delay and local tumor control after fractionated irradiation in human squamous cell carcinomas in nude mice. *Int J Radiat Oncol Biol Phys* 2005;61:908–914.

68. Zips D, Krause M, Hessel F et al. Experimental study on different combination schedules of VEGF-receptor inhibitor PTK787/ZK222584 and fractionated irradiation. *Anticancer Res* 2003;23:3869–3876.

## ■ FURTHER READING

69. Cengel KA, McKenna WG. Molecular targets for altering radiosensitivity: Lessons from Ras as a pre-clinical and clinical model. *Crit Rev Oncol Hematol* 2005;55:103–116.

70. Colevas AD, Brown JM, Hahn S, Mitchell J, Camphausen K, Coleman CN. Development of investigational radiation modifiers. *J Natl Cancer Inst* 2003;95:646–651.

71. Dent P, Yacoub A, Contessa J et al. Stress and radiation-induced activation of multiple intracellular signaling pathways. *Radiat Res* 2003;159:283–300.

72. Tofilon PJ, Saxman S, Coleman CN. Molecular targets for radiation therapy: Bringing preclinical data into clinical trials. *Clin Cancer Res* 2003;9:3518–3520.

# Biological individualisation of radiotherapy

## CATHARINE M.L. WEST, ROBERT G. BRISTOW AND ADRIAN C. BEGG

## 21.1 INTRODUCTION

Radiotherapy targeting and delivery have improved over the last two decades due to advances in medical physics, planning software and imaging for staging and delineation of tumour extent. Radiotherapy is now targeted with increased accuracy to tumours while minimising doses to surrounding healthy tissue. This improved delivery reduces toxicity and is leading to treatment intensification with a move towards isotoxic dose-escalated radiotherapy. To further improve clinical outcome, precision radiotherapy includes the established use of concurrent chemotherapy (see Chapter 19). There are also a number of molecularly targeted agents (see Chapter 20) to prescribe or investigate in combination with radiotherapy to improve tumour cell kill. Trials combining immunotherapy with (chemo)radiotherapy are also underway. Given the increased toxicity with multi-modality treatment, there is an increasing need to identify patients who are likely to benefit from these more aggressive (intensified) treatments using relevant biomarkers and spare those who are unlikely to benefit. Improvements with physical optimisation are now being realised and further gains in therapeutic ratio should be possible using biological optimisation.

Rapid and robust biomarkers are needed to understand enough about each patient and their tumour to choose the best treatment for that individual. At present, treatment choice is determined by clinicopathologic parameters such as tumour site, histological type, stage and performance status. These factors provide only broad prognostic groupings within which outcomes vary. There are different types of biomarkers and those that are prognostic or predictive are most relevant for clinical radiobiology research. A prognostic marker provides information on the risk of local or systemic outcome (e.g. recurrence) independent of treatment. A predictive marker provides information on outcome which is treatment dependent. Clinical radiobiology is particularly interested in the development of predictive biomarkers that identify patients who would benefit from a particular treatment: surgery versus radiotherapy for some cancers; the radiotherapy fractionation schedule (conventional, accelerated or hypofractionated); hypoxia modification; a molecularly targeted agent such as an epidermal growth factor receptor (EGFR) antagonist or temozolomide. As the interest is prediction rather than prognostication, the best way of identifying biomarkers is generally within the context

of randomised trials. The exceptions are when measuring radiosensitivity to predict for risk of toxicity (observational cohorts can be studied) or benefit of radiotherapy over surgery (both surgical and radiotherapy cohorts must be studied as randomisation between these two treatments is difficult).

There are many approaches for biomarker development that include investigation of functional assays, high-throughput technologies to derive DNA, RNA or protein profiles, and functional or molecular imaging. There are an increasing number of guidelines improving the quality of biomarker research (2,30,37,42,55,73). There is also an increasing emphasis on biomarker validation and qualification rather than solely on discovery, as this is important for the development of assays for widespread clinical use.

This chapter reviews predictive assay research and the development of approaches for the biological individualisation of radiotherapy.

## 21.2 MATERIALS AND METHODS FOR PREDICTIVE ASSAYS

Figure 21.1 summarises approaches for developing predictive assays for radiotherapy. The materials and methods are many and can be tumour site specific depending on the clinical question being addressed. The most widely studied tumour tissue is formalin fixed and paraffin embedded (FFPE) because relatively large retrospective studies can be carried out in stored material. Fresh frozen tissue is also used as some assays require enzymatic activity or post-translational protein modifications which can be lost during formalin fixation. Assays have also been developed using circulating tumour cells or DNA in blood. Whole blood can be collected (for DNA), or separated buffy coat (for lymphocyte assays), plasma or serum. Sometimes other normal tissue samples are taken, e.g. skin biopsies. Macromolecules taken for study can be DNA (including mitochondrial), RNA (coding and non-coding) or protein. Sequencing of the human genome and the development of high-throughput technologies are increasingly being used to derive both prognostic and predictive gene signatures. Methods for genome-wide analysis are widely used, e.g. there are arrays to analyse single nucleotide polymorphisms (SNPs), DNA methylation, large

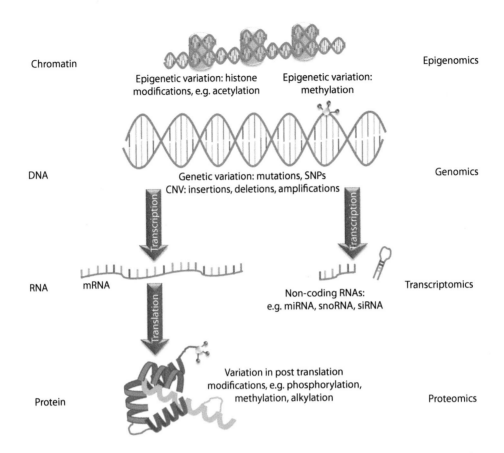

**Figure 21.1** Approaches for the development of predictive assays for radiotherapy. The approaches involve epigenomics, genomics, transcriptomics or proteomics to assess, respectively, chromatin, DNA, RNA or protein. The middle panel shows the relationships between the biological processes.

genome alterations via comparative genomic hybridisation (CGH) and activity via mRNA and non-coding RNAs (e.g. microRNAs). Although not feasible on a proteome-wide level, it is now possible to study a large number of proteins using proteomics. The development of tissue microarrays has facilitated the study of protein expression in large numbers of archival tissue samples. Application of these methods shows promise for developing biomarkers for tumour diagnosis, prognosis and prediction. Biomarkers for cancer treatment individualisation are now being used clinically; but none that specifically target outcome in radiotherapy patients.

## The DNA level

Individuals are genetically diverse, cancer occurs due to genetic alterations and genome instability is a feature of cancer. Individual genetic variation affects risks of developing cancer, treatment toxicity and tumour response. The heterogeneity of genetic alterations in cancer underlies variation in patient response to therapy. Mutation analyses are used clinically, e.g. the presence of *BRCA1/2* germline mutations in those with a family history of breast or ovarian cancer for response to poly(ADP-ribosylation)-polymerase inhibitors; lack of tumour *KRAS* mutations to predict benefit from cetuximab in EGFR-expressing colorectal cancer;

somatic mutations in *KIT* for benefit from imatinib. No mutation analyses are used specifically for radiotherapy patients. Individuals with homozygous germline mutations in *ATM* are hypersensitive to the damaging effects of radiation. Such mutations are so rare, and generally phenotypically obvious, that they have no role as a routine test to predict radiotherapy outcomes.

Mutations that are not deleterious become more prevalent in a population. SNPs are mutations seen in >1% of the population. As they are common, they are widely investigated for risk prediction. SNPs occur every ~300 bases with >10 million in the human genome. Current research in the area is possible because of consortium-driven sequencing and haplotype mapping of the human genome. Groups of SNPs are co-inherited as haplotypes and analysis of one SNP in a haplotype is used to infer others using data from the human haplotype map. Genome-wide analysis, therefore, involves ~500,000 rather than >10 million SNPs and is affordable. SNP profiling can look for germline (e.g. blood or saliva samples) or somatic (tumour samples) variation.

SNPs account for ~90% of genetic variation in humans. Copy number variation (CNV) – deletions or duplications of large regions of DNA – is another type of genetic variation. High-density arrays can detect genome-wide CNV in tumours, and the percent of genomic alterations used as a surrogate of genomic instability (47) to develop a prognostic genomic classifier (46). In addition to genetic sequence variation, there can be epigenetic variation that includes methylation, acetylation, phosphorylation, ubiquitylation, sumoylation and chromatin modification. DNA methylation is the most widely studied. There is good evidence that *MGMT* methylation predicts benefit from the addition of temozolomide to radiotherapy in patients with brain tumours (34,51,67). This evidence led to trial testing alternative chemotherapeutics to give with radiotherapy in patients with non-methylated *MGMT* (35), highlighting how trials are moving towards biomarker-selected or biomarker-enriched populations.

High-throughput next-generation sequencing methods enable rapid sequencing of large stretches of DNA base pairs spanning entire genomes. Next-generation sequencing is starting to transform laboratory approaches to extracting information on genomes, epigenomes (the group of modifications that occur in genomes) and transcriptomes (the set of RNA molecules, including mRNA, rRNA, tRNA and other non-coding RNA in a cell or sample). Sequencing the first human genome was a large collaborative project that took about 10 years to complete. The same data can now be obtained in a few days at a fraction of the cost and next-generation sequencing technology underpins the development of biomarkers assessing genetic heterogeneity (53,64). Cancer genome sequencing has potential to derive biomarkers for cancer diagnosis, prognosis and prediction of treatment response. The technology is also used in a targeted way to study specific regions such as exomes (the parts of the genome that are transcribed). Analysis of the mutational burden of tumours has revealed the diversity of mutational processes underlying cancer development (1), which should lead to refinement of pathology classifications and progression to greater individualisation of treatment.

Another method for detecting DNA in tumour samples is *in situ* hybridisation (ISH). ISH uses labelled cDNA (a probe) to identify a specific DNA sequence in a sample in tissue sections. For example, ISH is used to detect the integration of oncogenic human papilloma viruses (HPVs) into formalin-fixed, paraffin-embedded tumour cells. HPV testing in head and neck cancer is increasingly part of clinical diagnosis and a likely candidate for future risk stratification (3). Trials are investigating de-escalation of treatment in HPV-positive head and neck cancer with the aim of reducing radiotherapy side effects. Fluorescence *in situ* hybridisation (FISH) is also used on archival tissue, e.g. to study genomic imbalances associated with individual genes such as gain of *MYC*, *PTEN* and EGFR gain in relation to radiotherapy outcomes.

## The RNA level

ISH and FISH are also used to detect RNA in samples *in situ*. However, a more widely used approach is to use gene expression arrays to derive signatures or profiles or classifiers associated with prognosis or prediction of treatment outcome. Expression microarrays are small chips containing many thousands of DNA sequences in spots, one DNA sequence per spot. The DNA can be cDNA (messenger RNA back-translated into more stable complementary DNA [cDNA]) but more usually oligomers (short DNA chains) representing the partial sequence of a gene. Messenger RNA, representing all expressed genes, is extracted from a tumour or other sample of interest, then fluorescently labelled and added to the chip, where labelled RNA hybridizes only to the spot for that gene having the complementary DNA sequence. Highly expressed genes have bright spots on the array, while lowly expressed genes show low signals. After hybridization, the array is scanned automatically and rapidly to measure the expression of all genes.

Signatures are derived in different ways. A 'supervised' analysis can, for example, identify a set of genes with high or low expression associated with a specific treatment response (e.g. classify radiotherapy responders versus non-responders). Before such expression signatures are used in the clinic to select treatment options, they require rigorous testing and validation. Signatures are used in breast cancer patients to identify those with a high risk of recurrence (e.g. MammaPrint 70-gene signature) or who are likely to benefit from chemotherapy (e.g. Onco*type* DX 21-gene signature) and studies of both these tests show that their routine use is cost effective (62). The Oncotype DX Breast DCIS Score estimates 10-year local recurrence of ductal carcinoma *in situ* (DCIS) or invasive breast cancer. With the increased prevalence of DCIS due to screening programmes, the impact of the test on the need for adjuvant radiotherapy is being explored (52). 'Unsupervised' analyses use neural networking to identify commonalities between tumours to derive a set of co-expressed genes in a series of samples, which can then be tested post hoc to see if they are prognostic or predictive of outcomes. Signatures can be trained on a phenotype, e.g. hypoxia (71), and can be derived using data collected on cell lines, e.g. measurements of radiosensitivity (22).

Real-time or quantitative polymerase chain reaction (qPCR) is a technique used to amplify and simultaneously quantify a targeted DNA molecule. qPCR detects and quantifies RNA either as an absolute number of copies (e.g. NanoString methodology) or relative to normalising reference genes. Real-time reverse-transcription PCR (qRT-PCR) detects gene expression through creation of cDNA transcripts from RNA. qPCR is used in assessing expression of individual genes or signatures and has proven ability for clinical application (71). There are other approaches for measuring the expression of small signatures following whole genome profiling, e.g. Taqman low-density arrays (12). Technology is continually changing with new methods for multiplex detection of multiple genes, e.g. QuantiGene and Nanostring.

Non-coding RNAs are not translated into protein. Examples are microRNAs (miRNA), snoRNA and siRNA. miRNA are small non-coding RNAs of 19–24 nucleotides that generally downregulate gene expression by inhibiting protein translation. It is estimated that miRNAs affect expression of up to 30% of the genes in the mammalian genome. miRNAs play a role in development, differentiation, apoptosis and the initiation and progression of human cancers. miRNA profiling is showing potential to provide information on radiobiologically relevant features (e.g. hypoxia and radiosensitivity) and prognosis (27,32). Current research is moving away from microarray approaches for gene expression analyses to using next-generation sequencing technologies. RNA sequencing allows for quantification of absolute levels of normal and mutant transcripts and is used for gene expression profiling of different mRNA species, including small non-coding RNAs.

## The protein level

Since proteins (rather than mRNA) carry out the actual cellular functions, expression profiling at the protein level should in principle be better than at the mRNA level. However, proteins are an order of magnitude more diverse in structure and complexity (including post-translational modifications such as phosphorylation or acetylation) making such profiling more difficult. Despite this, rapid progress is being made including the development of antibody chips and mass spectrometry approaches. Proteomics using powerful mass spectrometry methods as clinical predictors has so far been restricted mainly to the study of serum proteins (50). There is increasing use of multi-analyte immunobead-based profiling using Luminex technology (19).

In addition, simple immunohistochemistry can be 'high throughput' by using tissue microarrays, in which hundreds of small paraffin-embedded tumour samples from different patients are placed on one microscope slide (45). Staining with a particular antibody can then be done simultaneously for all tumours in a clinical series. Scoring and registration of the data can also be automated. This is far from genome wide, since candidate protein targets (and the antibodies which detect them) must be chosen based on prior knowledge, and usually restricted to up to 30 markers. However, this method is ideal for testing potential predictive markers in retrospective series.

## 21.3 RADIOBIOLOGICAL DETERMINANTS OF RADIOTHERAPY OUTCOME

The radiobiological determinants of radiotherapy outcome can be categorised broadly as intrinsic radiosensitivity (tumour and individual), proliferation rate or the ability to undergo accelerated repopulation, and the extent of hypoxia. These are largely independent, e.g. radiosensitive tumours could have a range of proliferation rates and degrees of hypoxia; and tumours with high proliferation rates could have a range of radiosensitivities and degrees of hypoxia. These three key factors should thus be considered separately, and the goal is to measure them all to maximise the chance of accurately predicting response. In addition to these radiobiological parameters, there will be other factors that determine success or failure such as tumour size (reflecting

clonogen/stem cell number), propensity for angiogenesis, metastatic potential and immune response. Large tumours are harder to control than small tumours simply because there are more cells to kill which will require higher doses. In addition, they may be more genetically variable due to continuous mutations, increasing the likelihood of resistant subpopulations. Tumour size should therefore be taken into account when assessing the performance of a predictive assay, and multivariable analyses controlling for clinical stage and other factors should always be carried out to determine the added value of such tests. In general, the primary endpoint for tumour predictive assay research should be local control. Metastatic potential is clearly important for survival, but should initially be considered separately from factors affecting local tumour control.

## Tumour radiosensitivity

The term *radiosensitivity* is used in different contexts (cellular, tissue and clinical). It is classically measured using radiation survival curves (see Chapter 4) from which several parameters are derived, but different assays are used. Intrinsic radiosensitivity is that which is genetically determined. Actual radiosensitivity depends on the assay or cell type used. Work in the 1980s highlighted the importance of radiosensitivity as a factor influencing tumour response to radiotherapy (26) and showed that parameters derived from the initial part of radiation survival curves were the best measures of radiosensitivity: surviving fraction at 2 Gy (SF2), $\alpha$ and Dbar. Tumours vary in radiosensitivity both between and within different histological types. Primary human tumour SF2 was a significant and independent prognostic factor for radiotherapy outcome in both carcinoma of the cervix (77) and head and neck (13). However, findings from other studies were equivocal. The disadvantages of the colony assay are its poor success rate for human tumours (<70%) and the time needed to produce data (often up to 4 weeks). Subsequent studies evaluated alternative assays that generate results in less than a week. Examples include chromosome damage, DNA damage and apoptosis. However, comparing these assays with the 'gold standard' of clonogenic cell death in cell lines showed variable results. Most functional cell-based assays have limited clinical utility as predictive assays due to poor reproducibility, but have been useful in confirming one mechanism underlying differences in response of tumours to radiotherapy.

Attempts are being made to derive gene signatures associated with tumour radiosensitivity. The most developed signature was derived using measurements of SF2 in the NCI-60 panel of cell lines. A subsequent systems biology approach involved a network analysis to identify 10 genes. A radiosensitivity index (RSI) is calculated by ranking the expression of these 10 genes and using a ranked-based linear algorithm. RSI was prognostic in several data sets and predictive of benefit from radiotherapy over surgery in breast cancer patients (22) (Figure 21.2). The RSI has also been combined

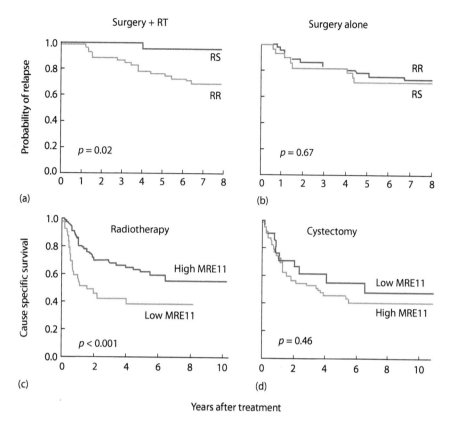

Figure 21.2 Prediction of benefit from radiotherapy over surgery. The upper graphs show a tumour radiosensitivity signature predicts benefit from adjuvant radiotherapy in breast cancer patients. Patients with radiosensitive tumours (RS) have a better outcome following with radiotherapy (RT) than those with radioresistant (RR) tumours (a). There is no difference in outcome for patients with RS and RR tumours treated with surgery alone (b). High tumour MRE11 expression is associated with a good outcome following radiotherapy (c) but is not prognostic for outcome following cystectomy (d). (From (18,22).)

with the linear-quadratic model to derive a genomic adjusted radiation dose (GARD), which was shown to be prognostic for radiotherapy outcomes in several tumour types (65).

An example of the use of supervised analyses to generate a signature that predicts benefit from radiotherapy is the work of Zhao et al. (79), who developed and validated a 24-gene predictor of response to postoperative radiotherapy in prostate cancer (80).

Studies also investigate protein expression of DNA damage response markers with a goal of predicting benefit from radiotherapy. A well-developed example showed that high protein expression of MRE11 in muscle-invasive bladder cancer predicted benefit from radiotherapy over cystectomy (18) (Figure 21.2). This study is highlighted as it involved both a discovery and a replication cohort, and it was subsequently reproduced by an independent group (48). A number of studies measured expression of DNA-PK associated proteins but high expression has been associated with both good and poor outcomes following radiotherapy. Contradictory findings are common in molecular marker studies and highlight the need to develop standardised methods, cut-offs and approaches (e.g. discovery and validation cohorts). The latter is crucial for the future development of predictive assays for radiotherapy.

## Tumour hypoxia

There is good evidence that measurements of tumour hypoxia are prognostic for outcomes following radiotherapy in several cancers. Evidence for an association between measurements of hypoxia in individual human tumours and response to radiotherapy are summarised in Chapters 17 and 18. Hypoxia has also been shown to be a negative prognostic factor after treatment with chemotherapy or surgery. The latter is consistent with data showing that hypoxia plays a key role in tumour progression by promoting both angiogenesis and metastasis.

Individualisation of radiotherapy requires methods to predict benefit from hypoxia modification (see Chapter 17). Many methods have been developed to measure tumour hypoxia. Although studies showed oxygen electrode measurements provide prognostic information, the approach has not been evaluated as a predictive test. The equipment is not widely available and the Eppendorf machine has not been made for a number of years. There is evidence that extrinsic hypoxia-specific chemical probes such as pimonidazole can predict benefit from the addition of carbogen and nicotinamide to radiotherapy (see Table 21.1). Pimonidazole is a nitroimidazole which undergoes bioreduction only under

Table 21.1 Measuring hypoxia to predict benefit from hypoxia modification of radiotherapy

| Method | Cancer | Treatment | n | p | Reference |
|---|---|---|---|---|---|
| Pimonidazole | HNC | AR ± CON | 38 | 0.010 | Kaanders et al. (40) |
| $^{18}$F-FMISO PET | HNC | CRT ± tirapazamine | 45 | 0.006 | Rischin et al. (61) |
| Osteopontin | HNC | RT ± nimorazole | 320 | 0.006 | Overgaard et al. (56) |
| CA9 | HNC | RT ± nimorazole | 320 | 0.800 | Eriksen et al. (20) |
| Pimonidazole | HNC | AR ± CON | 79 | 0.010 | Janssens et al. (39) |
| 15-gene | HNC | RT ± nimorazole | 323 | 0.003 | Toustrup et al. (71) |
| Osteopontin | HNC | CRT ± tirapazamine | 578 | 0.870 | Lim et al. (49) |
| 26-gene | HNC | AR ± CON | 157 | 0.009 | Eustace et al. (24) |
| 26-gene | Bladder | RT ± CON | 185 | 0.400 | Eustace et al. (24) |
| Necrosis | Bladder | RT ± CON | 231 | 0.001 | Eustace et al. (23) |
| CA9 | Bladder | RT ± CON | 189 | 0.030 | Eustace et al. (23) |
| EGFR low | HNC | AR ± CON | 272 | 0.009 | Nijkamp et al. (54) |
| $^{18}$F-FAZA PET | HNC | CRT ± tirapazamine | 24 | 0.004 | Graves et al. (29) |
| mir-210 | Bladder | RT ± CON | 183 | 0.070 | Irlam-Jones et al. (38) |
| 24-gene | Bladder | RT ± CON | 151 | 0.015 | Yang et al. (78) |

*Abbreviations:* HNC, head and neck cancer; AR, accelerated radiotherapy; CON, carbogen and nicotinamide; CRT, chemo-radiotherapy; RT, radiotherapy.

hypoxic conditions, followed by binding of reduced products to macromolecules. Bound adducts can be detected with an antibody and measured using immunohistochemistry. The approach requires prospective administration, which limits the ability to validate its predictive performance in multiple cohorts.

The most widely studied approach for assessing tumour hypoxia involves measuring hypoxia-inducible proteins (intrinsic hypoxia markers). These are mainly measured using immunohistochemistry on FFPE tumour biopsies. The most widely studied markers are CA9, HIF-1$\alpha$ and Glut-1. The best evidence for an association with a poor prognosis is for CA9 (60) but the results for prediction of benefit from adding hypoxia modification to radiotherapy are mixed (Table 21.1). Further work is required to standardise the methods used. Similarly mixed results have been found for studies looking at osteopontin levels in plasma samples (Table 21.1). Lack of standardisation and reproducibility of methods are issues for protein markers.

At the RNA level, gene expression signatures show promise as predictive markers (Table 21.1; Figure 21.3). There are an expanding number of signatures being derived using a variety of methods. A few signatures have been validated in multiple cohorts, shown to predict benefit from hypoxia modification of radiotherapy and have progressed to prospective qualification in clinical trials.

The use of fluorinated derivatives of bioreductive drugs allows their detection by non-invasive PET (5). This approach has the additional advantage of sampling the whole tumour and not just a small part of it. These drugs depend upon hypoxia for their reduction, although there are other factors that can influence their quantification and make them a less direct measure of hypoxia than is the case with electrodes. However, such agents are useful

for quantifying hypoxia in human tumours and changes during treatment, although they require administration of a drug. $^{18}$F-Fluoroazomycinarabinoside (FAZA) PET is currently of interest as a potential predictor of benefit from hypoxia modification of radiotherapy (29). Other imaging methods that are being evaluated to measure tumour hypoxia in the clinic include computed tomography and magnetic resonance imaging (36). Progress in this area is limited because studies are often small, replication is not carried out and there are many different imaging protocols.

## Tumour repopulation

The importance of tumour proliferation clinically is most clearly shown by the higher doses required to control a tumour when overall treatment time is increased (see Chapters 8 and 10). Further evidence comes from studies showing loss of local tumour control as a result of gaps in treatment, whether planned or unplanned. There is also evidence from randomised trials that accelerated regimens can improve outcome (see Chapter 11).

Methods for measuring tumour proliferation include counting the mitotic index (proportion of mitoses in tissue sections), determining the proportion of cells in the S-phase of the cell cycle by DNA flow cytometry, measuring the tumour potential doubling time, $T_{pot}$, with thymidine analogues such as IdUrd and BrdUrd, and using antibodies to detect proliferation-associated proteins. However, a multi-centre analysis of over 470 head and neck cancer patients treated with radiotherapy alone showed a lack of significance of $T_{pot}$ as a predictor (9). A number of other studies showed a significant although usually weak correlation between

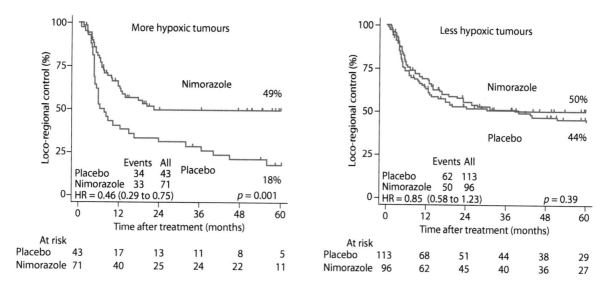

**Figure 21.3** Measurements of hypoxia predict benefit from hypoxia-modifying nimorazole in patients with head and neck cancer. (Reprinted from (71), with permission from Elsevier and the author.)

labelling index (LI) and radiotherapy outcome. Therefore, pre-treatment LI or $T_{pot}$ measurements are not sufficiently robust for determining tumour cell proliferation for prediction of radiotherapy outcome.

Nevertheless, there is evidence from several independent studies that it is possible to predict which patients benefit from accelerated rather than conventionally fractionated radiotherapy. As always, the strongest data are from randomised trials. Molecular marker profiles (protein expression) were derived in tumour material from patients enrolled in the randomised trial of conventional versus continuous hyperfractionated accelerated radiotherapy (CHART) in head and neck cancer. Tumours negative for p53 and Bcl-2 with a low but organised pattern of Ki-67 staining benefitted from CHART (16). A second study on the CHART trial showed high tumour-EGFR-expressing head and neck cancers benefitted from

accelerated radiotherapy (10) (Figure 21.4). This finding was confirmed in several independent studies (21,66,68). It was subsequently shown that high EGFR expression correlates with accelerated proliferation during radiotherapy in head and neck cancer (59). These findings warrant further study for biomarker development.

## Normal tissue radiosensitivity

The existence of individuals with extreme sensitivity to ionizing radiation was first highlighted by a study showing the hypersensitivity of fibroblasts cultured from a patient with ataxia telangiectasia (70). Then in the 1980s there was evidence for a range of radiosensitivities within the general population without known genetic syndromes. Further evidence for differences in cellular radiosensitivity as a

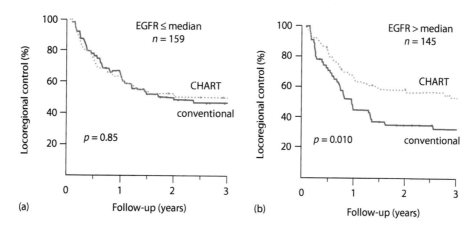

**Figure 21.4** High tumour EGFR expression predicts benefit from accelerated radiotherapy in patients enrolled in a randomised trial of continuous hyperfractionated accelerated radiotherapy (CHART). Tumours with low EGFR expression (a) show no benefit from the CHART whereas those with high EGFR expression (b) benefit from an accelerated regimen. (From (10), with permission of the author and reprinted with permission ©2005 American Society of Clinical Oncology. All rights reserved.)

determinant of normal tissue response to radiotherapy came from studies showing that inherent differences between individuals dominated normal tissue reactions more than other contributing factors (72).

In the 1990s, studies investigated whether the *in vitro* radiosensitivity of normal cells could predict risk of radiotherapy toxicity. Several small studies showed correlations between fibroblast radiosensitivity and the severity of late effects (17) but the findings were not confirmed in subsequent larger studies (58). Some studies showed that peripheral blood lymphocyte radiosensitivity correlated with the severity of late effects (76).

More rapid assays have also been evaluated, including the measurement of chromosome and DNA damage, and plasma proteins. Although some significant correlations with toxicity were reported, other studies showed no relationship. A general problem has been that experimental (assay) variability has been relatively large compared with inter-individual differences in radiosensitivity. Several groups have shown that low levels of radiation-induced apoptosis in pre-treatment lymphocytes predict increased risk of radiotherapy toxicity (14,15,33,57,63). The radiation-induced lymphocyte apoptosis (RILA) assay was validated in a prospective trial as a predictor of risk of breast fibrosis following radiotherapy (4). Expression profiling of patient lymphocytes irradiated *ex vivo* has also produced signatures correlating with the severity of normal tissue injury (69).

Radiosensitivity is a heritable trait and there are numerous candidate genes for radiotherapy toxicity (75). SNPs in these genes have been investigated in over 70 studies with many reporting positive associations (8). However, a large study failed to validate all reported SNP associations (7), and it is increasingly recognised that the reported effect sizes are generally unrealistically high. In 2009 an international Radiogenomics Consortium was established to encourage multi-centre cooperation and improve the quality of studies (74). Genome-wide association studies are identifying new candidate genes for radiotherapy toxicity (25,43) and risk of second cancer induction following radiotherapy (11). The advantage of the SNP approach is that easily accessible lymphocytes are ideal for the measurements and little biomarker development is required as clinical research laboratories for genetic testing are established. Once common variants (SNPs) have been identified, further studies need to explore other types of genetic variation (e.g. copy number variation and DNA methylation).

## 21.4 DEVELOPING TESTS FOR CLINICAL DECISION-MAKING

Development of a test for clinical decision-making involves three steps: discovery, validation and qualification. Most of the work published focuses on discovery. There are numerous tests and methods for assessing tumour hypoxia but none that have been validated and qualified for clinical use. Once a

test or marker or profile is identified, then detailed validation is required. For an assay or biomarker to have clinical utility, it must be precise and accurate. Progress in predictive assay research has been hampered because of insufficient effort assessing repeatability (intra-assay precision; multiple determinants of a sample in a single test), determining reproducibility (inter-assay variability) and establishing standardised assays that yielded reproducible results between laboratories. Intra-tumour/individual variability must also be studied in relation to inter-tumour/individual variability. Where relevant, the quantitation limit and linear range of a test should be given. If possible, sensitivity (number of true positives/[number of true positives + number of false negatives]) and specificity (number of true negatives/[number of true negatives + number of false positives]) should be determined. A receiver operating characteristic (ROC) curve should also be produced.

Many of the predictive assays studied in the past suffered from poor reproducibility because they were functional assays. RNA and plasma proteomics are very suited to detailed repeatability and reproducibility analyses. As signatures/profiles are derived, assay development becomes important. Faced with an increasing number of methods, a challenge in this area is in choosing which platform for assay development. For SNP testing in relation to prediction of risk of normal tissue toxicity, clinical laboratories are already established for genetic testing and the focus can be on discovery rather than assay development. However, the most widely studied biomarker is possibly protein expression using immunohistochemistry on FFPE tumour material. This type of biomarker is particularly challenging to reproduce because of the use of different antigen retrieval methods, antibodies, scoring methods and cut-off values. The breast cancer community put considerable effort into standardising methods for determining ER, PR and HER2 status (31) and the radiobiology community needs to follow their example. The promising results obtained using MRE11 (Figure 21.2) need to be followed by careful assay standardisation before the work is repeated in multiple cohorts using different methods and cut-off values for determining high expression, an approach likely to lead to conflicting findings and to hinder progress.

Once a predictive marker is discovered and validated, then qualification is required. It must be tested under standardised conditions in new cohorts of patients and preferably prospectively. This prospective testing might involve randomisation to standard or biomarker determined treatment.

## 21.5 INDIVIDUALISATION OF MOLECULARLY TARGETED AGENTS

For many cancers chemotherapy is now given concurrently with radiotherapy (see Chapter 19). There are also an increasing number of molecularly targeted agents to combine with radiation (see Chapter 20). These agents need to be targeted to those patients most likely to benefit. For example there is good evidence that *MGMT* methylation status predicts benefit from the addition of temozolomide to radiotherapy in patients with brain tumours (34,51,67). Temozolomide is hydrolysed in the body to form an active metabolite (3-methyl-[triazen-1-yl]imidazole-4-carboxamide) that produces approximately 12 base adducts in DNA including the cytotoxic lesion O6-methylguanine (O6-meG). *MGMT* encodes for O6-methylguanine-DNA methyltransferase that removes O6-meG from DNA and so the efficacy of temozolomide is increased when the gene is silenced following methylation. However, *MGMT* methylation testing is not used routinely in clinical decision-making because of poor precision. Temozolomide radiotherapy is not more effective than radiotherapy alone in some patients with *MGMT* promoter methylation and some patients whose tumours lack methylation appear to benefit from temozolomide. It is therefore likely that adducts in addition to O6-meG may affect treatment outcome.

A second example is EGFR antagonists. Cetuximab-treated patients with prominent cetuximab-induced rash (grade 2 or above) have better survival than patients with zero or grade 1 rash (6). In the future the presence or absence of a cetuximab-induced rash could be used to identify patients who might benefit from more prolonged treatment with cetuximab or treatment with other agents. However, there is currently no *a priori* predictive assay for the successful use of cetuximab in combination with radiotherapy as EGFR mutations are rare in head and neck cancers and EGFR expression does not predict cetuximab efficacy in this setting.

## 21.6 HPV AND RADIOTHERAPY INDIVIDUALISATION

The prevalence of HPV-associated head and neck cancer rose dramatically over the past 20 years and the first decade of the twenty-first century saw a rapid increase in studies of HPV in head and neck cancer. HPV is associated in particular with oropharyngeal cancers and a good prognosis. There is debate over the best way of assessing HPV positivity – the main approaches used are PCR assays, *in situ* hybridisation and immunohistochemistry for p16 expression. PCR is often considered the gold standard probably because of its use in cervical screening. PCR can measure DNA or E6/E7 mRNA, which indicate the presence of HPV but do not distinguish integrated and episomal forms of the virus. *In situ* hybridisation shows viral integration but is technically difficult. The p16 is a protein involved in cell-cycle regulation that is encoded by cyclin-dependent kinase inhibitor 2A (*CDKN2A*), which is a tumour suppressor gene. The immunohistochemistry of p16 is straightforward, widely available and considered a rapid screening method for HPV positivity. The p16 is considered to be a marker that could be used for individualisation of treatment possibly alone or

followed by PCR and/or *in situ* hybridisation to determine the presence of the virus.

There is a high level of evidence that HPV-associated head and neck cancers have a good prognosis. HPV status is the strongest independent prognostic factor for outcome following chemoradiotherapy (3). Patients with HPV positive versus negative head and neck cancers tend to be younger and less likely to smoke. Mutations in *TP53* are less common. Hypoxia might be less important, but this is debated. Although there are some conflicting data, evidence suggests enhanced radiosensitivity in HPV-positive head and neck cancer (44). A prognostic classifier was developed based on HPV status, smoking history and tumour stage that divided patients into low-, intermediate- or high-risk groups (3) and the classifier was subsequently validated in an independent cohort (28). Nevertheless, there is continuing debate over exactly how to individualise treatment based on HPV status. Some clinical trials are exploring de-escalation of treatment (41) and future trials will likely increasingly focus on selected populations with HPV-positive or HPV-negative cancers.

## 21.7 HOW SHOULD CLINICIANS RESPOND TO PREDICTION RESULTS?

There is now good evidence that patients that have (1) hypoxic tumours benefit most from combining hypoxia-modifying treatment with radiotherapy, (2) high EGFR-expressing tumours benefit from accelerated rather than conventional radiotherapy, (3) *MGMT* methylation in brain tumours benefits from the addition of temozolomide to radiotherapy, and (4) HPV-associated head and neck tumours have a good prognosis following radiotherapy. When reliable predictive assays are developed, their successful use must depend on the availability of alternative treatments. For example, patients with very hypoxic tumours could be assigned to treatments which include hypoxia-modifying or hypoxia-exploiting agents (e.g. CON, nimorazole or tirapazamine; see Chapter 17). Tumours with fast repopulation potential would be candidates for accelerated fractionation (including hypofractionation), or radiotherapy combined with drugs designed to combat proliferation (e.g. EGFR inhibitors).

In the short term, patients with radioresistant tumours may benefit from switching to an alternative therapeutic modality such as surgery or chemotherapy. Other strategies include the use of combined chemoradiotherapy or augmenting the radiation dose to the whole tumour using some form of conformal or high-LET therapy where possible or to specific areas of a tumour identified as radioresistant based on biopsies or imaging.

In the long term, the goal is to be able to obtain a complete genetic picture of each tumour, thereby understanding why a tumour is radioresistant, allowing a rational choice of tumour-specific radiosensitising drugs of the types described in Chapter 20. Continuing progress is being made in developing techniques for monitoring tumour genetics and this, coupled with the increasing pace of development of molecular-targeted drugs, should mean that more tumour-specific therapies with less toxicity should emerge in the not too distant future.

Last, if reliable information were available for predicting the risk of severe normal tissue effects, possible strategies would be to offer surgery rather than radiotherapy for some cancers (e.g. mastectomy rather than breast-conserving radiotherapy; surgery rather than radiotherapy for some bladder and head and neck tumours); to reduce the radiation dose for radiosensitive individuals; to offer a radioprotective agent (assuming the agent does not also protect tumours); or to use a post-radiotherapy strategy designed to reduce vascular and parenchymal consequences of irradiation, such as anti-TGF-$\beta$ and anti-inflammatory approaches (see Chapter 24).

In the short term, predictive assays could play an important role in enhancing patient populations in clinical trials to improve the detection of efficacy. For example, early phase trials of a new hypoxia-modifying agent could focus on patients identified as having the most hypoxic tumours. Also, therapy intensification could be trialled initially in sub-populations most likely to benefit, in order to reduce risk of additional toxicity in others. An example might be to select HPV-negative head and neck cancer for therapy intensification. The latter approach is less dependent on a high specificity for predicting, for example, good local control following radiotherapy. The development of new molecularly targeted agents focuses on specific pathways and it is increasingly common for pre-clinical studies to attempt to identify mutations that increase or decrease cytotoxicity. This work is likely to lead to an increase in trials focusing on particular sub-groups of patients.

## 21.8 SUMMARY

Designing treatments which are tailored to the individual patient requires (1) extensive knowledge of the genetics of that individual and of their tumour; (2) well-validated biomarkers that are reproducible; (3) the availability of alternative treatments and an array of agents which attack specific genes or pathways. With the rapid development of genome-wide screening approaches providing new information on tumour genetics, there has been considerable progress in the area of outcome prediction. It is hoped and anticipated that this will lead to more rational therapies.

### Key points

1. Once improvements with physical optimisation of radiotherapy are realised further gains in therapeutic ratio require biological optimisation.
2. Intrinsic tumour cell radiosensitivity is a significant and independent prognostic factor for radiotherapy outcome, but functional assays have limited clinical utility as predictive assays. Derivation of gene

signatures associated with tumour radiosensitivity is a promising approach.
3. Tumour hypoxia is an adverse prognostic factor after treatment with radiotherapy, chemotherapy or surgery and is predictive of benefit from hypoxia-modifying therapy. Derivation of gene signatures associated with tumour hypoxia is a promising approach.
4. Tumour proliferation, or repopulation, during fractionated radiotherapy is an important factor determining outcome. Several studies showed high tumour EGFR expression predicts benefit from accelerated radiotherapy in head and neck cancer.
5. An assay is needed that measures normal tissue radiosensitivity to spare undue toxicity in a subgroup of patients by dose reduction or applying alternative modalities. A radiation-induced lymphocyte assay has been validated and studies are identifying the common genetic variants (SNPs) associated with risk of toxicity.
6. HPV positivity is associated with a good outcome following radiotherapy in head and neck cancer and clinical trials are investigating de-escalated therapy and starting to select populations according to HPV status.
7. Tumour *MGMT* methylation is associated with a good response to temozolomide, but is not being used to individualise treatments.

## ■ BIBLIOGRAPHY

1. Alexandrov LB, Nik-Zainal S, Wedge DC et al. Signatures of mutational processes in human cancer. *Nature* 2013;500: 415–421.
2. Altman DG, McShane LM, Sauerbrei W, Taube SE. Reporting recommendations for tumor marker prognostic studies (REMARK): Explanation and elaboration. *PLoS Med* 2012;9: e1001216.
3. Ang KK, Harris J, Wheeler R et al. Human papillomavirus and survival of patients with oropharyngeal cancer. *N Engl J Med* 2010;363:24–35.
4. Azria D, Riou O, Castan F et al. Radiation-induced CD8 T-lymphocyte apoptosis as a predictor of breast fibrosis after radiotherapy: Results of the prospective multicenter french trial. *EBioMedicine* 2015;2:1965–1973.
5. Bachmann KA, Burkman AM. Phenylbutazone-warfarin interaction in the dog. *J Pharm Pharmacol* 1975;27:832–836.
6. Bar-Ad V, Zhang QE, Harari PM et al. Correlation between the severity of cetuximab-induced skin rash and clinical outcome for head and neck cancer patients: The RTOG Experience. *Int J Radiat Oncol Biol Phys* 2016;95:1346–1354.
7. Barnett GC, Coles CE, Elliott RM et al. Independent validation of genes and polymorphisms reported to be associated with radiation toxicity: A prospective analysis study. *Lancet Oncol* 2012;13:65–77.

8. Barnett GC, West CM, Dunning AM et al. Normal tissue reactions to radiotherapy: Towards tailoring treatment dose by genotype. *Nat Rev Cancer* 2009;9:134–142.

9. Begg AC, Haustermans K, Hart AA et al. The value of pretreatment cell kinetic parameters as predictors for radiotherapy outcome in head and neck cancer: A multicenter analysis. *Radiother Oncol* 1999;50:13–23.

10. Bentzen SM, Atasoy BM, Daley FM et al. Epidermal growth factor receptor expression in pretreatment biopsies from head and neck squamous cell carcinoma as a predictive factor for a benefit from accelerated radiation therapy in a randomized controlled trial. *J Clin Oncol* 2005;23:5560–5567.

11. Best T, Li D, Skol AD et al. Variants at 6q21 implicate PRDM1 in the etiology of therapy-induced second malignancies after Hodgkin's lymphoma. *Nat Med* 2011;17:941–943.

12. Betts GN, Eustace A, Patiar S et al. Prospective technical validation and assessment of intra-tumour heterogeneity of a low density array hypoxia gene profile in head and neck squamous cell carcinoma. *Eur J Cancer* 2013;49:156–165.

13. Bjork-Eriksson T, West C, Karlsson E, Mercke C. Tumor radiosensitivity (SF2) is a prognostic factor for local control in head and neck cancers. *Int J Radiat Oncol Biol Phys* 2000;46:13–19.

14. Bordon E, Henriquez-Hernandez LA, Lara PC, Pinar B, Rodriguez-Gallego C, Lloret M. Role of CD4 and CD8 T-lymphocytes, B-lymphocytes and natural killer cells in the prediction of radiation-induced late toxicity in cervical cancer patients. *Int J Radiat Biol* 2011;87:424–431.

15. Bordon E, Henriquez-Hernandez LA, Lara PC et al. Prediction of clinical toxicity in locally advanced head and neck cancer patients by radio-induced apoptosis in peripheral blood lymphocytes (PBLs). *Radiat Oncol* 2010;5:4.

16. Buffa FM, Bentzen SM, Daley FM et al. Molecular marker profiles predict locoregional control of head and neck squamous cell carcinoma in a randomized trial of continuous hyperfractionated accelerated radiotherapy. *Clin Cancer Res* 2004;10:3745–3754.

17. Burnet NG, Nyman J, Turesson I, Wurm R, Yarnold JR, Peacock JH. Prediction of normal-tissue tolerance to radiotherapy from in-vitro cellular radiation sensitivity. *Lancet* 1992;339:1570–1571.

18. Choudhury A, Nelson LD, Teo MT et al. MRE11 expression is predictive of cause-specific survival following radical radiotherapy for muscle-invasive bladder cancer. *Cancer Res* 2010;70:7017–7026.

19. Debucquoy A, Haustermans K, Daemen A et al. Molecular response to cetuximab and efficacy of preoperative cetuximab-based chemoradiation in rectal cancer. *J Clin Oncol* 2009;27:2751–2757.

20. Eriksen JG, Overgaard J; Danish Head and Neck Cancer Study Group (DAHANCA). Lack of prognostic and predictive value of CA IX in radiotherapy of squamous cell carcinoma of the head and neck with known modifiable hypoxia: An evaluation of the DAHANCA 5 study. *Radiother Oncol* 2007;83:383–388.

21. Eriksen JG, Steiniche T, Overgaard J; Danish Head and Neck Cancer Study Group (DAHANCA). The influence of epidermal growth factor receptor and tumor differentiation on the response to accelerated radiotherapy of squamous cell carcinomas of the head and neck in the randomized DAHANCA 6 and 7 study. *Radiother Oncol* 2005;74:93–100.

22. Eschrich SA, Fulp WJ, Pawitan Y et al. Validation of a radiosensitivity molecular signature in breast cancer. *Clin Cancer Res* 2012;18:5134–5143.

23. Eustace A, Irlam JJ, Taylor J et al. Necrosis predicts benefit from hypoxia-modifying therapy in patients with high risk bladder cancer enrolled in a phase III randomised trial. *Radiother Oncol* 2013;108:40–47.

24. Eustace A, Mani N, Span PN et al. A 26-gene hypoxia signature predicts benefit from hypoxia-modifying therapy in laryngeal cancer but not bladder cancer. *Clin Cancer Res* 2013;19:4879–4888.

25. Fachal L, Gomez-Caamano A, Barnett GC et al. A three-stage genome-wide association study identifies a susceptibility locus for late radiotherapy toxicity at 2q24.1. *Nat Genet* 2014;46:891–894.

26. Fertil B, Malaise EP. Intrinsic radiosensitivity of human cell lines is correlated with radioresponsiveness of human tumors: Analysis of 101 published survival curves. *Int J Radiat Oncol Biol Phys* 1985;11:1699–1707.

27. Gee HE, Camps C, Buffa FM et al. hsa-mir-210 is a marker of tumor hypoxia and a prognostic factor in head and neck cancer. *Cancer* 2010;116:2148–2158.

28. Granata R, Miceli R, Orlandi E et al. Tumor stage, human papillomavirus and smoking status affect the survival of patients with oropharyngeal cancer: An Italian validation study. *Ann Oncol* 2012;23:1832–1837.

29. Graves EE, Hicks RJ, Binns D et al. Quantitative and qualitative analysis of [(18)F]FDG and [(18)F]FAZA positron emission tomography of head and neck cancers and associations with HPV status and treatment outcome. *Eur J Nucl Med Mol Imaging* 2016;43:617–625.

30. Hall J, Jeggo PA, West C et al. Ionizing radiation biomarkers in epidemiological studies – An update. *Mutat Res* 2017;771:59–84.

31. Hammond ME, Hayes DF, Dowsett M et al. American Society of Clinical Oncology/College of American Pathologists guideline recommendations for immunohistochemical testing of estrogen and progesterone receptors in breast cancer. *J Clin Oncol* 2010;28:2784–2795.

32. He J, Zhang F, Wu Y et al. Prognostic role of microRNA-155 in various carcinomas: Results from a meta-analysis. *Dis Markers* 2013;34:379–386.

33. Henriquez-Hernandez LA, Carmona-Vigo R, Pinar B et al. Combined low initial DNA damage and high radiation-induced apoptosis confers clinical resistance to long-term toxicity in breast cancer patients treated with high-dose radiotherapy. *Radiat Oncol* 2011;6:60.

34. Herbert C, Williams M, Sawyer H, Greenslade M, Cornes P, Hopkins K. Treatment of glioblastoma multiforme with radiotherapy and concomitant and adjuvant temozolomide: Translation of randomised controlled trial evidence into routine clinical practice. *Clin Oncol (R Coll Radiol)* 2011;23:372–373.

35. Herrlinger U, Schafer N, Steinbach JP et al. Bevacizumab plus Irinotecan versus Temozolomide in newly diagnosed O6-methylguanine-DNA methyltransferase nonmethylated glioblastoma: The randomized GLARIUS trial. *J Clin Oncol* 2016;34:1611–1619.

36. Horsman MR, Mortensen LS, Petersen JB, Busk M, Overgaard J. Imaging hypoxia to improve radiotherapy outcome. *Nat Rev Clin Oncol* 2012;9:674–687.

37. Ilyas M, Grabsch H, Ellis IO et al. National Cancer Research Institute Biomarker Imaging Clinical Studies Group. Guidelines and considerations for conducting experiments using tissue microarrays. *Histopathology* 2013;62:827–839.

38. Irlam-Jones JJ, Eustace A, Denley H et al. Expression of miR-210 in relation to other measures of hypoxia and prediction of benefit from hypoxia modification in patients with bladder cancer. *Br J Cancer* 2016;115:571–578.

39. Janssens GO, Rademakers SE, Terhaard CH et al. Accelerated radiotherapy with carbogen and nicotinamide for laryngeal cancer: Results of a phase III randomized trial. *J Clin Oncol* 2012;30:1777–1783.

40. Kaanders JH, Wijffels KI, Marres HA et al. Pimonidazole binding and tumor vascularity predict for treatment outcome in head and neck cancer. *Cancer Res* 2002;62:7066–7074.

41. Kelly JR, Husain ZA, Burtness B. Treatment de-intensification strategies for head and neck cancer. *Eur J Cancer* 2016;68: 125–133.

42. Kerns SL, de Ruysscher D, Andreassen CN et al. STROGAR – Strengthening the reporting of genetic association studies in radiogenomics. *Radiother Oncol* 2014;110:182–188.

43. Kerns SL, Dorling L, Fachal L et al. Radiogenomics Consortium. Meta-analysis of genome wide association studies identifies genetic markers of late toxicity following radiotherapy for prostate cancer. *EBioMedicine* 2016;10:150–163.

44. Kimple RJ, Smith MA, Blitzer GC et al. Enhanced radiation sensitivity in HPV-positive head and neck cancer. *Cancer Res* 2013;73:4791–4800.

45. Kononen J, Bubendorf L, Kallioniemi A et al. Tissue microarrays for high-throughput molecular profiling of tumor specimens. *Nat Med* 1998;4:844–847.

46. Lalonde E, Alkallas R, Chua MLK et al. Translating a prognostic DNA genomic classifier into the clinic: Retrospective validation in 563 localized prostate tumors. *Eur Urol* 2017;72: 22–31.

47. Lalonde E, Ishkanian AS, Sykes J et al. Tumour genomic and microenvironmental heterogeneity for integrated prediction of 5-year biochemical recurrence of prostate cancer: A retrospective cohort study. *Lancet Oncol* 2014;15:1521–1532.

48. Laurberg JR, Brems-Eskildsen AS, Nordentoft I et al. Expression of TIP60 (tat-interactive protein) and MRE11 (meiotic recombination 11 homolog) predict treatment-specific outcome of localised invasive bladder cancer. *BJU Int* 2012;110:E1228–E1236.

49. Lim AM, Rischin D, Fisher R et al. Prognostic significance of plasma osteopontin in patients with locoregionally advanced head and neck squamous cell carcinoma treated on TROG 02.02 phase III trial. *Clin Cancer Res* 2012;18:301–307.

50. Maher SG, McDowell DT, Collins BC, Muldoon C, Gallagher WM, Reynolds JV. Serum proteomic profiling reveals that pretreatment complement protein levels are predictive of esophageal cancer patient response to neoadjuvant chemoradiation. *Ann Surg* 2011;254:809–816; discussion 16–17.

51. Malmstrom A, Gronberg BH, Marosi C et al. Nordic Clinical Brain Tumour Study Group. Temozolomide versus standard 6-week radiotherapy versus hypofractionated radiotherapy in patients older than 60 years with glioblastoma: The Nordic randomised, phase 3 trial. *Lancet Oncol* 2012;13:916–926.

52. Manders JB, Kuerer HM, Smith BD et al. Study Investigators and Study Participants. Clinical utility of the 12-gene DCIS score assay: Impact on radiotherapy recommendations for patients with ductal carcinoma *in situ*. *Ann Surg Oncol* 2017;24:660–668.

53. Mroz EA, Tward AD, Pickering CR, Myers JN, Ferris RL, Rocco JW. High intratumor genetic heterogeneity is related to worse outcome in patients with head and neck squamous cell carcinoma. *Cancer* 2013;119:3034–3042.

54. Nijkamp MM, Span PN, Bussink J, Kaanders JH. Interaction of EGFR with the tumour microenvironment: Implications for radiation treatment. *Radiother Oncol* 2013;108:17–23.

55. O'Connor JP, Aboagye EO, Adams JE et al. Imaging biomarker roadmap for cancer studies. *Nat Rev Clin Oncol* 2017;14:169–186.

56. Overgaard J, Eriksen JG, Nordsmark M, Alsner J, Horsman MR; Danish Head and Neck Cancer Study Group (DAHANCA). Plasma osteopontin, hypoxia, and response to the hypoxia sensitiser nimorazole in radiotherapy of head and neck cancer: Results from the DAHANCA 5 randomised double-blind placebo-controlled trial. *Lancet Oncol* 2005;6:757–764.

57. Ozsahin M, Crompton NE, Gourgou S et al. CD4 and CD8 T-lymphocyte apoptosis can predict radiation-induced late toxicity: A prospective study in 399 patients. *Clin Cancer Res* 2005;11:7426–7433.

58. Peacock J, Ashton A, Bliss J et al. Cellular radiosensitivity and complication risk after curative radiotherapy. *Radiother Oncol* 2000;55:173–178.

59. Pedicini P, Nappi A, Strigari L et al. Correlation between EGFR expression and accelerated proliferation during radiotherapy of head and neck squamous cell carcinoma. *Radiat Oncol* 2012;7:143.

60. Peridis S, Pilgrim G, Athanasopoulos I, Parpounas K. Carbonic anhydrase-9 expression in head and neck cancer: A meta-analysis. *Eur Arch Otorhinolaryngol* 2011;268:661–670.

61. Rischin D, Hicks RJ, Fisher R, Binns D, Corry J, Porceddu S, Peters LJ; Trans-Tasman Radiation Oncology Study Group. Prognostic significance of [18F]-misonidazole positron emission tomography-detected tumor hypoxia in patients with advanced head and neck cancer randomly assigned to chemoradiation with or without tirapazamine: A substudy of Trans-Tasman Radiation Oncology Group Study 98.02. *J Clin Oncol* 2006;24:2098–2104.

62. Rouzier R, Pronzato P, Chereau E, Carlson J, Hunt B, Valentine WJ. Multigene assays and molecular markers in breast cancer: Systematic review of health economic analyses. *Breast Cancer Res Treat* 2013;139:621–637.

63. Schnarr K, Boreham D, Sathya J, Julian J, Dayes IS. Radiation-induced lymphocyte apoptosis to predict radiation therapy late toxicity in prostate cancer patients. *Int J Radiat Oncol Biol Phys* 2009;74:1424–1430.

64. Schoenborn JR, Nelson P, Fang M. Genomic profiling defines subtypes of prostate cancer with the potential for therapeutic stratification. *Clin Cancer Res* 2013;19:4058–4066.

65. Scott JG, Harrison LB, Torres-Roca JF. Genomic-adjusted radiation dose – Authors' reply. *Lancet Oncol* 2017;18:e129.

66. Smid EJ, Stoter TR, Bloemena E et al. The importance of immunohistochemical expression of EGFr in squamous cell carcinoma of the oral cavity treated with surgery and postoperative radiotherapy. *Int J Radiat Oncol Biol Phys* 2006;65:1323–1329.

67. Stupp R, Hegi ME, Mason WP et al. European Organisation for Research and Treatment of Cancer Brain Tumour and Radiation Oncology Groups, National Cancer Institute of Canada Clinical Trials Group. Effects of radiotherapy with concomitant and adjuvant temozolomide versus radiotherapy alone on survival in glioblastoma in a randomised phase III study: 5-year analysis of the EORTC-NCIC trial. *Lancet Oncol* 2009;10:459–466.

68. Suwinski R, Jaworska M, Nikiel B et al. Predicting the effect of accelerated fractionation in postoperative radiotherapy for head and neck cancer based on molecular marker profiles: Data from a randomized clinical trial. *Int J Radiat Oncol Biol Phys* 2010;77:438–446.

69. Svensson JP, Stalpers LJ, Esveldt-van Lange RE et al. Analysis of gene expression using gene sets discriminates cancer patients with and without late radiation toxicity. *PLoS Med* 2006;3:e422.

70. Taylor AM, Harnden DG, Arlett CF et al. Ataxia telangiectasia: A human mutation with abnormal radiation sensitivity. *Nature* 1975;258:427–429.

71. Toustrup K, Sorensen BS, Lassen P, Wiuf C, Alsner J, Overgaard J; Danish Head and Neck Cancer Study Group (DAHANCA). Gene expression classifier predicts for hypoxic modification of radiotherapy with nimorazole in squamous cell carcinomas of the head and neck. *Radiother Oncol* 2012;102:122–129.

72. Turesson I, Nyman J, Holmberg E, Oden A. Prognostic factors for acute and late skin reactions in radiotherapy patients. *Int J Radiat Oncol Biol Phys* 1996;36:1065–1075.

73. Vandenbroucke JP. STREGA, STROBE, STARD, SQUIRE, MOOSE, PRISMA, GNOSIS, TREND, ORION, COREQ, QUOROM, REMARK... and CONSORT: For whom does the guideline toll? *J Clin Epidemiol* 2009;62:594–596.

74. West C, Rosenstein BS, Alsner J et al. Establishment of a radiogenomics consortium. *Int J Radiat Oncol Biol Phys* 2010;76:1295–1296.

75. West CM, Barnett GC. Genetics and genomics of radiotherapy toxicity: Towards prediction. *Genome Med* 2011;3:52.

76. West CM, Davidson SE, Elyan SA et al. Lymphocyte radiosensitivity is a significant prognostic factor for morbidity in carcinoma of the cervix. *Int J Radiat Oncol Biol Phys* 2001;51:10–15.

77. West CM, Davidson SE, Roberts SA, Hunter RD. The independence of intrinsic radiosensitivity as a prognostic factor for patient response to radiotherapy of carcinoma of the cervix. *Br J Cancer* 1997;76:1184–1190.

78. Yang L, Taylor J, Eustace A et al. A gene signature for selecting benefit from hypoxia modification of radiotherapy for high-risk bladder cancer patients. *Clin Cancer Res* 2017;23:4761–4768.

79. Zhao SG, Chang SL, Erho N et al. Associations of luminal and basal subtyping of prostate cancer with prognosis and response to androgen deprivation therapy. *JAMA Oncol* 2017;3:1663–1672.

80. Zhao SG, Chang SL, Spratt DE et al. Development and validation of a 24-gene predictor of response to postoperative radiotherapy in prostate cancer: A matched, retrospective analysis. *Lancet Oncol* 2016;17:1612–1620.

# Molecular image guided radiotherapy

## VINCENT GRÉGOIRE, KARIN HAUSTERMANS AND JOHN LEE

## 22.1 INTRODUCTION: MOLECULAR IMAGING AND ITS POTENTIAL USE IN MODERN RADIOTHERAPY

Molecular imaging, also referred to as biological imaging or functional imaging, is the use of non-invasive imaging techniques that enable the visualization of various biological pathways and physiological characteristics of tumours and/or normal tissues. In short, it mainly refers (but not only) to positron emission tomography (PET) and magnetic resonance imaging (MRI). In clinical oncology, molecular imaging offers the unique opportunity to allow an earlier diagnosis and staging of the disease to contribute to the selection and delineation of the optimal target volumes before and during (i.e. adaptive treatment) radiotherapy and to a lesser extent before surgery, to monitor the response early on during the treatment or after its completion, and to help in the early detection of recurrence. From the viewpoint of experimental radiation oncology, molecular imaging may bridge radiobiological concepts such as tumour hypoxia, tumour proliferation, tumour stem cell density and tumour radiosensitivity by integrating tumour biological heterogeneity into the treatment planning equation (Figure 22.1). From the viewpoint of experimental oncology, molecular imaging may also facilitate and speed up the process of drug development by allowing faster and cheaper pharmacokinetic and biodistribution studies.

For target volume selection and delineation, anatomic imaging modalities such as computed tomography (CT) and MRI remain the most widely used modalities. Over the last few years, however, the use of molecular imaging and in particular the use of PET and multi-parametric MRI (mpMRI) have become increasingly used. Providing appropriate tracers are used, molecular imaging with PET enables the visualization of the various molecular pathways in tumours including metabolism, proliferation, oxygen delivery and consumption, and receptor or gene expression, all of which may be important in the response to ionizing radiation.

The goal of radiotherapy treatment planning is to select and delineate target volumes (and organs at risk) based on all the available diagnostic information and on the knowledge of the physiology of the disease, i.e. the probability of local and nodal infiltration. This is done in part by using various imaging modalities, which depict more or less accurately the true tumour extent. The difficulty with using imaging modalities is that none of them has a sensitivity (no false negative) or a specificity (no false positive) of 100%. Thus, false negatives and false positives for depicting neoplastic processes occur. How the sensitivity and specificity of a particular imaging modality influences the radiotherapy planning process depends on the underlying objective of the treatment. If, for a particular disease, the objective is to avoid missing tumour at any expense, a highly sensitive approach needs to be selected. This will likely give a lower specificity, resulting in inclusion of non-neoplastic tissue into the target volume. However, this approach reduces the likelihood that neoplastic cells are missed. If, on the other hand, the aim is to avoid including non-neoplastic cells into the target volume to protect normal tissue, a highly specific approach will be selected with a very high specificity.

When incorporating PET and/or mpMRI into treatment planning, their sensitivity and specificity should be compared with CT and/or anatomic MRI, and with pathological verification of tumour extent from surgical sampling, if available. The potential impact of PET and/or mpMRI on treatment planning needs to be determined. For example, if an additional lymph node is visualized with a new imaging modality known to be more specific than the standard modality, it might be legitimate to increase the target volume(s) beyond what would have been the target volume using a standard procedure; conversely, if fewer nodes are visualized with a new imaging modality known to be more sensitive than the standard modality, it might be legitimate to decrease the target volume(s) below what would have been delineated using a standard procedure. Table 22.1 summarizes data on the specificity and sensitivity of fluorodeoxyglucose (FDG)-PET, CT, anatomic MRI and diffusion-weighted MRI (DW-MRI) for lymph node staging in lung cancer, head and neck cancer, cervical cancer, oesophageal cancer and colorectal cancer, comparing with surgical lymph node sampling as the gold standard.

In head and neck tumours, CT, MRI, DW-MRI and FDG-PET performed with a comparable diagnostic accuracy. A potentially interesting use of molecular imaging is in the staging of node-negative head and neck squamous cell carcinoma (HNSCC) patients (as assessed by other imaging modalities) where the issue could be to avoid treating the neck nodes if molecular imaging examination also turns out to be negative. However, in the node-negative neck, two

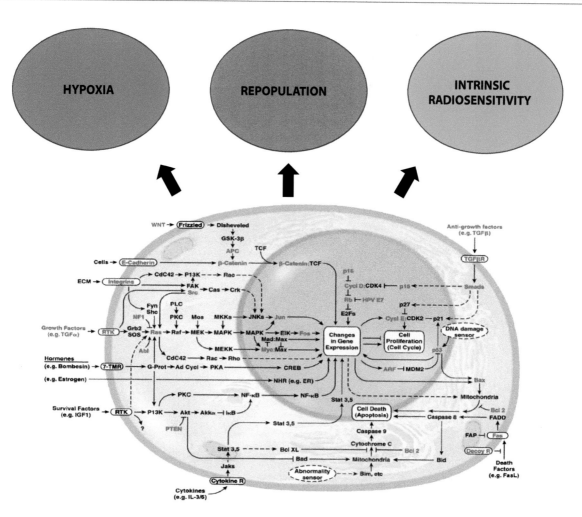

**Figure 22.1** Molecular imaging bridges radiobiological concepts such as tumour hypoxia, tumour proliferation and tumour radiosensitivity into the treatment planning equation.

meta-analyses reported that the sensitivity of FDG-PET, compared with the examination of the pathologic specimen after a neck node dissection, was only around 79% (51,56). DW-MRI performed a little better, but still its sensitivity only reached 84% (99). This is not surprising in light of the fact that in node-negative patients who underwent a prophylactic neck node dissection, microscopic nodal infiltration could be observed in up to 30% of cases (84). Thus, the rather low signal-to-background ratio of FDG and the limited spatial resolution of the cameras currently preclude the detection of microscopic disease with PET, and therefore compared with anatomic imaging modalities such as CT and MRI, it is unlikely that FDG-PET will be of any additional value in selecting prophylactic nodal target volumes in the neck. A similar conclusion appears true for the use of DW-MRI.

On the contrary, when evaluating the added value of FDG-PET in non-small cell lung cancer (NSCLC), the picture turns to be the opposite. The sensitivity and specificity for lymph nodes staging in lung cancer are significantly higher for FDG-PET and to a lower extent for DW-MRI compared to CT (36,105). This implies that a negative PET scan could result in substantially reduced target volumes and permit focusing on the primary tumour.

In oesophageal cancer, the specificity of FDG-PET is slightly better than that of CT (28,86,98). In particular, FDG-PET is specific for the staging of lymph nodes outside of the mediastinum, e.g. supra-clavicular or coeliac lymph nodes. If such lymph nodes are detected with FDG-PET, it is legitimate to enlarge the selection (thus the delineation) of the target volume (102).

In colorectal carcinoma, CT or MRI performs similarly to detect pelvic lymph nodes, and a slightly higher sensitivity of FDG-PET was observed (12,15). The consequence of such findings is however unclear for the clinical management of patients. No retrospective data have been published on the accuracy of DW-MRI for pelvic node staging.

For prostate cancer, $^{18}F$- or $^{11}C$-choline-PET have been shown to be more specific than CT or MRI, and may be of use to optimize the radiation dose prescription in those patients with positive pelvic nodes (27,44).

In para-aortic lymph nodes of patients with cervix carcinoma, FDG-PET is also reported to be more specific than CT and equally specific as MRI, whereas the sensitivity of these imaging modalities was poor (19,40).

The data in Table 22.1 were obtained with stand-alone PET cameras or with dual PET/CT systems. Few systematic

Table 22.1 Comparison between CT, MRI, FDG-PET and DW-MRI for nodal staging

| Site | Reference | Sensitivity (%)[a] | | | | Specificity (%) | | | |
| | | MRI | CT | FDG-PET | DW-MRI | MRI | CT | FDG-PET | DW-MRI |
| --- | --- | --- | --- | --- | --- | --- | --- | --- | --- |
| Head and neck cancer | 51[b] | 78 (54–92) | 74 (61–83) | 79 (72–85) | – | 80 (67–88) | 76 (68–83) | 86 (83–89) | – |
| | 56[b] | 65 (34–87) | 52 (39–65) | 66 (47–88) | – | 81 (64–91) | 93 (87–97) | 87 (77–93) | – |
| | 99 | 46 | | | 84 | 94 | | | 96 |
| Non-small cell lung cancer | 36[b] | – | 61 (50–71) | 85 (67–91) | – | – | 79 (66–89) | 90 (82–96) | – |
| | 105[b] | – | – | 75 (68–81) | 72 (63–80) | – | – | 89 (85–91) | 95 (68–81) |
| Oesophageal cancer | 98[b] | – | – | 51 (34–69) | – | – | – | 84 (76–91) | – |
| | 28 | – | 41 | 74 | – | – | 83 | 90 | – |
| | 86[b] | – | – | 62 (40–79) | – | – | – | 96 (93–98) | – |
| Colo-rectal carcinoma | 12[b] | 66 (54–76) | 55 (43–67) | – | – | 76 (59–87) | 74 (67–80) | – | – |
| | 15[b] | – | – | 85 (69–93) | – | – | – | 42 (23–67) | – |
| Prostate carcinoma | 44[b] | 39 (22–56) | 42 (26–56) | – | – | 82 (79–83) | 82 (80–83) | – | – |
| | 27 | – | – | 49 (40–58)[c] | – | – | – | 95 (92–97)[c] | – |
| Cervix carcinoma | 19[b] | 38 (32–43) | 52 (42–62) | 54 (46–61) | – | 97 (97–98) | 92 (90–94) | 97 (96–98) | – |

[a] Average value with range in parentheses.

[b] Meta-analysis.

[c] $^{18}$F-choline and $^{11}$C-choline.

comparisons between the diagnostic accuracy of stand-alone PET and integrated PET/CT have been performed. Overall, diagnostic accuracy might be slightly improved by the use of dual PET/CT cameras, but the overall conclusions about the compared diagnostic accuracy of these imaging modalities are not changed (1,7). It is, however, interesting to note that, although logistically more demanding, the performance of the side-by-side PET-CT comparison was almost as good as the dual cameras (1).

## 22.2 IMAGE ACQUISITION AND RECONSTRUCTION WITH PET

In oncology, PET has been used routinely as a diagnostic tool for detection of lesions. Volume delineation on PET images appears as a trendy move in radiotherapy, although its added value is not always demonstrated. In comparison with diagnosis, volume delineation requires greater care in acquisition, reconstruction and processing of PET images, in order to minimize the uncertainty about the tumour boundaries and reach acceptable volume accuracy.

First, it is useful to recall some inherent limitations of PET (91). For many physical reasons whose discussion is beyond the scope of this chapter, PET yields images with lower resolution than CT or MR (half a centimetre on average versus about 1 millimetre) (6). This explains the blurry aspect of PET images. Moreover, they suffer from a high level of statistical noise because PET is an emission modality: the activity of the injected dose must be limited for obvious radioprotective reasons and many positron disintegrations occur outside the field of view of the PET camera where they do not contribute to the image but can add additional noise (scattered events). Both the low resolution and the high noise level must be taken into account when selecting suitable acquisition protocols and reconstruction procedures. For instance, it is recommended to acquire images in three-dimensional mode and not in two-dimensional mode. If available, time-of-flight measurements also increase quality. Eventually, resolution recovery is a feature that can compensate (partly) for blur. In summary, there is a trade-off to attain between the injected tracer dose, the acquisition duration, patient comfort and image quality.

Regarding reconstruction protocols, iterative algorithms such as ordered subsets expectation maximization (OSEM) are preferred especially for accurate volumetric assessment. Iterative reconstruction is, however, slower than direct algebraic reconstruction and may not be suitable for routine diagnostic PET acquisition.

After the images have been reconstructed, denoising and deblurring filters can further improve image quality for target delineation. Denoising aims at reducing spurious random oscillations in the image that can affect contrast. When image quality is essential as it is for automatic segmentation, median filtering (2) or bilateral filtering (54) are preferred to usual Gaussian smoothing (66), which degrades resolution. A typical example of what image filtering does is shown in

Figure 22.2. Image deblurring aims at correcting images for their low resolution and partial volume effect (87). It restores sharp edges between regions of low and high tracer uptake. To some (limited) extent, they can also recover some of the uptake heterogeneities occurring within the tumour. Such methods, however, require an accurate knowledge of the resolution characteristics of the PET camera.

## 22.3 PET IMAGE SEGMENTATION

The accurate determination of the volume and shape of the tumour from PET images remains a challenging task and an incompletely resolved issue (53). A very widespread method consists of visual interpretation of the PET images and definition of the tumour contours by an experienced nuclear medicine physician or a radiation oncologist (e.g. [20]). Some aspects of this method appear highly debatable. First, the threshold level of the PET image, which depends on the window level, width and colour map chosen by the physician, influences strongly the visual perception of the tumour boundaries. Moreover, the visual delineation of objects is a subjective approach that will necessarily lead to substantial intra- and inter-observer variability (76,94). Highly trained physicians can develop an expertise that can be difficult to translate into an automatic method.

Factual variability in manual delineation has motivated the development of objective and reproducible methods of segmenting PET images. The simplest method relies on determining a fixed uptake threshold to distinguish between tumour and surrounding healthy tissues. It can be an absolute value, expressed in standardized uptake values (SUVs), or relative to some measured quantity, like the maximal uptake within the tumour ($SUV_{max}$) or some more elaborate statistic (e.g. $SUV_{peak}$). Common values are 2.5 SUV or about 40% of the $SUV_{max}$ (53). Using a fixed threshold of 50% of the maximal activity to automatically segment primary tumour of the head and neck region, tumour volumes delineated from PET images with FDG were larger than those delineated with CT in 25% of the cases (70). However, results from this study have to be taken with caution since the relevance of an arbitrary fixed threshold appears questionable. Indeed, it has been shown that the threshold required to match macroscopic laryngectomy specimens used as a 'gold standard' varied from one specimen to another between 36% and 73% of the maximal activity (37). Reinforced by the absence of validation studies, these data clearly illustrate that methods based on fixed thresholds are not adequate for accurately segmenting tumours from PET images.

Adaptive thresholding is an option that addresses some limitations of the methods described above. It relies on a model that determines the appropriate uptake threshold according to both the maximum uptake in the tumour and the average uptake in the surrounding background. This method has been shown to be accurate for segmenting PET images in a series of pharyngolaryngeal tumours (21). Although validated as a reliable segmentation method, it still

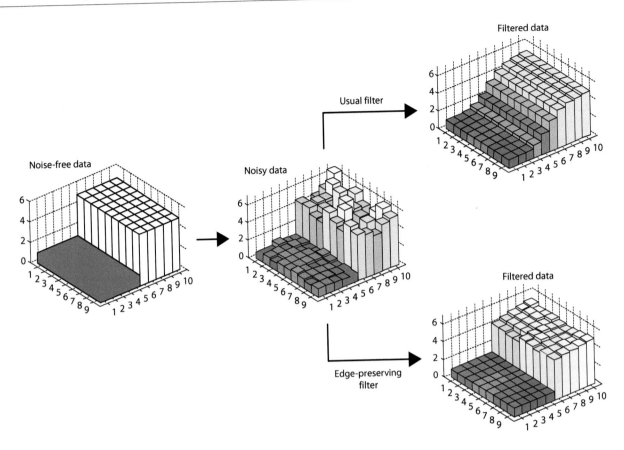

**Figure 22.2** The principle of edge-preserving filtering. An 'ideal' PET image consists of two regions, one with low activity and another with a higher activity (left panel). The activity is depicted with bars of varying height. 'Real' PET scanners do not yield noise-free images, and a simulation of a noisy 'real' image is depicted in the centre panel. From there, two different filters have been used. The top right image is obtained with a usual Gaussian filter, whereas the bottom right image results from the application of an edge-preserving filter. This 'real' image is much closer to the 'ideal' image.

has some limitations. For instance, it requires a calibration of its parameters for each different reconstruction protocol or PET camera model. Also, this method is not ideal for images with low signal-to-background ratios such as encountered in peritumoural inflammation induced by radiotherapy or in undifferentiated tumours. Other adaptive thresholding methods have been developed. Some of them subtract the background uptake from the $SUV_{max}$ instead of computing the ratio $SUV_{max}/SUV_{background}$. Iterative thresholding proceeds with successive refinements of the threshold, based on direct modelling of the camera resolution (95).

A large variety of methods relying on more complicated image segmentation techniques have been described and applied to PET data (53,85). They involve, e.g. probabilistic thresholds or (fuzzy) clustering techniques (9,41) that aim at addressing the issues of low resolution and partial volume effect. For instance, resolution blur has long prevented the application to PET of widespread segmentation techniques that associate object edges with ridges in the magnitude of the uptake gradient. Image restoration tools, like edge-preserving noise filters and deblurring algorithms (see Section 22.2 and Figure 22.2), partly overcome the problems of blur and noise and make gradient-based segmentation applicable to PET.

A method using these tools and segmenting the tumours with a watershed transform and a hierarchical cluster analysis has been successfully validated by comparison with surgical specimens in both HNSCC and NSCLC (32,103). The main advantage of this approach is that it accounts explicitly for all imperfections of PET images and does not need any calibration. Only the knowledge of the PET image resolution is necessary. Consequently, both the applicability of the method and its adoption could be increased since it could still yield a reasonable segmentation in difficult cases (e.g. an image with low signal-to-background ratio), where threshold-based methods usually fail. A typical example is the use of FDG-PET during radiotherapy (Figure 22.3). The combination of radio-induced mucositis, that increases the background signal, together with the reduction in tumour uptake secondary to the treatment response, leads to a drastic decrease in signal-to-background ratio. In this context, isolating the residual tumour from the surrounding inflammatory area requires powerful segmentation methods that are able to detect gradient-intensity crests of low magnitude and/or delayed imaging acquisition.

The difficulty of segmenting accurately PET images with rather low resolution has given rise to many different delineation methods, validated for specific tumour sites

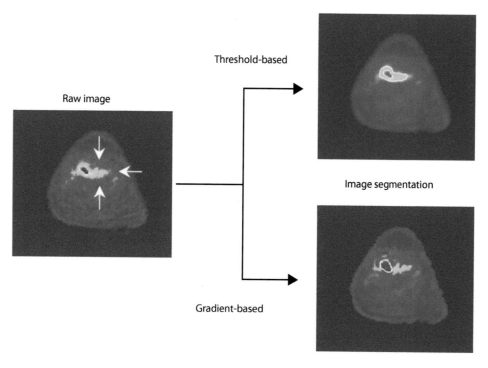

Threshold-based

Raw image

Image segmentation

Gradient-based

**Figure 22.3** Comparison between a threshold-based and a gradient-based method for the automatic segmentation of head and neck tumour during radiotherapy. The image is intrinsically noisier due to peri-tumoural radiation-induced mucositis. The gradient-based method led to more specific tumour segmentation.

and to various extents (versus phantoms, synthetic images, other imaging modalities like CT, or ground truth). Ongoing efforts attempt, however, to standardise image quality (not specifically for delineation purposes), survey existing or emerging developments in the field, emit recommendations and provide benchmarking tools.

## 22.4 IMAGE ACQUISITION AND RECONSTRUCTION WITH MRI

The basic requirements for signal generation with MRI are (1) the presence of a strong static magnetic field ($B_0$) aligning the protons with the longitudinal direction of the magnetic field and resulting in a net magnetization (M); (2) a superimposed radiofrequency (RF) pulse causing the net magnetization of protons to rotate away from the longitudinal magnetic field direction; and (3) – when the RF-pulse is turned off – a realignment of the net magnetization with the direction of $B_0$. The latter is called recovery or relaxation and it is during this recovery that the electromagnetic signal is generated (73).

Three forms of relaxation can be measured: (1) T1-recovery or longitudinal relaxation; (2) T2-decay or transverse relaxation; and (3) T2* (T2-star) decay, which is a decrease of the transverse magnetization because of magnetic field inhomogeneities. Differences in T1, T2 and proton density are pivotal for creating differences in MRI tissue contrast. This explains the complex relation between images and tissue characteristics on MRI compared to CT,

where contrast merely depends on atomic number and electron density. Consequently, sets of MR images need to be produced with various T1- and T2-weighting, contrast enhancement and functional sequences to allow true tissue characterization.

T1-weighted imaging is most beneficial for depicting anatomy but has low sensitivity for depicting disease entities unless paramagnetic contrast agents are administered. Typically, at T1-weighted imaging, fluid appears dark and fat appears bright. At T2-weighted images fluid appears bright and fat shows varying degrees of brightness. T2-weighted images best depict disease sites as most pathologic processes show higher water content compared to the surrounding tissue, appearing bright on T2-weighted images. However, it should be noted that the information provided by T2-weighting is often non-specific as the T2 signal is affected by many other parameters such as lesion vascularity and cellularity (see review [24]).

Diffusion-weighted MRI (DW-MRI) characterizes tissues by probing differences in the random mobility of water molecules related to tissue cellularity and cellular membrane integrity (see review [24]). A DW-MRI sequence is repeated with increasing strength of diffusion-sensitization of the magnetic gradients, categorized by $b$-values between 0 and 1000 s mm$^{-2}$. Crucially, high $b$-values allow perceiving water molecule movements at the cellular level. The signal decay with increasing $b$-value can be quantified using the apparent diffusion coefficient (ADC). Tissue with a relatively increased cellular density (e.g. tumour) will typically be bright on high $b$-value images and dark on the ADC map, while tissue with a relatively decreased cellular density (e.g. most benign tissues, inflammation and necrosis) will be dark on high *b*-value images and bright on the ADC map.

## 22.5 USING MOLECULAR IMAGES FOR TREATMENT PLANNING

### Brain tumours

Unlike other tissues, the brain almost exclusively metabolises glucose to meet its energy demands. Consequently, the accumulation of FDG in normal brain tissue is very high with a very limited contrast difference between normal white matter and viable tumour. Consequently, this limits the use of FDG-PET for brain tumour imaging. The most important PET tracers used for brain imaging are radiolabelled amino acid such as $^{11}$C-methionine (MET), $^{132}$I-methyl-tyrosine (IMT) and $^{18}$F-fluoroethyl-L-tyrosine (FET). Because uptake of MET in normal brain parenchyma is low, MET-PET is superior to FDG-PET in the assessment of tumour dimensions. The short half-life of $^{11}$C-MET limits its clinical usefulness to centres with on-site cyclotrons. FET is an attractive alternative, as it was shown that MET-PET and FET-PET were equal in their ability to diagnose vital glioma tumour tissue (104). The uptake of MET is correlated to prognosis and higher MET uptake has been seen in grade III or IV gliomas as compared to low-grade gliomas. Moreover, oligodendrogliomas tend to show a higher uptake of MET compared to astrocytomas, which is probably linked to oligodendroglial cellular differentiation (43). There are only few data available on the usefulness of MET-PET in radiotherapy treatment planning. In a recent review, Glaudemans et al. reported sensitivities and specificities of MET-PET to detect primary brain gliomas ranging from 75% to 100% (34), and the specificity of MET-PET was shown to be higher than that of MRI (39). Several studies have shown that the margins of tumours, as assessed by PET with amino acid tracers, were frequently wider than those assessed by MRI or CT (48). In this context, the use of MET-PET has been advocated in the post-operative setting for primary glioma gross tumour volume (GTV) delineation before radiotherapy, as being of superior value than MRI (see review [39]). The value of MET-PET has also been shown in planning recurrent tumours GTV delineation with an impact on patient outcome (39). Similar diagnostic accuracy has been reported for FET-PET to image glioma with a high specificity of 92% (74). This tracer has the advantage of longer half-life, but more data are needed to validate its usefulness in radiotherapy treatment planning. In meningiomas, difficulties in tumour delineation may occur as these tumours frequently infiltrate adjacent brain parenchyma and as MRI contrast enhancement in the normal tissues may be comparable to that of the tumour. Meningioma borders can be more accurately defined on the basis of MET-PET-CT (38,90). When it comes to anatomic imaging, MRI is firmly established as the superior imaging modality for diagnostic purposes when assessing cranial lesions. MRI provides better visualization of tumour and normal tissues (e.g. optic chiasm and cochlea) than CT, and significantly reduces intra-observer as well as inter-observer variability in target delineation of brain tumours (see review [24]). Malignant gliomas are typically hypo-intense on T1-spin echo images and due to breakdown of the blood-brain barrier, enhance heterogeneously following gadolinium contrast infusion. However, this may not be a reliable indicator of active tumour owing to the presence of non-enhancing tumour tissue or contrast-enhancing necrosis. As discussed earlier, in this respect, MET (or FET)-PET may have superior value to delineate the GTV. Ideally, T2-turbo spin echo or T2-FLAIR (fluid-attenuation inversion recovery) information, or both, should also be taken into account to estimate microscopic extension, especially if a low-grade component is suspected. With FLAIR sequences, the signal of fluid is suppressed, improving lesion delineation at the border of cerebrospinal fluid containing ventricles and sulci. However, the relative merit of MET-PET and MRI with appropriate sequences for the delineation of brain tumours is still not settled, and it is likely that the two modalities bring complementary information. For example, in this context, comparison between MET-PET and DW-MRI on a voxel basis did not show any correlation in a group of 31 patients with glioma (18).

Last, the use of diffusion tensor (DTI)-MRI have been proposed to image the paths of least resistance in the brain; anisotropic margins based on DTI in each individual patient could potentially be used to reduce unnecessary irradiation of normal brain tissue and at the same time improve disease control (50). This, however, requires some further validation.

### Head and neck squamous cell carcinoma

As discussed above, the value of FDG-PET for the selection of target volumes in the head and neck area has yet to be demonstrated. Indeed, its sensitivity and specificity for the assessment of head and neck node infiltration do not differ significantly from that of CT or MRI (Table 22.1). However, a study in 20 patients with mostly locally advanced disease, demonstrated an increase in sensitivity with the use of a hybrid PET/CT compared to CT alone and showed that PET/CT-based radiation treatment would have significantly changed the dose distribution (80). Although FDG-PET tends to be more routinely used in treatment planning, these findings should be confirmed prospectively in larger study populations before it can be implemented into routine use. Indeed, one does need to keep in mind that a positive node on FDG-PET does not automatically mean there is a presence of tumour cells, owing to the rather low specificity of this tracer.

FDG-PET has been shown to be of value for the delineation of the primary tumour GTV by comparing three-dimensional registration of CT, MRI and FDG-PET images of oropharyngeal, hypopharyngeal and laryngeal squamous cell carcinomas (21). In a subset of laryngeal tumours, the imaging modalities were also registered with the actual surgical specimen taken as a 'gold standard'. MRI did not provide any added value to CT, either in terms of volumetric GTV assessment or in terms of reduced inter-observer variability (30). FDG-PET demonstrated higher accuracy in delineating GTV with a statistically significant reduction in the target volumes. All three imaging modalities, however, failed to visualize the extent of superficial tumour, illustrating their limitation in spatial resolution. Interestingly, the differences observed between CT and FDG-PET for the GTV delineation translated into significant differences in clinical target volume (CTV) and planning target volume (PTV) delineation. When comparative three-dimensional conformal radiotherapy plans were made, FDG-PET-based plans were more conformal than the CT-based plans and reduction in the isodose volumes with subsequent reduction in the dose to the surrounding normal tissues were observed in the PET-based plans (31). In a prospective multicentric study which enrolled 40 patients, the use of FDG-PET for the delineation of primary tumour GTV and dose planning translated into more conformed dose distribution with more parotid sparing; in that study, tumour recurrences were all observed in the FDG-PET GTV and could not be explained by geographical miss (52). Such data have important consequences as they pave the way for possible dose escalation to the target volumes. In a phase I study on 21 patients with head and neck tumours, it was shown that an increase in dose per fraction (to 2.5 and 3 Gy per fraction) up to a median dose of 80.9 and 85.9 Gy, respectively, could be safely delivered to the FDG-PET-based PTV during part of the treatment (61). However, in that study, late

mucosal ulcers were observed in the highest radiation dose group. During a course of fractionated radiotherapy, it is anticipated that both anatomical and functional tumour changes will occur. Reassessment of the tumour during radiotherapy with subsequent adaptation of the plan might thus allow a much tighter dose distribution to the target volumes with consequent decrease of the total irradiated volume. In the hypopharynx, it has been shown (33) that the GTV progressively decreases during radiotherapy and that adaptive treatment could lead to a significant reduction in the high-dose volume in some cases (Figure 22.4).

## Non-small cell lung cancer

FDG-PET has a higher sensitivity and specificity for nodal staging than CT and might thus alter the GTV delineation either by detecting unnoticed metastatic lymph nodes, or by downstaging a CT false-positive mediastinal nodal station. Due to the particularly high sensitivity of FDG-PET, the latter is more frequent (Table 22.1). In a series of 44 patients, it was shown that FDG-PET altered the stage of the disease in 11 patients (25%) by downstaging 10 of these patients (23). As a consequence, the GTV based on FDG-PET was on average smaller than the GTV defined on CT. In a simulation study, it has been shown that for the same expected toxicity to lungs, spinal cord and oesophagus, the dose to the tumour could be increased by 25%, resulting in a potentially higher tumour control probability of 24% for PET-CT planning compared to 6.3% for CT alone (22).

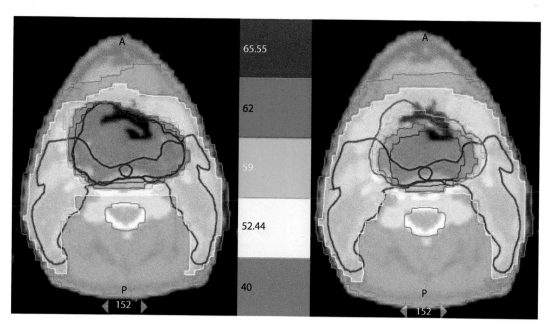

**Figure 22.4** Patient with a T4-N0-M0 squamous cell carcinoma of the hypopharynx. The patient was treated using a simultaneous integrated boost approach delivering a dose of **55.5 Gy (30 fractions of 1.85 Gy)** to the prophylactic PTV (dark blue) and a dose of 69 Gy (30 fractions of 2.3 Gy) to the therapeutic PTV (dark green). Comparison between a pre-treatment CT-based plan (left) and adaptive FDG-PET-based plan (right). On both plans, only the CT-based PTV are depicted. FDG-PET examination was performed before treatment and at 16, 24, 34 and 44 Gy. The dose distribution was adapted on the progressive reduction of the FDG-PET GTV.

In addition to a better detection of true positive lymph nodes, FDG-PET further alters the definition of GTV by discriminating tumour tissue from atelectasis or necrosis (Figure 22.5) (103,106). Other studies have reported that FDG-PET alters the GTV in 22%–62% of the patients (5), and PET, especially PET-CT, imaging has been shown to significantly reduce the inter-observer variability, as well as the intra-observer variability (4,29,94). In a modelling study, it was reported in 21 patients with N2-N3 NSCLC that the use of PET-CT for radiotherapy planning resulted in a lower radiation exposure of the oesophagus and the lungs, allowing a significant dose escalation to the tumour (96).

To date, only a few studies have prospectively included PET with FDG in radiotherapy planning and actually addressed its impact on local tumour control and survival. In a cohort of 153 patients with unresectable NSCLC, it was shown that the introduction of FDG-PET in the management impacted on staging, radiotherapy treatment and overall survival (60). These findings were recently confirmed in another series of patients from the same group (59). Also, selective mediastinal node irradiation based on PET with FDG has yielded a low rate of isolated nodal failure, suggesting that reducing the target volume indeed does not result in worse local control (23).

Some issues related to the use of PET in lung cancer radiotherapy remain unresolved. First, the optimal method for tumour delineation/contouring by PET is still a matter of debate among experts, and interdisciplinary cooperation including radiation oncologists and nuclear medicine specialists is likely to be beneficial for consistent contouring (25,67). Another important methodological issue in lung cancer radiation therapy is tumour motion during PET imaging. In this respect, four-dimensional-PET acquisition has been shown to improve tumour visualization by reducing image blurring and improve radiation treatment planning (3).

## Oesophageal tumour

As already mentioned, FDG-PET is particularly specific for lymph node detection outside of the mediastinum (Table 22.1). In an analysis of the additional value of FDG-PET for optimization of the CTV in 30 patients

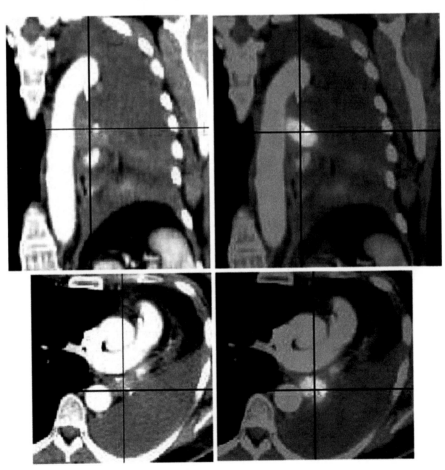

Figure 22.5 This example illustrates the role of FDG-PET for delineating the volume of a lung cancer. The left images represent sagittal (top) and axial (bottom) slices of a patient with a lung cancer located in the left hila region, with retro-obstructive atelectasis of the entire left lung, associated to a major pleural effusion. The metabolic information provided by FDG-PET (right images) shows that the tumour tissue is strictly located to the hilum. The delineation of the tumour margins is easier and more accurate with the help of FDG-PET, allowing for a significant modification of the target volume.

with advanced oesophageal cancer (102), discordances between conventional staging modalities, including CT and oesophageal endoscopic ultrasound (EUS), for the detection of lymph node involvement were found in 14 out of 30 patients (47%). In eight patients, the involved lymph nodes were only detected on CT/EUS, which would have led to a decrease in the CTV in three of them if PET alone had been used. PET with FDG was the only detector of lymph node involvement in six patients, resulting in a possible larger CTV in three of these patients (10%). The authors concluded that the high specificity of FDG-PET for lymph node detection justified its use for treatment volume adaptation in case of positive findings, while the low sensitivity of FDG-PET, i.e. false-negative lymph nodes, would give an erroneous reduction of the CTV. Whether the role of FDG-PET in oesophageal treatment planning will lead to a therapeutic gain without increasing the toxicity remains unanswered.

Another study evaluated the impact of CT and FDG-PET in conformal radiotherapy in 34 patients with oesophageal carcinoma referred for radical chemo-radiation (63). After manual delineation of the GTV on both modalities, CT and PET were coregistered. Image fusion (GTV-PET was used as overlay to GTV-CT) resulted in a reduction of the GTV in 12 patients (25%) and an increase in 7 patients (21%). Modification of the GTV affected the planning treatment volume in 18 patients and affected the percentage of lung volume receiving more than 20 Gy in 25 patients (74%), with a dose reduction in 12 patients and a dose increase in 13 patients. A similar study was performed with an integrated PET/CT scanner (55). Here, the GTV was enlarged in 9/10 (90%) patients by a median volume of 22% (range: 3%–100%) when PET with FDG information was added to the CT-based GTV. In three patients, the PET-avid disease was also excluded from the PTV defined on CT, which would have resulted in a geographical miss. In a study including 16 patients aiming to confirm the possible role of FDG-PET/CT in radiotherapy treatment planning for oesophageal cancer (45), CT-derived GTVs were compared with GTVs contoured on PET/CT images by means of a conformality index (CI). The mean CI was 0.46, suggesting a significant lack of overlap between the GTVs in a large proportion of patients. A subsequent study from the same group confirmed these data and indicated the influence of FDG PET-CT on radiotherapy planning (35). Another preliminary finding on incorporating EUS and PET scanning in the treatment planning process of 25 patients with oesophageal carcinoma showed that the measured tumour length was significantly longer on CT, compared to PET with FDG (49). The authors concluded that PET could be of additional help in the treatment planning. Although EUS measurements of the tumour length were as accurate as PET measurements, the results of EUS are difficult to translate into the planning process. A major drawback of this study was the lack of comparison with pathologic findings after surgery. A more recent study validated the use of FDG PET-CT after preoperative chemo-radiation in 63 patients with oesophageal cancer

from the correlation between pathological examination of the resected specimens. Macroscopic residual tumour was found outside the PET-GTV in 11% of the patients, and microscopic residual tumour was found outside the CTV in 14% of the patients (64).

Very few studies have supported the use of MRI for the detection of oesophageal cancer. This may be explained by technical shortcomings. Increased field strength, faster sequences and cardiac and respiratory gating might yield better image quality in the future.

In conclusion, despite encouraging data, the evidences from pathological and clinical validation are currently insufficient to support the routine use of FDG PET-CT in the radiotherapy planning process at least for the delineation of primary tumour. The use of FDG PET-CT may be of value for the delineation of the nodal target volume outside of the mediastinum.

## Rectal cancer

The potential use of FDG PET/CT in radiotherapy planning of rectal cancers has been studied by different groups. Buijsen et al. (17) compared primary tumour delineation on CT, diagnostic MRI and FDG PET-CT and correlated the tumour extent on all imaging techniques with pathology. They found that CT-based measurements were not correlated with pathology. MR-based measurements correlated significantly, while automatically generated FDG PET/CT-based contours provided the best correlation with the surgical specimen. Braendengen et al. (13) compared tumour volumes on CT, diagnostic MRI and PET-CT in 77 patients with advanced rectal cancer. They found that the median volume on MRI was larger than on PET-CT (111 cm$^3$ versus 87 cm$^3$, $p < 0.001$). In that study, unfortunately no comparison with the pathologic specimen was performed. In a study from Roels et al. (78), MRI and FDG-PET scans were acquired before, during and after neo-adjuvant chemo-radiotherapy in 15 patients with rectal cancer. In general, MRI showed larger target volumes than FDG-PET. There was an approximately 50% mismatch between the PET- and the MRI-based volumes at baseline and during chemo-radiotherapy. Another advantage of FDG PET/CT in the planning process was the possibility of automatic contouring which has been shown to reduce the inter-observer variability in delineation (17).

Although FDG-PET has a high sensitivity for colorectal cancer, there are some limitations in specificity, mainly due to FDG uptake by macrophages. This limitation becomes important when assessing tumour volume during treatment or when assessing response to chemo-radiation, as radiation induces mucositis of the rectal wall surrounding the tumour. In this regard, efforts are being made to develop new [18]F-labelled tracers that might be more tumour specific. Roels et al. (77) investigated the use of PET/CT with FDG, fluorothymidine (FLT) and fluoromisonidazole (F-MISO) for radiotherapy target definition and evolution in rectal cancer. Fifteen patients were scanned with the three tracers before and during chemo-radiotherapy. While FLT and FDG showed a good spatial correspondence, F-MISO seemed less reliable due to non-specific F-MISO uptake and tracer diffusion. These findings indicate that FDG, FLT and F-MISO-PET reflect different functional characteristics that change during chemo-radiotherapy for rectal cancer. From a pilot study with nine patients, Muijs et al. (65) concluded FLT-PET had limited value for the detection of pathologic lymph nodes and tumour delineation in rectal cancer. No other groups have reported on the value of F-MISO-PET in rectal cancer management.

Even if PET can provide additional functional information, its usefulness in the treatment of rectal cancer patients is still questionable and needs to be evaluated in prospective trials using a strict methodology. Its role may become more important when 'dose painting' to relevant biologic regions is achieved with simultaneous integrated boost techniques. Whether this in turn can improve patient outcome in terms of local control and/or sphincter preservation has to be tested in future trials. Moreover, there remain problems that require specific attention, like image coregistration and variations in patient setup, in organ motion (e.g. bowel movements) and in organ shape (e.g. bladder filling). The use of an integrated PET/CT is the modality of choice when it comes to more accurate registration in this site. However, there are still small variations possible, due to the elastic properties of the rectal wall, causing distortions of the rectum (and tumour) during the time of acquisition. Displacements of the rectal wall/tumour could also induce geographical misses when dose escalation to small volumes is planned.

DWI is another functional imaging technique, which is increasingly used in the assessment of patients with rectal cancer. It plays a role in tumour detection, in tumour characterization (cystic versus solid) and in the monitoring of response to treatment. In general, lower pre-treatment ADC values are associated with a better treatment response compared to tumours with high pre-treatment ADC values (see review [24]). Its role for target volume delineation has, however, not yet been demonstrated.

## Cervix cancer

Pelvic MRI has become the new standard for imaging gynecologic cancers due to its excellent soft tissue contrast resolution and its multi-planar capability. MRI is especially helpful in assessing parametrial, vaginal, uterine, bladder and recto-sigmoid invasion. The accuracy of staging of cervical cancer by MRI has been reported to be in the range of 75%–96% (79). Hricak et al. (47) correlated pre-operative MR with the surgical specimens and found the accuracy of MRI to be 81% when comparing imaging and histopathologic spread of disease, especially when assessing parametrial and vaginal spread. In a study aiming at comparing CT and MRI in pre-operative cervix cancer, inter-observer variation was

lower with the latter, and MRI was significantly better than CT for tumour visualization and detection of parametrial invasion (46). A volumetric study comparing CT and MRI for GTV delineation has, however, not been reported.

Regarding PET, in a series of 49 patients with stage Ib–IV cervix carcinoma, overall, a rather good correlation was observed between MRI-T2 and FDG-PET, although for larger tumours, MRI provided with better primary tumour visualization than FDG-PET (58). But in that study no correlation with the pathologic ground truth was performed. In a study conducted in 10 patients with stage I–II cervix cancer, the FDG-PET GTV correlated better to the GTV delineated on the pathological specimen than CT or MRI (107). As already discussed (Section 22.1 and Table 22.1), FDG-PET is of particular value in detecting para-aortic lymph node involvement, and based on that finding it influences target volume delineation and treatment (26).

Last, FDG-PET (40% of SUV) and DW-MRI have been compared in a small series of 20 patients with stage IB–IV cervix carcinoma, and a good concordance has been observed between these two imaging investigations (69).

In summary, FDG-PET or PET-CT has clinical value for the selection and delineation of the para-aortic lymph nodes, whereas the value of MRI to delineate the primary tumour target volume has not yet been unequivocally demonstrated.

## Prostate cancer

Contrary to other tumour types, the uptake of FDG is low in prostate cancer. The tracers that are most commonly used to visualize prostate cancer are $^{11}$C-choline and $^{11}$C-acetate. Choline PET-CT tends to underestimate local tumour extension. Conflicting results have been obtained when using these tracers to delineate the macroscopic tumour within the prostate (71). The high heterogeneity in metabolic rate between different prostate cancers and the reported overlap in uptake between regions of prostate cancer, benign prostate hyperplasia and healthy tissue certainly contribute to this conclusion. Promising results have been, however, obtained in the management of recurrent disease, where choline PET-CT may prove useful for the delineation of the sites of recurrence within the tumour bed and/or in the pelvic nodes (81).

While the routine use of MRI in the primary diagnosis and staging of prostate cancer is still being debated, its benefit for radiotherapy treatment planning is well recognized. Pelvic scans can be acquired in the treatment position using a flat tabletop and a posterior RF coil placed underneath it. Villeirs et al. have shown that the use of MRI in combination with CT improves the accuracy of prostate gland as well as OAR delineation, with decreased inter-observer variability (101). It should be noted that delineation of the prostatic apex is particularly difficult on CT. MRI can more reliably show the boundary between the high signal intensity peripheral zone tissue and the low signal intensity of the levator ani muscle,

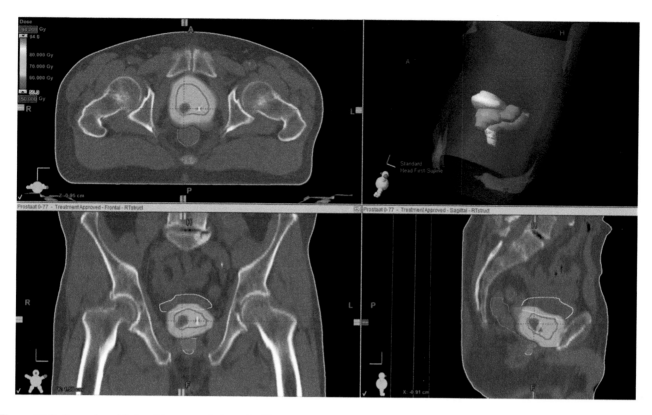

**Figure 22.6** Coronal, sagittal and transversal view of a CT scan in the treatment position. The prostate as CTV (red line) and the macroscopic tumour as GTV (light blue line) are delineated based on registration with a multiparametric MRI. A simultaneous integrated boost is given on the GTV. OARs are delineated (rectum in orange, bladder in yellow). The gold markers are used for daily positioning.

the rectum, the distal urethral sphincter and the fibrous tissue in the urogenital diaphragm (100). Steenbakkers et al. (89) studied the influence of MRI- versus CT-based prostate delineation using multiple observers on the dose to the prostate and OAR. They found that the dose delivered to the rectal wall and bulb of the penis was significantly reduced with plans based on MRI data, allowing a dose escalation of 2–7 Gy for the same rectal wall dose.

The development of high-precision radiation delivery techniques has paved the way for focal boost RT in prostate cancer. In this framework, DCE-MRI, DW-MRI and magnetic resonance spectroscopy have all been investigated for GTV detection. However, it seems unlikely that one imaging modality will be able to adequately detect all tumour targets, as illustrated by an increasing number of studies in which multi-parametric MRI is being explored (Figure 22.6) (see review [24]).

Last, the development of more accurate imaging methods for detection of lymph node metastases may allow the selection of patients for lymph node irradiation. In 36 surgical patients node negative on CT but with a high estimated risk of lymph node involvement, the role of $^{11}$C-choline PET-CT and DW-MRI was investigated (16). Almost half of the patients (47%) harboured regional disease, missed on conventional imaging. Disappointingly, sensitivity was extremely low for both investigational techniques (9.4% and 18.8%, respectively), confirming the substantial difficulty of reliably detecting lymph node disease through imaging

alone. Additional studies are thus still needed before using these methods for pelvic nodes delineation.

## 22.6 THERAGNOSTIC IMAGING FOR RADIATION ONCOLOGY

Throughout the first decades of cancer radiation therapy, the dosimetric challenge was to deliver a sufficiently high and homogeneous dose to the tumour. This was achieved with the use of cobalt-60 machine, thereafter with the use of high-energy linear accelerators (linacs). Target volumes delineation were progressively refined with the use of CT or MRI, which allowed to test the hypothesis that pushing up the dose could lead to higher local tumour control. This was achieved but only to some extent, as increased dose to the surrounding normal tissues was associated to increased late toxicity. This raised the question whether more advanced dose escalation strategies were more likely to provide a therapeutic gain.

Imaging-based dose painting, i.e. the prescription and delivery of a non-uniform dose to the clinical target volume (CTV) is a different paradigm for prescribing radiation therapy (11,57). The basic idea is to replace, completely or in part, the morphologically or anatomically defined target volumes with a map of the spatial distribution of a specific tumour phenotype that is hypothesized or has been shown to be related to local tumour control after radiotherapy. A dose prescription function is then used to transform this map into a map of prescribed doses that can be used as input to an inverse planning optimizer. Two prototypical strategies have been considered in the literature: sub-volume boosting also known as dose painting by volume (DPBV), where an imaging-defined discrete volume is given an additional 'boost' radiation dose, or dose painting by number (DPBN), where a dose is prescribed at the voxel level. In the latter case, the prescription function maps a range of image intensities onto a range of doses. Hybrids between the two strategies use a series of nested volumes, often about five or so, with a prescribed dose assigned to each of them.

Theragnostic imaging is the application of the quantitative information in biomedical images to produce a prescribed dose map, i.e. not just a map of where to treat but ideally also of the local dose fractionation that will optimize tumour control under specified normal tissue constraints (10). DPBN relies directly on theragnostic imaging, whereas sub-volume boosting could include morphologic as well as image intensities in the definition of the boost volume. However, in practice there is a continuum of dose prescription strategies ranging between these two ideal cases.

The dose painting paradigm is supported by several clinico-biological hypotheses: (1) local recurrences arise from cellular or micro-environmental niches that are (relatively) resistant at the radiation dose level that can safely be routinely delivered using a uniform dose distribution; (2) molecular imaging will allow spatio-temporal mapping of these regions of relative radioresistance; and (3) advances in radiation therapy planning and delivery technologies facilitate delivery of a graded boost to such regions which in turn should lead to improved local tumour control with acceptable side effects. Support for the dose-painting hypothesis comes in part from mathematical modelling studies. It has been shown that for a fixed integral dose to a tumour with a uniform spatial radiosensitivity distribution, delivering a uniform dose of radiation will maximize the tumour control probability; but for a non-uniform radiosensitivity distribution, a uniform dose distribution is inferior to a distribution that delivers a relatively higher proportion of the integral dose to the more resistant regions of the tumour, i.e. by dose painting (14).

## Dose painting targets

Validation of a dose-painting target does not necessarily require a mechanistic understanding of the relationship between dose response and expression of the target. It is sufficient that an empirical relationship has been demonstrated between target expression and worse local outcome of radiation therapy. The current interest focuses on three evidence-based causes of radiation therapy failure in the clinic: tumour burden or tumour cell density, tumour cell proliferation and hypoxia.

Regarding tumour burden, FDG uptake is commonly considered as a good surrogate for tumour cell density, although various parameters influence its accumulation, such as the rate of glycolysis and tumour perfusion, proliferation, inflammation and hypoxia (108). As mentioned previously (see Section 22.5), there are few 'proof-of-concept' planning studies that have demonstrated the feasibility of selective dose escalation based on FDG distribution in various tumour types (Figure 22.7), but only a few phase I trials have been already conducted (61). In prostate carcinoma, dose escalation modelling based on $^{11}$C-choline uptake has been

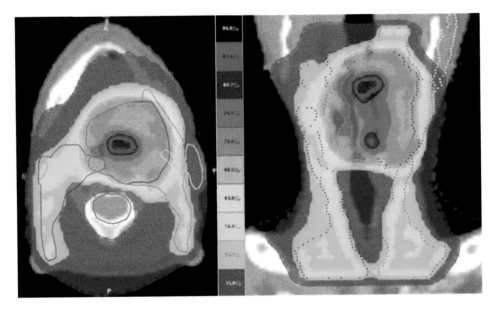

**Figure 22.7** Patient with a T4b-N0-M0 squamous cell carcinoma of the left oropharynx treated by concomitant chemo-radiotherapy. A prophylactic dose of 56 Gy (35 daily fractions of 1.6 Gy) was delivered on the bilateral level II to IV; a therapeutic dose of 70 Gy (35 daily fractions of 2 Gy) was delivered on the primary tumour PTV; within the primary tumour GTV the dose was 'painted' and escalated up to 86 Gy (35 fractions of 2.45 Gy) based on FDG-PET distribution.

reported, but with limited value (68). The use of DW-MRI appears as an attractive alternative imaging method to visualise tumour density, but no clinical dose painting study has been reported yet (24).

Regarding tumour cell proliferation, the use of the radiofluorinated thymidine analogue 3′-deoxy-3′-[18]F-fluorothymidine (FLT) has been investigated. It is a terminator of the growing DNA chain, which is therefore only incorporated into DNA during synthesis to a very limited extent, but it is retained in cells after phosphorylation by the thymidine kinase 1 (TK1) enzyme (75). FLT has been shown to be an imaging surrogate for tumour cell growth, which has enough sensitivity to detect various growth inhibition response (8). FLT-PET scans at baseline and 2 weeks into fractionated radiotherapy for HNSCC have been used to define targets for sub-volume boosting in a recent radiation therapy planning study (93). However, in the absence of direct clinical evidence for an association between these regions and a subsequent local treatment failure, the biological rationale for this boost strategy is still not completely clear, and further data are thus needed before using dose painting based on pre-treatment FLT distribution. Dose boosting based on residual FLT uptake is another possibility, but again further data are needed before embarking on that strategy. Probing the EGFR pathway with labelled cetuximab is another interesting avenue, which has been already tested in animal models but which needs clinical validation (97).

Tumour hypoxia has been observed in a wide variety of solid human tumours, and has been shown to be a strong factor for radioresistance and tumour failure after radiotherapy (see Chapter 17). Various non-invasive indirect methods have been developed to detect tumour hypoxia, and among them, positron-labelled tracers have been used in conjunction with PET camera. Typically, these tracers detect the presence of hypoxia when $pO_2$ drops below 10 mm Hg. Among the various PET tracers synthesized, [18]F-misonidazole (MISO) is the most commonly used, but more recently, other PET tracers such as [18]F-FAZA, [18]F-FETNIM, [18]F-EF3, [18]F-EF5 and [18]F-HX4 have also been introduced in the clinic (42). [18]F-FAZA has several advantages including an easy production with high specific activity, a chemical stability after injection, a specific metabolism in hypoxic cells and a rapid clearance of unbound tracer from non-hypoxic tissues leading to high tumour-to-background ratios compared to other tracers (72). Using FAZA, tumour hypoxia has been identified in 0%–51% of HNSCC cases (62,82). It varies both in intensity and in location throughout radiotherapy treatment, thus calling for adaptive treatment strategy. In a feasibility study, it has been shown that doses up to 86 Gy could be delivered to hypoxic voxels, without significantly exceeding the dose to the surrounding normal tissues (83). However, the magnitude of the required dose to control disease in PET hypoxic regions is still not clear. Simplistic back-of-an-envelope estimates based on *in vitro* oxygen-enhancement ratios are likely to be gross overestimates of the dose required in human tumours. In a proof-of-concept planning study using F-MISO-derived sub-GTV, it has been calculated that a 10% dose escalation (above 70 Gy) with dose redistribution could already be associated with significant increase in tumour control probability (92).

## Dose prescription and clinical implementation

The optimal mathematical form of the prescription function is unknown and may likely depend on the specific tracer of interest. The simplest, reasonable, voxel-based prescription function is a linear interpolation between a minimum dose and a maximum dose, as the voxel image intensity varies between its lower and upper bounds. However, it is likely that instead of a heterogeneous dose painting on top of a homogeneous minimal dose, that dose-painting prescription will be based on the concept of dose redistribution, which allows both dose increase and dose decrease to generate a similar integral dose as if the dose was homogeneously distributed throughout the target volume (88).

Irrespective of the dose prescription function, clinical implementation of dose painting strategies will require the conduct of phase I/II trials to look for toxicity and safety, that should be followed up by a phase III trial with loco-regional control probability and late toxicity as late endpoints. Although modelling has suggested large gains in tumour control from dose painting, the trials should have a sample size allowing detection of a 15% improvement in loco-regional control with 90% power. The trial sample size would be about 450 patients, but an adaptive design could be considered. Clearly, this would need a multicentre or cooperative group format to finish accrual within a reasonable time. Strong data from the early clinical trials will be required to motivate a phase III trial with this sample size and complexity of the intervention. We anticipate that such a trial will be initiated within the next few years.

---

## Key points

1. Molecular imaging is the use of noninvasive imaging techniques (e.g. PET, MRI) that enable the visualization of various biological pathways and physiological characteristics of tumours and normal tissues.
2. FDG-PET and multi-parametric MRI may be of benefit for the selection of target volumes depending on their sensitivity and specificity for various tumour types. Given the considerable range of accuracies across different tumour types, their role will not be identical in the different tumour locations.
3. In using PET for volume segmentation, image acquisition, reconstruction and analysis need new standards favouring image quality over reconstruction speed.

4. Observer-independent segmentation of PET images is required for automatic delineation of the GTV. Probabilistic thresholds or (fuzzy) clustering techniques appear more robust than threshold-based methods especially in difficult cases (low uptake and/or peritumoural inflammation) encountered during radiotherapy treatment.

5. The use of molecular imaging for treatment planning is under validation in various disease sites. It has shown encouraging results in head and neck and lung tumours.

6. 'Theragnostic' has been proposed to describe the use of molecular imaging to assist in prescribing the distribution of radiation dose in four dimensions, the three spatial dimensions plus time. It is a challenging concept at the frontier between radiation oncology, radiation biology and radiation physics that still requires thorough testing.

7. Before proper validation of the use of various PET tracers has been performed, and all methodological aspects have been fully optimized, it is reasonable to say that PET and/or multi-parametric MRI for treatment planning purposes should not be used on a routine basis, but should remain in the clinical research arena.

## ■ BIBLIOGRAPHY

1. Antoch G, Saoudi N, Kuehl H et al. Accuracy of whole-body dual-modality fluorine-18-2-fluoro-2-deoxy-D-glucose positron emission tomography and computed tomography (FDG-PET/CT) for tumor staging in solid tumors: Comparison with CT and PET. *J Clin Oncol* 2004;22:4357–4368.

2. Arias-Castro E, Donoho DL. Does median filtering truly preserve edges better than linear filtering? *Ann Stat* 2009;37: 1172–1206.

3. Aristophanous M, Berbeco RI, Killoran JH et al. Clinical utility of 4D FDG-PET/CT scans in radiation treatment planning. *Int J Radiat Oncol Biol Phys* 2012;82:e99–e105.

4. Ashamalla H, Rafla S, Parikh K et al. The contribution of integrated PET/CT to the evolving definition of treatment volumes in radiation treatment planning in lung cancer. *Int J Radiat Oncol Biol Phys* 2005;63:1016–1023.

5. Bachaud JM, Marre D, Dygai I et al. The impact of [18]F-fluorodeoxyglucose positron emission tomography on the 3D conformal radiotherapy planning in patients with non-small cell lung cancer. *Cancer Radiother* 2005;9:602–609.

6. Bailey DL, Townsend DW, Valk PE, Maisey MN (Eds). *Positron Emission Tomography. Basic Sciences.* London: Springer-Verlag; 2005.

7. Bar-Shalom R, Yefremov N, Guralnik L et al. Clinical performance of PET/CT in evaluation of cancer: Additional value for diagnostic imaging and patient management. *J Nucl Med* 2003;44:1200–1209.

8. Barwick T, Bencherif B, Mountz JM, Avril N. Molecular PET and PET/CT imaging of tumour cell proliferation using F-18 fluoro-L-thymidine: A comprehensive evaluation. *Nucl Med Commun* 2009;30:908–917.

9. Belhassen S, Zaidi H. A novel fuzzy C-means algorithm for unsupervised heterogeneous tumor quantification in PET. *Med Phys* 2010;37:1309–1324.

10. Bentzen SM. Theragnostic imaging for radiation oncology: Dose-painting by numbers. *Lancet Oncol* 2005;6:112–117.

11. Bentzen SM, Gregoire V. Molecular imaging-based dose painting: A novel paradigm for radiation therapy prescription. *Semin Radiat Oncol* 2011;21:101–110.

12. Bipat S, Glas AS, Slors FJ, Zwinderman AH, Bossuyt PM, Stoker J. Rectal cancer: Local staging and assessment of lymph node involvement with endoluminal US, CT, and MR imaging – A meta-analysis. *Radiology* 2004;232:773–783.

13. Braendengen M, Hansson K, Radu C, Siegbahn A, Jacobsson H, Glimelius B. Delineation of gross tumor volume (GTV) for radiation treatment planning of locally advanced rectal cancer using information from MRI or FDG-PET/CT: A prospective study. *Int J Radiat Oncol Biol Phys* 2011;81: e439–e445.

14. Brahme A, Agren AK. Optimal dose distribution for eradication of heterogeneous tumours. *Acta Oncol* 1987;26: 377–385.

15. Brush J, Boyd K, Chappell F et al. The value of FDG positron emission tomography/computerised tomography (PET/CT) in pre-operative staging of colorectal cancer: A systematic review and economic evaluation. *Health Technol Assess* 2011;15:1–192, iii–iv.

16. Budiharto T, Joniau S, Lerut E et al. Prospective evaluation of 11C-choline positron emission tomography/computed tomography and diffusion-weighted magnetic resonance imaging for the nodal staging of prostate cancer with a high risk of lymph node metastases. *Eur Urol* 2011;60:125–130.

17. Buijsen J, van den Bogaard J, Janssen MH et al. FDG-PET provides the best correlation with the tumor specimen compared to MRI and CT in rectal cancer. *Radiother Oncol* 2011;98:270–276.

18. Choi H, Paeng JC, Cheon GJ et al. Correlation of 11C-methionine PET and diffusion-weighted MRI: Is there a complementary diagnostic role for gliomas? *Nucl Med Commun* 2014;35:720–726.

19. Choi HJ, Ju W, Myung SK, Kim Y. Diagnostic performance of computer tomography, magnetic resonance imaging, and positron emission tomography or positron emission tomography/computer tomography for detection of metastatic lymph nodes in patients with cervical cancer: Meta-analysis. *Cancer Sci* 2010;101:1471–1479.

20. Ciernik IF, Dizendorf E, Baumert BG et al. Radiation treatment planning with an integrated positron emission and computer tomography (PET/CT): A feasibility study. *Int J Radiat Oncol Biol Phys* 2003;57:853–863.

21. Daisne JF, Duprez T, Weynand B et al. Tumor volume in pharyngolaryngeal squamous cell carcinoma: Comparison at CT, MR imaging, and FDG PET and validation with surgical specimen. *Radiology* 2004;233:93–100.

22. De Ruysscher D, Wanders S, Minken A et al. Effects of radiotherapy planning with a dedicated combined PET-CT-simulator of patients with non-small cell lung cancer on dose limiting normal tissues and radiation dose-escalation: A planning study. *Radiother Oncol* 2005;77:5–10.

23. De Ruysscher D, Wanders S, van Haren E et al. Selective mediastinal node irradiation based on FDG-PET scan data in patients with non-small-cell lung cancer: A prospective clinical study. *Int J Radiat Oncol Biol Phys* 2005;62:988–994.

24. Dirix P, Haustermans K, Vandecaveye V. The value of magnetic resonance imaging for radiotherapy planning. *Semin Radiat Oncol* 2014;24:151–159.

25. Doll C, Duncker-Rohr V, Rucker G et al. Influence of experience and qualification on PET-based target volume delineation. When there is no expert – Ask your colleague. *Strahlenther Onkol* 2014;190:555–562.

26. Esthappan J, Chaudhari S, Santanam L et al. Prospective clinical trial of positron emission tomography/computed tomography image-guided intensity-modulated radiation therapy for cervical carcinoma with positive para-aortic lymph nodes. *Int J Radiat Oncol Biol Phys* 2008;72:1134–1139.

27. Evangelista L, Guttilla A, Zattoni F, Muzzio PC, Zattoni F. Utility of choline positron emission tomography/computed tomography for lymph node involvement identification in intermediate- to high-risk prostate cancer: A systematic literature review and meta-analysis. *Eur Urol* 2013;63: 1040–1048.

28. Flamen P, Lerut A, Van Cutsem E et al. Utility of positron emission tomography for the staging of patients with potentially operable esophageal carcinoma. *J Clin Oncol* 2000;18:3202–3210.

29. Fox JL, Rengan R, O'Meara W et al. Does registration of PET and planning CT images decrease interobserver and intraobserver variation in delineating tumor volumes for non-small-cell lung cancer? *Int J Radiat Oncol Biol Phys* 2005;62:70–75.

30. Geets X, Daisne JF, Arcangeli S et al. Inter-observer variability in the delineation of pharyngo-laryngeal tumor, parotid glands and cervical spinal cord: Comparison between CT-scan and MRI. *Radiother Oncol* 2005;77:25–31.

31. Geets X, Daisne JF, Tomsej M, Duprez T, Lonneux M, Gregoire V. Impact of the type of imaging modality on target volumes delineation and dose distribution in pharyngo-laryngeal squamous cell carcinoma: Comparison between pre- and per-treatment studies. *Radiother Oncol* 2006;78:291–297.

32. Geets X, Lee JA, Bol A, Lonneux M, Gregoire V. A gradient-based method for segmenting FDG-PET images: Methodology and validation. *Eur J Nucl Med Mol Imaging* 2007;34:1427–1438.

33. Geets X, Tomsej M, Lee JA et al. Adaptive biological image-guided IMRT with anatomic and functional imaging in pharyngo-laryngeal tumors: Impact on target volume delineation and dose distribution using helical tomotherapy. *Radiother Oncol* 2007;85:105–115.

34. Glaudemans AW, Enting RH, Heesters MA et al. Value of 11C-methionine PET in imaging brain tumours and metastases. *Eur J Nucl Med Mol Imaging* 2013;40:615–635.

35. Gondi V, Bradley K, Mehta M et al. Impact of hybrid fluorodeoxyglucose positron-emission tomography/computed tomography on radiotherapy planning in esophageal and non-small-cell lung cancer. *Int J Radiat Oncol Biol Phys* 2007;67:187–195.

36. Gould MK, Kuschner WG, Rydzak CE et al. Test performance of positron emission tomography and computed tomography for mediastinal staging in patients with non-small-cell lung cancer: A meta-analysis. *Ann Intern Med* 2003;139: 879–892.

37. Gregoire V, Daisne JF, Geets X. Comparison of CT- and FDG-PET-defined GT. *Int J Radiat Oncol Biol Phys* 2005;63: 308–309.

38. Grosu AL, Lachner R, Wiedenmann N et al. Validation of a method for automatic image fusion (BrainLAB System) of CT data and 11C-methionine-PET data for stereotactic radiotherapy using a LINAC: First clinical experience. *Int J Radiat Oncol Biol Phys* 2003;56:1450–1463.

39. Grosu AL, Weber WA. PET for radiation treatment planning of brain tumours. *Radiother Oncol* 2010;96:325–327.

40. Haie-Meder C, Mazeron R, Magne N. Clinical evidence on PET-CT for radiation therapy planning in cervix and endometrial cancers. *Radiother Oncol* 2010;96:351–355.

41. Hatt M, Cheze le Rest C, Turzo A, Roux C, Visvikis D. A fuzzy locally adaptive Bayesian segmentation approach for volume determination in PET. *IEEE Trans Med Imaging* 2009;28: 881–893.

42. Haubner R. PET radiopharmaceuticals in radiation treatment planning – Synthesis and biological characteristics. *Radiother Oncol* 2010;96:280–287.

43. Herholz K, Holzer T, Bauer B et al. 11C-methionine PET for differential diagnosis of low-grade gliomas. *Neurology* 1998;50:1316–1322.

44. Hövels AM, Heesakkers RA, Adang EM et al. The diagnostic accuracy of CT and MRI in the staging of pelvic lymph nodes in patients with prostate cancer: A meta-analysis. *Clin Radiol* 2008;63:387–395.

45. Howard A, Mehta MP, Ritter MA et al. The value of PET/CT in gross tumor volume delineation in lung and esophagus cancer. *Int J Radiat Oncol Biol Phys* 2004;60(Suppl. 1): S536–S537.

46. Hricak H, Gatsonis C, Coakley FV et al. Early invasive cervical cancer: CT and MR imaging in preoperative evaluation – ACRIN/GOG comparative study of diagnostic performance and interobserver variability. *Radiology* 2007;245:491–498.

47. Hricak H, Lacey CG, Sandles LG, Chang YC, Winkler ML, Stern JL. Invasive cervical carcinoma: Comparison of MR imaging and surgical findings. *Radiology* 1988;166:623–631.

48. Jacobs AH, Winkler A, Dittmar C et al. Molecular and functional imaging technology for the development of efficient treatment strategies for gliomas. *Technol Cancer Res Treat* 2002;1:187–204.

49. Konski A, Doss M, Milestone B et al. The integration of 18-fluoro-deoxy-glucose positron emission tomography and endoscopic ultrasound in the treatment-planning process for esophageal carcinoma. *Int J Radiat Oncol Biol Phys* 2005;61:1123–1128.

50. Krishnan AP, Asher IM, Davis D, Okunieff P, O'Dell WG. Evidence that MR diffusion tensor imaging (tractography) predicts the natural history of regional progression in patients irradiated conformally for primary brain tumors. *Int J Radiat Oncol Biol Phys* 2008;71:1553–1562.

51. Kyzas PA, Evangelou E, Denaxa-Kyza D, Ioannidis JP. 18F-fluorodeoxyglucose positron emission tomography to evaluate cervical node metastases in patients with head and neck squamous cell carcinoma: A meta-analysis. *J Natl Cancer Inst* 2008;100:712–720.

52. Leclerc M, Lartigau E, Lacornerie T, Daisne JF, Kramar A, Gregoire V. Primary tumor delineation based on (18)FDG PET for locally advanced head and neck cancer treated by chemo-radiotherapy. *Radiother Oncol* 2015;116:87–93.

53. Lee JA. Segmentation of positron emission tomography images: Some recommendations for target delineation in radiation oncology. *Radiother Oncol* 2010;96:302–307.

54. Lee JA, Geets X, Gregoire V, Bol A. Edge-preserving filtering of images with low photon counts. *IEEE Trans Pattern Anal Mach Intell* 2008;30:1014–1027.

55. Leong T, Everitt C, Yuen K et al. A prospective study to evaluate the impact of coregistered PET/CT images on radiotherapy treatment planning for esophageal cancer. *Int J Radiat Oncol Biol Phys* 2004;60(Suppl. 1):S139–S140.

56. Liao LJ, Lo WC, Hsu WL, Wang CT, Lai MS. Detection of cervical lymph node metastasis in head and neck cancer patients with clinically N0 neck-a meta-analysis comparing different imaging modalities. *BMC Cancer* 2012;12:236.

57. Ling CC, Humm J, Larson S et al. Towards multidimensional radiotherapy (MD-CRT): Biological imaging and biological conformality. *Int J Radiat Oncol Biol Phys* 2000;47:551–560.

58. Ma DJ, Zhu JM, Grigsby PW. Tumor volume discrepancies between FDG-PET and MRI for cervical cancer. *Radiother Oncol* 2011;98:139–142.

59. Mac Manus MP, Everitt S, Bayne M et al. The use of fused PET/CT images for patient selection and radical radiotherapy target volume definition in patients with non-small cell lung cancer: Results of a prospective study with mature survival data. *Radiother Oncol* 2013;106:292–298.

60. Mac Manus MP, Hicks RJ, Ball DL et al. F-18 fluorodeoxyglucose positron emission tomography staging in radical radiotherapy candidates with nonsmall cell lung carcinoma: Powerful correlation with survival and high impact on treatment. *Cancer* 2001;92:886–895.

61. Madani I, Duprez F, Boterberg T et al. Maximum tolerated dose in a phase I trial on adaptive dose painting by numbers for head and neck cancer. *Radiother Oncol* 2011;101:351–355.

62. Mortensen LS, Johansen J, Kallehauge J et al. FAZA PET/CT hypoxia imaging in patients with squamous cell carcinoma of the head and neck treated with radiotherapy: Results from the DAHANCA 24 trial. *Radiother Oncol* 2012;105:14–20.

63. Moureau-Zabotto L, Touboul E, Lerouge D et al. Impact of CT and 18F-deoxyglucose positron emission tomography image fusion for conformal radiotherapy in esophageal carcinoma. *Int J Radiat Oncol Biol Phys* 2005;63:340–345.

64. Muijs C, Smit J, Karrenbeld A et al. Residual tumor after neoadjuvant chemoradiation outside the radiation therapy target volume: A new prognostic factor for survival in esophageal cancer. *Int J Radiat Oncol Biol Phys* 2014;88:845–852.

65. Muijs CT, Beukema JC, Widder J et al. 18F-FLT-PET for detection of rectal cancer. *Radiother Oncol* 2011;98:357–359.

66. Nagayoshi M, Murase K, Fujino K et al. Usefulness of noise adaptive non-linear gaussian filter in FDG-PET study. *Ann Nucl Med* 2005;19:469–477.

67. Nestle U, Kremp S, Schaefer-Schuler A et al. Comparison of different methods for delineation of 18F-FDG PET-positive tissue for target volume definition in radiotherapy of patients with non-small cell lung cancer. *J Nucl Med* 2005;46:1342–1348.

68. Niyazi M, Bartenstein P, Belka C, Ganswindt U. Choline PET based dose-painting in prostate cancer – Modelling of dose effects. *Radiat Oncol* 2010;5:23.

69. Olsen JR, Esthappan J, DeWees T et al. Tumor volume and subvolume concordance between FDG-PET/CT and diffusion-weighted MRI for squamous cell carcinoma of the cervix. *J Magn Reson Imaging* 2013;37:431–434.

70. Paulino AC, Koshy M, Howell R, Schuster D, Davis LW. Comparison of CT- and FDG-PET-defined gross tumor volume in intensity-modulated radiotherapy for head-and-neck cancer. *Int J Radiat Oncol Biol Phys* 2005;61:1385–1392.

71. Picchio M, Giovannini E, Crivellaro C, Gianolli L, di Muzio N, Messa C. Clinical evidence on PET/CT for radiation therapy planning in prostate cancer. *Radiother Oncol* 2010;96:347–350.

72. Piert M, Machulla HJ, Picchio M et al. Hypoxia-specific tumor imaging with 18F-fluoroazomycin arabinoside. *J Nucl Med* 2005;46:106–113.

73. Pooley RA. AAPM/RSNA physics tutorial for residents: Fundamental physics of MR imaging. *Radiographics* 2005;25:1087–1099.

74. Rapp M, Heinzel A, Galldiks N et al. Diagnostic performance of 18F-FET PET in newly diagnosed cerebral lesions suggestive of glioma. *J Nucl Med* 2013;54:229–235.

75. Rasey JS, Grierson JR, Wiens LW, Kolb PD, Schwartz JL. Validation of FLT uptake as a measure of thymidine kinase-1 activity in A549 carcinoma cells. *J Nucl Med* 2002;43:1210–1217.

76. Riegel AC, Berson AM, Destian S et al. Variability of gross tumor volume delineation in head-and-neck cancer using CT and PET/CT fusion. *Int J Radiat Oncol Biol Phys* 2006;65:726–732.

77. Roels S, Duthoy W, Haustermans K et al. Definition and delineation of the clinical target volume for rectal cancer. *Int J Radiat Oncol Biol Phys* 2006;65:1129–1142.

78. Roels S, Slagmolen P, Nuyts J et al. Biological image-guided radiotherapy in rectal cancer: Is there a role for FMISO or FLT, next to FDG? *Acta Oncol* 2008;47:1237–1248.

79. Sala E, Wakely S, Senior E, Lomas D. MRI of malignant neoplasms of the uterine corpus and cervix. *AJR Am J Roentgenol* 2007;188:1577–1587.

80. Schwartz DL, Ford EC, Rajendran J et al. FDG-PET/CT-guided intensity modulated head and neck radiotherapy: A pilot investigation. *Head Neck* 2005;27:478–487.

81. Schwarzenböck SM, Kurth J, Gocke C, Kuhnt T, Hildebrandt G, Krause BJ. Role of choline PET/CT in guiding target volume delineation for irradiation of prostate cancer. *Eur J Nucl Med Mol Imaging* 2013;40(Suppl 1):S28–S35.

82. Servagi-Vernat S, Differding S, Hanin FX et al. A prospective clinical study of (1)(8)F-FAZA PET-CT hypoxia imaging in head and neck squamous cell carcinoma before and during radiation therapy. *Eur J Nucl Med Mol Imaging* 2014;41:1544–1552.

83. Servagi-Vernat S, Differding S, Sterpin E et al. Hypoxia-guided adaptive radiation dose escalation in head and neck carcinoma: A planning study. *Acta Oncol* 2015;54:1008–1016.

84. Shah JP. Patterns of cervical lymph node metastasis from squamous carcinomas of the upper aerodigestive tract. *Am J Surg* 1990;160:405–409.

85. Shepherd T, Teras M, Beichel RR et al. Comparative study with new accuracy metrics for target volume contouring in PET image guided radiation therapy. *IEEE Trans Med Imaging* 2012;31:2006–2024.

86. Shi W, Wang W, Wang J, Cheng H, Huo X. Meta-analysis of 18FDG PET-CT for nodal staging in patients with esophageal cancer. *Surg Oncol* 2013;22:112–116.

87. Soret M, Bacharach SL, Buvat I. Partial-volume effect in PET tumor imaging. *J Nucl Med* 2007;48:932–945.

88. Søvik A, Malinen E, Bruland ØS, Bentzen SM, Olsen DR. Optimization of tumour control probability in hypoxic tumours by radiation dose redistribution: A modelling study. *Phys Med Biol* 2007;52:499–513.

89. Steenbakkers RJ, Deurloo KE, Nowak PJ, Lebesque JV, van Herk M, Rasch CR. Reduction of dose delivered to the rectum and bulb of the penis using MRI delineation for radiotherapy of the prostate. *Int J Radiat Oncol Biol Phys* 2003;57:1269–1279.

90. Sweeney RA, Bale RJ, Moncayo R et al. Multimodality cranial image fusion using external markers applied via a vacuum mouthpiece and a case report. *Strahlenther Onkol* 2003;179:254–260.

91. Tarantola G, Zito F, Gerundini P. PET instrumentation and reconstruction algorithms in whole-body applications. *J Nucl Med* 2003;44:756–769.

92. Thorwarth D, Eschmann SM, Paulsen F, Alber M. Hypoxia dose painting by numbers: A planning study. *Int J Radiat Oncol Biol Phys* 2007;68:291–300.

93. Troost EG, Bussink J, Hoffmann AL, Boerman OC, Oyen WJ, Kaanders JH. 18F-FLT PET/CT for early response monitoring and dose escalation in oropharyngeal tumors. *J Nucl Med* 2010;51:866–874.

94. van Baardwijk A, Bosmans G, Boersma L et al. PET-CT-based auto-contouring in non-small-cell lung cancer correlates with pathology and reduces interobserver variability in the delineation of the primary tumor and involved nodal volumes. *Int J Radiat Oncol Biol Phys* 2007;68:771–778.

95. van Dalen JA, Hoffmann AL, Dicken V et al. A novel iterative method for lesion delineation and volumetric quantification with FDG PET. *Nucl Med Commun* 2007;28:485–493.

96. van der Wel A, Nijsten S, Hochstenbag M et al. Increased therapeutic ratio by 18FDG-PET CT planning in patients with clinical CT stage N2-N3M0 non-small-cell lung cancer: A modeling study. *Int J Radiat Oncol Biol Phys* 2005;61:649–655.

97. van Dijk LK, Hoeben BA, Kaanders JH, Franssen GM, Boerman OC, Bussink J. Imaging of epidermal growth factor receptor expression in head and neck cancer with SPECT/CT and 111In-labeled cetuximab-F(ab')2. *J Nucl Med* 2013;54:2118–2124.

98. van Westreenen HL, Westerterp M, Bossuyt PM et al. Systematic review of the staging performance of 18F-fluorodeoxyglucose positron emission tomography in esophageal cancer. *J Clin Oncol* 2004;22:3805–3812.

99. Vandecaveye V, De Keyzer F, Vander Poorten V et al. Head and neck squamous cell carcinoma: Value of diffusion-weighted MR imaging for nodal staging. *Radiology* 2009;251:134–146.

100. Villeirs GM, De Meerleer GO. Magnetic resonance imaging (MRI) anatomy of the prostate and application of MRI in radiotherapy planning. *Eur J Radiol* 2007;63:361–368.

101. Villeirs GM, Van Vaerenbergh K, Vakaet L et al. Interobserver delineation variation using CT versus combined CT + MRI in intensity-modulated radiotherapy for prostate cancer. *Strahlenther Onkol* 2005;181:424–430.

102. Vrieze O, Haustermans K, De Wever W et al. Is there a role for FGD-PET in radiotherapy planning in esophageal carcinoma? *Radiother Oncol* 2004;73:269–275.

103. Wanet M, Lee JA, Weynand B et al. Gradient-based delineation of the primary GTV on FDG-PET in non-small cell lung cancer: A comparison with threshold-based approaches, CT and surgical specimens. *Radiother Oncol* 2011;98:117–125.

104. Weber WA, Wester HJ, Grosu AL et al. O-(2-[18F]fluoroethyl)-L-tyrosine and L-[methyl-11C]methionine uptake in brain tumours: Initial results of a comparative study. *Eur J Nucl Med* 2000;27:542–549.

105. Wu LM, Xu JR, Gu HY et al. Preoperative mediastinal and hilar nodal staging with diffusion-weighted magnetic resonance imaging and fluorodeoxyglucose positron emission tomography/computed tomography in patients with non-small-cell lung cancer: Which is better? *J Surg Res* 2012;178:304–314.

106. Yang RM, Li L, Wei XH et al. Differentiation of central lung cancer from atelectasis: Comparison of diffusion-weighted MRI with PET/CT. *PLOS ONE* 2013;8:e60279.

107. Zhang Y, Hu J, Li J et al. Comparison of imaging-based gross tumor volume and pathological volume determined by whole-mount serial sections in primary cervical cancer. *Onco Targets Ther* 2013;6:917–923.

108. Zhao S, Kuge Y, Mochizuki T et al. Biologic correlates of intratumoral heterogeneity in 18F-FDG distribution with regional expression of glucose transporters and hexokinase-II in experimental tumor. *J Nucl Med* 2005;46:675–682.

# Retreatment tolerance of normal tissues

## WOLFGANG DÖRR, DOROTA GABRYŚ AND FIONA A. STEWART

## 23.1 INTRODUCTION

Improvements in cancer treatment in general and radiotherapy in particular, based on advances in medical radiation physics and radiation biology, have resulted in a substantial prolongation of survival times and significantly increased survival rates for a variety of malignancies over the past two decades. This has led to a transition from a perception of cancer patients to a recognition of and attention for cancer survivorship (e.g. [38]). Surviving cancer patients are, however, at an increased risk of developing secondary neoplasms (see Chapter 27). The most important reason for this is that patients cured of one cancer have a chance to grow older and hence underlies an increasing risk of 'naturally' occurring (then second) cancer with older age. Second, compared to the general population, they still retain more risk (e.g. molecular predisposition) to develop a (second) tumour than any other person of similar age, gender, lifestyle, etc., who had not previously experienced the disease. Third, the etiologic factors associated with the first tumour, e.g. smoking for lung and head and neck tumours, or alcohol consumption for tumours of the head and neck or the oesophagus, or exposure to other carcinogens, in many cases do continue and hence promote the manifestation of a second malignancy. Of more than 30,000 irradiated patients with a primary head and neck tumour, more than 20% developed a second neoplasm (14), out of which more than 80% were found in the head and neck region, the oesophagus and the lung. Fourth, the therapy itself, radiation exposure as well as chemotherapy and more recently exposure to biologically targeted agents ('biologicals'), is associated with an increased risk for second tumours. This is of particular importance for children and younger adults; childhood cancer survivors are at an up to 19-fold increased risk for developing another malignancy (11).

In many instances, *second primary tumours* occur without a relation to the initial radiation treatment volumes, thus their treatment may be considered similar to a primary therapy. However, second primary tumours may also be observed within, or – even more frequently – close to the initial high-dose treatment volume (12). Moreover, *recurrent tumours* can develop within or close to the original gross tumour volume.

Both second primary tumours and recurrences must be treated adequately, which frequently involves radiotherapy.

Decisions regarding safe retreatment are very complex; for example, surgical options are frequently compromised by local responses (e.g. fibrosis) to the first treatment. Hence, for the development of curative or even palliative reirradiation strategies, a number of parameters must be considered:

- Initial radiotherapy: dose (equieffective dose, e.g. EQD2), volume, spatial relationship to the required reirradiation fields and volumes
- Additional treatments for the first tumour (e.g. chemotherapy, 'biologicals')
- Time interval between therapy courses
- Organs and tissues at risk (OAR) involved
- Alternative treatment options

These considerations must include scenarios of possible long-term recovery, potential (stable) residual damage after longer time periods or even progression of (subclinical) damage over time. There are examples for all these settings, depending on the OAR under consideration. Based on the risk factors mentioned above, the potential tissue-specific morbidity caused by the second treatment, and its impact on the patient's quality of life, must be weighed against the expected benefits in terms of tumour response and survival.

This chapter focuses on scenarios where the initial radiation treatment was in the range of *sub-tolerance* doses, with the induction of only sub-clinical or minimal clinically manifest changes. The main findings from experimental and clinical studies on the reirradiation tolerance of various normal tissues are summarized. Clinical studies that provide information on one specific side effect and more general descriptions for entire tumour entities are also reviewed. In order to compare data from studies with different fractionation regimes, we have recalculated the doses administered in these studies to obtain the *equieffective dose in 2 Gy fractions*, $EQD2_{\alpha/\beta}$, according to Bentzen et al. (5); using the linear-quadratic approach with $\alpha/\beta$ values of 10 Gy for early reactions and 3 Gy for late reactions (see Chapters 9 and 10). Tolerance doses, here defined as threshold doses above which specified grades of morbidity are observed at a specified incidence rate, are referred to as the $EQD2_{tol}$. The contribution of both the initial treatment and the retreatment can hence be specified as a percentage of the total $EQD2_{tol}$.

It should be mentioned that the vast majority of the increasing number of clinical reports on reirradiation do not include data from simultaneous control groups with primary irradiation of the same site, and hence do not provide quantitative information. It must also be emphasised that most of the clinical studies have enrolled patients over long time periods, and therefore only provide limited information due to changes, for example, in irradiation techniques and side effect classification. Moreover, many studies include highly variable radiotherapy (and chemotherapy) protocols and treatments with curative as well as palliative intent. These studies will receive minor attention in this review.

## 23.2 EARLY TISSUE REACTIONS

Early tissue reactions are usually found in fast proliferating, turnover tissues (see Chapter 14). Based on surviving stem cells within the irradiated volume or area, or on stem cells migrating into the irradiated tissue from non-irradiated sites, regeneration and restitution of tissue architecture and cellularity occur, which should result in complete or partial restoration of the radiation tolerance.

### Epidermis

Reports on the reirradiation tolerance for early epidermis-based skin reactions in rodents are consistent in demonstrating very good recovery from the initial damage with restoration of the radiation tolerance (Figure 23.1). Recovery is faster after lower initial doses and is inversely proportional to the extent of (stem) cell kill (see Figure 14.3). After single radiation doses that induce clinical desquamation of the epidermis, complete restitution of the

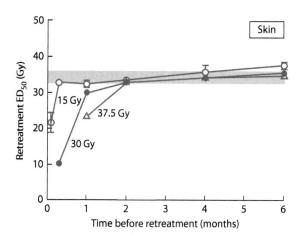

**Figure 23.1** Retreatment tolerance of mouse skin at different times after initial treatments with 15–37.5 Gy. The vertical scale gives the retreatment dose required for a specified level of skin damage (ED$_{50}$ for desquamation). The shaded area shows the range of ED$_{50}$ doses for the same level of skin damage for previously untreated mice. (Adapted from (57), with permission.)

initial tolerance has been observed after 2 months in mice (57). In another study with fractionated irradiation, high initial doses, causing severe early damage, resulted in some residual damage even after 6 months, with the consequence of reduced tolerance ($\approx$80% EQD2$_{tol}$ after 10 $\times$ 5 Gy pre-treatment) as demonstrated by increased early responses, particularly to high retreatment doses (6).

### Oral and oesophageal mucosa

No pre-clinical animal data are available on reirradiation effects in oral and oesophageal mucosa. However, in patients with head and neck cancer, oral mucositis has been quantified after repeated radiotherapy courses with treatment breaks (60). If these breaks were in the range of 2 weeks, then mucositis developed with an identical time course and severity after each of three treatment cycles. If the breaks are shorter, around 10 days, then the severity of oral mucositis can even be lower after a second cycle (28), as the repopulation response (see Chapter 12) is still maximally active and can effectively counteract the (stem) cell kill right from the onset of reirradiation.

However, early reactions after short treatment breaks do not necessarily fully reflect the responses to reirradiation. Patients subject to reirradiation in the head and neck region after longer time intervals of 2–3 years may present with mucosal erythema (mucositis grade 1 according to RTOG/EORTC), or even focal lesions, already before the start of the second radiotherapy course. More severe mucosal reactions (confluent: grade 3) are frequently observed at earlier time points after reirradiation than in the first radiation series (Figure 23.2). This may be a consequence of chronic mucosal atrophy, i.e. reduced cell numbers, resulting in an increased vulnerability and a reduction in the time required for total cell depletion (see Chapter 14).

### Bone marrow

The potential and extent of long-term recovery in bone marrow is clearly dependent on the toxicity of the initial treatment. At high doses, in the range used for total-body irradiation as a conditioning regimen for bone marrow/stem cell/progenitor cell transplantation, the stem cell pool is irreversibly damaged and no recovery is possible without an external supply of stem cells. At more moderate doses, the first response of the bone marrow is the stimulation of transit divisions (see Chapter 14), i.e. an increase in the number of transit generations resulting in an increased output of differentiated cells per stem cell division. This counteracts cell depletion in the peripheral blood at early time points (Figure 23.3). However, it needs to be emphasised that regeneration at the stem cell level may take much longer (16). The toxicity of the initial treatment must therefore be considered carefully for reirradiation, independently of peripheral blood cell counts, as the latter may be critically misleading.

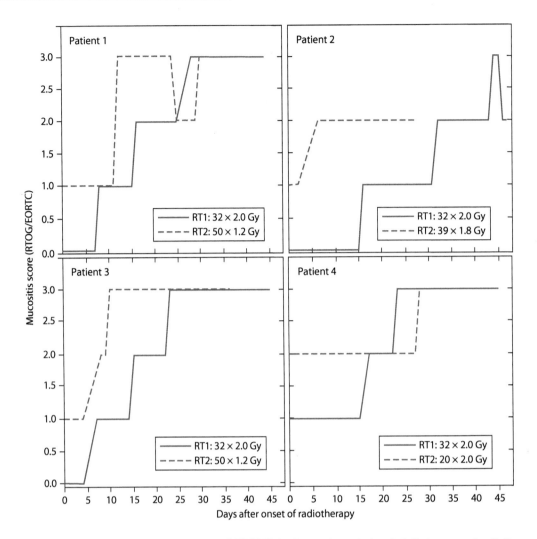

**Figure 23.2** Clinical scores of oral mucositis according to RTOG/EORTC for four patients during their first course of radiotherapy (solid lines) and during reirradiation (dashed lines). (Dörr et al., unpublished data.)

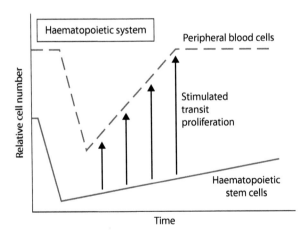

**Figure 23.3** Changes in peripheral blood cell counts (dashed line) versus number of haematopoietic stem cell numbers in bone marrow (solid line). Earlier recovery of the peripheral cell number is based on stimulated transit proliferation, and does not reflect recovery of the stem cell population, i.e. restoration of radiation tolerance.

Restitution of stromal elements, which closely interact with the stem-progenitor cell system in the bone marrow, may take even longer than for the haematopoietic system itself. At higher doses, no regeneration occurs and the marrow is irreversibly converted into fatty tissue. Thus – in mice – irradiation with 6.5 Gy resulted in persistent damage in the stromal and the progenitor compartment after 1 year; the effect was even more pronounced when the initial exposure was fractionated over 15 days. It has also been demonstrated in mice and dogs that this residual injury is more pronounced in neonates and younger animals compared to adults (16), indicating a lower reirradiation tolerance of the bone marrow and its stroma.

## Urinary bladder

The early response of the urinary bladder, presenting as a reduction in storage capacity, is independent of urothelial cell depletion, which would not be expected during or shortly after radiotherapy, based on long turnover times of several months in this tissue (see Chapter 14). Reirradiation tolerance of the urinary bladder with regard to early reactions, assessed as a more than 50% reduction in compliance capacity during the first 4 weeks after treatment, has been studied in mice. After an initial treatment with $5 \times 5.3$ Gy (inducing reduced compliance in $\approx$30% of the animals), the original tolerance was restored between 25 and 50 days (Figure 23.4). Longer intervals were required after higher initial doses. At later time points, reduced tolerance was found, presumably due to an overlap between the early response to the reirradiation and the onset of late damage from the first treatment.

## Rectum

For the reirradiation tolerance of the rectum, clinical data are available. Reirradiation for rectal cancer was carried out in 103 patients after an initial median dose of 50.4 Gy with fractionated doses of 15–49.2 Gy, plus 5FU-based chemotherapy, after a median interval of 19 months (36). Cumulative (initial plus retreatment) doses were 70.6–108 Gy. During reirradiation, early rectal toxicity comprised $\geq$grade 3 diarrhoea and mucositis, requiring treatment breaks (8% of patients) or even cessation of the therapy (15%). Relatively low toxicity was found by Valentini et al. (58), who studied retreatment after initial doses of $\leq$55 Gy (median interval 27 months). Reirradiation doses were 30 Gy plus a hyperfractionated boost of 10.8 Gy ($2 \times 1.2$ Gy/day) with concurrent chemotherapy. Grade $\leq$3 gastrointestinal early toxicity was 5.1%; 10.2% of the patients had temporary treatment interruption and the therapy was terminated early in 3.4%.

Well tolerated was also hyperfractionated radiotherapy delivered twice a day with 1.2 Gy per fraction concurrent

with capecitabine chemotherapy in 72 patients treated for recurrent and irresectable rectal cancer (54). Patients were evaluated for resectability after 36 Gy and radiotherapy was continued to 51.6–56.4 Gy in inoperable cases. Grade 3–4 toxicity as diarrhoea was present in 9.7% and granulocytopenia in 8.3% of patients. Diarrhoea was the cause of interruption in two patients who subsequently refused to resume radiotherapy.

## 23.3 LATE EFFECTS

### Skin and subcutaneous tissue

Using hind limb deformation as an endpoint for late subcutaneous fibrosis (6), there is a clear reduction in tolerance for reirradiation after 6 months (Figure 23.5). The effect of reirradiation was much more pronounced after more aggressive initial radiation protocols ($10 \times 5$ Gy versus $10 \times 4$ Gy). Also, this effect was markedly more prominent than for early skin reactions in the same animals (cf. epidermis in Section 23.2). Further studies similarly suggest a significantly poorer retreatment tolerance for late compared to early skin reactions. In general, a reduction in retreatment tolerance to 50%–70% of the $EQD2_{tol}$ is seen. However, there are also contradictory studies, where very good retreatment tolerance has been demonstrated for late deformity endpoints, e.g. in pig skin (49). In some mouse studies, the reduced reirradiation tolerance for late damage may have been influenced by the high severity of early epidermal reactions in response to the first treatment, which are associated with the development of consequential late effects (see Chapter 14).

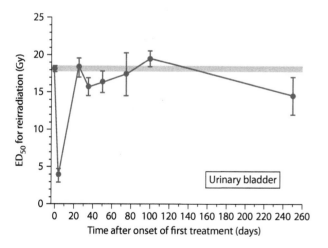

Figure 23.4 Retreatment tolerance of mouse urinary bladder (early damage) at different times after irradiation with $5 \times 5.3$ Gy over 1 week. The ordinate indicates the retreatment $ED_{50}$ required for a 50% reduction in bladder storage capacity (at 1–3 weeks after reirradiation). The shaded area shows the $ED_{50}$ for the effect in previously untreated mice. (Satthoff and Dörr, unpublished data.)

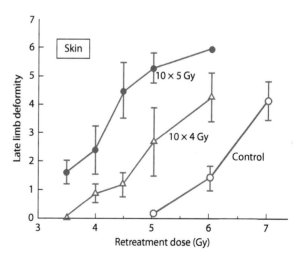

Figure 23.5 Retreatment tolerance for late hind-limb deformity in mice, as measured by fibrosis. Reirradiation was with 10 fractions at the dose per fraction indicated on the abscissa, administered at 6 months after an initial treatment with $10 \times 4$ Gy or $10 \times 5$ Gy, or without previous irradiation. (Redrawn from (6), with permission.)

## Head and neck tissues

The major organ at risk that needs to be considered with regard to reirradiation of head and neck cancer is the *carotid artery*. Carotid rupture is an infrequent but serious complication, as e.g. shown by McDonald et al. (32): among 1554 patients receiving salvage head and neck reirradiation, 41 (2.6%) experienced carotid rupture, 76% of which were fatal. The authors suggest that accelerated hyperfractionated reirradiation was associated with a higher risk of carotid rupture compared to conventional or exclusively hyperfractionated reirradiation.

Kasperts et al. (18) reviewed 27 retreatment studies of head and neck cancer, where the second irradiation was performed as teletherapy or brachytherapy, in combination with chemotherapy or after surgery. Major late complications were *fibrosis, mucosal ulceration/necrosis* and *osteoradionecrosis*, with substantial variation in the incidence rates between the individual studies. Despite the treatment-related morbidity, they recommended high-dose reirradiation. Similar side effects were reported by De Crevoisier et al. (10) in a series of 169 patients reirradiated to cumulative doses of 120 Gy (reirradiation dose 60–65 Gy). After initial irradiation with 68 Gy, plus 67 Gy in the second series, Salama et al. (46) found grade 4–5 late reactions (osteoradionecrosis, carotid haemorrhage, myelopathy, neuropathy) in a total of 18% of the patients, with more than 16% fatalities.

Lee et al. (25) reirradiated 105 patients with nasopharyngeal tumours with 59.4 Gy after initial doses of 62 Gy. Severe early and late complications were found in 23% and 15% of the patients; the latter comprised mainly *temporal lobe necrosis, hearing loss, dysphagia* and *trismus*. Lee et al. (24) compared late complications (excluding xerostomia) in more than 3600 patients given only a single course of radiotherapy and 487 patients given a second course of radiotherapy for nasopharyngeal carcinoma. The observed incidence of normal tissue injury in the retreatment series was clearly lower than expected, based on the sum of initial and retreatment doses, indicating partial long-term recovery of the head and neck tissues, particularly with intervals ≥2 years.

In a report on 291 recurrent nasopharyngeal tumours (69), gross recurrent tumour volume (TV) was shown to be a significant prognostic factor for outcome and toxicity-related death. In patients with TV <22 cm³, tumour progression, especially loco-regional failure, was the leading cause of death, whereas in patients with TV ≥22 cm³, radiation-induced injuries including mucosa necrosis or massive haemorrhage, radiation encephalopathy, feeding difficulty and other radiation injuries became more frequent and generated half of deaths in this group. The 5-year treatment-related death was brought to 39.5%.

Results of two prospective phase II trials of reirradiation and chemotherapy, RTOG 9610 and RTOG 9911, were reported by Spencer et al. (50) and by Langer et al. (22), respectively. In both studies, patients received reirradiation to a total dose of 60 Gy (1.5 Gy per fraction bid, 5 days/week).

In RTOG 9610, four weekly cycles of 5FU-bolus and oral hydroxyurea were applied. The median radiation dose in the first treatment series was 65.2 (45–73.8) Gy, the median time to reirradiation was 2.5 (0.6–19.8) years. Early morbidity grade ≥4 occurred in 25.3%, late adverse events grade ≥3 in 22.4% of the patients, six patients died of early treatment-related causes, but no late grade 5 toxicity was reported. In RTOG 9911, cisplatinum and paclitaxel were administered. The median radiation dose in the initial treatment series was 65.4 (45–75) Gy, the median time between the courses was 3.3 (0.5–26.5) years. Grade ≥4 general early complications occurred in 28%, grade ≥4 early hematologic toxicity in 21% of the patients. Eight treatment-related deaths (8%) occurred: five associated with early effects, three in the late phase (including two carotid haemorrhages).

In another randomized phase III trial on postoperative reirradiation combined with chemotherapy in head and neck carcinoma (17), disease-free survival was improved, while no difference was observed in overall survival. Yet, 28% and 39% of the patients experienced early and late grade ≥3 morbidity after 2 years follow-up, respectively, with 8% treatment-related deaths.

Thus, in head and neck tumours, local control rates of >30% can be achieved with total retreatment doses of at least 50–60 Gy; lower doses are ineffective. Severe complications, observed in up to 60% of long-term survivors, are generally associated with higher cumulative total doses and shorter intervals before retreatment.

Stereotactic reirradiation may be a promising but still developing treatment modality in managing recurrent head and neck cancer and rare carotid rupture is a major concern. Careful patient selection without tumour encasement of less than one-third of the carotid artery may decrease the risk of complication. In the study of Lartigau et al. (23), when stereotactic reirradiation was combined with cetuximab they recorded only one such case. More detailed analysis was performed by Yamazaki et al. (70) in a multi-institutional matched-cohort analysis. They identified factors predisposing to carotid blowout as the presence of ulceration, and irradiation to lymph node. Moreover, only patients with carotid invasion of more than 180° developed carotid blowout.

Toxicity related to salvage stereotactic reirradiation in the head and neck region may also be related to the localization of recurrence. In their retrospective study on 291 patients, Ling et al. (26) showed that those treated for a recurrence in the larynx/hypopharynx experienced significantly more severe late toxicity compared with other primary tumour sites and nodal recurrence. In fact half of the patients with laryngeal/hypopharyngeal recurrence experienced severe late toxicity, compared with 6%–20% for other sites. In the whole group grade ≥3 late toxicities were found in 43 patients (18.9%), with grade 5 late in 3% consisting of carotid blowout syndrome, dysphagia, laryngeal oedema and mucosal bleeding. The median primary dose was 68.4 (20.4–170.7) Gy, and median stereotactic body radiation therapy (SBRT) dose was 44 (16–52.8) Gy. Reirradiation dose ≥44 Gy was significantly correlated with more patients presenting grade ≥3 early and late toxicity.

The potential of targeted therapies ('biologicals') to reduce morbidity compared to conventional chemotherapy also remains unclear. Similarly, the option to improve efficacy and reduce late complications by innovative irradiation technologies needs to be explored. As clearly indicated by Wong et al. (66), further well-designed and powered clinical studies are required to answer these open questions.

## Breast

Reirradiation for breast cancer, applied as partial breast irradiation, can be delivered either as conformal external beam irradiation (e.g. with electrons), interstitial brachytherapy or intraoperative radiation therapy (IORT), with or without chemotherapy. These procedures are associated with an acceptable incidence of side effects, such as fibrosis, pain, rib fracture, infection, lymphedema, but less acceptable results with regard to cosmesis.

Siglin et al. (48) reviewed seven studies with repeated breast-conserving therapy for local recurrences. One study did not report complications. Only 2/6 studies reported morbidity grade ≥3 (10%–17%), the remainder did not observe any such complications. Another review by Datta et al. (9) analysed 34 studies treating locally recurrent breast cancers with hyperthermia and radiotherapy but without surgery or concurrent chemotherapy. Studies varied in the radiotherapy dose and hyperthermia schedules. The mean reirradiation dose was 38.2 (24–60) Gy, delivered with a dose per fraction 1.8–4 Gy and in the majority of cases hyperthermia was delivered after radiotherapy (76.5%). The scoring of the toxicities was quite heterogeneous because these studies were carried out during a 34-year period. Mean acute and late grade 3/4 toxicities with reirradiation and hyperthermia were 14.4% and 5.2%, respectively.

Wahl et al. (61) reported on reirradiation to the chest wall (median cumulative doses of 106 [74.4–137.5] Gy; median initial dose 60 Gy; median reirradiation dose 48 Gy). The majority of patients (54%) also received concurrent hyperthermia, 20% received hyperfractionation and 54% received concurrent chemotherapy. Only 5% of patients developed late grade ≥3 morbidity; no treatment-related deaths occurred. The development of late complications was not associated with any reirradiation therapy variables.

Müller et al. (37) applied post-operative (30 patients) or definitive reirradiation (12 patients) as a second curative approach, with concurrent hyperthermia in 29 patients. Patients were reirradiated to a median cumulative dose of 110 (85–126) Gy (initial median dose 54 Gy, median retreatment dose 60 Gy). No patient experienced complications grade ≥4. In conclusion, reirradiation can be administered with acceptable early and late morbidity for recurrent breast cancer.

In a prospective trial of partial breast reirradiation for locally recurrent breast cancer with pulsed dose-rate (PDR) brachytherapy in 39 patients, Kauer-Dorner et al.

(19) reported 5-year actuarial local control rates of 93%. Morbidity, cosmetic outcome and health-related quality of life (QoL) were assessed in 24/39 patients. Late side effects grade 1–2 were observed in 20/24 patients and grade 3 in 4/24 patients after a mean follow-up of 30 (±18) months. Cosmetic outcome was excellent to fair in 76% of women. Overall, QoL was comparable to a healthy control group. It was concluded that morbidity is moderate and cosmetic outcome and QoL are good for accelerated PDR-brachytherapy following breast-conserving surgery for local recurrences.

In 234 breast cancer patients (41), reirradiation plus hyperthermia resulted in long-term local control (70% at 5 years). Median total primary dose was 50 (30–92.7) Gy, median retreatment dose was 46.9 (20–58.6) Gy delivered with 4 or 3 Gy for fraction, giving median cumulative dose 66.7 (40–95.7) Gy. A dose per fraction of 4 Gy resulted in a significantly ninefold higher risk of rib fractures compared to 3 Gy, detected in 16 of 234 patients (actuarial risk: 7% at 5 years). The majority of rib fractures were located in the photon/electron abutment area, emphasizing the disadvantage of field overlap. No other individual factors were found. Good retreatment tolerance was also shown in 127 female breast cancer patients treated with radiotherapy and hyperthermia (43). Fifty-four were reirradiated and the remaining 73 were irradiated for the first time. Grade 3–4 desquamation was the most common adverse event (24.4% of the patients) followed by ulceration (6.7%), fibrosis (6.3%) and telangiectasia (4.7%). One patient had abscess formation. There was no significant difference in grade 3–4 adverse events among patients who had prior radiotherapy (43.8%) versus those who did not (46.3%).

Heterogeneity of acute and late toxicity reporting together with variability of applied schedules composed of different radiotherapy total and fractional doses, hyperthermia schemas and surgical and systemic treatment, does not allow the creation of a clear consensus on the optimal treatment schedule for advanced recurrent breast cancer to achieve best survival with minimum toxicity. Nevertheless, the available data present reirradiation as an effective and safe modality for the management of recurrent breast cancer.

## Lung

The response of the lung to irradiation occurs in two waves, pneumonitis as a delayed early effect, followed by late fibrosis. These endpoints, however, are not independent (see Chapter 14), indicating a strong consequential component. Moreover, the underlying (molecular) pathogenetic processes appear to be associated with continuous (subclinical) changes starting from the time of the initial radiation exposure.

In a mouse study using death from pneumonitis to evaluate lung reirradiation tolerance (56), there was complete recovery from an initial single dose of 6–8 Gy (approximately 30%–50% of the tolerance dose). The time to restitution was – depending on the initial dose – in the range of 1–2 months (Figure 23.6). After higher initial doses (≥70%

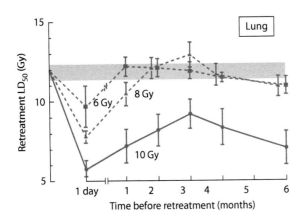

Figure 23.6 Retreatment tolerance of the mouse lung. The ordinate indicates $LD_{50}$ values due to pneumonitis for retreatment at the indicated times after priming treatment with 6, 8 or 10 Gy. The shaded area shows the $LD_{50}$ value for previously untreated animals. (Adapted from (56), with permission.)

of the total tolerance), reirradiation tolerance increased from 1 day to 3 months, to approximately 75% of the tolerance in previously untreated mice. Yet, at 6 months after the initial irradiation, a clear decline in retreatment tolerance was observed, probably as the result of developing fibrosis from the initial irradiation, complicating the analysis of pneumonitis retreatment tolerance. No later time points were studied, and hence it is unclear if this trend continued, or if it also occurred at later times after lower initial doses. Thus, the reirradiation tolerance of the lung demonstrated in these experimental studies only applies for the pneumonitis phase. It is likely that retreatment tolerance for late lung fibrosis may be poorer, although no conclusive evidence is available.

In recurrent lung cancer, reirradiation with fractionated doses of 10–70 Gy (median 50 Gy, 1.8–3 Gy per fraction) after an initial treatment with 30–80 Gy (median 60 Gy, 1.5–2 Gy per fraction) was studied in 34 patients (40). Major morbidities were symptomatic pneumonitis (56% of the patients) and esophagitis (18%); no radiation myelopathy was observed. Wu et al. (67) analysed 23 lung carcinoma patients with loco-regional recurrence after a first course of irradiation with a median dose of 66 (30–78) Gy, and a median reirradiation dose of 51 (46–60) Gy. Pneumonitis grade 1–2 was observed in 22%, pulmonary fibrosis grade 2–3 in 26% of the patients. Early esophagitis grade 1–2 occurred in 9%. No other severe late complications were observed.

With regard to reirradiation of lung tumours, the location of the tumour must be taken into account, in particular if stereotactic radiotherapy is applied. Peulen et al. (42) found pneumonitis grade 2–3 developed in 12% of the patients, fibrosis grade 2 in 22% and pain grade 2 in 16% (mainly after treatment for peripheral tumours). Three patients with central tumours died due to bleeding, and one patient presented with a vena cava superior stenosis and a fistula between the trachea and the gastric tube. Larger target volumes and central tumours were associated with more

severe complications. This indicates that a careful selection of patients for reirradiation is required, also demonstrated by Meijneke et al. (35).

In-field or out-of-field relapse may also play an important role in reirradiation toxicity as shown by Kelly et al. (20) in their study on stereotactic reirradiation. The most common side effect was symptomatic pneumonitis seen in 50% of patients, but no grade 3 pneumonitis was seen in reirradiated patients who had an in-field relapse. Opposite, the chest wall pain was more common in the group undergoing SBRT for in-field relapse.

Protons may also provide an option for reirradiation of lung cancer. McAvoy et al. (31) showed 27% pulmonary and 12% oesophageal complications grade 3–4 after reirradiation of NSCLC with protons. Proton therapy must be incorporated into the reirradiation very carefully, because it can be associated with significant toxicity as shown by Chao et al. (7), where six grade 5 toxicities were reported, with acute toxicity developing in 39%, and late toxicity developing in 12%. They confirmed that increased overlap with the central airway region was associated with significantly higher rates of grade $\geq 3$ together with other factors such as mean oesophagus and heart doses and concurrent chemotherapy.

In one of the largest (102 patients) studies on NSCLC reirradiation with median initial EQD2 dose 70 (33–276) Gy and median EQD2 reirradiation dose 60.5 (25.2–155) Gy, the median cumulative EQD2 dose was 131.2 (60–360) Gy. Despite the application of high radiation doses, toxicity was acceptable although higher than reported by others with 7% grade $\geq 3$ oesophageal toxicity and 10% of grade $\geq 3$ pulmonary toxicity. Concurrent chemotherapy increased oesophageal but not lung toxicity. Lung toxicity was increased with larger reirradiated lung V10, V20 and mean lung dose (MLD). Surprisingly, there was no association between oesophageal or pulmonary toxicity and treatment technique (intensity modulated radiation therapy versus proton beam therapy (PBT)), time to reirradiation (<6 months versus $\geq 6$ months), tumour location (central versus peripheral) or EQD2 at reirradiation (30).

In lung cancer, the retreatment doses are generally lower than the initial doses (palliative treatment intent) and most patients will succumb to their disease before late normal tissue sequelae become clinically manifest. In addition, all clinical studies suffer from a small number of highly inhomogeneous patients. This prevents any clear conclusions on the options and the potential of reirradiation in this particular tumour site but available research results suggest that reirradiation can be safely administered.

## Heart and large vessels

The heart is one of the most radiosensitive organs. However, the responses, e.g. cardiovascular disease and myocardial infarction, are only seen after long to very long time intervals up to decades after radiation exposure. In experimental studies in rats, local heart irradiation with a single dose caused a progressive decrease in cardiac function in a dose-dependent manner, depending on both the time interval between subsequent doses and the size of the initial dose. A decreased tolerance of the heart to reirradiation was observed at time intervals >6 months (63). In patients reirradiated for thoracic tumours (13), a 25% incidence of grade 5 aortic complications was found in patients receiving cumulative doses ≥120 Gy to 1 cm³ of the aorta.

Currently, the reirradiation tolerance of the heart and large blood vessels (information restricted to the carotid artery, see section on head and neck tissues) remains unclear, but the available data suggest that there may be weak long-term recovery or even progression of damage, and hence poor retreatment tolerance.

## Kidney

The kidneys are also among the most radiosensitive of organs, although the latent period before expression of clinically manifest radiation effects may – as in the heart – be very long, particularly after low doses. Progressive, dose-dependent development of functional damage, without apparent recovery, has been clearly demonstrated in rodents (51,53). This is consistent with clinical observations of slowly progressive renal damage, which develops over many years after irradiation. Based on the known dose-dependence of renal radiation, moderate initial doses (≥14 Gy) will result in complete loss of function after longer intervals, and hence reirradiation cannot cause any further damage.

After sub-tolerance doses, however, the absence of any *clinically measurable* renal dysfunction at the time of retreatment certainly cannot be interpreted in terms of remaining retreatment tolerance, because of progression of the subclinical effects. Experimental studies demonstrate that doses of radiation too low to produce overt renal damage nevertheless significantly reduce the tolerance to retreatment (51); none of these studies has demonstrated any long-term functional recovery of the kidney. After an initial dose as low as 6 Gy (25% of the $EQD2_{tol}$), the tolerance for retreatment actually decreases with time between 2 weeks and 26 weeks (Figure 23.7). This is consistent with continuous progression of occult damage in the interval between treatments and implies that reirradiation of the kidneys after *any* previous irradiation should be approached with extreme caution, if still existing function needs to be preserved.

## Urinary bladder

Studies on the reirradiation tolerance of mouse urinary bladder, similarly to the kidney, have not demonstrated any recovery from late, functional damage (as measured by increased urination frequency or reduced bladder compliance) for retreatment intervals of 12 or 40 weeks compared with short (1 day) intervals (Figure 23.8). The latent period before expression of permanent functional

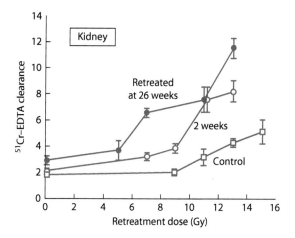

**Figure 23.7** Dose-response curves for renal damage in mice at 35 weeks after reirradiation. Retreatment was administered either 2 weeks (open circles) or 26 weeks (closed circles) after the initial treatment with 6 Gy. The response of age-matched control animals without previous irradiation (open squares) is also shown. Renal damage was worse for retreatment with the longer 26 week interval than for a shorter interval, indicating progression of sub-threshold damage rather than recovery. (From (51), with permission.)

damage was also much shorter in animals that were reirradiated compared to a single course of treatment, even after low, sub-tolerance initial doses (52).

## Pelvic tissues

The early experience of retreatment for recurrent *cervical cancer* was not encouraging. Local control and survival rates were generally poor (10%–20% long-term survival) and complication rates were high (30%–50%). Several more recent

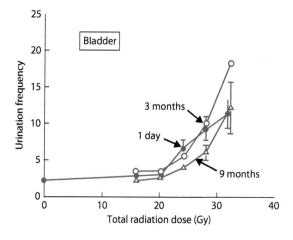

**Figure 23.8** Dose-response curves for late urinary bladder damage in mice after irradiation with two doses separated by 1day (closed circles), 3 months (open circles) or 9 months (open triangles). The total dose for a given effect did not increase with increasing time from first treatment. (From (52), with permission.)

studies, in which patients were carefully selected on the basis of volume and location of the cancer, have demonstrated much better results, particularly for retreatment using brachytherapy. In these studies, long-term survival rates of ≥60% could be achieved after full-dose retreatment, with a severe complication rate less than 15%. Favourable conditions were small tumour volume, second primary malignancies and retreatment with brachytherapy, while recurrent cancer, large tumour volume and retreatment with external-beam therapy were clearly discouraging.

Reirradiation, mainly by brachytherapy, of *vaginal recurrences* of carcinomas of the cervix has been tried with 20–40 Gy in three to five fractions in 3–4 weeks (68). Side effects were severe, with rectal changes (14%), haematuria (12%) and fistula (12%). In another study on 22 patients re-treated with brachytherapy (3), the incidences of vesicovaginal or rectovaginal fistula and soft tissue necrosis were low (<5%), although most patients had vaginal fibrosis, two experienced rectal bleeding and one had urinary tract bleeding. In a retreatment series in 20 patients with cervical or vaginal cancer (71), a cumulative median EQD2 of 133.5 Gy (range: 96.8–164.2 Gy) was applied to the tumour; the $D_{2cm3}$ in the bladder was 99.3 Gy (70.4–122.3 Gy). Grade ≥3 late genitourinary morbidity was observed in two patients (International Commission on Radiation Units and Measurements [ICRU] bladder point EQD2 137.6 Gy, $D_{2cm3}$ 122.3 Gy); grade 3 late gastrointestinal complications (requiring laser coagulation) were observed in one patient (ICRU rectal point EQD2 101.3 Gy). Mabuchi et al. (27) re-treated 52 women with recurrent cervical cancer with HDR brachytherapy; grade ≥3 late adverse events were observed in 13 (25%) of the patients.

Reirradiation of patients with *rectal cancer* led to the development of chronic diarrhoea (17% of patients), fistula (4%), skin ulceration (2%) and small bowel obstruction (15%) as reported by Mohiuddin et al. (36). Late morbidity was significantly reduced in patients re-treated with hyperfractionated regimen and after intervals between treatments more than 24 months. Valentini et al. (58) concluded that hyperfractionation retreatment resulted in acceptable late toxicities, i.e. skin fibrosis and urinary complications requiring nephrostomy. Safety of hyperfractionated accelerated reirradiation for rectal cancer was also confirmed by others (54,55). Although a significantly higher rate of grade 3–4 late toxicity was found in patients who underwent surgery compared to those without surgery (54% versus 16%) leading to a high (34%) actuarial 3-year rate of toxicity, in this study (55) patients were treated with hyperfractionated reirradiation with or without chemotherapy to a median total dose of 39 (30–45) Gy delivered twice a day with 1.5 Gy per fraction after a primary median dose of 50.4 (25–63) Gy.

## Brain

Over the last decades, improved irradiation conformality and radiosurgery have led to an increase in radiation doses,

without increased risk of brain radionecrosis. These studies, however, provide information on brain reirradiation tolerance. Mayer and Sminia (29) reviewed the information on reirradiation of brain tumours by stereotactic radiotherapy or radiosurgery. There was no correlation between the time interval between the radiation courses and the incidence of radionecrosis. Necrotic reactions were observed at cumulative EQD2 exceeding 100 Gy. Kohshi et al. (21) reported that combined conformal radiotherapy and hyperbaric oxygen retreatment of brain tumours resulted in a high incidence of necrosis (28%), even when the cumulative EQD2 was as low as 86 Gy. We still need much more information on interaction between brain reirradiation and drugs used. In a study on reirradiation and bevacizumab for recurrent glioma there was no significant difference in toxicity between patients who did and did not receive adjuvant bevacizumab (8).

## Spinal cord

Spinal cord has been studied most extensively with regard to retreatment, in various rodent species and in non-human primates. Moreover, clinical data are available. There is evidence for substantial long-term recovery, indicating that retreatment is feasible.

Analyses of data obtained on reirradiation of rodent spinal cord, using paralysis as an endpoint, are illustrated in Figure 23.9. In juvenile animals, long-term recovery starts early and maximum retreatment tolerance is observed after 1–2 months; the maximum total dose (initial plus reirradiation) is 120% of the tolerance for previously untreated animals (44) and the higher the initial dose is, the lower is the tolerance to reirradiation. In adult animals, restitution starts with a delay of several months and reaches a maximum of ≈140% of the original tolerance after 5–6 months (59,62). These data were

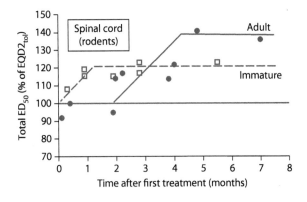

**Figure 23.9** Long-term recovery after irradiation of rodent cervical cord. The total cumulative isoeffective dose (for 50% paresis) is expressed as a percentage of $EQD2_{tol}$ and as a function of the interval between initial and reirradiation dose. Data are for 3-week-old (open squares) and adult (closed circles) rats. (Adapted from (44,62,59), with permission.)

confirmed in an extensive study in rats for different levels of initial damage (64).

An extensive reirradiation study was performed in non-human primates (1,2). In these experiments, an 8 cm length of the cervical cord was initially irradiated with 20 fractions of 2.2 Gy, which is equivalent to about 60% of the $ED_{50}$ for a 50% incidence of paralysis (76 Gy in 2.2 Gy fractions). After 1, 2 or 3 years, the non-symptomatic monkeys were reirradiated with graded doses in fractions of 2.2 Gy. Only a few animals developed paralysis with the retreatment doses administered; therefore, the data were compared at a 10% incidence level of paralysis, rather than at 50%. The reirradiation $ED_{10}$ increased from 55 Gy after 1 year, to 59 Gy after 2 years to 66 Gy after 3 years. The total $EQD2_{tol}$ for initial and retreatment doses amounted to 150%, 156% and 167% for retreatment after 1, 2 or 3 years (Figure 23.10). Hence, despite a different time course in rodents and primates, the extent of long-term recovery in spinal cord, using paralysis as an endpoint, may be adopted for reirradiation of patients.

Some clinical analyses of radiation myelopathy after reirradiation of spinal cord are available. Nieder et al. (39) summarised data from a total of 78 patients reirradiated to the spinal cord with various regimens. Their conclusion was that if the interval between the two radiotherapy courses was longer than 6 months, and the EQD2 in each course was ≤48 Gy, the risk for myelopathy was small after a total EQD2 of 68 Gy. In a smaller series, no myelopathies were seen after cumulative $EQD2_{tol}$ of 125%–172%, with intervals between the series of 4 months to 13 years.

For calculation of the reirradiation tolerance for spinal cord, the initial tolerance must be defined. Both human and primate data (4,47) demonstrate that at an EQD2 of 55 Gy, the incidence of myelopathy is less than 3%. At a dose of 60 Gy, the incidence of myelopathy is about 5% for doses per fraction <2.5 Gy and for one fraction per day. This level of risk may be acceptable in a reirradiation situation, which is frequently the last curative option for the patient. Assuming, for example, that a patient received an initial dose to the spinal cord of 40 Gy, this leaves 20 Gy tolerance from the first irradiation. Restitution of 40% of the initial dose amounts to an EQD2 of 16 Gy, hence reirradiation with a dose of 36 Gy can probably be administered to the spinal cord in 2 Gy fractions. However, the dose to the spinal cord is usually less than the dose to the planning target volume, which must be included in the calculation of the equieffective initial dose (EQD2). Moreover, the pronounced fractionation effect of the spinal cord can be exploited by administering reirradiation in a hyperfractionated protocol. Based on these considerations, reirradiation with a curative intent is often possible.

In an analysis of clinical cases of myelopathy (65), the mean latent time before clinical symptoms became manifest after a single course of radiotherapy (EQD2 of 60.5 Gy) was 18.5 months ($n = 24$). After reirradiation to a total EQD2 of 74 Gy ($n = 11$), myelopathies were observed after a significantly shorter mean latent time of 11.4 months. These data are in line with results from the pre-clinical studies.

In the era of radiosurgery and stereotactic treatments, there is increasing interest in the effects of high single doses to the spinal cord, also with regard to reirradiation. In a pig model (33,34) radiosurgery was applied at 1 year after fractionated spinal cord irradiation (10 × 3 Gy). Retreated animals had more extensive histological tissue changes, including infarction of the gray matter, but only at radiosurgery doses >20 Gy. Pigs retreated after fractionated radiotherapy were not at increased risk of developing motoric deficits compared to radiosurgery alone. Saghal et al. (45) reviewed the data for radiation myelopathy after stereotactic reirradiation with one to five fractions. They concluded that reirradiation is safe if the cumulative $EQD2_{2Gy}$ does not exceed approximately 70 Gy, the interval between treatments is at least 5 months and the maximum reirradiation EQD2 constitutes less than approximately 50% of the cumulative EQD2.

Safe spinal reirradiation with SBRT was also shown in a multi-institutional pooled study on 215 patients with 247 spinal target volumes (15). The median cumulative dose delivered to critical neural tissues (CNTs), $EQD2_{2Gy}$ $D_{max}$ was 60.8 (14.0–107.6) Gy. The median SBRT total dose was 18 (8–50) Gy with median SBRT CNT $EQD2_{2Gy}$ $D_{max}$ 24.6 (0–70.1) Gy. There were no cases of radiation myelopathy, or radiculopathy. Eleven vertebral compression fractures (VCFs) were observed (rate of 4.5%): five formed *de novo* and six were fracture progression with rates of 2.1% and 2.5%, respectively.

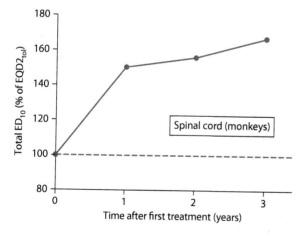

**Figure 23.10** Total tolerance (initial plus retreatment) of monkey spinal cord. Retreatment was performed after 1–3 years after an initial dose of 44 Gy (i.e. 60% of $EQD2_{tol}$). All treatments were given with 2.2 Gy per fraction. (Data from (1), with permission.)

## 23.4 SUMMARY OF EXPERIMENTAL AND CLINICAL DATA

Figure 23.11 summarises results from experimental studies for reirradiation tolerance in tissues where recovery following a range of initial treatments has been evaluated. Both the initial and the retreatment radiation exposures are shown

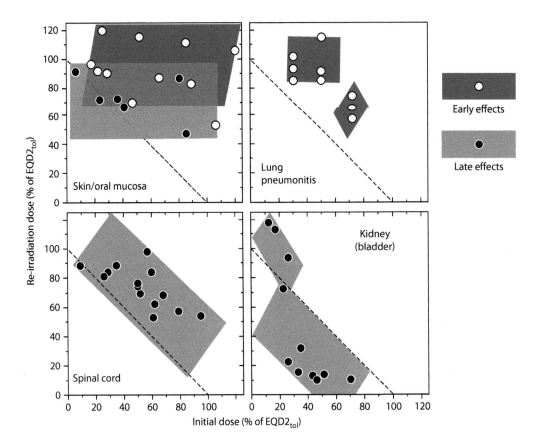

**Figure 23.11** Summary of retreatment tolerance from experimental studies reported in the literature. Both the initial and retreatment doses have been calculated as a percentage of EQD2$_{tol}$. The dashed line indicates the residual tissue tolerance if no long-term restitution occurred. Data points above the dashed line (in skin, lung and cord) indicate some long-term recovery, while data below this line (kidney, bladder) point towards a progressive reduction of tissue tolerance with time after the initial irradiation.

as a percentage of the tolerance dose for a defined endpoint or level of damage, calculated in terms of EQD2$_{tol}$ using the appropriate $\alpha/\beta$ value for each tissue. The dashed lines indicate the relationship that would be expected if neither long-term reconstitution of tolerance nor progression of damage would occur. Data points for retreatment above the dashed line (in skin, lung and cord) indicate some long-term recovery in the tissue. Where the data points fall below the dashed line (kidney), this indicates a progressive reduction of tissue tolerance with time after the initial irradiation rather than recovery.

The general conclusion is that, on the basis of studies in experimental animals and the still limited information from clinical observations and studies, several normal tissues are able to tolerate considerable retreatment with radiation. The phenomenon is not, however, universal.

These experimental and – more importantly – clinical data also clearly indicate that reirradiation is an option for some selected patients with recurrent or second tumours. However, the risk of normal tissue damage and impact on the quality of life, as well as possible alternative therapeutic approaches, must be taken into account. If a second course of radiotherapy has to be administered, this should be done with maximum care and accuracy. Optimum conformation of the planning target volume is required. For

radiobiological reasons – in order to reduce the risk of late effects – hyperfractionation protocols should be considered for curative treatments.

---

### Key points

1. If the tolerance within a given tissue volume has already been exceeded during the first treatment, and loss of function is present or expected soon, then reirradiation is not possible without loss of function.

2. For early effects, restitution of the original tolerance may be complete after low to moderate doses, after tissue-specific and dose-dependent time intervals. At high doses, residual damage may remain for longer time intervals, particularly at the stem cell level, which is not necessarily reflected by the number of differentiated cells in the functional tissue compartments (e.g. blood cell counts for bone marrow).

3. For some late responding tissues, partial (CNS, lung) or complete (skin) restoration of tolerance is observed after low and moderate initial doses ($\leq$60% of the initial tolerance).

4. In some late responding tissues (e.g. kidney, heart), progression of damage at a subclinical level must be expected, thus precluding reirradiation without exceeding tolerance.

5. Alternative treatment options must be considered before reirradiation.

6. If (curative) reirradiation is to be administered, optimum treatment planning (dose conformation) and a proper choice of fractionation protocol (hyperfractionation) are required.

## ■ BIBLIOGRAPHY

1. Ang KK, Jiang GL, Feng Y, Stephens LC, Tucker SL, Price RE. Extent and kinetics of recovery of occult spinal cord injury. *Int J Radiat Oncol Biol Phys* 2001;50:1013–1020.

2. Ang KK, Price RE, Stephens LC et al. The tolerance of primate spinal cord to re-irradiation. *Int J Radiat Oncol Biol Phys* 1993;25:459–464.

3. Badakh DK, Grover AH. Reirradiation with high-dose-rate remote afterloading brachytherapy implant in patients with locally recurrent or residual cervical carcinoma. *J Cancer Res Ther* 2009;5:24–30.

4. Baumann M, Budach V, Appold S. Radiation tolerance of the human spinal cord. *Strahlenther Onkol* 1994;170: 131–139.

5. Bentzen SM, Dörr W, Gahbauer R et al. Bioeffect modeling and equieffective dose concepts in radiation oncology – Terminology, quantities and units. *Radiother Oncol* 2012;105: 266–268.

6. Brown JM, Probert JC. Early and late radiation changes following a second course of irradiation. *Radiology* 1975;115: 711–716.

7. Chao HH, Berman AT, Simone CB 2nd et al. Multi-institutional prospective study of reirradiation with proton beam radiotherapy for locoregionally recurrent non-small cell lung cancer. *J Thorac Oncol* 2017;12:281–292.

8. Cuneo KC, Vredenburgh JJ, Sampson JH et al. Safety and efficacy of stereotactic radiosurgery and adjuvant bevacizumab in patients with recurrent malignant gliomas. *Int J Radiat Oncol Biol Phys* 2012;82:2018–2024.

9. Datta NR, Puric E, Klingbiel D, Gomez S, Bodis S. Hyperthermia and radiation therapy in locoregional recurrent breast cancers: A systematic review and meta-analysis. *Int J Radiat Oncol Biol Phys* 2016;94:1073–1087.

10. De Crevoisier R, Bourhis J, Domenge C et al. Full-dose reirradiation for unresectable head and neck carcinoma: Experience at the Gustave-Roussy Institute in a series of 169 patients. *J Clin Oncol* 1998;16:3556–3562.

11. Dickerman JD. The late effects of childhood cancer therapy. *Pediatrics* 2007;119:554–568.

12. Dörr W, Herrmann T. Second primary tumors after radiotherapy for malignancies. Treatment-related parameters. *Strahlenther Onkol* 2002;178:357–362.

13. Evans JD, Gomez DR, Amini A et al. Aortic dose constraints when reirradiating thoracic tumors. *Radiother Oncol* 2013;106: 327–332.

14. Hashibe M, Ritz B, Le AD, Li G, Sankaranarayanan R, Zhang ZF. Radiotherapy for oral cancer as a risk factor for second primary cancers. *Cancer Lett* 2005;220:185–195.

15. Hashmi A, Guckenberger M, Kersh R et al. Re-irradiation stereotactic body radiotherapy for spinal metastases: A multi-institutional outcome analysis. *J Neurosurg Spine* 2016;25:646–653.

16. Hendry JH, Yang F. Response of bone marrow to low LET irradiation. In: Hendry JH and Lord BI, editors. *Radiation Toxicology: Bone Marrow and Leukaemia*. London: Taylor & Francis Group; 1995. pp. 91–116.

17. Janot F, de Raucourt D, Benhamou E et al. Randomized trial of postoperative reirradiation combined with chemotherapy after salvage surgery compared with salvage surgery alone in head and neck carcinoma. *J Clin Oncol* 2008;26: 5518–5523.

18. Kasperts N, Slotman B, Leemans CR, Langendijk JA. A review on re-irradiation for recurrent and second primary head and neck cancer. *Oral Oncol* 2005;41:225–243.

19. Kauer-Dorner D, Pötter R, Resch A et al. Partial breast irradiation for locally recurrent breast cancer within a second breast conserving treatment: Alternative to mastectomy? Results from a prospective trial. *Radiother Oncol* 2012;102: 96–101.

20. Kelly P, Balter PA, Rebueno N et al. Stereotactic body radiation therapy for patients with lung cancer previously treated with thoracic radiation. *Int J Radiat Oncol Biol Phys* 2010;78:1387–1393.

21. Kohshi K, Yamamoto H, Nakahara A, Katoh T, Takagi M. Fractionated stereotactic radiotherapy using gamma unit after hyperbaric oxygenation on recurrent high-grade gliomas. *J Neurooncol* 2007;82:297–303.

22. Langer CJ, Harris J, Horwitz EM et al. Phase II study of low-dose paclitaxel and cisplatin in combination with split-course concomitant twice-daily reirradiation in recurrent squamous cell carcinoma of the head and neck: Results of Radiation Therapy Oncology Group Protocol 9911. *J Clin Oncol* 2007;25:4800–4805.

23. Lartigau EF, Tresch E, Thariat J et al. Multi institutional phase II study of concomitant stereotactic reirradiation and cetuximab for recurrent head and neck cancer. *Radiother Oncol* 2013;109: 281–285.

24. Lee AW, Foo W, Law SC et al. Total biological effect on late reactive tissues following reirradiation for recurrent nasopharyngeal carcinoma. *Int J Radiat Oncol Biol Phys* 2000;46:865–872.

25. Lee N, Chan K, Bekelman JE et al. Salvage re-irradiation for recurrent head and neck cancer. *Int J Radiat Oncol Biol Phys* 2007;68:731–740.

26. Ling DC, Vargo JA, Ferris RL et al. Risk of severe toxicity according to site of recurrence in patients treated with stereotactic body radiation therapy for recurrent head and neck cancer. *Int J Radiat Oncol Biol Phys* 2016;95:973–980.

27. Mabuchi S, Takahashi R, Isohashi F et al. Reirradiation using high-dose-rate interstitial brachytherapy for locally recurrent cervical cancer: A single institutional experience. *Int J Gynecol Cancer* 2014;24:141–148.

28. Maciejewski B, Zajusz A, Pilecki B et al. Acute mucositis in the stimulated oral mucosa of patients during radiotherapy for head and neck cancer. *Radiother Oncol* 1991;22:7–11.

29. Mayer R, Sminia P. Reirradiation tolerance of the human brain. *Int J Radiat Oncol Biol Phys* 2008;70:1350–1360.

30. McAvoy S, Ciura K, Wei C et al. Definitive reirradiation for locoregionally recurrent non-small cell lung cancer with proton beam therapy or intensity modulated radiation therapy: Predictors of high-grade toxicity and survival outcomes. *Int J Radiat Oncol Biol Phys* 2014;90:819–827.

31. McAvoy SA, Ciura KT, Rineer JM et al. Feasibility of proton beam therapy for reirradiation of locoregionally recurrent non-small cell lung cancer. *Radiother Oncol* 2013;109:38–44.

32. McDonald MW, Moore MG, Johnstone PA. Risk of carotid blowout after reirradiation of the head and neck: A systematic review. *Int J Radiat Oncol Biol Phys* 2012;82: 1083–1089.

33. Medin PM, Boike TP. Spinal cord tolerance in the age of spinal radiosurgery: Lessons from preclinical studies. *Int J Radiat Oncol Biol Phys* 2011;79:1302–1309.

34. Medin PM, Foster RD, van der Kogel AJ, Sayre JW, McBride WH, Solberg TD. Spinal cord tolerance to reirradiation with single-fraction radiosurgery: A swine model. *Int J Radiat Oncol Biol Phys* 2012;83:1031–1037.

35. Meijneke TR, Petit SF, Wentzler D, Hoogeman M, Nuyttens JJ. Reirradiation and stereotactic radiotherapy for tumors in the lung: Dose summation and toxicity. *Radiother Oncol* 2013;107:423–427.

36. Mohiuddin M, Marks G, Marks J. Long-term results of reirradiation for patients with recurrent rectal carcinoma. *Cancer* 2002;95:1144–1150.

37. Müller AC, Eckert F, Heinrich V, Bamberg M, Brucker S, Hehr T. Re-surgery and chest wall re-irradiation for recurrent breast cancer: A second curative approach. *BMC Cancer* 2011;11:197.

38. National Cancer Institute. Survivorship. 2016; https://www.cancer.gov/about-cancer/coping/survivorship

39. Nieder C, Grosu AL, Andratschke NH, Molls M. Update of human spinal cord reirradiation tolerance based on additional data from 38 patients. *Int J Radiat Oncol Biol Phys* 2006;66: 1446–1449.

40. Okamoto Y, Murakami M, Yoden E et al. Reirradiation for locally recurrent lung cancer previously treated with radiation therapy. *Int J Radiat Oncol Biol Phys* 2002;52: 390–396.

41. Oldenborg S, Valk C, van Os R et al. Rib fractures after reirradiation plus hyperthermia for recurrent breast cancer: Predictive factors. *Strahlenther Onkol* 2016;192: 240–247.

42. Peulen H, Karlsson K, Lindberg K et al. Toxicity after reirradiation of pulmonary tumours with stereotactic body radiotherapy. *Radiother Oncol* 2011;101:260–266.

43. Refaat T, Sachdev S, Sathiaseelan V et al. Hyperthermia and radiation therapy for locally advanced or recurrent breast cancer. *Breast* 2015;24:418–425.

44. Ruifrok AC, Kleiboer BJ, van der Kogel AJ. Reirradiation tolerance of the immature rat spinal cord. *Radiother Oncol* 1992;23:249–256.

45. Sahgal A, Ma L, Weinberg V et al. Reirradiation human spinal cord tolerance for stereotactic body radiotherapy. *Int J Radiat Oncol Biol Phys* 2012;82:107–116.

46. Salama JK, Vokes EE, Chmura SJ et al. Long-term outcome of concurrent chemotherapy and reirradiation for recurrent and second primary head-and-neck squamous cell carcinoma. *Int J Radiat Oncol Biol Phys* 2006;64:382–391.

47. Schultheiss TE. The radiation dose-response of the human spinal cord. *Int J Radiat Oncol Biol Phys* 2008;71:1455–1459.

48. Siglin J, Champ CE, Vakhnenko Y, Anne PR, Simone NL. Radiation therapy for locally recurrent breast cancer. *Int J Breast Cancer* 2012;2012:571946.

49. Simmonds RH, Hopewell JW, Robbins ME. Residual radiation-induced injury in dermal tissue: Implications for retreatment. *Br J Radiol* 1989;62:915–920.

50. Spencer SA, Harris J, Wheeler RH et al. Final report of RTOG 9610, a multi-institutional trial of reirradiation and chemotherapy for unresectable recurrent squamous cell carcinoma of the head and neck. *Head Neck* 2008;30: 281–288.

51. Stewart FA, Luts A, Lebesque JV. The lack of long-term recovery and reirradiation tolerance in the mouse kidney. *Int J Radiat Biol* 1989;56:449–462.

52. Stewart FA, Oussoren Y, Luts A. Long-term recovery and reirradiation tolerance of mouse bladder. *Int J Radiat Oncol Biol Phys* 1990;18:1399–1406.

53. Stewart FA, Oussoren Y, Van Tinteren H, Bentzen SM. Loss of reirradiation tolerance in the kidney with increasing time after single or fractionated partial tolerance doses. *Int J Radiat Biol* 1994;66:169–179.

54. Sun DS, Zhang JD, Li L, Dai Y, Yu JM, Shao ZY. Accelerated hyperfractionation field-involved re-irradiation combined with concurrent capecitabine chemotherapy for locally recurrent and irresectable rectal cancer. *Br J Radiol* 2012;85:259–264.

55. Tao R, Tsai CJ, Jensen G et al. Hyperfractionated accelerated reirradiation for rectal cancer: An analysis of outcomes and toxicity. *Radiother Oncol* 2017;122:146–151.

56. Terry NH, Tucker SL, Travis EL. Residual radiation damage in murine lung assessed by pneumonitis. *Int J Radiat Oncol Biol Phys* 1988;14:929–938.

57. Terry NH, Tucker SL, Travis EL. Time course of loss of residual radiation damage in murine skin assessed by retreatment. *Int J Radiat Biol* 1989;55:271–283.

58. Valentini V, Morganti AG, Gambacorta MA et al. Study Group for Therapies of Rectal Malignancies. Preoperative hyperfractionated chemoradiation for locally recurrent rectal cancer in patients previously irradiated to the pelvis: A multicentric phase II study. *Int J Radiat Oncol Biol Phys* 2006;64:1129–1139.

59. van der Kogel AJ, Sissingh HA, Zoetelief J. Effect of X rays and neutrons on repair and regeneration in the rat spinal cord. *Int J Radiat Oncol Biol Phys* 1982;8:2095–2097.

60. van der Schueren E, van den Bogaert W, Vanuytsel L, van Limbergen E. Radiotherapy by multiple fractions per day (MFD) in head and neck cancer: Acute reactions of skin and mucosa. *Int J Radiat Oncol Biol Phys* 1990;19:301–311.

61. Wahl AO, Rademaker A, Kiel KD et al. Multi-institutional review of repeat irradiation of chest wall and breast for recurrent breast cancer. *Int J Radiat Oncol Biol Phys* 2008;70:477–484.

62. White A, Hornsey S. Time dependent repair of radiation damage in the rat spinal cord after X-rays and neutrons. *Eur J Cancer* 1980;16:957–962.

63. Wondergem J, van Ravels FJ, Reijnart IW, Strootman EG. Reirradiation tolerance of the rat heart. *Int J Radiat Oncol Biol Phys* 1996;36:811–819.

64. Wong CS, Hao Y. Long-term recovery kinetics of radiation damage in rat spinal cord. *Int J Radiat Oncol Biol Phys* 1997;37:171–179.

65. Wong CS, Van Dyk J, Milosevic M, Laperriere NJ. Radiation myelopathy following single courses of radiotherapy and retreatment. *Int J Radiat Oncol Biol Phys* 1994;30:575–581.

66. Wong SJ, Bourhis J, Langer CJ. Retreatment of recurrent head and neck cancer in a previously irradiated field. *Semin Radiat Oncol* 2012;22:214–219.

67. Wu KL, Jiang GL, Qian H et al. Three-dimensional conformal radiotherapy for locoregionally recurrent lung carcinoma after external beam irradiation: A prospective phase I-II clinical trial. *Int J Radiat Oncol Biol Phys* 2003;57:1345–1350.

68. Xiang EW, Shu-mo C, Ya-qin D, Ke W. Treatment of late recurrent vaginal malignancy after initial radiotherapy for carcinoma of the cervix: An analysis of 73 cases. *Gynecol Oncol* 1998;69:125–129.

69. Xiao W, Liu S, Tian Y et al. Prognostic significance of tumor volume in locally recurrent nasopharyngeal carcinoma treated with salvage intensity-modulated radiotherapy. *PLOS ONE* 2015;10:e0125351.

70. Yamazaki H, Ogita M, Himei K et al. Carotid blowout syndrome in pharyngeal cancer patients treated by hypofractionated stereotactic re-irradiation using CyberKnife: A multi-institutional matched-cohort analysis. *Radiother Oncol* 2015;115:67–71.

71. Zolciak-Siwinska A, Bijok M, Jonska-Gmyrek J et al. HDR brachytherapy for the reirradiation of cervical and vaginal cancer: Analysis of efficacy and dosage delivered to organs at risk. *Gynecol Oncol* 2014;132:93–97.

## ■ FURTHER READING

72. Morris DE. Clinical experience with retreatment for palliation. *Semin Radiat Oncol* 2000;10:210–221.

73. Nieder C, Milas L, Ang KK. Tissue tolerance to reirradiation. *Semin Radiat Oncol* 2000;10:200–209.

74. Stewart FA. Re-treatment after full-course radiotherapy: Is it a viable option? *Acta Oncol* 1999;38:855–862.

75. Stewart FA, van der Kogel AJ. Retreatment tolerance of normal tissues. *Semin Radiat Oncol* 1994;4:103–111.

# Biological response modification of normal tissue reactions: Basic principles and pitfalls

## WOLFGANG DÖRR

## 24.1 INTRODUCTION

Modulation of radiation effects in normal tissues is closely related to the pathogenetic cascade of radiation-induced changes at the molecular level, which eventually results in a loss of tissue function within the exposed volume, with regard to specific clinical endpoints (see Chapters 14, 15 and 16). The sequence of changes at the subcellular ('molecular'), cellular and tissue levels, and their functional and clinical consequences, are illustrated in Figure 24.1. Options for interventions are given at any of these pathomechanistic steps, from the very early induction of free radicals to the delayed proliferative changes in early reacting tissues or even the late oxidative stress and fibrotic remodelling in late responding organs. It should be emphasized, however, that any sensible strategy for modulation of adverse events of radiotherapy in normal tissues must

- Be highly dependent on the endpoint under consideration, even in the same organ at risk (OAR)
- Require (more or less) precise knowledge of the (molecular) pathogenetic mechanisms underlying the respective endpoint
- Be tested for selectivity, i.e. a potential effect on tumours (originated from the tissues under consideration) needs to be excluded

Over the last decade, there has been a plethora of new ideas on biology-based modulation of radiation-related morbidity, but in general with only minor knowledge about the details of mechanistic pathways. In consequence, many of the approaches turned out to be ineffective or in some cases even toxic, and hence had to be terminated. A better understanding of the mechanisms underlying specific morbidity endpoints will be instrumental in the development of novel, more promising strategies for biological targeting.

This chapter will therefore summarise some of the principles that can be applied to modulate radiation effects in normal tissues in general, and present selected investigations as examples to illustrate the efficacy of the different strategies. The status of targeted radioprotection and radiation injury mitigation and treatment agents has also been reviewed by Kalman et al. (29). It must be emphasized, however, that the vast majority of approaches to modifying normal tissue side effects have been experimental and not validated in clinical studies. Moreover, most strategies are aiming at modification of early normal tissue reactions, as these are usually better assessed and documented compared to late sequelae, and patients are way more compliant to accept mitigative or even prophylactic biology-based activities during their time of treatment as compared to their asymptomatic post-therapeutic time interval before clinically manifest late radiogenic symptoms occur.

This chapter does not focus on modification of normal tissue effects by radiotherapy treatment planning, i.e. dose fractionation or modification of overall treatment time (for this, see Chapters 9, 10 and 12), or by a modulation of the exposed volume (see Chapter 16). Moreover, only those strategies for biological response modification are reviewed, which have already been tested in pre-clinical investigations in experimental animals or in first clinical trials; there will be no reference to any *in vitro* only investigations, as their relevance with regard to the applicability to patients is at least unclear, uncertain or even clearly doubted for many of those studies. Moreover, the clinical *prophylaxis* or *symptomatic* management of already clinically manifest normal tissue reactions is excluded; this is dealt with in various guidelines of the scientific associations, e.g. the Multinational Association of Supportive Care in Cancer (MASCC) and quite a number of reviews for supportive care in radiation oncology.

One major prerequisite for the reasonable clinical application of normal tissue response modifiers is their association with a *therapeutic gain*, i.e. a clear and significant benefit regarding a reduction of normal tissue endpoints ('morbidity') as compared to a potential tumour protective effect. This can be achieved either by selectivity for normal tissues and their specific endpoints, and hence exclusion of similar effects in tumours, or by a relatively greater effect on the normal tissue endpoint compared to tumour cure in curative clinical protocols. The latter, definitely, has to be demonstrated not only in pre-clinical studies, but eventually in well-designed, prospective clinical trials.

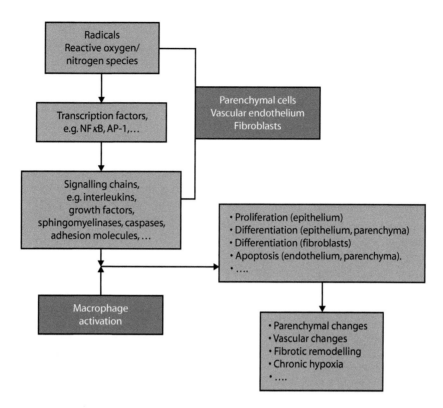

**Figure 24.1** The 'molecular' pathogenetic cascade of normal tissue effects. Radiation primarily induces free radicals, which then generate reactive oxygen and other reactive molecular species. Indirectly, this results in the activation of nuclear transcription factors, which consequently leads to modulation of various signalling chains. The orchestrated response of all tissue components, plus the contribution of macrophages, results in various changes at the cellular and tissue level.

## Terminology

According to the conclusions of a National Cancer Institute workshop on normal tissue protection (52), interventions in the development of radiation effects should be termed as

- *Prophylaxis/protection:* If applied pre-exposure
- *Mitigation:* If applied during or shortly after exposure before clinically manifest symptoms occur, i.e. during the latent time (see Chapter 14)
- *Treatment/management/therapy:* In the eventual symptomatic phase

This obviously applies to short-term exposure, e.g. during radiation accidents or stereotactic treatments, but must be modified for conventional, fractionated radiotherapy, as the latter is given over a course of several weeks (Figure 24.2). In the latter scenario, prophylactic approaches must comprise not only interventions before exposure, but also during the time interval of ongoing radiotherapy until the threshold dose for a specific side effect is reached (see Chapter 14). However, it must be emphasized that some signalling cascades are activated already by the first radiation dose(s) of radiotherapy (Figure 24.1), and they may be interrupted or modulated already at very early time points of radiotherapy (or even before, such as radical induction).

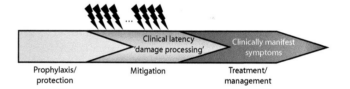

**Figure 24.2** A terminology for intervention strategies in normal tissue radiation effects. Based on the terminology developed for accidental radiation exposure (52), in radiotherapy *prophylaxis* or *protection* is defined as any measure applied before the threshold dose for the specific side effect is reached. Subsequently, but before the manifestation of clinical symptoms, *mitigation* strategies are used. Afterwards, in the symptomatic phase, *treatment* or *management* of side effects is required.

These radiation-induced activations or modulations of signalling cascades become only clinically relevant if the tissue-specific tolerance doses are exceeded, or in a case of retreatment (see Chapter 23). Hence, in radiotherapy, there is a clear overlap between *prophylaxis*, defined clinically, and *mitigation*, in terms of interaction with early processes at a molecular level. *Prevention* is a term frequently used to describe interventions that are applied before the onset of clinical symptoms, and hence may refer to prophylaxis as well as mitigation.

## Study protocols and endpoints

Most of the (*in vivo*) studies on biological response modification in normal tissues have been performed with single-dose irradiation. Aside from radiological accidents or attacks, there are only a few situations where this is really relevant for radiation oncology. These include stereotactic radiotherapy, intraoperative irradiation, brachytherapy with few high-dose fractions, and perhaps treatments given over very short time periods, such as total-body irradiation as a conditioning treatment in preparation for stem/progenitor cell transplantation.

For application to standard external-beam radiotherapy, protection and mitigation strategies must be tested pre-clinically using experimental fractionation protocols as close to the clinical situation as possible, i.e. comprising daily fractionation with doses in the clinical range, administered over several weeks. The latter is required, for example, in order to investigate potential interactions, beneficial or counterproductive, with repopulation processes in early responding normal tissues, but also potentially in tumours, in order to guarantee for the selectivity of the normal tissue-protective strategies (see Chapters 11 and 12).

Modification approaches must also be investigated particularly for endpoints that are clinically relevant. For example, studies into modulation of skin or mucosal *erythema* are only appropriate if the associated pain reaction is concomitantly assessed, and may be entirely irrelevant for the epithelial, ulcerative response, and hence the clinical situation. The same applies – even more importantly – for the relevance of endpoints used in studies of late effects. Because of the highly dynamic development and compilation of information from research into individual organ/symptom modulation strategies, this chapter does not summarise the accumulated knowledge in any detail, but focuses mainly on general aspects. It demonstrates, with a few examples, some potential applications – but prominently also potential pitfalls – of studies on modulation of normal tissue radiation effects particularly in *in vivo* models of radiation adverse events. This follows the sequence of radiation effects in tissues as illustrated in Figure 24.1.

## 24.2 MODIFICATION OF NORMAL TISSUE OXYGEN LEVELS

The oxygen partial pressure in normal tissues, with few exceptions (e.g. cartilage), is normally above the range where the oxygen effect is important (see Chapter 17). Therefore, any reduction in oxygen levels, i.e. by induction of hypoxia, could be expected to reduce radiosensitivity. This has been demonstrated experimentally for total-body hypoxia as well as for local hypoxia.

### Systemic hypoxia

A *systemic* reduction of oxygen partial pressure can be achieved by breathing air with a reduced oxygen concentration. The *protection factor* is defined as the dose required for a specific effect with reduced oxygen compared to the dose resulting in the same effect with normal oxygen breathing. In single-dose studies, protection factors in the range of 1.2–1.4 have been observed. An increase in the binding of oxygen to haemoglobin, e.g. by the drug BW12C, developed as an agent for the treatment of sickle cell anaemia, results in reduced availability of oxygen in normal tissues, with protection factors between 1 and 1.3.

Yet, importantly, in radiotherapy the induction of systemic hypoxia must also be expected to be associated with an increase in the fraction of hypoxic cells within the tumour, and hence an increase in tumour radioresistance (see Chapters 17 and 18). Therefore, this strategy is inherently precluded for the amelioration of radiotherapy complications.

### Local hypoxia

*Local* hypoxia in skin, by a pressure-induced reduction of blood flow, was one of the first instances where the radiobiological oxygen effect was described (see Chapter 17). Alternatively, in radiotherapy for head and neck tumours, 'cryotherapy', i.e. oral cooling, may be applied (51) and patients are asked to chew ice chips before irradiation, in order to reduce the blood flow in the oral mucosa via vasoconstriction. Experimental studies have also demonstrated mucoprotective effects of local administration of vasoconstricting drugs in the rectum and skin. If such approaches are considered, however, care must be taken to ensure that the target oxygenation and hence response, particularly of superficial tumours, is not affected.

## 24.3 RADICAL SCAVENGING AND CELLULAR DETOXIFICATION

The induction of free radicals is one of the earliest intracellular events after radiation exposure (Figure 24.1). Administration of radical scavenging agents or, alternatively, the stimulation of endogenous detoxification mechanisms, has therefore been proposed to reduce the subsequent damage of biomolecules and consequently cellular and tissue radiation effects. The administration of antioxidants in combination with radiotherapy remains controversial, particularly with regard to the selectivity of the many individual approaches. However, reviews have concluded that antioxidants do not counteract the effectiveness of cytotoxic therapies (4,28,34). Clinical studies are available for the use of $\alpha$-tocopherol (vitamin E), other vitamins, beta-carotene, melatonin, retinol palmitate and others, and with few exceptions, a beneficial effect of these drugs has been concluded (e.g. [49]). The most prominent example of all the drugs proposed for radical scavenging is WR2271 (Amifostine). Intracellular detoxification strategies also include superoxide dismutase (SOD) and glutathione peroxidase stimulation via selenium.

## Amifostine (WR2721, Ethyol)

Amifostine is an organic thiophosphate compound that has been suggested for amelioration of radiation effects in a variety of normal tissues. The most promising application appears to be in reducing radiation-induced xerostomia. With regard to radiation-induced early oral mucositis, some analyses have demonstrated a beneficial effect (e.g. [24]) although the results are conflicting (reviewed in [15]), which may be partly attributed to differences in dosing and timing of the drug in different studies, and the inclusion of unblinded studies in meta-analyses (e.g. [6]). At least one phase III study even reported a marginally significant *increase* in severe mucositis in the amifostine arm (3).

Intravenous administration of amifostine is associated with significant side effects, such as nausea and hypotension, as well as skin reactions. Therefore, subcutaneous or topical applications have been suggested as alternative routes, and have been shown to be effective in experimental studies. With *single-dose irradiation* in a mouse model, no effect with subcutaneous irradiation was observed, in contrast to intravenous administration (15). In clear contradiction, in combination with clinically relevant, daily fractionation protocols, amifostine – in both administration pathways – was effective in reducing oral mucositis in the first treatment week only, but not in the second week of fractionation (Figure 24.3). If radical scavenging were the only or dominating

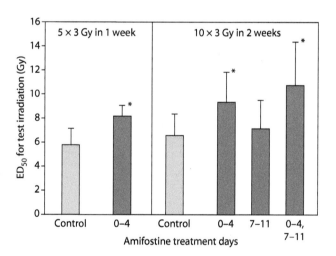

**Figure 24.3** Modulation of oral mucositis in mice by amifostine, using radiation fractionation studies. Mouse tongue mucosa was irradiated with 5 × 3 Gy per week over 1 or 2 weeks, and each protocol was terminated by graded test doses to generate complete dose-effect curves. The $ED_{50}$ for test irradiation (the dose at which an ulceration is expected in 50% of the animals) therefore represents a read-out of the residual radiation tolerance of the tissue at the time of test irradiation. Amifostine administered in the first week of fractionation consistently resulted in a significant increase in mucosal tolerance (*$p < 0.05$). In contrast, administration of amifostine in the second week of the 2-week fractionation protocol had no significant effect. (Data from (15).)

mechanism of action, similar effects in both treatment weeks would be expected, and therefore at least additional mechanisms must be postulated, such as a shortening of the latent time to the onset of repopulation processes (see Chapter 12). Importantly, these data demonstrate the importance of pre-clinical studies with clinically relevant fractionation protocols, as the results from any single-dose studies may be entirely misleading.

The selectivity of amifostine for normal tissues is controversial, and tumour effects cannot be excluded (1). Hence, further clinical trials are still required to determine the indications and the optimum application protocols of this drug. In general, amifostine is recommended for only a very limited panel of indications.

## Selenium

Selenium stimulates glutathione peroxidase, which is supposed to reduce the level of toxic oxygen compounds in irradiated cells. Only few data are available on potential tumour effects of selenium which, however, do not suggest any detrimental outcome (8). After total-body irradiation of rats, a clear increase in animal survival was found after administration of sodium selenite. Also, protection of salivary glands by sodium selenite has been found in rats (44).

In a study on the effects of selenium on oral mucositis (19), a significant effect was found for both systemic and local administration in combination with single-dose irradiation, with protection factors of 1.3–1.4. With 1 week of fractionation, a significant increase in isoeffective doses for oral mucositis (mouse) was observed for both routes of administration, equivalent to compensation of two to three dose fractions. With administration of selenium in the first week of a 2-week fractionation protocol, an effect similar to that seen for only 1 week of fractionation was observed. However, selenium given in week 2 alone, or in weeks 1 and 2 together, did not result in any significant change in isoeffective doses compared to irradiation alone, similar to the results with amifostine (see previous discussion). If the effects of selenium were based only on increased radical scavenging by activation of glutathione peroxidase, then a similar effect of administration in either week would be expected. Therefore, as with amifostine, mechanisms independent of the antioxidative effects have been suggested, e.g. a shortening of the lag phase to effective repopulation. Clinical data have not provided a basis for any recommendation either in favour or against selenium supplementation in cancer patients.

## 24.4 GROWTH FACTORS

For modulation of radiotherapy-associated morbidity by growth factors or cytokines, two general aspects must be considered. First, exogenous growth factors may be applied in order to activate or stimulate tissue-specific endogenous protective, or to inhibit endogenous detrimental signalling cascades. Second, growth factor signalling has been shown to change due to radiation exposure to single doses and – more importantly – during fractionated radiotherapy, and hence inhibition of upregulated or stimulation of downregulated signalling cascades may be applied. This can be achieved by either antibodies against the growth factor or the respective receptors, or by downstream interaction, for example by receptor tyrosine kinase inhibitors. Again, it needs to be emphasized that the signalling responses, and hence the intervention strategies, may be strongly dependent on the equieffective dose and fractionation delivered. Therefore, single-dose pre-clinical *in vivo* studies may be misleading with regard to the real efficacy of the investigated strategies, both agents and administration protocols, during actual clinical radiotherapy.

## Exogenous growth factors

A variety of growth factors have been studied for their potential to modulate normal tissue effects of radiotherapy. Most prominent examples are haematopoietic growth factors (granulocyte colony-stimulating factor [G-CSF] or granulocyte-monocyte colony-stimulating factor [GM-CSF]) to ameliorate radiation effects in the bone marrow, but also in other tissues, such as oral mucosa.

For bone marrow, at all levels of the cellular differentiation sequence, the respective growth factors that trigger cells into the next differentiation step are known (37). Stimulation of progenitor cells by G-CSF or GM-CSF has been demonstrated in numerous pre-clinical and clinical studies. The administration was initially established for the management of leukopenia in cancer patients (18). *Erythropoietin* (EPO) was introduced for the treatment of cancer- or therapy-related anaemia (2). Other factors, e.g. including c-mpl ligand (megakaryocyte growth and development factor, thrombopoietin), are under investigation.

GM-CSF and G-CSF – besides their undoubted beneficial effect on bone marrow hypoplasia – have also repeatedly been tested for their potential to ameliorate oral mucositis. Guidelines strongly recommend not to apply GM-CSF mouthwashes for the prevention of oral mucositis in the transplant setting. In head-and-neck patients undergoing radiotherapy, a placebo-controlled, randomized study has demonstrated no significant effect of systemic administration of GM-CSF on the severity or duration of oral mucositis (43), and their use is therefore not recommended in head-and-neck patients (30). It should also be noted that tumour protective effects of haematopoietic growth factors have also been demonstrated experimentally for various tumour types, and as this cannot yet be excluded in clinical applications, great caution is required in any use of these agents (37).

*Keratinocyte growth factor* (KGF-1) is synthesized predominantly by mesenchymal cells (fibroblasts). The target cells are epithelial cells in a variety of tissues. KGF-1 has been tested in pre-clinical models for its potential to ameliorate radiation effects in oral mucosa, skin, intestine, lung and urinary bladder. Positive effects have been found consistently in all studies. The most extensive studies have been carried out in mouse oral mucosa with palifermin, a truncated recombinant form of KGF-1 (7). In single-dose studies, the dose modification factors observed were between 1.7 and 2.3, depending on the KGF treatment protocol. In combination with single-dose irradiation, repeated KGF administration is required to achieve a significant effect. However, the treatment with KGF is even effective if given *after* irradiation, which offers some options for scenarios with accidental radiation exposure. In contrast, KGF treatment during fractionated irradiation, given as only a single injection at the beginning of the first or second weekend break, was as effective as repeated applications over the entire weekend. An increase in the effect was observed with up to four repeated treatments at consecutive weekends (Figure 24.4), starting before the onset of radiotherapy (12).

In a large, randomised, placebo-controlled, double-blinded phase III study in patients receiving total-body irradiation and high-dose chemotherapy in preparation for peripheral blood progenitor cell transplantation, treatment with palifermin resulted in a highly significant reduction in the incidence and duration of oral mucositis (50). Two phase III studies in patients with radio(chemo)therapy

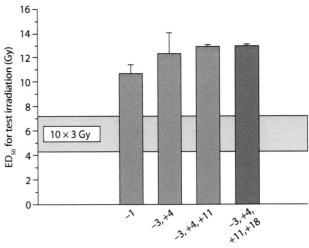

**Figure 24.4** The effect of repeated applications of palifermin over subsequent weekends, on the incidence of oral mucosal ulcerations in the mouse. Mouse tongue mucosa was irradiated with 10 × 3 Gy over 2 weeks. Palifermin was given before the onset of radiotherapy (day −1), or over 2, 3 or 4 subsequent weekends. Each protocol was terminated by graded test doses to generate complete dose-effect curves. The $ED_{50}$ for test irradiation can be regarded as a measure of the mucosal tolerance at the time of test irradiation. Palifermin resulted in a highly significant increase in mucosal tolerance in all protocols tested. However, addition of a third palifermin injection on day +11 only yielded a minor increase in $ED_{50}$ values, and a further injection on day +18 had no further effect. (Data from (12).)

– post-operative or primary – for head and neck tumours have also revealed a substantial and significant reduction of the mucositis response (26,32).

The mechanisms through which KGF acts remain unclear, and appear to be multifactorial (e.g. [14]). One component is the stimulation of proliferation and the modification of differentiation (reduction of cell loss) in the epithelial tissues (7). However, KGF has been demonstrated to also modulate the response of vascular endothelial cells and macrophages to irradiation, which appears to contribute to a complex mechanism of action. Probably because of this uncertainty as to the exact mechanism of action, KGF has not been recommended in various guidelines for prevention of radiotherapy-induced oral mucositis (e.g. [42]).

With regard to late complications in the lung, conflicting data have emerged from various studies using *fibroblast growth factor-2*. In the central nervous system and the kidney, insulin-like growth factor-1 (IGF-1) as an anti-apoptotic factor for oligodendrocytes and their progenitor cells, and platelet-derived growth factor (PDGF) as a survival factor of progenitor cells, have been suggested as strategies to prevent the development of radiation-induced necrosis. Several interleukins, as well as angiogenic growth factors, such as FGF-1 and FGF-2 and vascular endothelial growth factor (VEGF) and others, have been proposed for the modification of gastrointestinal reactions to irradiation. However, at present there is no convincing evidence for the efficacy of any of these approaches in a clinical setting.

## Inhibition of growth factor signalling

Among the most prominent growth factor signalling cascades where regulation in early responding normal tissues after irradiation has been observed are the epidermal growth factor pathway (upregulation of the receptor EGFR) and the tumour necrosis factor-$\alpha$ (TNF-$\alpha$) pathway (upregulation of the growth factor). For late responding tissues, a significant stimulation of transforming growth factor-ß (TGF-ß) has been reported. These processes therefore might be targeted in order to modify normal tissue radiation effects.

## Epidermal growth factor signalling

The epidermal growth factor receptor (EGFR) is over-expressed in a variety of tumours and hence may represent one specific target for improving the tumour effects of radiotherapy (see Chapter 20). However, in animal models, upregulation of EGFR expression in early responding tissues by irradiation has also been shown. Therefore, targeting of EGFR may also modify normal tissue effects to radiotherapy, independent of the radiation-independent side effects of some of the drugs used, such as skin changes. In mouse oral mucosa, EGFR inhibition by a specific tyrosine kinase inhibitor (BIBX1382BS) during fractionated irradiation did not have a significant effect (13). However, preliminary results (Dörr, unpublished) using another tyrosine kinase inhibitor as well as an anti-EGFR antibody, suggest that the normal tissue effects may be drug specific.

## Tumour necrosis factor-$\alpha$ signalling

TNF-$\alpha$ is a growth factor with a profound role in inflammatory processes, and upregulation in normal tissues by irradiation has been demonstrated in a number of pre-clinical studies. These processes are usually considered to promote the radiation response of these normal tissues. Therefore, inhibition of TNF-$\alpha$ signalling might be beneficial for the reduction of some radiation-induced morbidity endpoints. Drugs directed against TNF-$\alpha$ signalling (e.g. infliximab) are already used clinically for treating Crohn disease, rheumatoid arthritis and psoriasis. However, in mouse kidney, treatment with infliximab significantly *exacerbated* radiation nephropathy (38).

In a set of pre-clinical studies on oral mucositis in an established mouse model (25), it has been clearly demonstrated that anti-TNF-$\alpha$ strategies did not impact on the *epithelial* response of the oral mucosa, i.e. ulceration. However, beneficial effects on the inflammatory effects, including pain, of the radiation response, cannot be excluded from these pre-clinical studies (e.g. [16]).

These examples, again, clearly illustrate that the hypotheses underlying any strategy for intervention into the biological processes associated with the response of normal tissues to irradiation must be carefully tested in relevant pre-clinical models, before clinical testing is undertaken.

## Transforming growth factor-$\beta$ signalling

Although the essential role of TGF-$\beta$ for the development of radiation-induced fibrosis has been well documented (see Chapter 14), approaches to inhibit TGF-$\beta$ signalling have only emerged more recently (e.g. [53]). One strategy is to inhibit the activation of TGF-$\beta$ from its latent form, which, at least in the lung, is regulated by the integrin $\alpha(v)\beta6$. Treatment of irradiated mice with a monoclonal antibody against this integrin has prevented fibrosis (41).

## 24.5 ANTI-INFLAMMATORY TREATMENTS

### Glucocorticoids

Standard anti-inflammatory approaches with glucocorticoids are frequently applied as symptomatic, supportive treatment in order to manage oedema and pain associated with the inflammatory component of radiation-induced side effects, e.g. in central nervous system, lung or skin. However, no conclusive results are available for this class of drugs for any specific targeting of inflammatory processes in order to prevent radiotherapy side effects.

## Non-steroidal anti-inflammatory drugs

As with corticoids, non-steroidal anti-inflammatory drugs (NSAIDs), particularly acetylic salicylic acid (ASA), are frequently used for the symptomatic management of inflammatory signs of (early) radiation side effects. However, some pre-clinical studies have addressed the potential of ASA to specifically target the biological mechanisms of normal tissue complications. In a first study in mouse kidney, ASA was administered as an *anti-thrombotic agent* (54). This treatment resulted in a significant prolongation of the latent time to development of renal failure. In a further study in mouse urinary bladder (9), where ASA was applied in order to reduce the increase in detrusor muscle tone during the early response phase, which is mediated through arachidonic acid metabolites, the treatment yielded significant restoration of the bladder storage capacity.

## Others

### ESSENTIAL FATTY ACIDS

Essential fatty acids (EFAs) are known to interact with the arachidonic acid metabolism by shifting the end products into an anti-inflammatory direction. In pig skin, oral administration of EFA resulted in a clear reduction of the severity of both early and late skin reactions (27). Similarly, in mouse urinary bladder, EFA treatment has yielded a reduction of the incidence of late effects (Dörr, unpublished).

### INHIBITORS OF CYCLOOXYGENASE-2 (COX-2)

Similar to EGFR inhibitors (see Section 24.4), COX-2 inhibitors have been proposed as drugs that specifically target the metabolism of tumours, where COX-2 is frequently upregulated. However, upregulation of COX-2 is also seen in normal tissues, particularly during the early response; the relevance of these changes regarding the manifestation of morbidity is unknown. In studies on mouse tongue mucosa, no clear decrease in epithelial radiation effects is seen when the COX-2 inhibitor Celecoxib is administered during daily fractionated radiotherapy (25).

### PENTOXIFYLLINE (PTX)

PTX is an unspecific phosphodiesterase inhibitor, with rheological and anti-inflammatory activities. With systemic administration of PTX in combination with fractionated irradiation, early oral mucositis is reduced significantly in pre-clinical studies, presumably based on an inhibition of the expression of TNF-$\alpha$ and interleukin-1$\beta$ (IL-1$\beta$) and improved local tissue perfusion (22,23).

### DERMATAN SULFATE (DS)

Glycosaminoglycans, such as dermatan sulfate (DS), interact with growth factors and cytokines. Pre-clinical studies indicate significant reduction in radiation-induced oral mucositis with single-dose as well as fractionated irradiation (Gruber, personal communication).

## 24.6 MODULATION OF MACROPHAGE ACTIVITY

The relevance of macrophage responses to normal tissue side effects is discussed controversially. For late effects, such as radiation pneumopathy, a contribution of alveolar macrophages to the orchestrated reaction of the tissue has been clearly demonstrated (see Chapter 14). Also, for early radiation reactions, changes in macrophage activation have been observed. However, their relevance to the clinical manifestation of the respective side effects – although very likely – has remained obscure.

Selective modulation of macrophage activity has been tested in a rat model of radiation proctitis (45). Tetrachlorodecaoxide (TCDO, WF10) is a drug that activates macrophages, but then regulates their activity at an intermediate level. Treatment of rats at early time points after irradiation results in a clear prolongation of the time to onset of late proctitis. Administration at later time points also significantly reduces the severity of the response. For early radiation-induced oral mucositis in the mouse, local administration of TCDO appears to reduce the response to daily fractionated irradiation, while no effect is observed with single-dose irradiation (Schmidt and Dörr, unpublished). Similarly, the experimental immunomodulator JBT3200, a bacterial wall component, seems to reduce the oral mucosal response only during fractionated irradiation, but is largely ineffective in combination with single-dose irradiation (Dörr, unpublished).

## 24.7 STIMULATION OF PROLIFERATION IN EARLY RESPONDING TISSUES

The severity of early radiation effects during fractionated irradiation is clearly related to the regeneration response of the tissue, a complex reaction to the damage induced that is depicted as repopulation (see Chapter 12). Therefore, stimulation of cell production in epithelial tissues has been tested for its potential to reduce early complications of radiotherapy. Besides the administration of growth factors (Section 24.4), removal of the superficial epithelia layers may increase the normal trigger for proliferation in the germinal compartment. In skin this can, for example, be achieved by 'tape stripping' or hair plucking which however has only been tested in combination with single-dose irradiation. In accordance with the more rapid turnover of the stimulated epidermis, epidermal reactions started earlier than in unstimulated skin.

Similar observations, with single-dose irradiation, have been made in mouse oral mucosa after ablation of the superficial keratin layers by mild silver nitrate solution as an adstringent (11). However, when fractionated irradiation was applied, stimulated proliferation translated into an increased radiation tolerance, which was attributed to an earlier onset of repopulation processes. These data have been validated in a clinical study with accelerated radiotherapy for head and neck tumours, but – although the proliferative effect was demonstrated in mucosal biopsies – its consequences on the clinical manifestation of oral mucositis could not be confirmed with conventional fractionation protocols (10). It was concluded, that for effective stimulation of repopulation, an early switch from asymmetrical to symmetrical divisions (see Chapter 12) is required in addition to stimulated proliferation, which is only achieved during accelerated but not during conventional fractionation. Alternatively, low-level laser treatment – termed *photobiomodulation* (PBM) – can be successfully administered to oral mucosa in head-and-neck cancer patients for the management of oral mucositis and also for other treatment-associated morbidities (58). However, a variety of other mechanisms may contribute to the morbidity-reducing activities of PBM (59).

## 24.8 STRATEGIES TO REDUCE CHRONIC OXIDATIVE STRESS

For late effects in normal tissues, a long-lasting perpetuation of the production of reactive oxygen and nitrogen species appears to play an essential role. Therefore, strategies have been developed to interrupt this chronic oxidative stress cascade and have been tested for fibrotic changes in skin, using a combination of pentoxifylline (PTX) and tocopherol (vitamin E) as anti-oxidative agents.

In breast cancer patients ($n = 24$) with manifest radiation skin fibrosis, a clear regression of the fibrotic lesions was observed at 6 months after treatment with PTX and tocopherol in a randomised, placebo-controlled trial (5). These results, however, were not confirmed in a larger, double-blind placebo-controlled trial in breast cancer patients (21), or in a further trial in patients after pelvic radiotherapy (20). Nevertheless, some practical guidelines suggest this approach for the reduction of fibrosis (56).

## 24.9 INTERVENTION IN THE ANGIOTENSIN PATHWAY

The angiotensin system appears to be involved in the development of fibrosis, at least in the lung, presumably through interactions with TGF-$\beta$ signalling, but appears also to be involved in cardiovascular radiation effects. In the kidney, angiotensin-converting enzyme (ACE)-induced hypertension also contributes to the development of the radiation response. Therefore, ACE inhibitors, such as Captopril, and antagonists of the angiotensin II type 1- (AT1-) and type 2- (AT2-) receptors, have been tested for their potential to mitigate or treat late radiation effects particularly in the kidney and lung, and are also suggested to mitigate radiation-induced cardiovascular disease (55,57).

In a rat model of total-body irradiation and bone marrow transplantation, resulting in nephropathy, ACE inhibitors have been shown to effectively prevent kidney sequelae of irradiation (35). These drugs also were effective in the treatment of kidney damage. Obviously, different modes of action are relevant at different time periods, i.e. for mitigation and management of morbidity. As a hypothesis for kidney morbidity, mitigation may be based on the suppression of the renin-angiotensin system, but treatment of established nephropathy is based on (additional) blood pressure control.

It has to be noted that most studies so far were done with high single doses of radiation, given locally (lung) or as total-body irradiation in combination with chemotherapy, which may alter the pathobiology of the radiation effects. Therefore, validation of the results in studies with conventional fractionation protocols is still desirable.

## 24.10 STEM CELL THERAPY

A novel, potentially selective approach for the amelioration of normal tissue radiation effects is the treatment with (adult) stem cells. This includes the administration of bone marrow (i.e. haematopoietic plus mesenchymal stem cells) or mesenchymal stem cells, or the mobilisation of autologous stem cells by growth factors, e.g. G-CSF. These strategies have been tested in pre-clinical models of radiation injury in skin, salivary glands, intestine and oral mucosa.

### Transplantation of bone marrow

Transplantation of (syngeneic) bone marrow has been studied for its potential to ameliorate oral mucositis in the mouse (46,47). Following single-dose irradiation, transplantation between days 0 to 10 did not result in any change in the mucosal response. In contrast, transplantation during daily fractionated irradiation resulted in a reduction in mucosal reactions, particularly if the stem cell treatment was administered at time points later in the irradiation regimen.

### Transplantation of mesenchymal stem cells

Systemically administered mesenchymal stem cells (MSCs) appear to home in specifically on (radiation) injured tissues. Systemic administration of human MSCs reduced the severity of the response and improved healing in human skin transplanted onto nude mice (17). Similarly, in the intestine, intravenous MSC transplantation accelerated crypt regeneration in a mouse model (48). In mouse oral mucosa, intravenous administration of MSC at various time points during daily fractionated irradiation significantly reduced the incidence of confluent oral mucositis (47). Mesenchymal stem cell therapy has also been applied successfully as part of the therapy of skin lesions in patients after radiation accidents (e.g. [31]).

## Mobilisation of bone marrow stem cells

Release of stem cells from the bone marrow can be stimulated by growth factors, such as G-CSF, and other drugs, like inhibitors of the receptor for the stromal cell derived factor 1 (SDF-1, CXCL12), which regulates the retention of the stem cells in the bone marrow. It must be noted that mobilisation of stem cells by G-CSF (at least in the mouse) affects both haematopoietic and mesenchymal stem cells.

Treatment of mice with G-CSF induced the homing of bone marrow cells to irradiated submandibular glands (33), and was associated with increased gland weight, number of acinar cells and salivary flow rates. In mouse oral mucosa (46), administration of G-CSF has resulted in a clear reduction of radiation-induced mucositis after single-dose irradiation, particularly when the maximum number of stem cells in the circulation was induced at a time when the mucosal regeneration phase was about to start. Similarly, during daily fractionated irradiation, a maximum number of circulating stem cells was most effective at the time when radiation-induced repopulation processes (see Chapter 12) were effective (Figure 24.5). In histological studies,

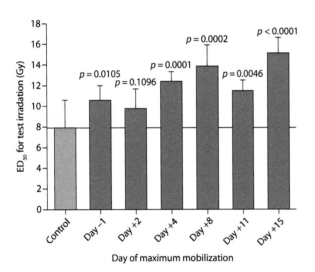

**Figure 24.5** The effect of the mobilisation of bone marrow stem cells on oral mucosal tolerance in mice. Daily fractionated irradiation was given with 5 × 3 Gy per week over 3 weeks, and the protocols were terminated by graded test doses in order to generate dose-effect curves, using the $ED_{50}$ values as a measure of the residual tissue tolerance. Bone marrow stem cells were mobilised by two daily injections of G-CSF over 4 days. This protocol has been shown to result in a maximum number of circulating stem cells at day 10 after the first injection. This maximum mobilisation effect was adjusted to various time points during the fractionation protocol, shown on the abscissa. With the exception of day +2, all mobilisation protocols yielded a significant reduction in the incidence of oral mucosal ulcerations. The effect was most pronounced at later time points, when mucosal repopulation processes (see Chapter 12) were maximally stimulated. (Data from Dörr, unpublished.)

only individual haematopoietic cells were found in the submucosal and mucosal tissues, without any indication of clonal expansion or trans-differentiation.

## Administration of tissue-specific stem cells

Transplantation of bone marrow stem or progenitor cells is known to restore the bone marrow after myeloablative treatments. However, reliable methods to identify stem cells specific for other tissues and, more importantly, to stimulate these cells to proliferate *in vitro*, are in only the early stages of development. These are prerequisites in order to achieve cell numbers sufficient for transplantation. For the prevention, mitigation or management of radiation-induced xerostomia, stem cell therapy has been proposed (36,40). In pre-clinical investigations, administration of tissue-specific stem cells has resulted in long-term restoration of salivary gland morphology and function (39).

## Mechanisms of action

In rat salivary glands, improved morphology and function are not associated with any trans-differentiation of bone marrow cells into salivary gland cells. Similarly, the reduction in oral mucosal reactions to single-dose or fractionated irradiation in mouse oral mucosa is not linked to any clonal expansion of either mesenchymal or haematopoietic cells or to trans-differentiation into an epithelial cell type. For irradiated skin, the data are less consistent, with some indication of trans-differentiation processes. Two alternative mechanisms of action must hence be considered: (1) homing of stem cells into radiation-damaged sites and production of paracrine factors that locally stimulate tissue regeneration, or (2) release of such factors by stem cells which are still in the circulation. In contrast to bone marrow stem cells, tissue-specific stem cells (including haematopoietic stem cells in the bone marrow) do appear to differentiate into functional cells, for example in salivary glands (39).

## 24.11 CONCLUSIONS

A variety of approaches for the prophylaxis, mitigation or treatment of radiation side effects have been suggested, based on the specific biology of the response of different tissues to irradiation. These interventions are still mostly experimental though in a few instances, described previously, they have been translated into clinical studies.

Moreover, it must be noted that many experimental studies have been carried out only in combination with single-dose irradiation. This could reflect clinical scenarios of stereotactic irradiation, brachytherapy or myeloablative conditioning for stem cell transplantation. However, it clearly lacks relevance for fractionated radiotherapy given over several weeks where, for example, repopulation processes in early responding tissues are a factor dominating the radiation tolerance of these tissues (see Chapter 12), but also for late-tissue reactions a repeated stimulus of the radiopathological pathways occurs. Parallel studies with single and fractionated doses of radiation have clearly demonstrated that the results can be highly contradictory, e.g. for bone marrow transplantation in oral mucosa (see Section 24.10). During fractionated irradiation, intervention at intervals before the onset of repopulation can result in effects that are different from intervention at later times, as has been demonstrated for administration of amifostine or selenium to ameliorate oral mucositis (see Section 24.3).

Some approaches, such as stimulation of proliferation for a reduction of early epithelial radiation effects, or a reduction of the chronic oxidative stress response in irradiated tissues for the prophylaxis or treatment of late radiation sequelae in skin or lung, have been tested in clinical trials, but with conflicting results. A number of 'targeted' interventions, e.g. administration of growth factors or stem cell therapy, appear to act through several different mechanisms, which deserve further investigation.

In general, modification of normal tissue responses to radiation exposure requires thorough pre-clinical testing, with

- Appropriate *in vivo* (animal) models
- Analysis of clinically relevant endpoints after irradiation
- Adequate (fractionation) protocols

The mechanisms of action of effective interventions must then be clarified in order to develop optimal clinical strategies.

In order to guarantee a clinical benefit, possible tumour effects of the normal tissue modification strategies must also be assessed. This must be done under the same premises with regard to suitability of the *in vivo* models, relevance of treatment protocols and endpoints. A therapeutic gain is only achieved if the target normal tissue demonstrates significantly greater radioprotection compared with any reduction of the radiation effect in the tumour being treated.

## Key points

1. Strategies for modification of normal tissue responses to irradiation must be based on the underlying pathobiology.
2. Interventions in the processing of radiation damage can be directed against any step of the pathogenetic cascade from early production of free radicals to late tissue changes. The mechanisms of action underlying the protective effects must be clarified in order to design optimum clinical protocols.

3. Before clinical application, modification approaches must be thoroughly tested in animal models, with relevant irradiation protocols and endpoints. Results from single-dose and fractionation studies can be divergent.
4. Comparison with potential tumour effects is essential in order to achieve a therapeutic gain.
5. Most promising, with the first clinical studies, are the interaction with growth factor signalling, the interruption of chronic oxidative stress cascades in late tissue reactions, and the treatment (mobilisation, transplantation) with stem cells, haematopoietic or mesenchymal.

## ■ BIBLIOGRAPHY

1. Andreassen CN, Grau C, Lindegaard JC. Chemical radio-protection: A critical review of amifostine as a cytoprotector in radiotherapy. *Semin Radiat Oncol* 2003;13: 62–72.
2. Bokemeyer C, Aapro MS, Courdi A et al. EORTC guidelines for the use of erythropoietic proteins in anaemic patients with cancer: 2006 update. *Eur J Cancer* 2007;43:258–270.
3. Buentzel J, Micke O, Adamietz IA, Monnier A, Glatzel M, de Vries A. Intravenous amifostine during chemoradiotherapy for head-and-neck cancer: A randomized placebo-controlled phase III study. *Int J Radiat Oncol Biol Phys* 2006;64:684–691.
4. Citrin D, Cotrim AP, Hyodo F, Baum BJ, Krishna MC, Mitchell JB. Radioprotectors and mitigators of radiation-induced normal tissue injury. *Oncologist* 2010;15:360–371.
5. Delanian S, Porcher R, Balla-Mekias S, Lefaix JL. Randomized, placebo-controlled trial of combined pentoxifylline and tocopherol for regression of superficial radiation-induced fibrosis. *J Clin Oncol* 2003;21:2545–2550.
6. Devine A, Marignol L. Potential of amifostine for chemora-diotherapy and radiotherapy-associated toxicity reduction in advanced NSCLC: A meta-analysis. *Anticancer Res* 2016;36: 5–12.
7. Dörr W. Oral mucosa: Response modification by keratinocyte growth factor. In: Nieder C, Milas L and Ang KK, editors. *Modification of Radiation Response: Cytokines, Growth Factors and Other Biological Targets*. Berlin: Springer-Verlag; 2003. pp. 113–122.
8. Dörr W. Effects of selenium on radiation responses of tumor cells and tissue. *Strahlenther Onkol* 2006;182:693–695.
9. Dörr W, Eckhardt M, Ehme A, Koi S. Pathogenesis of acute radiation effects in the urinary bladder. Experimental results. *Strahlenther Onkol* 1998;174(Suppl 3):93–95.
10. Dörr W, Jacubek A, Kummermehr J et al. Effects of stimu-lated repopulation on oral mucositis during conventional radiotherapy. *Radiother Oncol* 1995;37:100–107.
11. Dörr W, Kummermehr J. Increased radiation tolerance of mouse tongue epithelium after local conditioning. *Int J Radiat Biol* 1992;61:369–379.

12. Dörr W, Reichel S, Spekl K. Effects of keratinocyte growth factor (palifermin) administration protocols on oral mucositis (mouse) induced by fractionated irradiation. *Radiother Oncol* 2005;75:99-105.

13. Fehrmann A, Dörr W. Effect of EGFR-inhibition on the radiation response of oral mucosa: Experimental studies in mouse tongue epithelium. *Int J Radiat Biol* 2005;81:437-443.

14. Finch PW, Mark Cross LJ, McAuley DF, Farrell CL. Palifermin for the protection and regeneration of epithelial tissues following injury: New findings in basic research and pre-clinical models. *J Cell Mol Med* 2013;17:1065-1087.

15. Fleischer G, Dörr W. Amelioration of early radiation effects in oral mucosa (mouse) by intravenous or subcutaneous administration of amifostine. *Strahlenther Onkol* 2006;182:567-575.

16. Fox BS, Sonis S. TNF and oral mucositis. Letter to the editor, responding to 'Effect of selective inhibitors of inflammation on oral mucositis: Preclinical studies' in *Radiother Oncol* 2009; 92:472-476. *Radiother Oncol* 2010;94:123.

17. Francois S, Mouiseddine M, Mathieu N et al. Human mesenchymal stem cells favour healing of the cutaneous radiation syndrome in a xenogenic transplant model. *Ann Hematol* 2007;86:1-8.

18. Ganser A, Karthaus M. Clinical use of hematopoietic growth factors. *Curr Opin Oncol* 1996;8:265-269.

19. Gehrisch A, Dörr W. Effects of systemic or topical administration of sodium selenite on early radiation effects in mouse oral mucosa. *Strahlenther Onkol* 2007;183:36-42.

20. Gothard L, Cornes P, Brooker S et al. Phase II study of vitamin E and pentoxifylline in patients with late side effects of pelvic radiotherapy. *Radiother Oncol* 2005;75:334-341.

21. Gothard L, Cornes P, Earl J et al. Double-blind placebo-controlled randomised trial of vitamin E and pentoxifylline in patients with chronic arm lymphoedema and fibrosis after surgery and radiotherapy for breast cancer. *Radiother Oncol* 2004;73:133-139.

22. Gruber S, Hamedinger D, Bozsaky E et al. Local hypoxia in oral mucosa (mouse) during daily fractionated irradiation - Effect of pentoxifylline. *Radiother Oncol* 2015;116:404-8.

23. Gruber S, Schmidt M, Bozsaky E et al. Modulation of radiation-induced oral mucositis by pentoxifylline: Preclinical studies. *Strahlenther Onkol* 2015;191:242-247.

24. Gu J, Zhu S, Li X, Wu H, Li Y, Hua F. Effect of amifostine in head and neck cancer patients treated with radiotherapy: A systematic review and meta-analysis based on randomized controlled trials. *PLOS ONE* 2014;9:e95968.

25. Haagen J, Krohn H, Rollig S, Schmidt M, Wolfram K, Dorr W. Effect of selective inhibitors of inflammation on oral mucositis: Preclinical studies. *Radiother Oncol* 2009;92:472-476.

26. Henke M, Alfonsi M, Foa P et al. Palifermin decreases severe oral mucositis of patients undergoing postoperative radiochemotherapy for head and neck cancer: A randomized, placebo-controlled trial. *J Clin Oncol* 2011;29:2815-2820.

27. Hopewell JW, van den Aardweg GJ, Morris GM et al. Amelioration of both early and late radiation-induced damage to pig skin by essential fatty acids. *Int J Radiat Oncol Biol Phys* 1994;30:1119-1125.

28. Johnke RM, Sattler JA, Allison RR. Radioprotective agents for radiation therapy: Future trends. *Future Oncol* 2014;10:2345-2357.

29. Kalman NS, Zhao SS, Anscher MS, Urdaneta AI. Current status of targeted radioprotection and radiation injury mitigation and treatment agents: A critical review of the literature. *Int J Radiat Oncol Biol Phys* 2017;98:662-682.

30. Lalla RV, Bowen J, Barasch A et al. Mucositis Guidelines Leadership Group of the Multinational Association of Supportive Care in Cancer/International Society of Oral Oncology. MASCC/ISOO clinical practice guidelines for the management of mucositis secondary to cancer therapy. *Cancer* 2014;120:1453-1461.

31. Lataillade JJ, Doucet C, Bey E et al. New approach to radiation burn treatment by dosimetry-guided surgery combined with autologous mesenchymal stem cell therapy. *Regen Med* 2007;2:785-794.

32. Le QT, Kim HE, Schneider CJ et al. Palifermin reduces severe mucositis in definitive chemoradiotherapy of locally advanced head and neck cancer: A randomized, placebo-controlled study. *J Clin Oncol* 2011;29:2808-2814.

33. Lombaert IM, Wierenga PK, Kok T, Kampinga HH, deHaan G, Coppes RP. Mobilization of bone marrow stem cells by granulocyte colony-stimulating factor ameliorates radiation-induced damage to salivary glands. *Clin Cancer Res* 2006;12:1804-1812.

34. Maier P, Wenz F, Herskind C. Radioprotection of normal tissue cells. *Strahlenther Onkol* 2014;190:745-752.

35. Moulder JE, Fish BL, Cohen EP. Treatment of radiation nephropathy with ACE inhibitors and AII type-1 and type-2 receptor antagonists. *Curr Pharm Des* 2007;13:1317-1325.

36. Nevens D, Nuyts S. The role of stem cells in the prevention and treatment of radiation-induced xerostomia in patients with head and neck cancer. *Cancer Med* 2016;5:1147-1153.

37. Nieder C, Jeremic B, Licht T, Zimmermann FB. Hematopoietic tissue II: Role of colony-stimulating factors. In: Nieder C, Milas L and Ang KK, editors. *Modification of Radiation Response: Cytokines, Growth Factors and Other Biological Targets*. Berlin: Springer-Verlag; 2003. pp. 103-112.

38. Nieder C, Schnaiter A, Weber WA et al. Detrimental effects of an antibody directed against tumor necrosis factor alpha in experimental kidney irradiation. *Anticancer Res* 2007;27:2353-2357.

39. Pringle S, Maimets M, van der Zwaag M et al. Human salivary gland stem cells functionally restore radiation damaged salivary glands. *Stem Cells* 2016;34:640-652.

40. Pringle S, Van Os R, Coppes RP. Concise review: Adult salivary gland stem cells and a potential therapy for xerostomia. *Stem Cells* 2013;31:613-619.

41. Puthawala K, Hadjiangelis N, Jacoby SC et al. Inhibition of integrin α(v)β6, an activator of latent transforming growth factor-β, prevents radiation-induced lung fibrosis. *Am J Respir Crit Care Med* 2008;177:82-90.

42. Raber-Durlacher JE, von Bultzingslowen I, Logan RM et al. Mucositis Study Group of the Multinational Association of Supportive Care in Cancer/International Society of Oral

Oncology. Systematic review of cytokines and growth factors for the management of oral mucositis in cancer patients. *Support Care Cancer* 2013;21:343–355.

43. Ryu JK, Swann S, LeVeque F et al. The impact of concurrent granulocyte macrophage-colony stimulating factor on radiation-induced mucositis in head and neck cancer patients: A double-blind placebo-controlled prospective phase III study by Radiation Therapy Oncology Group 9901. *Int J Radiat Oncol Biol Phys* 2007;67:643–650.

44. Sagowski C, Wenzel S, Jenicke L, Metternich FU, Jaehne M. Sodium selenite is a potent radioprotector of the salivary glands of the rat: Acute effects on the morphology and parenchymal function during fractioned irradiation. *Eur Arch Otorhinolaryngol* 2005;262:459–464.

45. Sassy T, Breiter N, Trott KR. Effects of tetrachlorodecaoxide (TCDO) in chronic radiation lesions of the rat colon. *Strahlenther Onkol* 1991;167:191–196.

46. Schmidt M, Haagen J, Noack R, Siegemund A, Gabriel P, Dorr W. Effects of bone marrow or mesenchymal stem cell transplantation on oral mucositis (mouse) induced by fractionated irradiation. *Strahlenther Onkol* 2014;190:399–404.

47. Schmidt M, Piro-Hussong A, Siegemund A, Gabriel P, Dorr W. Modification of radiation-induced oral mucositis (mouse) by adult stem cell therapy: Single-dose irradiation. *Radiat Environ Biophys* 2014;53:629–634.

48. Semont A, Francois S, Mouiseddine M et al. Mesenchymal stem cells increase self-renewal of small intestinal epithelium and accelerate structural recovery after radiation injury. *Adv Exp Med Biol* 2006;585:19–30.

49. Singh VK, Beattie LA, Seed TM. Vitamin E: Tocopherols and tocotrienols as potential radiation countermeasures. *J Radiat Res* 2013;54:973–988.

50. Spielberger R, Stiff P, Bensinger W et al. Palifermin for oral mucositis after intensive therapy for hematologic cancers. *N Engl J Med* 2004;351:2590–2598.

51. Stokman MA, Spijkervet FK, Boezen HM, Schouten JP, Roodenburg JL, de Vries EG. Preventive intervention possibilities in radiotherapy- and chemotherapy-induced oral mucositis: Results of meta-analyses. *J Dent Res* 2006;85:690–700.

52. Stone HB, Moulder JE, Coleman CN et al. Models for evaluating agents intended for the prophylaxis, mitigation and treatment of radiation injuries. *Report of an NCI Workshop, December 3–4, 2003. Radiat Res* 2004;162:711–728.

53. Straub JM, New J, Hamilton CD, Lominska C, Shnayder Y, Thomas SM. Radiation-induced fibrosis: Mechanisms and implications for therapy. *J Cancer Res Clin Oncol* 2015;141:1985–1994.

54. Verheij M, Stewart FA, Oussoren Y, Weening JJ, Dewit L. Amelioration of radiation nephropathy by acetylsalicylic acid. *Int J Radiat Biol* 1995;67:587–596.

55. Westbury CB, Yarnold JR. Radiation fibrosis – Current clinical and therapeutic perspectives. *Clin Oncol (R Coll Radiol)* 2012;24:657–672.

56. Wong RK, Bensadoun RJ, Boers-Doets CB et al. Clinical practice guidelines for the prevention and treatment of acute and late radiation reactions from the MASCC Skin Toxicity Study Group. *Support Care Cancer* 2013;21:2933–2948.

57. Zagar TM, Cardinale DM, Marks LB. Breast cancer therapy-associated cardiovascular disease. *Nat Rev Clin Oncol* 2016;13:172–184.

58. Zecha JA, Raber-Durlacher JE, Nair RG et al. Low-level laser therapy/photobiomodulation in the management of side effects of chemoradiation therapy in head and neck cancer: Part 2: Proposed applications and treatment protocols. *Support Care Cancer* 2016;24:2793–2805.

59. Zecha JA, Raber-Durlacher JE, Nair RG et al. Low level laser therapy/photobiomodulation in the management of side effects of chemoradiation therapy in head and neck cancer: Part 1: Mechanisms of action, dosimetric, and safety considerations. *Support Care Cancer* 2016;24:2781–2792.

# ■ FURTHER READING

60. Bentzen SM. Preventing or reducing late side effects of radiation therapy: Radiobiology meets molecular pathology. *Nat Rev Cancer* 2006;6:702–713.

61. Coleman CN, Stone HB, Moulder JE, Pellmar TC. Medicine. Modulation of radiation injury. *Science* 2004;304:693–694.

62. Moulder JE, Cohen EP. Future strategies for mitigation and treatment of chronic radiation-induced normal tissue injury. *Semin Radiat Oncol* 2007;17:141–148.

# Hadron therapy: The clinical aspects

## VINCENT GRÉGOIRE, JAY W. BURMEISTER, MICHAEL C. JOINER AND WOLFGANG DÖRR

## 25.1 INTRODUCTION

Hadron therapy, often referred to as 'particle therapy', includes the use of protons, carbon ions as well as other less common hadrons such as pions, neutrons, helium, lithium, oxygen and silicon ions to treat tumours. In this chapter, we only describe the use of protons and carbon ions, the charged hadrons for which the largest clinical experience, although still modest, has been accumulated.

Robert Wilson is considered 'the father' of hadron therapy from his seminal description in 1946 that the depth-dose profile of protons in matter had significant increase at the end of their path, the 'Bragg peak', and that this might be used to treat deeply located tumours more accurately than with X-rays. The differentiating factor between hadron therapy and electron therapy is this favourable depth-dose distribution which results from the fact that hadrons are much more massive than electrons. While all charged particles have a significant increase in energy deposition per unit distance near the end of their path, electrons are so light that they scatter through tortuous paths and stop at various depths in the patient (see Figure 6.1). Conversely, the more massive hadrons are more difficult to scatter, meaning that they all come to rest together at approximately the same depth, a phenomenon which we observe as the familiar Bragg peak. The technical challenge is therefore to be able to accelerate these hadrons to the very high energies required to reach the necessary depth in human patients. The development of hadron therapy was intimately associated with the development of cyclotrons and synchrotrons, accelerators originally built for fundamental nuclear physics research. The 160 MeV cyclotron at Harvard University (Boston, Massachusetts) was one of the first machines used to treat malignant tumours with protons in the early 1960s. Almost 10,000 patients were treated on this machine until 2002 when a newer generation hospital-based 230 MeV cyclotron with a rotating gantry was commissioned. In 2015, close to 45 proton therapy facilities were in operation across the world and it was estimated that more than 110,000 cancer patients had been treated then with protons worldwide (4). Carbon ions are 12 times heavier than protons, and therefore more difficult to accelerate to therapeutic energies. In addition to providing similar (or even slightly better) dose distributions than protons, carbon ions are high linear energy transfer (LET) radiation and thus offer a potential differential biological advantage related to differences in relative biological effectiveness (RBE) between tumour and normal tissues (see Chapter 6). The heavy ion medical accelerator (HIMAC) in Chiba (Japan) was the first machine to treat patients with carbon ions in a medical environment. From 1994 until the present, over 9000 patients with 'radioresistant tumours' have been treated in this facility. In 1997, clinical trials began at the carbon ion facility in the research centre in Darmstadt (Germany) where around 400 patients were treated. In 2009, this facility closed, and patients were transferred to the Heidelberg (Germany) ion-beam therapy (HIT) centre. This facility is equipped with a rotating gantry enabling carbon ion therapy with geometric delivery capabilities similar to that of proton therapy. As of 2016, at least seven other facilities are treating patients with carbon ions in Italy (CNAO), Austria (MedAustron), China (Lanzhou; Shanghai) and Japan (HIBMC, Hyogo; GHMC, Gunma; SAGA-HIMAT, Tosu; i-ROCK, Yokohama), and several projects are being discussed in the United States. Altogether, more than 15,000 patients have already been treated with carbon ions (4).

## 25.2 PHYSICAL BASIS FOR CHARGED PARTICLE THERAPY

With conventional X-ray therapy, absorbed dose increases very rapidly within the short distance in which electronic equilibrium ('build-up') occurs, and then decreases exponentially with increasing penetration. Neutrons are also uncharged and their depth-dose characteristics are therefore similar. In contrast, charged hadron beams deposit a relatively constant dose as a function of depth until they approach the end of their range, where their rate of energy deposition increases dramatically resulting in a large increase in dose called the Bragg peak (15,17) as shown in Figure 25.1. Such beams can therefore maximize the ratio of tumour-to-normal-tissue dose compared with conventional photon therapy. Moreover, almost no dose is deposited beyond the Bragg peak, allowing the possibility of significant reduction in the dose to tissues distal to the target. It should be noted that for carbon ions, however, because of nuclear interactions of carbon ions with atoms of the irradiated tissue, fragmentation of carbon ions can occur producing low-energy ions of boron, beryllium, lithium and helium,

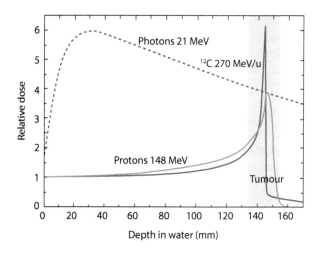

Figure 25.1 Comparison of depth–dose curves for 21 MeV photons, 148 MeV protons and 270 MeV u$^{-1}$ carbon ions.

which will deposit their energy beyond the range of carbon in the 'fragmentation tail'.

Since the Bragg peak is very narrow, in order to cover the full tumour width, several beams of different intensities and ranges need to be superimposed to produce the 'spread-out Bragg peak'. As of 2016, most centres were still using passive techniques with modulators, collimators and compensators to spread out protons and carbon ions for treatment. This can be achieved by passing the primary beam through a rotating wheel with sectors of different thicknesses of plastic sheet. Passive beam delivery allows simpler treatment planning and is more robust, particularly in the treatment of a moving target. Nevertheless, the dose to the normal tissue in the entrance path is higher than with active techniques. Active beam delivery is becoming more common, using spot scanning or raster scanning techniques in which focused pencil beams are deflected laterally by magnetic dipoles. Using different energy levels and various gantry angles, three-dimensional intensity-modulated hadron therapy can be delivered (Figure 25.2). Active scanning techniques result in high conformity with less dose in the entrance path. Because of the scanning delivery, however, the active techniques are more sensitive to interfractional and intrafractional movement of the target volume.

## 25.3 DIFFERENTIAL BIOLOGICAL EFFECT OF PROTONS AND CARBON IONS

While protons do become what we would consider 'high-LET' particles having RBE $\gg$ 1 near the end of their range, this does not happen until the distal edge of a Bragg peak. Since a spread-out Bragg peak is created by the summation of multiple Bragg peaks of varying energy, some high-LET dose is therefore distributed throughout the target volume. As such, the net RBE of proton therapy will differ slightly from conventional photon and electron radiotherapy. The RBE for proton radiotherapy is generally estimated to be approximately 10% higher than that for conventional high-energy photon radiotherapy (approximately the same as that for 250 kVp X-rays) and a uniform RBE value of 1.1 is generally applied to absorbed doses in proton radiotherapy (14). This RBE value is an average for conventionally fractionated delivery and is similar for both existing *in vitro* and *in vivo* data. However, there is significant variation in this value between different tissues and for different fractionation regimens. These variations, along with the rapid change in stopping power near the end of the proton track, mean that even though proton radiotherapy does not have an average RBE substantially higher than conventional photon radiotherapy, there are still potentially significant uncertainties in the assignment of an RBE as a function of location in the beam and tissue type. These uncertainties should ideally be considered in the treatment planning and clinical application of proton radiotherapy.

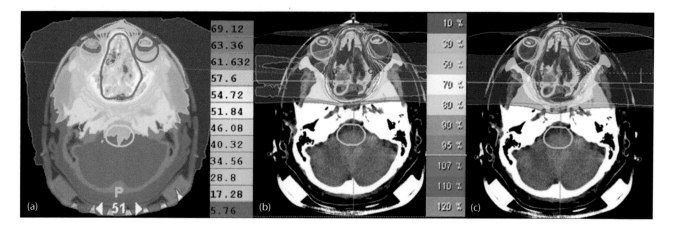

Figure 25.2 Comparison of dose distributions between IMRT (a: IMRT: 6 MeV, tomotherapy, 57.6 Gy in 32 fractions), IMPT (b: IMPT: 160 MeV, 57.6 Gy equivalent in 32 fractions) and carbon ions (c: 60 Gy equivalent in 20 fractions) for the treatment of an ethmoid sinus meningioma. The same beam arrangements were used for carbon ion and proton plans. These plans consisted of two lateral beams and one cranial beam. (From (9), with permission.)

In contrast to proton radiotherapy, carbon ion therapy is high-LET with RBE significantly greater than 1 throughout its entire range in tissue. As a result, the RBE of carbon ion radiotherapy will be typically on the order of 1.5–2 in the plateau region of a spread-out Bragg peak, increasing to approximately 3 near the distal edge of the Bragg peak. Thus, carbon ions can have a relative biological effectiveness similar to fast neutron therapy but with dose-shaping characteristics potentially even better than proton radiotherapy. As indicated in Chapter 6, one of the radiobiological rationales for the use of high-LET radiation beams such as carbon ions is the reduction of the relative radioresistance of certain tumour types compared to photons. A tumour resistant to photons will be likely more responsive to carbon ions, and thus more amenable to local tumour control. If the radiosensitivity of normal tissues is also increased, but to a relatively lower extent than the tumour, carbon ion therapy will provide an even more favourable differential biological effect (Figure 25.3). Furthermore, with the use of highly conformal dose distributions such as achieved with carbon ions, substantially less radiation dose can be delivered to critical surrounding normal tissues, thus creating a physical dose sparing effect in addition to the differential biological effect. This is a clear advantage of carbon-ion therapy over neutron therapy. Neutron therapy was extensively tested from the 1960s to the 1980s, and while favourable radiobiological differentials for some tumour types were achieved, these were countered by the poorer dose distributions achievable with neutron therapy (e.g. [8]).

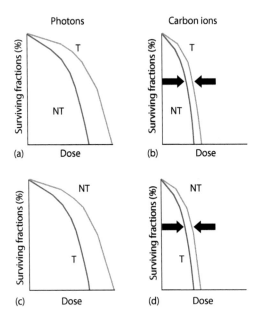

Figure 25.3 The differential biological effect. For tumours (T) more radioresistant to photons than normal tissue (NT) (a), the use of carbon ions could be beneficial by decreasing the unfavourable difference in radiosensitivity between tumour and normal tissue (b). For tumours more radiosensitive to photons than normal tissue (c), the use of carbon ions could be detrimental by decreasing the favourable difference in radiosensitivity between normal tissue and tumour (d).

The definition of 'radioresistant tumour' is not straightforward, and it is probably easier to list those tumours for which a treatment with carbon ions is not likely to be required. Patients with lymphoma (e.g. Hodgkin lymphoma) or seminoma, for which cure rates on the order of 90% or greater have been reported with relatively moderate doses (e.g. 30–40 Gy) using photon radiotherapy, will not benefit from carbon ions. In contrast, patients with sarcoma (e.g. chondrosarcoma, soft-tissue sarcoma or osteosarcoma), and melanoma who are not amenable to surgery for medical or technical (i.e. tumour location and/or extension) reasons could potentially benefit from carbon ion treatment. But even tumours not definitively categorized as 'resistant tumours' such as squamous cell carcinomas have been treated with carbon ions in the head and neck, lung and oesophagus. A more detailed review of the clinical indications for carbon ions is presented in Section 25.6.

## 25.4 FRACTIONATION WITH HADRON THERAPY

In Chapter 6 it is shown that radiations with higher LET (hence higher RBE) will demonstrate higher $\alpha/\beta$ values which reflects less fractionation effect. Nevertheless, even with overall higher $\alpha/\beta$ across the board, the rank order of fractionation effect between early reactions, late reactions and the different tumour types and sites will still hold so that for each tumour type and site the fractionation strategies which prove more successful with 6 MV radiotherapy (e.g. conventional or SBRT) are likely to also be most successful with high-LET hadron therapy using carbon ions. However, differences in outcome seen between much versus little fractionation with high-LET radiation will be less than seen with low-LET radiation and may be judged as being not important when set against the increased complexity, uncertainty and cost associated with delivering many versus few high-LET fractions. Thus, Figure 25.4 from Withers et al. (18) demonstrates the situation with the high LET and RBE values that were found with lower energy clinical neutron therapy. Although neutrons are no longer used in routine clinical practice, these data show that even with high LET and RBE there can be some normal tissue sparing from giving at least two fractions but much less benefit in fractionating much further. It should also be noted that even at these high-LET values, there can still be some hypoxia-mediated radioresistance (see Chapters 17 and 18) and that this would manifest worst with single-dose delivery which is therefore best avoided with carbon ions.

Protons are effectively low LET at the high energies required for clinical delivery at depth, so in principle, radiobiologically, require fractionation for the same reasons as we fractionate conventional photon radiotherapy. However, in some sites we may select hypofractionation because we can gain precision with intensity modulation and better imaging (see Chapters 9 through 11). With protons we also achieve greater precision because of the

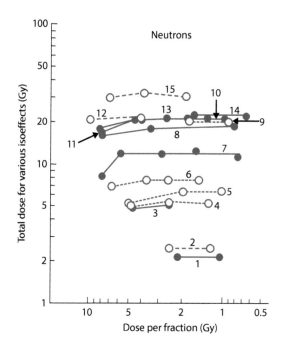

**Figure 25.4** Summary of published data on isoeffect curves for neutrons (high-LET radiation) as a function of dose per fraction in various tissues of mice and rats. Broken lines indicate data on acute-responding tissues; full lines are for late-responding tissues. Compare with Figure 9.1. Key: 1, thyroid function; 2, haemopoietic colonies; 3, vertebral growth; 4, spermatogenic colonies; 5, fibrosarcomas; 6, jejunum colonies; 7, lung $LD_{50}$; 8, lumbar nerve root function; 9,12, skin desquamation; 10, skin contraction; 11, skin late changes; 13, spinal cord; 14, oral mucosa necrosis; 15, skin necrosis. (From (18), with permission.)

inherent depth-dose distribution (Figure 25.2). So with proton delivery we may also select fewer fractions, e.g. in lung or liver tumours. But the same reasons for avoiding a small number of large fractions in some sites, for example head and neck, will also apply to protons. This flexibility is needed in some sites because of the requirement to include locally disseminated or microscopic disease in the treatment plan.

To summarise the hadron fractionation discussion, it is sound clinical radiobiology to deliver all carbon-ion (or neutron) therapy in at least two fractions. Proton therapy fractionation regimes should be similar to those used in treating the same site with photon radiotherapy, thus conventional, hyper- or hypo-fractionation as appropriate.

## 25.5 POTENTIAL CLINICAL INDICATIONS OF PROTONS

As discussed in Section 25.2, protons can provide a better dose distribution compared to photons. When intensity modulated proton therapy (IMPT) is compared to IMRT with photons, the planned dose distribution is typically similar in the planning target volume (PTV), whereas medium- and low-dose volumes to organs at risk (OAR) are substantially

smaller with IMPT. Does this observation suffice to promote a wide use of protons on the basis of the ALARA principle (as low as reasonably achievable)? Challengers to this point of view put forward that in many clinical situations, the complications of IMRT are already extremely low, that the dose reduction may occur in normal tissues which may have a low relevance in terms of complications, and that for some patients their life expectancies, irrespective of the treatment efficacy, are small in relation to the time line of complications. In addition, the potential benefit of IMPT may be extremely sensitive to daily variations in dose distribution that may occur due to subtle daily anatomic variations, thus calling for robust adaptive treatment delivery. Indeed, the effects of such anatomic variations on the delivered dose distribution can be profoundly greater in proton radiotherapy than in photon radiotherapy. Last, in times of economic pressure, the question of cost-effectiveness must be raised. The cost of a proton therapy treatment may be as high as five times the cost of an IMRT treatment, and our societies may not be able to afford any longer the use of expensive treatments for all patients (12).

In 2012, De Ruysscher et al. published a systematic review of all the clinical data available for proton and carbon ion therapy at that time (3). This review is a 5-year update of a previous report published in 2007 (13). In summary, they individualized 39 clinical studies with protons and by the end of 2010, still only one randomized trial on locally advanced prostate carcinoma was available (16). This study reported a significant increase in local control in patients with poorly differentiated tumours without any difference in overall survival or disease-specific survival, and at an expense of a higher complication rate. Although no definite conclusion can be drawn from this review, there are however clinical indications for which proton therapy could be accepted based only on a more favourable dose distribution, i.e. ocular melanoma, paediatric solid tumours and to a lower extent some orphan diseases such as chordoma and chondrosarcoma of the skull base, optic nerve meningioma and retroperitoneal sarcoma.

Choroidal melanoma is a rare tumour occurring with a frequency of 0.7 per 100,000 population. Few retrospective studies of patients with choroidal melanoma treated with low energy (around 70–80 MeV) protons have been reported, and for medium size to large tumours local control up to 90% at 10 years has been reported with a high rate of eye retention. Controversy, however, still exists on how protons perform in comparison with brachytherapy (e.g. ruthenium or iodine seeds) especially for small tumours, and it is unlikely that randomized studies will ever be performed to settle this issue.

Paediatric solid tumours represent a heterogeneous mix of various clinical entities originating mainly in the brain (e.g. medulloblastoma, craniopharyngioma, astrocytoma and ependymoma), soft tissues (e.g. rhabdomyosarcoma), kidney (i.e. Wilms tumour), neural crest tissue (i.e. neuroblastoma), eye (i.e. retinoblastoma) or bone (i.e. osteosarcoma or Ewing sarcoma). For these tumours, the main concern with the use of radiotherapy is the long-term side effects, such as growth retardation, neuro-cognitive deficit and radiation-induced second malignancies. Retrospective series with protons show that local control rates are in the same range to those achieved after conventional radiotherapy. The potential benefit of protons in reducing late side effects for this patient group, including secondary cancer induction, is yet unclear and will require in-depth studies of large cohorts of children with much longer follow-up durations (1,11). Regarding radiation-induced cancer, it was shown that after photon irradiation, second cancers typically arose within 5–10 mm from the edge of the irradiated volume, i.e. in the high to medium dose range, which might not be dramatically reduced with protons (5). Also, with protons, although the medium to low radiation dose range outside of the target is drastically reduced, most of the existing facilities (as of 2016) still use passive scattering, which leads to an increase in the neutron production from the head of the machine, thus irradiating the whole body with low doses of high-LET radiation. Such neutron dose production is however not observed with the more modern facilities using IMPT with pencil beam scanning technology. Last, regarding other long-term toxicities, current data are scarce and do not yet provide definitive evidence for decreased toxicity from proton therapy.

For the orphan diseases such as chordoma and chondrosarcoma of the skull base, optic nerve meningioma and retroperitoneal sarcoma, proton therapy could be envisaged on the basis of the high dose required and the proximity of radiosensitive normal tissues such as the optic nerve, the brain stem, the brain parenchyma and kidneys. But clinical evidence is scarce and it is likely that only prospective non-randomized studies will be conducted.

The field of proton therapy is however moving quickly and in July 2015, the National Cancer Institute (NCI) clinical database (http://www.cancer.gov/about-cancer/treatment/clinical-trials/search) mentioned three ongoing randomized studies comparing IMRT with IMPT: in stage II-IIIB non-small cell lung cancer (RTOG 1308 trial), in low- or intermediate-risk prostate adenocarcinoma (NCI 11–497 trial) and in HPV-positive oropharyngeal squamous cell carcinoma (MD Anderson Cancer Center trial 2012-0825).

There is no doubt that proton therapy will gain wider acceptance in the radiation oncology community if its indications can be based on results from randomized phase III studies comparing the best of IMRT to the best of IMPT. For technology assessment, however, some authors advocate the use of model-based indications relying on *in silico* comparative dose distribution analysis and calculation of tumour control probability (TCP) and normal tissue complication probability (NTCP) (e.g. [10]). Such analyses are based on TCP and/or NTCP models derived from retrospective clinical series with photons, which may not take into account all the parameters influencing tumour and normal tissue response to ionizing radiation, such as predisposing genetic disorder (e.g. heterozygote for ataxia telangiectasia, scleroderma pigmentosum), concomitant disease (e.g. diabetic patients), tumour microenvironment (e.g. tumour hypoxia) or the volume of normal tissue irradiated. Furthermore, the concern for some late complications, although theoretically valid, may not be a critical factor in a given patient population, e.g. radiation-induced cancer in elderly prostate carcinoma patients. Also, given their beam properties, protons are more sensitive to geometric variations during treatment than photons, e.g. due to setup inaccuracies, tumour shrinkage, weight loss and organ motion, which over the course of a fractionated treatment may lead to underdosage in the tumour and/or overdosage in an OAR. Different strategies will have to be applied to account for these uncertainties, such as robust treatment planning techniques, multicriteria optimization, computed tomography-based image guidance, adaptive proton therapy and online verification techniques (e.g. prompt gamma). Taken altogether, such issues might compromise the intrinsically advantageous dose distribution from proton therapy.

In this context, model-based indications could be used to triage patients with an anticipated better outcome with protons who should be included in randomized trials. Because of the active pre-selection, such a study could be run with a much lower number of patients, thus limiting the cost, but not the need for a sufficient follow-up period. For the other indications for which randomized studies will never be performed, patients should be carefully followed for efficacy and toxicity assessment using validated scales, and their data should be included in large prospective databases.

## 25.6 POTENTIAL CLINICAL INDICATIONS OF CARBON IONS

As discussed in Sections 25.2 and 25.3, carbon ion beams not only have better dose distributions resulting from the Bragg peak, but they also have a differential biological efficacy. The translation of the latter into indisputable clinical selection criteria remains however poorly defined, and the 'intrinsically radioresistant tumours' are typically considered as good indications. Unfortunately, similar to what was previously discussed for protons, there is yet no completed randomized study that has employed heavy ion therapy using either photons or protons as the comparative arm. Only retrospective studies mainly coming from HIMAC (Chiba, Japan), GSI (Darmstadt, Germany) and HIT (Heidelberg, Germany) including selected patients have been reported so far. Reviews of the clinical experiences acquired in these centres have been reported (2,7). In a nutshell, these centres have treated almost all tumour types, with the exception of only osteosarcoma in paediatric patients, with carbon ions. In almost all studies, the clinical results reported for carbon ion therapy have been better than that anticipated with photons, while toxicity was comparatively low. It is however impossible to determine whether these observations result from selection biases or clearly reflect a clinical advantage of carbon ions. Until prospectively validated, carbon ion treatment should still be considered as experimental, and clinical recommendations are thus impossible to formulate.

Inoperable adenoid cystic carcinoma originating from major or minor salivary glands of the head and neck area are probably one of the best possible tumour candidates. For this tumour type, a randomized study was conducted in the 1980s to compare neutrons (a high-LET radiation therapy with similar RBE) and photon beams, and local control was significantly improved with neutrons (6). However, no randomized data are yet available for adenoid cystic carcinoma treated with carbon ions. Base of skull chordoma, chondrosarcoma and meningioma are other tumours for which a benefit could be anticipated based on their relative 'tumour resistance' and the proximity of surrounding sensitive normal structures to avoid such as the optic path, the brainstem and the brain parenchyma. Prospective randomized trials are ongoing for these tumours at HIT. A clinical benefit could also be anticipated for soft-tissue sarcomas and non-resectable osteosarcomas (including children), but again no randomized data are yet available to support such indications. Limited (T1 and T2, node negative) non-small cell lung carcinoma has been treated with carbon ions at HIMAC, but it is still unclear whether the excellent reported local control of the order of 80%–90% is better than with IMPT or even IMRT (SBRT). This is especially true as motion management presents significant challenges in the delivery of carbon-ion therapy, especially for scanning beam delivery, and there are significant potential differences in the accurate delivery of dose distributions in the lung in comparison to photon IMRT. Carbon ions have also been used for gastrointestinal malignancies including hepatocellular carcinoma, and in prostate carcinoma, but again no conclusion can be yet drawn from these studies. For all the clinical indications mentioned above, combined treatment using carbon ions with photons or even protons has been proposed, giving photon-equivalent doses per fraction higher than typically possible with photon IMRT alone.

## 25.7 CONCLUSIONS

The exquisite dose distributions from hadrons compared with photons makes them an attractive treatment modality to further increase local tumour control and/or decrease the treatment morbidity. For carbon, in addition to the dose distribution advantage, a differential radiobiological effect can be expected which might be beneficial for conventionally radioresistant tumours. However, no randomized study has ever been reported to demonstrate the clinical benefit of hadrons, and clinical indications are thus only based on clinical judgment. Randomized studies are nevertheless ongoing, and it is expected that they will pave the way for evidence-based hadron therapy. For carbon ions, considering the current enormous financial investment (e.g. 100–200 million euros depending on the size of the facility),

it is recommended to open only a limited number of centres to which patients would be referred and treated under strict protocol conditions.

---

### Key points

1. Hadrons (e.g. protons and carbon ions) allow for dose deposition with steep dose gradients.
2. Although no randomized data are available, the accepted clinical indications for proton therapy (IMPT) based on a more favourable dose distribution are ocular melanoma, paediatric solid tumours and to a lesser extent some orphan diseases such as chordoma and chondrosarcoma of the skull base, optic nerve meningioma and retroperitoneal sarcoma.
3. For the other adult tumours, model-based indications could be used to triage patients with an anticipated better outcome with protons who should be included in randomized trials.
4. In children, the potential benefit of protons in reducing late side effects, including secondary cancer induction, is yet unclear and will require in-depth studies of large cohorts of children with much longer follow-up durations.
5. For tumours more radioresistant to photons than normal tissue, the use of carbon ions would be beneficial as it decreases the relative difference in radiosensitivity between tumour and normal tissue. However, no randomized clinical data are available to formulate clinical recommendations and thus carbon ion treatment should still be considered as experimental.

---

## ■ BIBLIOGRAPHY

1. Bekelman JE, Schultheiss T, Berrington De Gonzalez A. Subsequent malignancies after photon versus proton radiation therapy. *Int J Radiat Oncol Biol Phys* 2013;87:10–12.
2. Combs SE, Debus J. Treatment with heavy charged particles: Systematic review of clinical data and current clinical comparative trials. *Acta Oncol* 2013;52:1272–1286.
3. De Ruysscher D, Lodge M, Jones B et al. Charged particles in radiotherapy: A 5-year update of a systematic review. *Radiother Oncol* 2012;103:5–7.
4. Degiovanni A, Amaldi U. History of hadron therapy accelerators. *Phys Med* 2015;31:322–332.
5. Diallo I, Haddy N, Adjadj E et al. Frequency distribution of second solid cancer locations in relation to the irradiated volume among 115 patients treated for childhood cancer. *Int J Radiat Oncol Biol Phys* 2009;74:876–883.
6. Griffin TW, Pajak TF, Laramore GE et al. Neutron vs photon irradiation of inoperable salivary gland tumors: Results of an RTOG-MRC Cooperative Randomized Study. *Int J Radiat Oncol Biol Phys* 1988;15:1085–1090.

7. Kamada T, Tsujii H, Blakely EA et al. Carbon ion radiotherapy in Japan: An assessment of 20 years of clinical experience. *Lancet Oncol* 2015;16:e93–e100.

8. Koh WJ, Griffin TW, Laramore GE, Stelzer KJ, Russell KJ. Fast neutron radiation therapy. *Results of phase III randomized trials in head and neck, lung, and prostate cancers. Acta Oncol* 1994;33:293–298.

9. Kosaki K, Ecker S, Habermehl D et al. Comparison of intensity modulated radiotherapy IMRT with intensity modulated particle therapy (IMPT) using fixed beams or an ion gantry for the treatment of patients with skull base meningiomas. *Radiat Oncol* 2012;7:44.

10. Langendijk JA, Lambin P, De Ruysscher D, Widder J, Bos M, Verheij M. Selection of patients for radiotherapy with protons aiming at reduction of side effects: The model-based approach. *Radiother Oncol* 2013;107:267–273.

11. Leroy R, Benahmed N, Hulstaert F, Van Damme N, De Ruysscher D. Proton therapy in children: A systematic review of clinical effectiveness in 15 pediatric cancers. *Int J Radiat Oncol Biol Phys* 2016;95:267–278.

12. Lievens Y, Pijls-Johannesma M. Health economic controversy and cost-effectiveness of proton therapy. *Semin Radiat Oncol* 2013;23:134–141.

13. Lodge M, Pijls-Johannesma M, Stirk L, Munro AJ, De Ruysscher D, Jefferson T. A systematic literature review of the clinical and cost-effectiveness of hadron therapy in cancer. *Radiother Oncol* 2007;83:110–122.

14. Paganetti H. Relative biological effectiveness (RBE) values for proton beam therapy. Variations as a function of biological endpoint, dose, and linear energy transfer. *Phys Med Biol* 2014;59:R419–R472.

15. Rong Y, Welsh J. Basics of particle therapy II biologic and dosimetric aspects of clinical hadron therapy. *Am J Clin Oncol* 2010;33:646–649.

16. Shipley WU, Verhey LJ, Munzenrider JE et al. Advanced prostate cancer: The results of a randomized comparative trial of high dose irradiation boosting with conformal protons compared with conventional dose irradiation using photons alone. *Int J Radiol Oncol Biol Phys* 1995;32: 3–12.

17. Welsh JS. Basics of particle therapy: Introduction to hadrons. *Am J Clin Oncol* 2008;31:493–495.

18. Withers HR, Thames HD, Peters LJ. Biological bases for high RBE values for late effects of neutron irradiation. *Int J Radiat Oncol Biol Phys* 1982;8:2071–2076.

## ■ FURTHER READING

19. Alpen EL. *Radiation Biophysics*. 2nd ed. San Diego, CA: Academic Press; 1998.

20. Suit H, DeLaney T, Goldberg S et al. Proton vs carbon ion beams in the definitive radiation treatment of cancer patients. *Radiother Oncol* 2010;95:3–22.

# Tissue response models

PETER VAN LUIJK, WOLFGANG DÖRR AND ALBERT J. VAN DER KOGEL

## 26.1 INTRODUCTION

The risk of radiation effects to normal tissues is an important factor, both in the process of considering radiotherapy and in the optimization of personalized radiotherapy for individual patients. Severe toxicity may cause a lifelong reduction in quality of life and sometimes the risk of morbidity even limits dose and efficacy of the treatment.

Developments in treatment technology have increased the possibilities to reduce dose to normal tissues. Moreover, the same developments have also increased the number of ways to influence numerous characteristics of the three-dimensional (3D) dose distribution. For example, multi-leaf collimators offer increased control of beam shapes. Increasing computation power improves the ability of treatment planning systems to handle an increasing number of beams, or even rotational techniques. Finally, the availability of particle therapy offers beams with entirely new dose-depth curves and for heavier ions even variations in the biological effects of dose (see also Chapters 6 and 25).

Optimal use of these technologies requires criteria with respect to which treatment planning can be optimized. At present, treatment planning is most often steered based on dose constraints and dose objectives. However, in parallel to these technological developments, the field of modelling morbidity risk has developed strongly. The advantage of using risk models over dose metrics is that it provides insight into the clinical consequences of a change in dose. Being able to appraise these risk models and their clinical utility requires knowledge of the methods and data that were used to construct the risk model. Therefore, in this chapter a brief overview of normal tissue response data and methodologies for risk modelling are given.

## 26.2 EXPERIMENTAL AND CLINICAL DATA FOR VOLUME EFFECTS IN INDIVIDUAL ORGANS

In this section, volume effects are described for selected organs: skin, spinal cord, parotid gland, lung, heart, liver, intestinal tract and kidney. Pre-clinical studies of the volume effect, if available, are summarized for these organs. The literature on clinical dose-volume effects is expanding rapidly and examples of relevant clinical data are cited where possible.

### Skin

The skin shows an 'area' effect similar to oral mucosa. In studies in pig skin (15), no effect of the irradiated area was observed for early epidermal changes when the field diameter was larger than 20 mm, and for late effects when the diameter was larger than 10 mm. At smaller diameters, a steep rise in isoeffective doses was found (Figure 26.1). In the orthovoltage era, this area effect of small fields used to be exploited by using a 'sieve technique', where part of the skin was shielded with the bridges of a lead sieve, and hence tolerable reactions only occurred in the small irradiated fields, but did not get to confluency. This allowed for curative tumour doses despite the unfavourable depth-dose distribution of these low-energy X-rays.

### Spinal cord

#### LENGTH OF IRRADIATED SPINAL CORD

A marked volume effect for irradiation of very short lengths of spinal cord (<1 cm), and less pronounced or no volume effects for cord lengths >2 cm, have been demonstrated in rats, pigs, monkeys and dogs. This suggests migration of tissue-restoring cells, with only a limited migration distance, from outside the irradiated volume (Chapter 16).

In *rat* spinal cord, a very steep rise in $ED_{50}$ (i.e. the radiation dose at which white-matter necrosis and myelopathy are expected in 50% of treated animals) was observed when the irradiated cord length was reduced below 10 mm (Figure 26.2). For irradiation of cord lengths between 10 and 30 mm, little change in $ED_{50}$ was found. This observation was confirmed by more detailed studies, exploiting a high-precision proton beam for irradiation (4): rats were irradiated with either a single field of 8 mm or two fields of 4 mm, separated by an unirradiated length of cord of 8 or 12 mm (Figure 26.2). The $ED_{50}$ for myelopathy with $2 \times 4$ mm fields was 42–45 Gy, which is less than 54 Gy for a single field of 4 mm, but considerably greater than the $ED_{50}$ for $1 \times 8$ mm (25 Gy).

Single radiation doses given to 2.5, 5 and 10 cm lengths of *pig* spinal cord showed only a small (~1 Gy) decrease in $ED_{50}$ for induction of white-matter necrosis with increasing field size. At low probabilities of injury,

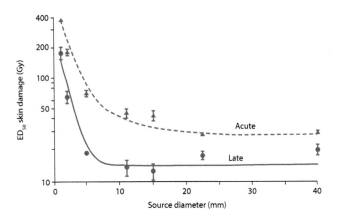

**Figure 26.1** The influence of field diameter on the dose required to induce acute and late skin reactions in 50% of pigs after single-dose irradiation with small fields. A steep rise in ED50 is seen below a diameter of 20 mm for early reactions and 10 mm for late sequelae, respectively. At larger field sizes, the ED50 is independent of the area exposed. (From (16), with permission.)

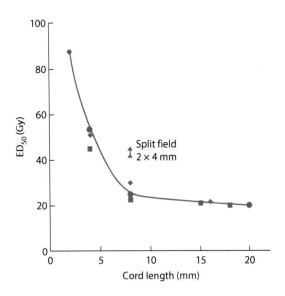

**Figure 26.2** The influence of field size on biological response in rat spinal cord after single-dose irradiation with small fields. A steep rise in ED50 occurs as field size is reduced below 10 mm, with very little change in ED50 for larger field sizes. The single fields were focused on C4, the two concomitant 4 mm fields were at C1/C2 and C7/T1, separated by ~10 mm. Data show the ED50 for induction of white-matter necrosis. (From (16,3,6), with permission.)

which are clinically relevant, this difference was no longer significant (43), similar to the results in the kidney (see the following text).

The irradiated cord length also influenced the incidence of myelopathy in *monkeys*, given fractionated irradiation (39). The incidence of myelopathy after a total dose of 70.2 Gy (2.2 Gy/fraction) increased from 15%, to 20% to 37.5% for field sizes of 4, 8 and 16 cm, respectively.

In an extensive study in *dogs* (34), irradiation of 4 and 20 cm lengths of spinal cord were compared using a fractionated schedule of 4 Gy per fraction. For functional, neurological symptoms, such as thoracic pain or paresis, a large increase in ED50 from 54 Gy for the large field to 78 Gy for the small field was found. In contrast, a much less pronounced increase was observed for morphological, necrotic lesions (Figure 26.3). This again indicates the relevance of the endpoint studied for volume effects.

## INFLUENCE OF DOSE SURROUNDING THE HIGH-DOSE VOLUME

The marked volume effect for irradiation of only very short lengths of spinal cord is clearly compromised, when a small dose is given to the surrounding tissue. This has been demonstrated for rat spinal cord in 'bath-and-shower' experiments (4), where graded subtolerance doses ('bath') were given to a large segment (20 mm) of spinal cord, and a high dose ('shower') was given to small segments of 2–8 mm in the centre of the low-dose volume (Figure 26.4). The ED50 for a 4 mm field given 53 Gy alone was reduced to 39 Gy with a bath dose of only 4 Gy. For a 2 mm high-dose segment, the ED50 was reduced from 88 to 61 Gy. Paralysis was based on necrotic lesions in the high-dose region, whereas no histological changes were seen in the bath volume. The hypothesis to describe these observations was that migration of presumptive stem cells into the high-dose region was compromised by the bath dose.

In further experiments with the same model (4), the shower dose was placed at the edge rather than the centre of the low-dose segment. Assuming migration phenomena, the tolerance in this setup should be similar to that with high-dose irradiation alone (88 Gy) for a 2 mm shower segment. However, the observed ED50 was intermediate, at 69 Gy,

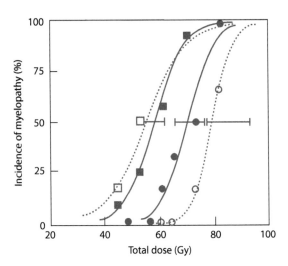

**Figure 26.3** Influence of change in field size on spinal cord damage in dogs. Increasing the field size from 4 cm (circles) to 20 cm (squares) had a more marked influence on the development of neurological signs of injury (dotted lines) than on the occurrence of severe pathological lesions (solid lines). (Redrawn from (34), with permission.)

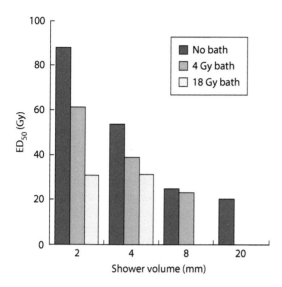

Figure 26.4 The influence of a surrounding low dose on the tolerance of a small high-dose volume ('bath and shower' irradiations) in the rat cervical spinal cord. The high-dose volumes of 2, 4 or 8 mm ('shower') were focused at C5, while the remainder of the 20 mm cervical cord was irradiated with a 'bath' dose of 4 Gy or 18 Gy. (From (4,6).)

indicating additional mechanisms underlying the volume effect for small cord lengths. It is important to note that none of the existing normal tissue complication probability (NTCP) models take these non-local effects into account.

### LATERAL DOSE DISTRIBUTION

With conformal radiotherapy, variations not only in the *length* of spinal cord irradiated, but also in the *lateral* distribution of the dose can occur. These effects have also been studied in rats irradiated with high-precision proton beams (5). The left lateral half of the spinal cord was irradiated with a penumbra (20%–80% isodose) of 1.1 or 0.8 mm, or the midline of the cord with a penumbra of 0.8 mm. The irradiated length of spinal cord was 20 mm in all experiments. The resulting $ED_{50}$ values for paralysis were 29 and 33 Gy for lateral irradiation, respectively, and 72 Gy for midline irradiation; the corresponding homogeneous irradiation of a 20 mm cord segment resulted in an $ED_{50}$ of 20 Gy. Hence, the gray matter is highly resistant to radiation: no lesions observable by light microscopy were induced, even after a single dose as high as 80 Gy; all lesions were restricted to white matter structures.

Although these experiments in rats suggested a higher tolerance of the cord when irradiating the lateral half compared to a homogeneous irradiation of the same length of cervical spine, this does not seem to be present in the pig spinal cord. In these studies the $ED_{50}$ for uniform irradiation of the cervical cord was 20.2 Gy, while for a non-uniform lateral beam the $ED_{50}$ was 20 Gy (30).

In summary, there is a clear volume effect for severe lesions in the spinal cord, which lead to irreversible signs of myelopathy; this is most pronounced at high levels of injury. At low probabilities of injury (<5%), which usually define clinical tolerance doses, a volume effect may not be detectable and should have minimal impact on the clinical practice of maintaining spinal cord dose below 55 Gy. However, when clinical conditions require the choice of higher dose levels closer to tolerance, such as in a re-irradiation situation (Chapter 23), the existence of a volume effect might be taken into consideration. The volume effect in the spinal cord is complex, with an impact of the surrounding dose as well as of the lateral dose distribution across the tissue. It must be emphasized that none of the existing NTCP models take this complexity into account.

## Parotid gland

### EXPERIMENTAL DATA

Parotid gland response to irradiation has been investigated extensively in rats and mice. In a mouse model, transplantation of mouse (28) or human (35) stem cells (capable of self-renewing and differentiating into all functional cells of the salivary gland) was found to rescue the gland function after irradiation with an ablative dose. This indicates that the salivary gland stem cell is a target for radiation-induced loss of function. Besides depending on irradiated volume, significant regional variations in response to irradiation were observed in the rat (24). The response after irradiation of the cranial 50% of the gland resulted in a much stronger response than irradiation of the caudal 50%. Interestingly, irradiation of the cranial 50% was associated with degeneration of the non-irradiated caudal 50%. This was explained by the non-uniform distribution of stem cells over the organ. In mice, rats and patients the salivary gland stem cells were found to be localized in the largest ducts. These ducts are concentrated in a limited sub-volume of the gland. In rats it was shown that inclusion of this region rich in stem cells into the radiation fields changed the dependence of damage from being proportional (Figure 26.5a) to become unrelated to irradiated volume (Figure 26.5b). Moreover, dose to this region predicted the degeneration of non-irradiated gland tissue in rats as well as post-treatment function in patients (45).

### CLINICAL DATA

The parotid glands are important dose-limiting organs in treatment of the head and neck with conventional radiation techniques, as they often cannot be spared. Doses above 40–50 Gy lead to permanent loss of function contributing to xerostomia (parotid glands produce approximately 60% of the saliva) and impairment of quality of life by dryness of mouth and its consequences. One of the major advantages of the introduction of 3D-conformal techniques in the head and neck area is the possibility to limit the irradiated volume to parts of the parotids and this has resulted in a reduction of permanent xerostomia. Pooling of two large prospective

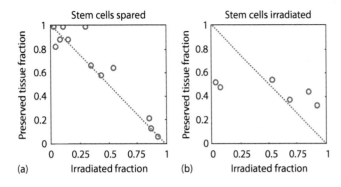

(a) Stem cells spared — Irradiated fraction / Preserved tissue fraction

(b) Stem cells irradiated — Irradiated fraction / Preserved tissue fraction

**Figure 26.5** The relation between irradiated volume and preserved tissue fraction in the rat parotid gland. The amount of tissue lost is proportional to the irradiated volume if the sub-volume that is rich in stem cells is spared (a). In contrast, the damaged volume is not related to irradiated volume if the sub-volume rich in stem cells is irradiated (b). (Modified from (45).)

studies showed preservation of >25% salivary flow at 1 year after mean doses to the parotid of up to ~40 Gy (9).

## Lung

### EXPERIMENTAL DATA

The influence of irradiated lung volume on structural and functional changes has been investigated experimentally in mice, rats, dogs and pigs. All studies demonstrate a pronounced volume effect for total lung function, with little or no symptomatic pneumonitis for small irradiated volumes. These volume effects depend on the spare capacity of the non-irradiated tissue, which enables overall function to be maintained despite destruction of a substantial part of one lung (14).

The induction of local structural lung changes varies between different pathologies. The inductions of e.g. inflammation and vascular damage were also found to depend on irradiated volume (7,12). However, as assessed by radiology, histology and collagen content, fibrosis induction within the irradiated volume does not depend on the volume irradiated (Figure 26.6).

Besides depending on irradiated volume, in the mouse (42) and rat (32) the response of the lung was observed to depend on which sub-volume was irradiated. In the rat this response was found to relate to inclusion of the heart in the radiation portal (44) (Figure 26.7). This finding was explained by the tight functional connection of the lung to the heart. The lung requires blood supply from the right ventricle and needs to be able to feed it back into the left atrium of the heart. Irradiation of the lung was found to damage the pulmonary microvasculature, leading to increased pulmonary vascular resistance and consequent pulmonary hypertension (12) (Figure 26.8). Conversely, heart irradiation reduced left ventricle diastolic function leading to congestion and increasing inflammation in the pulmonary vasculature (13).

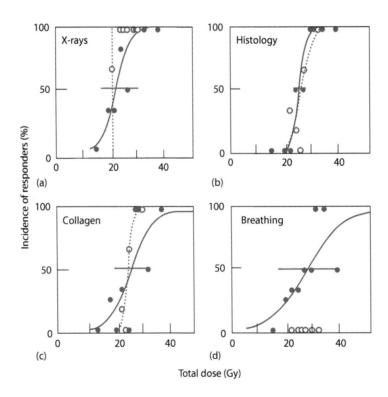

**Figure 26.6** Dose-response curves for radiation-induced lung damage in pigs after irradiation with five fractions, given to half of the right lung (o) or to the whole right lung (●). Damage was assessed from radiographic changes (a), histological evidence of fibrosis (b), elevated hydroxyproline (collagen) levels (c), or increased breathing rate (d). Only the functional endpoint demonstrated a volume effect. (From (14), with permission.)

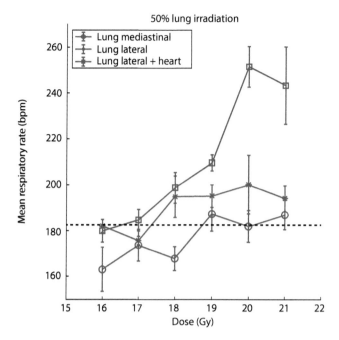

Figure 26.7 Dose-response relation of the lung. The response of the lung depends on which sub-volume is irradiated. Irradiation of the lateral parts of the lung leads to more loss of function than irradiation of the mediastinal parts. Co-irradiation of the heart further aggravates function loss. (Modified from (44).)

Taken together these results demonstrate that pulmonary toxicity may be subject to regional variations in response to radiation as well as interactions between heart and lung. Moreover, the tight functional integration of heart and lung can cause irradiation of either of them to result in damage to both and lead to changes in the cardiopulmonary physiology as a whole. As such, pulmonary and cardiac morbidity observed after thoracic irradiation should be regarded as integrated entities.

## CLINICAL DATA

Also in patients regional variations in response have been observed, with differences between anterior and posterior

parts of the lung explained by regional variations in lung perfusion (40). However, in a prospective test, a model based on mean perfusion-weighed dose did not adequately separate patients developing radiation pneumonitis from those that did not (23). In addition to an anterior-posterior variation, irradiation of caudally located lung tumours resulted in a greater risk of radiation pneumonitis than irradiation of tumours located in other parts of the lungs (40). Though the exact cause of this variation has not been found, caudally located tumours were associated with higher doses in the heart, which in rats increases the risk and severity of radiation pneumonitis (44).

Several prospective clinical studies have described the influence of a change in irradiated lung volume on local lung damage and on NTCP (reviewed in [31]). The incidence of radiation-induced pneumonitis can be related to the dose volume histogram (DVH) for the irradiated lung. For this analysis, the 3D physical dose distribution is converted into a mean biological dose to the whole lung, after a normalisation procedure using the linear-quadratic model with $\alpha/\beta$ values of 2.5–3 Gy. This parameter, the 'mean normalised total lung dose', which does not include any critical-volume parameter, correlates well with the incidence of pneumonitis, as for example shown by Kwa et al. (26) in a large series of 540 patients treated for malignant lymphoma, lung or breast cancer in five different institutes (Figure 26.9). Further studies have focused on other, simple parameters such as the percentage of total lung volume irradiated with defined doses, i.e. >20 or >30 Gy, which hence incorporate a critical-volume component. These parameters can be used to predict the probability of radiation pneumonitis. However, it has been demonstrated that the ideal parameter for estimation of the NTCP for pneumonitis from DVH, despite ample data and studies, has not yet been identified (29,37). As indicated by several studies (e.g. [18]), additionally considering *heart* dose in a multi-variable approach may lead to improvements.

Regarding lung fibrosis as a biological endpoint of lung morbidity, data are scarce. This is partly related to the constriction and thus the change in anatomy of the lung due to the fibrotic changes, which complicates the reference to the irradiated volume.

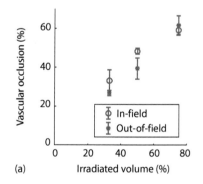

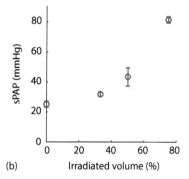

(a)  (b)

Figure 26.8 Physiological effects of lung irradiation. Irradiation of the lung causes vascular remodelling leading to occlusion of the pulmonary microvasculature (a). The resulting reduction in flow capacity of the pulmonary vascular bed leads to an increase in pulmonary artery pressure (b). This effect is strongly dependent on irradiated volume. (Modified from (12).)

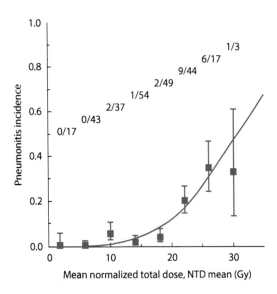

**Figure 26.9** Incidence of radiation pneumonitis as a function of mean normalised total dose to the whole lung. Pooled data are shown from a group of 264 patients with lung cancer, breast cancer or malignant lymphoma, treated in five different centres. The absolute number of patients contributing to each dose level is indicated. (From (26), with permission.)

## Liver

The liver is usually regarded as a prime example of a parallel-type organ, with liver acini as functional subunits. Like in the lung, structural damage, i.e. loss of function within the irradiated volume, can be demonstrated with scintigraphy and other methods. Whole-liver irradiation with doses around 30 Gy (2 Gy/fraction) is generally associated with the induction of 5%–10% hepatitis. Until the introduction of 3D treatment planning, the relationship between tolerance dose and partial volume irradiation was very conservatively interpreted. However, extensive clinical data on liver tolerance to partial organ irradiation was accumulated at the University of Michigan for more than 200 patients (8). Lyman Kutcher Burman (LKB)-NTCP analyses resulted in a large volume effect parameter (the $n$-exponent in the power law function) of 0.97, demonstrating that the liver indeed behaves as a parallel-type organ with a large reserve capacity. No cases of radiation-induced liver disease grade 3 according to Radiation Therapy and Oncology Group/European Organisation for Research and Treatment of Cancer (RTOG/EORTC) were observed when the mean liver dose was <31 Gy. Estimates of tolerance doses associated with 5% risk of liver disease after uniform irradiation to partial volumes were 47 Gy for two-thirds and >90 Gy for one-third of the total volume. A negligible complication risk, regardless of dose, is associated with irradiation of a partial volume of ≤25%. An analysis in 105 patients with hepatocellular carcinoma revealed that the total liver volume receiving ≥30 Gy also appears to be a useful dose-volumetric parameter for predicting the risk of hepatic toxicity and should be limited to ≤60% (22).

The tolerance of patients with primary liver cancer is lower than of patients with liver metastases or without liver tumours (8). However, the functionality of the unirradiated liver volume, which may be impaired by chemotherapy, alcohol consumption or other trauma, has to be taken into consideration. The presence of liver cirrhosis is known to be the predominant risk factor for hepatic toxicity following radiotherapy.

## Intestinal tract

The results of several trials have been published relating the bowel volume irradiated, e.g. during treatment for prostate, rectal or cervix cancer, to the incidence of complications, particularly with conformal irradiation, to various DVH parameters. Restricting dose conformation to the planning target volume can substantially decrease the normal tissue volumes exposed to significant doses. For example, a study from the Royal Marsden Hospital in London showed that the volume of small bowel irradiated to >90% of the prescribed dose could be reduced from 24% using conventional fields, to 18% for 3D conformal therapy and 5%–8% for intensity modulated radiation therapy (IMRT), depending on the number of fields used. For the rectum, the high-dose irradiated volumes could be reduced from 89%, to 51% and 6%–16%, respectively (33). It has to be noted that early complications in the intestine result in an increased incidence of late effects, thus representing a consequential component (see Chapter 14). Therefore, volume effect studies on late complications may be affected by a varying influence of early effects.

### ORAL MUCOSA

The clinical consequences of oral mucositis are closely related to the mucosal area, but importantly also to the localisation where the reaction occurs. For example, complications can be significantly reduced, if the lips are excluded from the irradiated volume. Also, changes in taste acuity can be prevented by a reduction of the tongue volume included in the high-dose volume (21).

### OESOPHAGUS

A study on 215 patients treated for non-small cell lung cancer (47) revealed that early oesophageal symptoms were dominated by DVH parameters, such as the mean dose, or the relative volume treated to doses above 20 Gy (rV20), but were independent of clinical factors.

### SMALL BOWEL

The mobility of the small intestine largely prevents irradiation of the same segment or loop during subsequent fractions. Hence, the dose to individual loops can vary over wide ranges, and usually is lower than the dose to the target volume. However, previous surgery, related to or independent of the oncological disease, as well as inflammatory changes in the abdominal cavity, can compromise mobility and hence significantly increase the dose to bowel segments fixed in the high-dose volume. These uncertainties appear to be one of the reasons for the conflicting data for a correlation of dose and volume with the incidence of small bowel symptoms.

Volume effects for small-bowel obstruction have been demonstrated in patients treated with extended field radiotherapy (bowel volumes $>800$ cm³), as reviewed by Letschert et al. (27). No volume effects for bowel obstruction were observed in patients receiving postoperative radiotherapy for rectal carcinoma. In these patients, the incidence of chronic diarrhoea was 31% for volumes $<77$ cm³, compared to 42% for volumes $>328$ cm³. The type of surgery was a strong influence on the incidence of chronic diarrhoea and malabsorption.

## Rectum

The incidence of late rectal bleeding and other chronic changes has generally been found to correlate with irradiated volume exposed to high doses, as quantitated by DVH parameters. Some studies have demonstrated a significant dose-volume relationship for late rectal bleeding using a single cut-off value for the rectal volume irradiated to certain doses (Figure 26.10). Other studies describe a more complex relationship with several cut-off levels which significantly discriminated between a high or low risk of severe rectal bleeding, or a continuous relationship between rectal bleeding and dose-volume parameters. A study on rectal mucosal changes assessed by rectoscopy using a specific score in 35 patients receiving external beam radiotherapy and high dose rate brachytherapy for carcinoma of the cervix has revealed $ED_{50}$ values for irradiated volumes of 2, 1 or 0.1 cm³ of 68, 73 and 84 Gy (Figure 26.11). The corresponding doses for changes according to late effects normal tissue task force (LENT)/ Subjective, Objective, Management, Analytic (SOMA) were 73, 78 and 97 Gy.

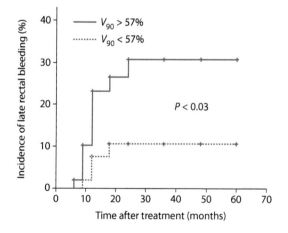

**Figure 26.10** Actuarial incidence of rectal bleeding in patients with rectal volumes irradiated to at least 90% of the isodose (~60 Gy) of greater than 57% or less than 57%. (From (46), with permission.)

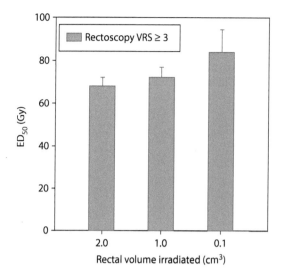

**Figure 26.11** $ED_{50}$ values (doses at which a response is expected in 50% of the patients) for rectoscopic mucosal changes (Vienna Rectoscopy Score $\geq 3$) in patients receiving tele- and brachytherapy for cervical cancer in rectal volumes of 2, 1 or 0.1 cm³. (Data from (11), with permission of the authors.)

One aspect to be considered for highly conformal radiotherapy, particularly for the rectum, is the dose distribution through the cross section of the organ. Gross clinical symptoms are observed only if a larger part or the entire circumference is exposed to significant doses. In rats, it was demonstrated that shielding of half the circumference completely prevented late bowel obstruction, which occurred with increasing dose in animals with irradiation of the entire rectal wall. The incidence (but not the area) of mucosal ulceration was similar in both groups. Similarly, an intrarectal balloon can be applied for displacement of the posterior rectal wall and hence for a reduction in dose to this part, which results in a decrease in side effects. In contrast, emptying of the rectum before irradiation increases dose homogeneity and reduces variations of DVH parameters for the planning target volume, but may increase the risk of rectal complications.

As with other organs, such as the lung (see previous text), the functional status of the rectum can influence the volume tolerance. Thus, Huang et al. (17) demonstrated that an individual history of haemorrhoids clearly correlated with the incidence of rectal bleeding at a given volume irradiated.

It has to be noted that the individual endpoints, such as bleeding, obstruction, frequency or incontinence, are related to the dose administered to different sub-volumes of the rectum, and for these, the dose-volume relationship is largely unclear.

## Kidney

Volume effects in the irradiated kidney are strongly influenced by the duality of this organ and by its mainly parallel organisation, with a large reserve capacity.

Unirradiated parts of one kidney and the contralateral kidney are able to undergo drastic post-irradiation hypertrophy and increase their performance to compensate for functional impairment within another part of the organ and thus maintain renal function.

Studies in pigs (36) demonstrated that the individual function of a kidney after unilateral irradiation can actually be poorer than after irradiation of both kidneys with the same dose. Total renal function is, however, much less reduced after irradiation of only one kidney (Figure 26.12). Interestingly, if the unirradiated kidney is removed after unilateral irradiation, the previously non-functional irradiated kidney may be capable of partial restoration of glomerular filtration rate and effective renal plasma flow to maintain a viable level of total renal function. These experiments demonstrate that the functional response of a unilaterally irradiated kidney depends on the compensatory response in the unirradiated, contralateral organ. The presence and increased function of the unirradiated kidney may actually promote functional impairment, or inhibit functional recovery, in the irradiated kidney.

A pronounced volume effect was also observed in scintigraphic studies in 91 patients who received abdominal irradiation with various doses and to varying volumes (25), but only at higher incidence levels for the loss of kidney function. The dose for a 5% incidence was in the range of 3–6 Gy, independent of volume, due to uncertainties in the dose-effect analysis. However, the doses estimated for a 50% incidence clearly increased with decreasing kidney volume, from approximately 8 Gy for 100% to 27 Gy for 10% of the volume.

In a study in 44 patients receiving radiochemotherapy for gastric cancer (20), where the left kidney was included in the high-dose radiotherapy volume, the V20 (left kidney) and mean left kidney dose were identified as parameters associated with decreased kidney function.

## 26.3 MODEL DEVELOPMENT

The development of a model to predict treatment outcome involves data, a modelling formalism/methodology and methods to combine them to yield a predictive model. Based on assumptions, the formalism/methodology defines how the risk of a complication depends on e.g. dose metrics and other factors. In this section a brief overview of modelling formalisms and methods is given. In addition, the criticality of various properties of the data used in modelling are discussed.

### Choice of endpoint: Relevance versus specificity and accuracy

For the evaluation of toxicity, numerous different endpoints are available. These vary from measurements of changes in organs or tissues or their function to their overall effect on quality of life. The choice of endpoint is subject to a number of considerations. The endpoint must be relevant clinically to justify including it in a dose optimization process. From that perspective quality-of-life endpoints would seem the ideal choice. However, since health-related quality of life is the final result of a complex mixture of disease, treatment and other factors, it is a very unspecific type of endpoint in terms of optimization of the dose distribution. In contrast, the relation between dose to organs and resulting changes measured by imaging or functional assays may be much more specific, the direct relevance to the well-being of the patient is often less clear. In conclusion, choosing an endpoint involves a trade-off between model specificity and relevance of the endpoint.

Many controversies and pitfalls also exist for the 'outcomes' input data and the model fitting itself (38). Most mathematical NTCP models assume dichotomous (yes or no) endpoints, but in practice complications are usually graded, with their severity subject to interpretation. In addition it is important to have a sufficient number of solid data points (complications) to yield quantitative results. A lack of events can lead to lumping together of infrequent but severe complications (i.e. those that we would like to model and then avoid) with more frequent but less severe ones (that in many cases could be effectively treated, but whose 'numbers' help in model parameterization). All of this can lead to large confidence limits on model parameters.

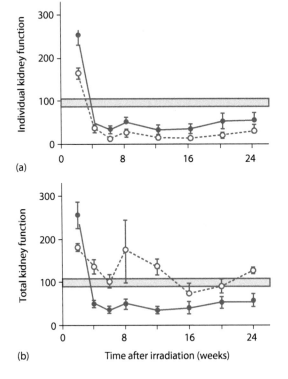

**Figure 26.12** Time-related changes in glomerular filtration rate in pigs in which one (o) or both (●) kidneys were irradiated with a single dose of 12.6 Gy. (a) Change in individual kidney function, as a percentage of control values. (b) Total renal function in the same pigs. (Redrawn from (36), with permission.)

## From 3D dose distribution to potential predictors

In radiation therapy, uninvolved organs and other normal tissues are non-uniformly irradiated during attempts to conform the dose to the target volume. Since it is not possible to directly interpret a 3D dose distribution in terms of population tolerance, dose distributions are often summarized into a DVH (see Chapter 7). The differential DVH is a frequency distribution of the dose levels for the organ or tissue of interest, showing how often (in e.g. % or $cm^3$ of the volume) each dose value occurs. However, it is more common to display 'cumulative' DVHs. Rather than showing the volume that receives a certain dose, this shows the volume that receives at least that dose. It is obtained by summing the volumes of all dose bins of the direct DVH starting at the high dose end, down to the specified dose level. Besides individual points of the dose-volume histogram, other summarizing statistics such as mean, minimum and maximum dose are used.

The main limitation of a DVH compared to the 3D dose distribution is that all spatial information is discarded. As such, one can use a DVH to read off, for example, $D_{3\%}$, the minimum dose to the hottest 3% of the volume, but one cannot determine from the DVH where this dose is located and how it is distributed.

The quality of data is an important factor determining the quality of models that can be developed based on them. However, though treatment planning dose calculation algorithms are much improved, significant differences can exist between those treatment plans and what the patient actually received over the full treatment course. That is, due to patient setup uncertainties, organ motion and anatomical changes during the treatment course, it can be difficult to track which volume received what dose (19).

## Selection of a formalism

For close to a century it has been recognized that the dose dependence of 'poisoning can be described by an S-shaped curve, and that such a curve is properly conceived as an expression of the variation, either in sensitiveness or in resistance, of organisms, tissues or cells toward a given poison' (41). However, though a dose of 'poison' can usually be characterized by a single number, normal tissues are generally not receiving a uniform radiation dose. Therefore, one of the challenges in modelling tissue responses is to recognize which predictive factor(s) best characterizes the variation of the resistance to the treatment (population tolerance distribution).

Reduction of a dose distribution into e.g. a dose-volume histogram results in a large pool of candidate predictors, one or more of which could be predictive of a specific morbidity. Historically two branches of modelling exist in radiotherapy. First, a number of fixed-form models have been developed (see Chapter 7). In this philosophy, the optimal predictors are identified by assuming basic mechanisms underlying the endpoints that are modelled. As such, here the selection of the formalism is done prior to analysing the data. Second, data-driven variable selection methods are available that use the data themselves as a guide for model building (10). In these methods, the selection procedure is part of the analysis of the data.

### DATA-DRIVEN FORMALISMS AND METHODS: LOGISTIC REGRESSION

The starting point of data-driven formalisms is that the data themselves can show which (combination of) factors are most capable of predicting the desired endpoint. The generally used example of this in medicine is logistic regression analysis. The logistic function is a sigmoid curve and can be written as

$$NTCP = \frac{1}{1 + \exp(-z)}$$

Here $z$ is a function of predictive factors. The parameter $z$ represents a dosage with respect to which tolerance can be defined. In the logistic model it is assumed that the population distribution of tolerance for $z$ follows a bell-shaped curve, leading to the sigmoid logistic curve for the incidence of complications as a function of $z$. For $z$ usually a linear combination of predictors is used:

$$z = \beta_0 + \beta_1 \cdot x_1 + \beta_2 \cdot x_2 + \cdots$$

Note that, even though this is a linear function, the parameters $x_1...x_n$ may represent non-linear functions of dose, volume, clinical factors or other patient characteristics. Principally one could even include the predictors used in the fixed-form formalisms in this logistic regression analysis. The challenge of this formalism, however, is to identify the combination of predictors that provides the best prediction. Methods used for this are described in the following general section on model development.

## Techniques in model development

The development of predictive models requires the use of various techniques. A comprehensive and detailed overview of these methods is beyond the scope of this chapter. Rather, an overview of essential steps required to understand the strengths and weaknesses of models will be given.

### MODEL FITTING

Model formalisms generally consist of (candidate) predictors and parameters. For these parameters, values need to be found that yield the best correspondence between the model and data. The LKB formalism (see Equation 7.7), for example, uses the DVH, but still requires values for $n$, $m$ and $D_{50}$. In the logistic regression model, the values of $\beta_0...\beta_n$ need to be determined that yield the best description of the data. The most frequently used method to perform this fit is the maximum-likelihood fit. This method selects the parameter values that maximize the likelihood that the experimental data would occur, given the predictions of the fitted model. Besides parameter values it provides the likelihood as a measure for correspondence between model and data.

## PARAMETER SELECTION

The aim of the parameter selection procedure is to identify the model that provides the best description of the data, or has the best predictive performance. However, a dose-volume histogram will typically consist of at least 10 dose-volume points. In addition to aggregate parameters such as the equivalent uniform dose, minimum dose and maximum dose, a plethora of clinical parameters and patient characteristics could be considered. Taken together this quickly adds up to dozens of candidate predictors for post-treatment toxicity. Already for a dozen parameters the number of combinations is half a billion! As such, the number of candidate models that can be constructed is too large to be able to test them all. Therefore, strategies have been developed to limit testing to the most likely candidates (for an overview see [10]). Briefly, these methods add or remove parameters based on their contribution to the performance of the model. As such, sequential forward selection repeatedly adds the predictor to the model that improves its performance most. In this procedure, addition of a new parameter from a pool of 12 only requires 12 tests. Alternatively, sequential backward elimination starts with a model that contains all candidate predictors and repeatedly removes the one, loss of which has the lowest impact on model performance. In this strategy the maximum number of tests is given by the current number of parameters.

## MODEL ORDER DETERMINATION AND SELECTION OF ROBUST PREDICTORS: CROSS-VALIDATION TECHNIQUES

When selecting predictors from a pool of candidate predictors, an important question is: How many predictors should be included in the model? Inclusion of more predictors will often improve the fit to the data set in which the model is developed, visible in e.g. an improvement in the likelihood obtained in a likelihood fit. However, when exceeding a certain optimum number of parameters, this increased precision of the model will not result in improved ability to predict outcome in new data sets. At some point, adding more predictors will only help the model to fit the random (statistical) variations in the data that are not representative of the mean expected outcome. This process is called over-fitting. Therefore, rather than selecting parameters based on the quality of a fit to the data, such selection should be based on performance in data that was not used to fit the model (10). Cross-validation techniques provide a means to do this. These techniques work by dividing the available data into independent test and validation sets.

The most general type of cross validation is $k$-fold validation. The data are divided in $k$ equal-sized sub-samples. The candidate model is then fitted to such sub-sample (training set). Subsequently, the performance of the resulting model is evaluated in the remainder of the data (test set.) Since the data were divided in $k$ sub-samples, this procedure can be repeated $k$ times. Each of these repetitions yields information on the performance. This can be combined (e.g. averaged) to determine optimal number and combination of predictors.

## MODEL?? DATA, DATA, DATA: VALIDATION AND USE OF A MODEL

Careful studies of the partial organ tolerance of normal tissues to therapeutic ionizing radiation are emerging, as are attempts to model these data (2). This, however, deserves cautious consideration. Most published model fitting is phenomenological and 'descriptive' rather than predictive. Model parameters derived from a specific cohort of patients may not apply to other irradiation conditions and fractionation schedules (e.g. few fields versus many fields, large fields followed by boost fields versus IMRT with a simultaneous integrated boost).

Principally, a model represents a description or an efficient summary of the data it originated from. As such, any application fundamentally represents an extrapolation from these data. Therefore, it is important that one always critically assesses the extent to which such extrapolation is possible for the application at hand. For instance, the shapes of dose distributions made by 3D conformal radiotherapy techniques differ from those obtained with intensity-modulated radiotherapy (IMRT) techniques. While the first often introduces relatively uniform irradiated sub-volumes in normal tissues, the latter produces more gradual dose distributions. As a result, for e.g. a fixed mean dose to an organ (often included in predictive models), dose distributions in the organ can differ a lot. The effects of such different non-uniformity may not be predicted by a model that was based on data that did not contain information on these specific non-uniformities. Similarly, a model for pulmonary complications, developed in a relatively healthy breast cancer population, may not predict well in a less-healthy population, such as lung cancer patients. Though these are rather obvious examples, one should be aware of the less-obvious ones, such as regional differences between patient populations, institutional differences in treatment techniques (i.e. what exactly *is* IMRT?) and temporal changes in populations due to changing indications for radiotherapy. After model development, information on the model's reliability is limited to the extent to which the model corresponds to the data it was fitted to. Safe clinical use of a model, however, rather requires information on its predictive performance. Taken together, these examples show that the applicability of a model is fully determined by the data it was based on. Validation analysis provides a means to assess whether these data justify use of the model for specific applications.

The design of a validation analysis depends on the intended application of the model, since this defines what data are required to validate it. In other words, a validation analysis does not yield a validated model, but validates it for a specific application. Performance of the model can be measured in many ways (1). Measures for model performance that can be considered are agreement between model and data, the amount of variance in outcome explained by the model and discriminative ability.

## 26.4 RELATION OF NTCP MODELS TO MORBIDITY: ANIMAL MODELS

Several model formalisms have been developed and are used to describe data. However, a model can only be expected to be capable of predicting responses in a new patient population if it is validated for that population. Currently most available models are not validated. Moreover, for those that were validated to the extent which such validation justifies use for treatment optimization is not always clear, since additional model-based optimization will change the dose distribution, raising the question whether the doses received by a population getting this optimized treatment are similar to the population in which the model was validated. Therefore, optimization of a treatment using a risk model is only guaranteed to optimize the dose metric(s) on which the model was based.

Whether this also yields a predictable improvement in the associated biological endpoint depends on whether the association resulted from a causal relation between the metric and the endpoint, rather than from, e.g. multi-collinearity. Yet, this potential of making a valid prediction of the effect of a change in dose distinguishes NTCP model–based treatment optimization from dose-based optimization. Proving the desired causal relation between models and biological endpoints is often not easily realized due to obvious limitations of clinical studies. However, in animal studies one can compare dose-volume effects in normal tissue damage with dose metrics that are currently used in risk models.

Common to most current models/modelling formalisms is that they are based on predictors derived from whole-organ dose-volume histograms, lacking information on the spatial distribution of dose over the organ. For these predictors to be predictive of the biological endpoint the underlying biological processes should not need this spatial information. This assumption is not easily tested in patients. Therefore, a large number of animal studies have been dedicated to testing whether radiation damage in normal tissues and consequent symptoms can be described without using such spatial information. Interestingly, as described in Section 26.2, there is considerable evidence from animal studies that normal tissue responses result from damage to specific sub-structures of the organ or even interactions between organs. Examples of these are non-local responses observed in the parotid gland (45) and spinal cord, and

damage to heart and lungs secondary to initial damage in each of them separately (13).

As such, there are clear discrepancies between the observed dependence on the spatial dose distribution of biological responses in various animal models, and the lack of spatial information in current risk models. This suggests that, though the dose metrics on which these models are based are associated to toxicity in current patient data, they are not related to the underlying biology with respect to which treatments really need to be optimized.

As discussed in Section 26.3, the extent to which predictions can be made based on an association depends on the similarity of the treatments in which the model was developed with the treatments in which the model is applied. The ability of the model to make predictions depends on the strength of the relation between the dose metric related to the underlying biology and dose metric used in the model. If this relation changes due to changes in treatment technique, model predictions will be biased and lose precision. Such a model is likely to produce accurate predictions when used for treatment plan evaluation purposes in a population identical to the one used for model development. However, any other use, such as further optimization of a technique or extrapolation to other populations, techniques or modalities should be considered hypothesis generating and requires validation. Therefore, routine use of models for such purpose should be preceded by a properly designed validation study.

---

### Key points

1. Dose-volume effects in normal tissues are highly dependent on the organ and endpoint, and the related organ sub-volume.
2. Clinical consequences of exposure of a certain volume to a certain dose are largely determined by the functional status of the organ volume receiving no or low doses.
3. The translation from initial tissue damage into changes in organ function or clinical morbidity is determined by organ- and function-specific processes such as cell migration, non-uniform distribution of stem cells or function and functional connections between organs.
4. Two modelling frameworks can be distinguished. First, fixed-form model formalisms have been derived based on hypothesized organ structures. Second, in a more data-driven approach, models can be designed using multivariable regression methods including a variable selection procedure.
5. Published risk models in general represent correlations between treatment and patient-related features. Consequently, their clinical utility needs to be proven by validation in independent data.

# ■ BIBLIOGRAPHY

1. Beetz I, Schilstra C, van Luijk P et al. External validation of three dimensional conformal radiotherapy based NTCP models for patient-rated xerostomia and sticky saliva among patients treated with intensity modulated radiotherapy. *Radiother Oncol* 2012;105:94–100.

2. Bentzen SM, Constine LS, Deasy JO et al. Quantitative analyses of normal tissue effects in the clinic QUANTEC: An introduction to the scientific issues. *Int J Radiat Oncol Biol Phys* 2010;76:S3–S9.

3. Bijl HP, van Luijk P, Coppes RP, Schippers JM, Konings AW, van der Kogel AJ. Dose-volume effects in the rat cervical spinal cord after proton irradiation. *Int J Radiat Oncol Biol Phys* 2002;52:205–211.

4. Bijl HP, van Luijk P, Coppes RP, Schippers JM, Konings AW, van der Kogel AJ. Unexpected changes of rat cervical spinal cord tolerance caused by inhomogeneous dose distributions. *Int J Radiat Oncol Biol Phys* 2003;57:274–281.

5. Bijl HP, van Luijk P, Coppes RP, Schippers JM, Konings AW, van Der Kogel AJ. Regional differences in radiosensitivity across the rat cervical spinal cord. *Int J Radiat Oncol Biol Phys* 2005;61:543–551.

6. Bijl HP, van Luijk P, Coppes RP, Schippers JM, Konings AW, van der Kogel AJ. Influence of adjacent low-dose fields on tolerance to high doses of protons in rat cervical spinal cord. *Int J Radiat Oncol Biol Phys* 2006;64:1204–1210.

7. Coppes RP, Muijs CT, Faber H et al. Volume-dependent expression of in-field and out-of-field effects in the proton-irradiated rat lung. *Int J Radiat Oncol Biol Phys* 2011;81:262–269.

8. Dawson LA, Ten Haken RK. Partial volume tolerance of the liver to radiation. *Semin Radiat Oncol* 2005;15:279–283.

9. Dijkema T, Raaijmakers CP, Ten Haken RK et al. Parotid gland function after radiotherapy: The combined Michigan and Utrecht experience. *Int J Radiat Oncol Biol Phys* 2010;78:449–453.

10. El Naqa I, Bradley J, Blanco AI et al. Multivariable modeling of radiotherapy outcomes, including dose-volume and clinical factors. *Int J Radiat Oncol Biol Phys* 2006;64:1275–1286.

11. Georg P, Kirisits C, Goldner G et al. Correlation of dose-volume parameters, endoscopic and clinical rectal side effects in cervix cancer patients treated with definitive radiotherapy including MRI-based brachytherapy. *Radiother Oncol* 2009;91:173–180.

12. Ghobadi G, Bartelds B, van der Veen SJ et al. Lung irradiation induces pulmonary vascular remodelling resembling pulmonary arterial hypertension. *Thorax* 2012;67:334–341.

13. Ghobadi G, van der Veen S, Bartelds B et al. Physiological interaction of heart and lung in thoracic irradiation. *Int J Radiat Oncol Biol Phys* 2012;84:e639–e646.

14. Herrmann T, Baumann M, Voigtmann L, Knorr A. Effect of irradiated volume on lung damage in pigs. *Radiother Oncol* 1997;44:35–40.

15. Hopewell JW, Coggle JE, Wells J, Hamlet R, Williams JP, Charles MW. The acute effects of different energy beta-emitters on pig and mouse skin. *Br J Radiol* 1986;Suppl 19:47–51.

16. Hopewell JW, Trott KR. Volume effects in radiobiology as applied to radiotherapy. *Radiother Oncol* 2000;56:283–288.

17. Huang EH, Pollack A, Levy L et al. Late rectal toxicity: Dose-volume effects of conformal radiotherapy for prostate cancer. *Int J Radiat Oncol Biol Phys* 2002;54:1314–1321.

18. Huang EX, Hope AJ, Lindsay PE et al. Heart irradiation as a risk factor for radiation pneumonitis. *Acta Oncol* 2011;50:51–60.

19. Jaffray DA, Lindsay PE, Brock KK, Deasy JO, Tome WA. Accurate accumulation of dose for improved understanding of radiation effects in normal tissue. *Int J Radiat Oncol Biol Phys* 2010;76:S135–S139.

20. Jansen EP, Saunders MP, Boot H et al. Prospective study on late renal toxicity following postoperative chemoradiotherapy in gastric cancer. *Int J Radiat Oncol Biol Phys* 2007;67:781–785.

21. Kamprad F, Ranft D, Weber A, Hildebrandt G. Functional changes of the gustatory organ caused by local radiation exposure during radiotherapy of the head-and-neck region. *Strahlenther Onkol* 2008;184:157–162.

22. Kim TH, Kim DY, Park JW et al. Dose-volumetric parameters predicting radiation-induced hepatic toxicity in unresectable hepatocellular carcinoma patients treated with three-dimensional conformal radiotherapy. *Int J Radiat Oncol Biol Phys* 2007;67:225–231.

23. Kocak Z, Borst GR, Zeng J et al. Prospective assessment of dosimetric/physiologic-based models for predicting radiation pneumonitis. *Int J Radiat Oncol Biol Phys* 2007;67:178–186.

24. Konings AW, Cotteleer F, Faber H, van Luijk P, Meertens H, Coppes RP. Volume effects and region-dependent radiosensitivity of the parotid gland. *Int J Radiat Oncol Biol Phys* 2005;62:1090–1095.

25. Köst S, Dörr W, Keinert K, Glaser FH, Endert G, Herrmann T. Effect of dose and dose-distribution in damage to the kidney following abdominal radiotherapy. *Int J Radiat Biol* 2002;78:695–702.

26. Kwa SL, Lebesque JV, Theuws JC et al. Radiation pneumonitis as a function of mean lung dose: An analysis of pooled data of 540 patients. *Int J Radiat Oncol Biol Phys* 1998;42:1–9.

27. Letschert JG, Lebesque JV, Aleman BM et al. The volume effect in radiation-related late small bowel complications: Results of a clinical study of the EORTC Radiotherapy Cooperative Group in patients treated for rectal carcinoma. *Radiother Oncol* 1994;32:116–123.

28. Lombaert IM, Brunsting JF, Wierenga PK et al. Rescue of salivary gland function after stem cell transplantation in irradiated glands. *PLOS ONE* 2008;3:e2063.

29. Marks LB, Bentzen SM, Deasy JO et al. Radiation dose-volume effects in the lung. *Int J Radiat Oncol Biol Phys* 2010;76:S70–S76.

30. Medin PM, Foster RD, van der Kogel AJ, Sayre JW, McBride WH, Solberg TD. Spinal cord tolerance to single-session uniform irradiation in pigs: Implications for a dose-volume effect. *Radiother Oncol* 2013;106:101–105.

31. Mehta V. Radiation pneumonitis and pulmonary fibrosis in non-small-cell lung cancer: Pulmonary function, prediction, and prevention. *Int J Radiat Oncol Biol Phys* 2005;63:5–24.

32. Novakova-Jiresova A, van Luijk P, van Goor H, Kampinga HH, Coppes RP. Pulmonary radiation injury: Identification of risk factors associated with regional hypersensitivity. *Cancer Res* 2005;65:3568–3576.

33. Nutting CM, Convery DJ, Cosgrove VP et al. Reduction of small and large bowel irradiation using an optimized intensity-modulated pelvic radiotherapy technique in patients with prostate cancer. *Int J Radiat Oncol Biol Phys* 2000;48:649–656.

34. Powers BE, Thames HD, Gillette SM, Smith C, Beck ER, Gillette EL. Volume effects in the irradiated canine spinal cord: Do they exist when the probability of injury is low? *Radiother Oncol* 1998;46:297–306.

35. Pringle S, Maimets M, van der Zwaag M et al. Human salivary gland stem cells functionally restore radiation damaged salivary glands. *Stem Cells* 2016;34:640–652.

36. Robbins ME, Hopewell JW. Effects of single doses of X-rays on renal function in the pig after the irradiation of both kidneys. *Radiother Oncol* 1988;11:253–262.

37. Rodrigues G, Lock M, D'Souza D, Yu E, Van Dyk J. Prediction of radiation pneumonitis by dose-volume histogram parameters in lung cancer – A systematic review. *Radiother Oncol* 2004;71:127–138.

38. Schultheiss TE. The controversies and pitfalls in modeling normal tissue radiation injury/damage. *Semin Radiat Oncol* 2001;11:210–214.

39. Schultheiss TE, Stephens LC, Ang KK, Price RE, Peters LJ. Volume effects in rhesus monkey spinal cord. *Int J Radiat Oncol Biol Phys* 1994;29:67–72.

40. Seppenwoolde Y, De Jaeger K, Boersma LJ, Belderbos JS, Lebesque JV. Regional differences in lung radiosensitivity after radiotherapy for non-small-cell lung cancer. *Int J Radiat Oncol Biol Phys* 2004;60:748–758.

41. Shackell LF, Williamson W, Deitchman MM, Katzman GM, Kleinman BS. The relation of dosage to effect. *J Pharmacol Exp Ther* 1924;24:53–65.

42. Travis EL, Liao ZX, Tucker SL. Spatial heterogeneity of the volume effect for radiation pneumonitis in mouse lung. *Int J Radiat Oncol Biol Phys* 1997;38:1045–1054.

43. van den Aardweg GJ, Hopewell JW, Whitehouse EM. The radiation response of the cervical spinal cord of the pig: Effects of changing the irradiated volume. *Int J Radiat Oncol Biol Phys* 1995;31:51–55.

44. van Luijk P, Novakova-Jiresova A, Faber H et al. Radiation damage to the heart enhances early radiation-induced lung function loss. *Cancer Res* 2005;65:6509–6511.

45. van Luijk P, Pringle S, Deasy JO et al. Sparing the region of the salivary gland containing stem cells preserves saliva production after radiotherapy for head and neck cancer. *Sci Transl Med* 2015;7:305ra147.

46. Wachter S, Gerstner N, Goldner G, Potzi R, Wambersie A, Pötter R. Rectal sequelae after conformal radiotherapy of prostate cancer: Dose-volume histograms as predictive factors. *Radiother Oncol* 2001;59:65–70.

47. Wei X, Liu HH, Tucker SL et al. Risk factors for acute esophagitis in non-small-cell lung cancer patients treated with concurrent chemotherapy and three-dimensional conformal radiotherapy. *Int J Radiat Oncol Biol Phys* 2006;66:100–107.

■ **FURTHER READING**

48. Chaikh A, Docquiere N, Bondiau PY, Balosso J. Impact of dose calculation models on radiotherapy outcomes and quality adjusted life years for lung cancer treatment: Do we need to measure radiotherapy outcomes to tune the radiobiological parameters of a normal tissue complication probability model? *Transl Lung Cancer Res* 2016;5:673–680.

49. Crispin-Ortuzar M, Jeong J, Fontanella AN, Deasy JO. A radiobiological model of radiotherapy response and its correlation with prognostic imaging variables. *Phys Med Biol* 2017;62:2658–2674.

50. Geng C, Paganetti H, Grassberger C. Prediction of treatment response for combined chemo- and radiation therapy for non-small cell lung cancer patients using a bio-mathematical model. *Sci Rep* 2017;7:13542.

# Second cancers after radiotherapy

KLAUS RÜDIGER TROTT AND WOLFGANG DÖRR

## 27.1 INTRODUCTION

The progress of cancer treatments – both in medical and radiation oncology – over recent decades has led to a significant increase in local control and overall survival rates. An obvious consequence is a steep rise in the prevalence of cancer survivors in the general population. A recent report by the National Cancer Institute of the United States estimated that 3.5% of the individuals in the population are cancer survivors. Inevitably, this also increases the frequency of second cancers as an age-related disease. Second or even third cancers account for 17% of cancers newly diagnosed and reported to the cancer registries (36). It goes without saying that patients and physicians are curious about the cause of those new malignancies after cure from an initial malignant disease.

*Age* is the most important risk factor for developing and dying from cancer. At a given age, the risk of developing cancer within the subsequent year changes little between the end of childhood and the age of 40. In women the risk increases earlier than in men, yet in both sexes the most dramatic increase is observed after the age of 60, as demonstrated in Figure 27.1. Table 27.1 shows the risk of developing a second cancer within 5 years after treatment of a malignancy – i.e. within the commonly practised follow-up time after radio(chemo) therapy – for patients treated at the age of 50, 55, 60, 65, 70 or 75, assuming that cancer rates follow those found in the general population as shown in Figure 27.1. Since there is neither convincing evidence, nor any plausible reason, that the development of one cancer protects against the development of another cancer, we may conclude that during the typical follow-up period of a patient radically and successfully treated for cancer, a relatively large proportion of patients will present with a second cancer purely based on the age distribution. This frequency will vary between 1% and more than 10%, depending on gender and age at treatment. The results of epidemiological studies described in the following text indicate that in cancer patients, after successful curative radiotherapy, the increased lifespan is by far the most important risk factor leading to second cancers. This risk estimate, determined from cancer registry data which cover entire populations, may be further increased by individual factors, such as specific carcinogen exposure or genetic predisposition.

It is generally accepted that the majority of cancers are causally related to exposure of the individual to common carcinogens – the most important being dietary factors and smoking – which, together, cause more than 50% of all cancer deaths (11). Importantly, most carcinogens are known to be related to more than one cancer entity. Smoking, for example, is causally related to cancer of the lung and head and neck, but also of bladder and breast. This means that a patient cured from lung or head and neck cancer, independent of the treatment modality, consequently will have a greater risk than other members of the general population to develop, for example, bladder cancer. The dimension of this increase in the individual risk, however, is difficult to determine. For the quantification of treatment-related second cancer risks in epidemiological studies, the potential bias related to specific carcinogen exposure has to be eliminated or reduced. The best approaches are the determination of radiation dose dependence of the risk or, alternatively, the comparison of different curative treatment modalities for the same type and stage of cancer.

The risk of a person developing specific cancers is also influenced by the individual genetic predisposition. The impact of this predisposition varies with the underlying genetic background. Well-known examples of a strong genetic predisposition are mutations of the Rb gene (predisposing for retinoblastoma and osteosarcoma) and of the *BRCA1/2* genes (predisposing for early breast and ovarian cancer). In many instances, moreover, the genetic basis of an increase in cancer risk as assessed by anamnesis ('family history') is unknown. The fact that the known, and probably most other, predisposing factors are associated with more than one type of cancer, also means that people cured from one of those cancers have a higher than the population average probability to develop other cancers associated with the respective genetic aberration. It must be emphasized that the impact of genetic predisposition on the risk of developing a second cancer after cure from the first cancer is difficult to assess at the present state of knowledge. The most obvious example is the high risk of children treated with radiotherapy for retinoblastoma to develop osteosarcomas in the irradiated volume. Some of the modalities used to effectively treat cancer have a proven carcinogenic potential. A large number of studies have explored the impact of various chemotherapy and radiotherapy schedules, as well as their combination, on the incidence of second cancers. The most detailed and comprehensive analysis of such studies carried out up to 2010 was published by the National Council of Radiation Protection and Measurements (see [36]).

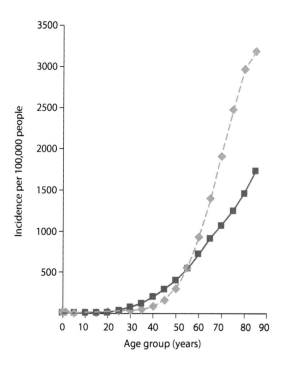

Figure 27.1 Average annual cancer incidence in the United Kingdom by sex and attained age. Diamonds, male; squares, female. (Data from (42).)

There is increasing evidence in long-term survivors who were treated as children or young adults for cancers such as Hodgkin or non-Hodgkin lymphoma, testicular cancer or paediatric malignancies, that the most important cause of death is second cancers causally related to the treatment of the first cancer. Radiotherapy and chemotherapy are both implicated in the induction of those second malignancies. In general, chemotherapy is mostly related to the induction of leukaemia, in particular acute myelogenous leukaemia, most of which occur within 10 years after the primary treatment. Radiotherapy, in contrast, is more related to the induction of solid cancers. The latter are associated with a significantly longer latency, with the risk persisting for several decades or maybe even lifelong (27). There are strong indications that

Table 27.1 The spontaneous cancer incidence risk within a follow-up period of 5 years, in patients treated at different ages

| Age at treatment (years) | Cancer risk within the next 5 years (%) | |
| --- | --- | --- |
| | Males | Females |
| 50 | 1.5 | 2.0 |
| 55 | 2.5 | 2.7 |
| 60 | 5.0 | 3.6 |
| 65 | 7.0 | 4.6 |
| 70 | 10.0 | 5.4 |
| 75 | 12.5 | 6.3 |

Data from United Kingdom, England and Wales 1983–1987 (see Figure 27.1).

radiotherapy also is a co-factor for second leukaemias and, vice versa, chemotherapeutic drugs also co-increase the risk of solid cancers.

The risk of treatment-related second cancers is commonly determined by the comparison of the frequency of second cancers after different treatment modalities, such as surgery versus radiotherapy, or with the general population. This way, a ratio of frequencies is calculated which indicates relative risks* (RR) of cancers caused by a specific treatment. These RR values tend to vary greatly between different second cancers for the same primary cancer and, in many cases such as leukaemia after treatment of Hodgkin lymphoma, may assume very high values. Although RR values form the basis of epidemiological and statistical analyses, they may be entirely misleading with regard to the dimension of the clinical problem. Since many treatment-related cancers (particularly those with high RR values) are rare in the general population, a high RR may still translate into a low absolute risk. For example, a high RR of 4 for a tumour with a baseline incidence rate of $2/10^5$ person/year indicates an increase in the absolute excess incidence by just 6 cases in 10,000 people per year. Therefore, the excess absolute risk (EAR), which estimates the excess number of second malignancies per 10,000 patients per year, clearly reflects the second malignancy burden of treated patients better than relative risk values (40).

## 27.2 RADIATION-INDUCED SECOND CANCERS AFTER CURATIVE RADIOTHERAPY OF CANCERS IN ADULT PATIENTS

Radiation is a well-established carcinogen. Therefore, it has to be assumed that successful curative radiotherapy of cancer may also cause a new, second cancer in addition to age-related cancer risks. The incidence rate of these second, radiation-induced cancers, however, remains obscure. In radiation protection, estimation of radiation-induced cancer follows a method which has been developed by the International Commission on Radiological Protection (ICRP) for preventive purposes in radiation worker populations (18,19). It is largely based on the determination of the 'effective dose' and thus on data derived from epidemiological studies in larger populations exposed to (1) whole body and (2) low doses of radiation, in particular the Life Span Study of the Japanese atomic bomb survivors. The method of risk estimation involves three steps:

1. Calculation of the mean organ dose equivalent, i.e. absorbed dose adjusted by a radiation quality factor, for the different organs at risk such as lung, stomach, colon, bone marrow and others (based on specific dosimetric procedures, which also may be subject for controversies).

* Absolute risk (AR): incidence, prevalence; relative risk (RR): incidence in exposed versus non-exposed individuals; excess absolute/relative risk (EAR/ERR): AR/RR over baseline.

2. Multiply the mean organ dose equivalent with the respective organ weighting factor, which ranges from 0.01 for skin to 0.12 for the four most critical organs, i.e. lung, bone marrow, colon and stomach.

3. Add the weighted mean organ doses for all organs at risk. This weighted total body dose is called 'effective dose'. This effective dose is then multiplied with the appropriate risk factor that varies between 4% and 10% per Gy, depending on age and exposure dose rate, to calculate the lifetime cancer risk from the respective radiation exposure. Gender is not considered here.

In many published studies, this approach has also been applied to determine the risks from radical radiotherapy and to compare different treatment plans in radiotherapy. Yet, the risk estimates derived using this method in general yield very high values, which may be up to two orders of magnitude higher than the risk derived directly from the epidemiological studies described below. The reasons for this discrepancy are the extraordinary dose inhomogeneities within individual organs and between organs in a scenario of therapeutic administration of radiation. Epidemiological and experimental evidence actually shows that the probability of cancer induction decreases dramatically as the dose inhomogeneity in any irradiated organ increases. It is mainly for this reason that the ICRP strongly advises *not* to use the effective dose approach to estimate the risks of radiation-induced cancer in situations of very large dose inhomogeneities with peak doses well above doses which would cause acute or chronic radiation effects (i.e. doses >5 Gy), e.g. in ICRP 60 (18) and ICRP 103 (19). ICRP also very clearly recommends that data derived directly from epidemiological investigations on radiotherapy patients should be used to estimate the risk of induction of second cancers by the radiation treatment of the first cancer.

Such data can best be collected by the comparison of the rate of second cancers in large patient cohorts who have been cured from the first cancer by protocols with either radiotherapy or, e.g. surgery. In this respect, conditions of suitability are

- The first cancer has to be common.
- The first cancer has to have a good chance of cure (≥50%).
- The chance of cure from surgery and radical radiotherapy has to be similar and the decision of treating by radiotherapy or surgery should be largely independent of factors affecting cancer risks.
- The life expectancy of a large proportion of the cured patients has to be long enough, preferably more than 10 years.

Two entities of malignancies fulfil these conditions particularly well: cancer of the cervix and the prostate. For both these cancers, large epidemiological studies have been conducted which currently provide the main source of data and basis of conclusions on second cancer risks after radiotherapy in patients of advanced age.

In addition, important information can also be derived from studies on the topographical relationship of primary cancer and second cancer in symmetrical organs, in particular in patients with a primary breast cancer developing second lung cancer. Moreover, studies on second cancers after radiotherapy of young people and their comparison with age-matched healthy populations also provide important information, since they permit very long follow-up. Yet their interpretation is sometimes difficult and may be misleading because of strong genetic susceptibility factors influencing risks, and because of other, confounding carcinogenic treatment modalities such as chemotherapy, which render any identification of radiation risks difficult. However, in some cancers, in particular Hodgkin lymphoma, testicular cancer and paediatric malignancies, it has been possible to separate out the contributions of radiotherapy and chemotherapy and their interaction.

## Carcinoma of the cervix

The first analysis on the risk of second cancers after radical radiotherapy of primary cancers was a multi-institutional study on long-term survivors of cancer of the cervix. The study of Kleinerman et al. (21) was a cohort study of the incidence of second cancers in 66,541 patients with cervical cancer reported to 13 population-based cancer registries in five countries. Out of this patient group, 49,828 (75%) were treated with radiotherapy and 16,713 (25%) were treated surgically. The average follow-up was 10.4 years. More than 2000 second cancers were recorded and analysed. The results of this study are remarkable in several aspects. In contrast to the UNSCEAR studies on the Japanese atomic bomb survivors (39), the greatest risk occurs in the bladder and in the rectum (both of which received high radiation doses close to the target dose). The colon, which obviously also received considerable doses in radiotherapy of cervix cancer, did not show any increased second cancer rates. Only two organs included in the low-dose volumes showed significantly increased cancer rates: stomach (exposed to mean doses of 2 Gy) and bone marrow (mean dose 4.5 Gy). The leukaemia risk per gray derived from these data was less than 10% of the risk per gray estimated from the atomic bomb survivor study, demonstrating the overriding importance of dose inhomogeneity on second malignancy risks.

## Carcinoma of the prostate

Several small studies on the risks of second cancers after radical radiotherapy of prostate cancer have yielded inconclusive results. Yet, the results of the very large cohort study on 122,123 prostate cancer patients registered in the SEER program (the National Cancer Institute's Surveillance, Epidemiology and End Results program) who had either surgery or radiotherapy (5) clearly demonstrate the dimension of the problem in clinical radiotherapy. The

Table 27.2 Results of the study of second cancers after radiotherapy of prostate cancer

| | Surgery only | Radiotherapy |
|---|---|---|
| Number of patients | 70,539 | 51,584 |
| Person-years at risk | 312,499 | 218,341 |
| Mean survival time (years) | 4.4 | 4.2 |
| Mean age at therapy (years) | 71.4 | 70.3 |
| Mean age at second cancer (years) | 77 | 75.3 |
| Percentage (%) of persons at risk after: | | |
| 5–10 years | 35.8 | 33.5 |
| >10 years | 10.8 | 9.8 |
| Number of second malignancies: | | |
| At all times after treatment | 5055 | 3549 |
| After >5 years | 1646 | 1185 |
| After >10 years | 393 | 305 |

Data from (5).

study was a cohort study on patients with prostate cancer. The results of this study are summarised in Table 27.2.

By comparing second cancer rates of patients treated either with radiotherapy or surgery at different follow-up times, the risk of radiation-induced second cancer and its dependence on follow-up can be calculated. Results are shown in Table 27.3. Out of the approximately 17,000 prostate cancer patients who survived more than 5 years after radical radiotherapy, 1185 (7%) developed a second cancer. More than 1000 of those second cancers (>85%) have been attributed to the increased lifespan as a consequence of cure from the first cancer. Importantly, just about 120–150 of those second cancers among 51,584 prostate cancer patients (0.3%) were related to radiotherapy, i.e.

- Approximately 50 cases of bladder cancer
- Approximately 15 cases of cancer of the rectum
- Approximately 50 cases of lung cancer
- Approximately 12 cases of leukaemia

Table 27.3 Risk of radiation-induced second cancer after radiotherapy of prostate cancer

| | Relative risk | |
|---|---|---|
| | After >5 years | After >10 years |
| All second cancers: | 1.11 ($p < 0.007$) | 1.27 ($p < 0.002$) |
| Bladder | 1.55 ($p < 0.0001$) | 1.77 ($p < 0.01$) |
| Rectum | 1.35 ($p < 0.06$) | 2.05 ($p < 0.03$) |
| Lung | 1.22 ($p < 0.01$) | 1.42 ($p < 0.02$) |
| Leukaemia in the first 10 years: | | |
| Surgery patients | Irradiated patients | Relative risk in 10 years |
| 39 in 343,690 person-years | 25 in 112,422 person years | 2 ($p < 0.05$) |

Data from (5).

As was observed in the cervix studies, bladder and rectum cancers found in the high-dose volume are most frequent. The unexpected large number of radiotherapy-associated lung cancers is probably related to the older treatment techniques, using large fields, administered mostly with cobalt-60 units. A mean lung dose of 0.5 Gy has been estimated resulting from scattered radiation. This is in agreement with the risk of radiation-induced lung cancer from the atomic bomb survivor studies. Modern conformal treatment protocols may result in a much lower lung exposure of about 10% of the doses estimated in the Brenner et al. study (5). However, lung doses from some modern techniques, such as intensity modulated radiotherapy (IMRT) of prostate cancer, may be close to those (ancient) doses and may hence possibly be associated with similar risks of second lung cancer. This is due to the use of more treatment fields and higher number of monitor units.

The most important result of the prostate cancer study is that half of all radiation-induced second cancers occur in the high-dose volumes and only the other half in the volumes exposed to those radiation doses commonly associated with radiation carcinogenesis. It is very likely that two entirely different mechanisms are involved (or interact) in the high- and low-dose volumes. In the low-dose volumes, we may assume the same molecular and cellular mechanisms as in other situations of low-dose radiation carcinogenesis which have been extensively explored in radiation protection research (39). Radiation doses given to the bladder and the rectum often lead to chronic radiation injury which is characterised by progressive micro-vascular damage, parenchymal atrophy and chronic inflammation (see Chapter 14). This condition has been recognised for more than 100 years as a pre-cancerous lesion. Therefore, one may classify the radiation-induced second cancers in the high-dose organs as secondary to chronic radiation injury, thus combining a dose-dependent, deterministic probability of a tissue reaction and a probabilistic carcinogenicity risk. This combination and interaction has a very pronounced impact on the overall dose-risk relationship. In consequence, optimisation of treatment plans has to be adjusted as discussed in the concluding paragraph.

## Breast cancer

Patients treated with post-operative radiotherapy for breast cancer may receive significant radiation doses of more than 5% of the target dose to the contralateral breast. Since second cancers in the contralateral breast occur more frequently than expected – although this may be partially attributed to a genetic/anamnestic predisposition – and comprise nearly half of all second cancers in women with breast cancer, a causal relationship with the radiation exposure from the treatment of the first cancer has been suggested. However, a case control study by Stovall et al. (31) embedded into the WECARE study with 708 women with asynchronous bilateral breast cancer and 1399 women with unilateral breast cancer (controls) demonstrated that women older than 40 years of age who received >1 Gy to the specific quadrant of the contralateral breast had a 2.5-fold greater risk for contralateral breast cancer than unexposed women. No excess was observed in women older than 40 years of age.

Patients treated with post-operative radiotherapy for breast cancer receive very different doses to the ipsilateral compared to the contralateral lungs. Darby et al. (8) reported a cohort study on 308,861 women, included in the SEER program, who were treated for breast cancer between 1973 and 2001 and of which 115,165 (37%) received radiotherapy as part of their primary treatment. Of these women treated, 482 women (0.4%) later died from lung cancer for which the affected side was clearly defined in the records. The main endpoint of the study was, which side of the lung, in relation to which breast was originally treated, developed a second cancer. More than 1000 cases of lung cancer (0.5%) occurred in women who did not receive radiotherapy, and there was no difference between the rates of ipsilateral and contralateral lung cancers. Of the 482 cases of lung cancer which occurred in women who received radiotherapy, 283 cases (59%) were ipsilateral and 199 (41%) were contralateral. From these findings, the risk of radiation-induced lung cancer could be estimated. The proportion of ipsilateral second lung cancers in women who had received radiotherapy increased with increasing follow-up time from a ratio of 1.2 less than 10 years after treatment to 2.7 more than 15 years after treatment (Table 27.4).

Grantzau et al. (15) analysed the long-term risk of second primary solid non-breast cancers in the Danish national population-based cohort of more than 46,000 patients treated according to national guidelines of the Danish Breast Cancer Cooperative Group for early breast cancer between 1982 and 2007. About half of the study population received postoperative radiotherapy and were compared to those not receiving radiotherapy. Altogether, 2358 second cancers occurred during the (median) follow-up of 5 years after radiotherapy and 8 years without radiotherapy. The hazard ratio was not increased for sites distant from the treatment volume; however, it progressively increased with duration of follow-up for sites in the thorax, in particular the lungs (Table 27.5). These results are compatible with those of the study by Darby et al. (8). The estimated attributable risk of developing a secondary cancer in the thorax (excluding contralateral breast) translates into one radiation-induced second cancer in every 200 women treated with radiotherapy.

**Table 27.4** Ipsilateral and contralateral second lung cancers in patients treated with post-operative radiotherapy of breast cancer

| Duration of follow-up (years) | Number of second cancers | | Lung cancer mortality ratio |
| --- | --- | --- | --- |
| | Ipsilateral | Contralateral | |
| <10 | 161 | 134 | 1.2 |
| 10–15 | 65 | 44 | 1.5 |
| >15 | 57 | 21 | 2.7 |

Data from (8).

**Table 27.5** Hazard ratio for secondary lung cancer in irradiated and nonirradiated early breast cancer patients in the Danish cohort

| Latency (years) | 23,627 irradiated women | | 22,549 unirradiated women | | HR (9% C.I.) |
| --- | --- | --- | --- | --- | --- |
| | Observed | Person–years | Observed | Person–years | |
| 1–4 | 52 | 68,678 | 88 | 71,902 | 0.72 (0.5–1.1) |
| 5–9 | 57 | 39,034 | 84 | 57,926 | 1.17 (0.8–1.7) |
| 10–14 | 41 | 15,780 | 70 | 33,001 | 1.40 (0.9–2.1) |
| >15 | 36 | 7,273 | 50 | 20,661 | 1.94 (1.2–3.1) |
| All | 186 | 139,765 | 292 | 183,490 | 1.27 (1.0–1.6) |

Data from (15).

Studies such as these provide good evidence that women cured from breast cancer using radiotherapy of the chest wall – with significant exposure also of lung tissue – have an increased risk of developing radiation-induced lung cancer and that the risk increases with increasing mean lung dose. However, this information is of little help in the optimization of treatment planning in radiation oncology practice. This would require information on the dependence of lung cancer risk on local radiation dose and dose distribution. Such information can only be obtained by performing case-control studies. Grantzau et al. (16) performed such a study on the 151 secondary lung cancer cases of her first study (15), comparing them with 443 matched controls. Individual dose reconstructions were performed and the dose delivered to the position of the centre of the lung cancer was determined (and in the same location in controls). She obtained a dose-risk relationship which was compatible with a linear-non-threshold relationship between a few gray and 40 Gy, with an increase in relative risk of 8.5% per gray.

## Conclusions: The risk of second cancer induced by radiotherapy of first cancers in adult patients

A considerable number of studies published in recent years clearly demonstrated that definitive radiotherapy may, in cured patients who survive the first cancer for more than 5–10 years, increase the risk of developing a second cancer. This risk is small but significant in adult patients (in the order of 1%). In a comprehensive analysis of data stored in the U.S. Surveillance, Epidemiology and End Results (SEER) Cancer Registries, Berrington de Gonzalez et al. (3) determined the proportion of second cancers which are attributable to radiotherapy treatments in 647,672 adults who survived their first cancer for more than 5 years and were followed up for another 7 years: 60,271 (9%) developed a second solid cancer between 5 and 12 years after treatment of the first cancer (Table 27.6). The relative risk of second cancer and the proportion of cancers attributable

Table 27.6 Estimated number of excess second solid cancers attributable to radiotherapy of first cancer sites

| First cancer site | Observed second cancers | Excess number | Percentage (%) attributable to radiotherapy |
|---|---|---|---|
| Brain | 314 | 28 | 9 |
| Testes | 628 | 150 | 24 |
| Prostate | 11,292 | 1131 | 10 |
| Lung | 2,395 | 152 | 6 |
| Head and neck | 7,166 | 375 | 5 |
| Breast | 12,450 | 660 | 5 |
| All | 42,294 | 3266 | 8 |

Data from (3).

to radiotherapy were calculated by comparing cancer rates for patients receiving radiotherapy versus patients not receiving radiotherapy in the definitive treatment of 15 types of first malignancy. In total, an estimated 3266 excess solid cancers could be related to radiotherapy in these 5-year survivors, i.e. 8% of the total second cancers diagnosed in the cancer survivors who had received radiotherapy, while >90% were related to the increased lifespan of the cancer patient who was cured. The authors estimated that for every 1000 patients treated with radiotherapy there were an estimated three excess cancers by 10 years after first cancer diagnosis which increased to five excess cases by 15 years. Over half of the excess cases occurred in organs likely to have received >5 Gy. Moreover, more than half of the excess cases were determined in patients who had been treated and cured from prostate cancer and breast cancer using radiotherapy.

Dörr and Herrmann (13) determined the anatomical relationship between the location of the planned target volume of radiotherapy and the location of second cancers. They found that the majority of second cancers occurred outside of but close to the planning target volume (PTV) of radiotherapy. This observation which has been confirmed in further studies, has important implications for estimating the role of local dose, irradiated volume and organs at risk on the induction of second cancers by radiotherapy and may suggest modifications of radiotherapy treatment planning criteria to reduce the small but significant risk even further. This is discussed in the paragraph on dose response relationships of second cancer induction.

## 27.3 RADIATION-INDUCED SECOND CANCERS AFTER COMBINED RADIOCHEMOTHERAPY OF MALIGNANCIES IN YOUNG ADULTS

### Hodgkin lymphoma

The treatment results of Hodgkin lymphoma have improved significantly since the introduction of intensive, large-field radiotherapy which was mainly based on the work of

Kaplan at Stanford (e.g. [20]). As a result, today thousands of long-term survivors of Hodgkin lymphoma are at risk for late effects of therapy including second cancers and cardiovascular diseases.

Wolden et al. (41) described the incidence of second cancers in 697 patients who were less than 21 years old at the time of treatment in Stanford, some followed up for more than 35 years. Eighty patients (11%) developed 85 new malignant tumours. Twenty-five (31%) were non-melanoma skin cancers. The second most frequent second cancer was breast cancer (16 patients), followed by sarcoma (13 patients). Eight second leukaemias occurred, all but one within 10 years and all eight patients had received chemotherapy with alkylating agents. The actuarial risk of second cancer at 20 years after treatment for Hodgkin lymphoma, at a mean attained age of 36 years, was 9.7% for males and 16.8% for females with more than half of their risk being due to breast cancer (9.2%). The most remarkable finding of this important single institution study was that among the 48 solid second cancers, 43 (90%) occurred within the high-dose radiotherapy treatment field or in the penumbra region, and 40 (83%) developed in volumes that had received at least 35 Gy. The authors stress that treatment policies for Hodgkin lymphoma have changed dramatically over the past 30 years, putting more emphasis on multi-agent chemotherapy and reduced radiation doses and treatment volumes to involved sites. Thus, the second malignancy rates seen after long follow-up in this study do not represent the risk for patients treated in the modern era. It should be noted that death of the patients from their primary Hodgkin lymphoma was more than twice as likely as from a second cancer (11% versus 4%).

Dores et al. (12) reported results of a large international study on 32,591 Hodgkin lymphoma patients with 2861 patients followed-up for more than 20 years and 1111 patients for more than 25 years. Mean age at treatment was 37 years. Second malignancies developed in 2153 patients (7%) which, compared to the age- and gender-adjusted general population, was an increase of more than a factor of 2. The risk of late-developing solid cancers was particularly increased after radiotherapy, while second leukaemias were mostly related to chemotherapy. The highest excess absolute second cancer risk was for cancers of the lung and breast. While the relative risk of all second cancers decreased with increasing age at diagnosis of Hodgkin lymphoma, the excess absolute risk of second cancers increased with increasing age from 30 cases per 100,000 person-years for less than 21-year-old patients to 107 cases per 100,000 person-years in 51- to 60-year-old patients. This was not seen for second breast cancer, where the risk was highest in patients treated less than 30 years. The authors calculated a 25 years cumulative risk of treatment-induced second cancers of 11.7%, most of which was related to radiotherapy.

In a case control study of British patients, Swerdlow et al. (32) demonstrated that also chemotherapy leads to a dose-dependent elevated risk of lung cancer, and that this risk was not further increased if also radiotherapy was given.

In their review of late effects after treatment for Hodgkin lymphoma, Swerdlow and van Leeuwen (33) concluded that the substantial increase in solid tumour risk with time since diagnosis necessitated careful, lifelong medical surveillance of all patients. Women treated with mantle field irradiation before the age of 30 are at greatly increased risk of breast cancer. In many centres, from 8 years after irradiation on, the follow-up program of these women includes yearly breast palpation and mammography; however, the efficacy of these measures in this specific population has not been demonstrated yet.

## Testicular cancer

In a large international study on nearly 29,000 patients with testicular cancer who survived more than 1 year, Travis et al. (35) analysed the dependence of 1406 observed second cancers (which was an overall excess of 43%) on time since treatment and on treatment modality, with special emphasis on the histology of first and of second tumour. The 25 years cumulative second cancer risk after treatment of seminoma was 18% and that of non-seminomatous testicular cancer was 11% compared to 6% in an age-matched normal population. Compared to the general population, the excess cancer risk increased steadily for at least 30 years. The most pronounced, significantly increased second cancer rates among the 3306 patients surviving more than 20 years were related to cancer of the bladder, which receives the highest radiation dose of all organs at risk. Seventy bladder cancers were diagnosed among the total of 276 cancer cases in this group, mostly related to radiotherapy with a relative risk of greater than three. In a later study, Travis et al. (34) related the risk of treatment-induced leukaemia to the type of treatment. Both radiotherapy and cisplatinum-based chemotherapy increased leukaemia risk in a dose-dependent way: After cisplatinum-based chemotherapy, leukaemia risk was nearly twice that of radiotherapy. However, the absolute risk was small after both treatment modalities (15 years cumulative risk about 0.1%) compared to the risk of treatment-induced solid second cancers, most of which was attributed to radiotherapy.

## 27.4 RADIATION-INDUCED SECOND CANCERS AFTER TREATMENT OF PAEDIATRIC MALIGNANCIES

The probability of children with cancer being cured and having a near normal life expectancy has currently reached a level which was unimaginable 30 years or longer ago. However, the price for this progress – in terms of second cancer risk – is high. Importantly, the epidemiological studies on second malignancies after radiotherapy of children and adolescents demonstrate that the majority of second, radiotherapy-induced cancers occur in tissues and organs not commonly considered in radiation protection, such as connective tissue.

In the largest cohort of childhood cancer survivors in the Scandinavian countries, comprising nearly 50,000 long-term survivors treated between 1943 and 2005, a total of 1180 asynchronous second primary cancers were observed. The relative risk was significantly increased in all age groups, even in the sub-cohort treated in childhood now approaching the age of 70 years (25). Repeated analyses of several large childhood cancer survivor studies (CCSSs), in particular the U.S. CCSS and the French-British CCSS, demonstrated that both radiotherapy and chemotherapy, and in particular the combination of both, caused a significant risk of developing a second malignancy. Leukaemia predominates in the first ten years, whereas various solid cancers develop later in life, which is in accordance with the atomic bomb survivor observations and others.

Neglia et al. (23) investigated a cohort of 13,581 children from the CCSS registry in the United States who survived at least 5 years, with a median follow-up of 15 years. A total of 298 second malignancies were observed after a mean latency of 12 years. Whereas the risk of secondary leukaemia (altogether 24 cases) increased to a peak after 5–9 years, the risk of solid second cancers, in particular breast (60 cases), thyroid (43 cases) and central nervous system (36 cases) was significantly elevated during the entire follow-up period of up to 30 years. The authors concluded that second malignant neoplasms are 'infrequent but extremely serious events following therapy for primary cancers'. In particular, female survivors of childhood cancer are at a high risk of developing secondary breast cancer. Yet the authors also warned not to compromise the effectiveness of treatment of the first cancer because of the low risk of second cancers. In their analysis, only less than two excess malignancies (0.2%) were recorded per 1000 patient-years of follow-up.

Neglia et al. (24) reported a case control study in children from the CCSSs who developed secondary glioma ($n = 40$) or meningioma ($n = 66$), respectively, after mean intervals of 9 or 17 years after primary radiotherapy. Local radiation dose at the site of the second brain tumour was the most important risk factor. No cases were observed at <10 Gy, and the maximal risk (RR >10) was related to a mean brain dose of >30 Gy. The risk of secondary glioma was particularly high in children given radiotherapy at age <5 years, which may be attributed to greater susceptibility of the developing brain to radiation.

The study of de Vathaire et al. (9) on the French-British CCSS analysed the second cancer risk in 4400 3-year survivors treated in eight centres in France and the United Kingdom, 3109 (71%) of whom received radiotherapy. For 2831 (91%) of these children, individual radiation doses at 151 points of the body were determined, based on the individual treatment plans using an age and body-size adaptable computer phantom. A total of 113 patients (4%) developed a solid second malignant tumour (non-melanoma skin cancers excluded). The cumulative incidence of treatment-associated second solid tumours increased dramatically as the patient progressed into their age older than 30. Twenty-five years after treatment of the primary malignancy, the cumulative risk was about 5%, 5 years later it approached 8%. In 543 patients who had already attained an age older than 30 years, 16 second cancers were diagnosed, while only 3.3 were expected, a fivefold increase.

In conclusion, the most critical organs for radiation-induced second cancers in paediatric radiotherapy are breast, brain, bone, soft tissues and thyroid. More than 80% of all second solid tumours occurred in those organs and tissues – yet there were great differences in sensitivity with age and in dose dependence: sarcomas and brain tumours tended to develop in the high-dose volumes, while carcinomas tended to occur in the intermediate- to low-dose volumes.

More recent studies on this particular, well-documented cohort of childhood cancer survivors added important information. Diallo et al. (10) analysed the anatomical relationship between the location of (fatal) second cancers and the PTV for sarcomas, brain tumours, breast cancer and thyroid cancer (Table 27.7). The most important information from this study is that two-thirds of all fatal second cancers occurred at the margins of the border. The uncertainty of local dose and dose distribution in this region, however, urgently needs to be resolved. This poses one of the greatest challenges in current clinical research, as it may be the key to develop methods to reduce second cancer rates in childhood cancer survivors. Tukenova et al. (38) reported that sarcomas occurred earlier than carcinomas but stayed constant after 20 years while the rate of carcinomas continues to increase steadily with increasing follow-up time.

In a study on 102 second cancers among 930 children treated for Hodgkin disease, Constine et al. (7) reported a three times higher risk of female children compared to male children treated for Hodgkin disease to develop second cancers. This is mainly due to the high rate of second cancers of the breast, but also of thyroid carcinomas and of sarcomas in females. These three cancer types comprise three-quarters of all second cancers in female Hodgkin survivors. Apparently, second cancers in childhood cancer survivors are a particularly serious problem in females.

This high sensitivity of the developing breast in female children was the topic of a particularly important study by Schellong et al. (28). In long-term follow-up of 590 female children treated in childhood for Hodgkin disease, within five consecutive randomized clinical trials in which the radiation dose was systematically reduced, 26 primary breast cancers were diagnosed between 14 and 31 years after radiotherapy with doses between 20 and 45 Gy. The cumulative incidence of breast cancer at an attained age of 40 years was 10%, the standard incidence ratio was 25. The development of breast cancer followed a similar pattern as in women who carry a *BRCA-2* mutation. All breast cancers occurred in those (480) children who were between 9 and 16 years at radiotherapy, none occurred in the 74 children who were younger than 9 at radiotherapy.

The progress in the efficiency of the treatment in paediatric oncology is associated with rapidly changing treatment schedules, both regarding chemotherapy (drugs, their combination and dosage) and radiotherapy (with a tendency to decrease target volumes and doses). The epidemiological data on the risk of second cancers are therefore, inevitably, resulting from outdated treatment techniques. Whether the methods used today are associated with a lower or higher risk of second cancers cannot be directly answered and any conclusions appear premature and speculative. The short latency of leukaemias may permit the investigation of this problem for relatively recent chemotherapy schedules since chemotherapy is mainly associated with secondary leukaemia arising within <10 years. Identifying the criteria determining risk in radiotherapy may be more difficult due to the long latency periods of solid cancers. The location of these second solid cancers, matched to the patient's individual dose-volume distributions, must be in the focus of future studies of this risk of second malignancies after childhood cancer treatment.

As a caveat, it should be emphasized that all studies on treatment-induced second cancers after radiotherapy of paediatric malignancies, so far, show only the tip of the iceberg. The vast majority of study members are still under the age of 50, yet from the atomic bomb survivor studies we may conclude that, even though relative risk may decrease with time, most radiation-induced cancers will occur only when the cured patients reach an age older than 60 years. For this reason, it is of utmost importance for paediatric radiation oncology that these studies be continued for at least another 20 years.

## 27.5 THE DEPENDENCE OF SECOND CANCER RISKS ON DOSE, DOSE DISTRIBUTION AND AGE AT EXPOSURE: HOW TO REDUCE RISK?

Considering the evidence presented in this chapter, there can be no doubt that radical radiotherapy of malignant diseases may cause second cancers, but many years later. The risk of radiotherapy-induced second cancers varies considerably with the type of primary cancer (paediatric malignancies posing the highest risk) and treatment technique. Though by necessity, all data on second cancer risks after radiotherapy of first cancers relate to techniques which are more than 20 years old, and most are outdated. This poses two important questions:

Table 27.7 Location of fatal second cancers in relation to dose

| Site | Number | Location | | |
| --- | --- | --- | --- | --- |
| | | In beam | Border | Distant |
| Sarcomas | 52 | 10 | 36 | 6 |
| Breast cancer | 13 | 1 | 9 | 3 |
| CNS malignancies | 10 | 0 | 4 | 6 |
| Thyroid cancer | 17 | 2 | 11 | 4 |
| All | *115* | *14* | *76* | *25* |

Data from (10).

1. *Is the risk of radiotherapy-induced second cancers too high a price to be acceptable in the decision-making process for treating the first cancer?*

The absolute risk of radiotherapy-induced second cancers is below or at 1% after radical radiotherapy of most adult cancers. The risk of dying from uncontrolled disease within months to years after radiotherapy is much higher than the risk of developing a second cancer, which – even more important – usually develops 10 or 20 years later. This conclusion also applies to post-operative radiotherapy of breast cancer.

With regard to juvenile and childhood malignancies, the answer has to be more guarded. Certainly, radiotherapy has made a great impact on long-term survival in these patients. After a 20-year follow-up, the risk of recurrence of the primary cancer is higher than the risk of developing a radiotherapy-induced second cancer (22). However, if this relative risk persisted throughout the remaining lifespan that those patients have been granted by the success of the radiation treatment in the first place, the risk of radiotherapy-induced second cancers would rise to levels which might cause serious concern. These considerations have been supported by the results of the large and well-documented study of Schellong et al. (28), and can no longer be considered as speculation. Yet, the peculiar dependence of risk on age and the uncertainty on anatomical dose distribution and the influence of the biology of breast development all require further investigations. The results of ongoing epidemiological studies may uncover the true picture in 10 or 20 years from now.

2. *Can the risk of radiotherapy-induced second cancer be reduced by optimising the treatment techniques and the dose-volume distributions?*

It is very likely and it can be deduced from the evidence presented that different treatment techniques are associated with different risks of radiation-induced second cancers. These variations in risk would be primarily due to differences in dose-volume distributions. The findings of the epidemiological studies in patients treated for cervix and prostate cancers suggest that two different mechanisms, leading to radiation-induced second cancers, may exist which show very different relationships with radiation dose. One mechanism is the induction of DNA mutations that cause malignant transformation of the cells which subsequently, after promoted proliferation and acquisition of further mutations, gain the potential to uncontrolled, unlimited proliferation. This 'classical' mechanism is favoured in radiation protection research and related to low doses in tissue volumes distant from the therapeutic target. This is of particular importance for highly conformal radiotherapy techniques, such as multiple-field irradiation of IMRT, where the second tumour risk still has to be evaluated. As this classical mechanism of radiation-induction of second tumours may be counteracted by a reduction of the low-dose volume, a certain potential of proton radiotherapy – particularly in paediatric cancer – can be assumed to be explored.

A second, similarly important mechanism is related to consequential and chronic radiation sequelae after moderate to very high radiation doses in certain tissues, such as the rectum, bladder or skin. Atrophy as a hyper-proliferative disorder is a well-known precancerous lesion, in particular if associated with chronic inflammation. In the epidemiological studies on second cancers after radiotherapy for cervix and prostate cancer, about half of all radiation-induced second cancers are probably caused by this mechanism. In consequence, treatment optimisation which aims at reducing the risk of severe chronic radiation damage would also reduce the risk of second cancer on the basis of this mechanism.

We conclude that there are different mechanisms of radiation carcinogenesis after radiotherapy, each of which is critical at different dose levels, in different organs and in different age groups. It seems inconceivable that a single dose-volume risk relationship would be suitable to estimate the treatment-related cancer risk in all clinical situations.

The most critical organs in the low-dose volume with regard to radiation-induced second cancers are the breast of girls and young women, and lung and thyroid in both sexes. The dose-dependence of this risk has repeatedly been discussed. Based on the results of *in vitro* experiments determining malignant transformation in suitable cell models as well as some *in vivo* experiments in mice, a 'mechanistic' dose-response relationship has been proposed with a linear or linear-quadratic increase at doses <6–10 Gy (the induction mechanism) followed at higher doses by a decrease caused by the sterilisation of potential target cells (tissue-specific stem cells?). For a mixture of second cancers after radiotherapy for benign or malignant diseases, this has been demonstrated by Dörr and Herrmann (13,14). Schneider et al. (29,30) developed this concept further proposing the 'organ equivalent dose' – not to be confused with the organ dose equivalent in radiation protection – as a measure of second cancer risk. In this concept, cancer induction is assumed to be proportional to the number of cells in the tissue and the number of original cells is reduced by 'cell kill' as defined by the linear-quadratic cell-survival model (see Chapter 4), yet the number of killed original cells is (partially) reconstituted by proliferation ('repopulation') of surviving cells. By fitting this mathematical model to clinical data or epidemiological data from the atomic bomb survivors, parameters can be derived to describe the dose dependence of risk. However, it needs to be emphasized that these parameters have very large confidence intervals.

The 'mechanistic' model of radiation-induced second cancers, which is based on concepts of cellular radiobiology, may not (entirely) conform to the complexity of the various biological processes elicited by the very inhomogeneous dose distributions in radiotherapy patients, and the intra- and inter-tissue interaction of the associated events. Fundamental for this and other, comparable models is the assumption that risk increases to a maximum at a certain dose and then decreases with a further increase in dose (30). This hypothesis has been severely challenged by a case control meta-analysis performed by Berrington de Gonzalez et al. (4) who evaluated the dose-dependence data of the induction of 11 types of cancers from 28 studies with 3434 second cancer patients with individual dosimetric data. Overall, they concluded that there was little evidence that the dose-response curve was nonlinear in the direction of a downturn in risk at higher doses, not even at organ doses of over 60 Gy. Thyroid cancer was the only exception, with evidence of a decrease in risk at doses from 20 Gy. Also, Grantzau et al. (16) did not show a decrease of risk at local doses >20 Gy. Moreover, for all cancers, the calculated excess relative risk per gray from these studies of second malignancies after radiotherapy was 5–10 times lower than the risk of exposures of <2 Gy among the Japanese atomic bomb survivors.

Precise information on the shape of the dose-cancer induction relationship would be invaluable in the development of second cancer risk projection models for novel radiation therapy techniques with particular dose distributions, such as stereotactic radiotherapy and ion radiotherapy. However, such studies require precise information on the anatomical distributions of radiation doses within the critical organs (for cancer induction) of the individual patients as well as on the anatomical location of the respective, potentially radiation-induced second cancers. These are prerequisites in order to perform case control studies, which are the exclusive approach to generate sound information on which to base treatment plan optimisation algorithms.

Another critical issue arises from the frequent observation that most radiation-induced second cancers were found in the border region of the primary high-dose volume (e.g. [13]), where due to physical factors and organ motion, dose definition is notoriously difficult. Progress in this field is urgently required to base considerations on the reduction of second cancer risks on a sound scientific basis. A more pragmatic conclusion is that improved conformity of the PTV to the gross tumour volume might not only reduce late normal tissue complications but also the risk of this ('high' dose) mechanism of radiation-induction of second cancers, with, however, a price to pay in the form of an increase in the low-dose volume due to multiple beam directions. This is the basis for the current discussion on the possible benefits (as well as the potential risks) offered by radiotherapy using ion beams, e.g. protons in particular in paediatric radiotherapy.

A first report comparing second cancer rates in mostly adult (median age 59 years) patients treated with scattered protons at MGH Boston with expected second cancer rates based on data of individually matched patients from the SEER database was published by Chung et al. (6). Only 29 of 558 proton patients but 42 of 558 photon patients developed a second primary cancer after a median follow-up of 6–7 years. The reduction of second cancer rates was only seen in the first five years of follow-up which may indicate selection artefacts. The authors cautiously concluded that their findings suggested that the use of proton radiotherapy was not associated with a significantly increased risk of second malignancies compared with photon therapies, yet longer follow-up was needed to determine if there is a *decrease* in second malignancies from proton radiotherapy. In an editorial to this paper, Bekelman et al. (2) drew attention to several deficiencies in the MGH study, and argued that hypotheses about the relative benefits or harms of proton therapy remain two-sided; i.e. that proton therapy may be associated with increased as well as decreased rates of subsequent malignancies compared with photon therapy. The important question of whether proton therapy is associated with fewer or more second malignancies than photon therapy can be answered only with careful study design and the commitment of the international radiation oncology community. A European study has looked at the optimal design and the feasibility of such a prospective study, but concentrating on paediatric patients (26).

The only option for the radiation oncologist to reduce the risk of treatment-induced second cancer is the optimisation of the anatomical distribution of radiation doses in and out of the treated volumes. From the data presented here, it appears reasonable to consider both the 'high' dose volumes and the low dose volumes as important targets for optimisation of radiotherapy treatment planning, i.e. the reduction and best conformity of the dose distribution (irradiated volume) to the gross tumour volume (GTV) on the one hand and the reduction of exposure of large parts of the body from scatter and entrance and exit beams on the other hand. Protons appear particularly attractive since they offer realistic possibilities of achieving both aims. This is in clear contrast to photons, where approaching one of these aims in almost all instances is associated with a loss at the other. Therefore, protons have been advocated as the treatment of choice particularly for paediatric cancer patients. However, high-energy protons on interaction with matter produce a certain amount of neutrons which may be more carcinogenic, at a given absorbed dose, than photons and protons. There are no human cohorts in whom the relative biological effectiveness (RBE) could be directly determined, and various animal experiments gave widely differing RBE values ranging from less than 2 to more than 100 (37). The distribution of neutron doses in and out of the irradiated volumes differs significantly between the two different modalities of proton delivery, i.e. pencil beam scanning or passive modulation (17). Whereas the neutron doses in the high dose volumes are similar, the neutron doses at distant sites are much higher in treatment with passive modulation than with pencil scanning. The consequences of this fact for clinical practice are controversially discussed. The European project ANDANTE (1) investigated relevant problems such as neutron dose and energy spectrum distribution in clinical settings and the RBE of those particular neutron spectra and doses on the process of radiation carcinogenesis in humans. In conclusion, since out-of-field 'effective' neutron doses from proton therapy are smaller than the photon stray doses whichever (reasonable) RBE is chosen for comparison, and since the absolute risk of radiation-induced second cancer rates is in the order of 1% in the cohorts of adult patients who have been treated in the past with methods which caused relatively high out-of-field doses to large body volumes, it is highly unlikely that such patients treated in the future with highly conformal particle therapy are at a higher radiation-induced second cancer risk than those patients treated with photons with modern conformal techniques. However, any such statements on this topic must be considered premature, until results of dedicated studies become available.

## Key points

1. More than 90% of second cancers occurring after radiotherapy are the consequence of increased life expectancy due to cure from the first cancer.
2. In radical radiotherapy, the radiation exposure of non-involved organs and tissues may cause second cancers several decades later.
3. Increased cancer rates may persist lifelong.
4. The risk of radiation-induced second cancers is much smaller than the risk of recurrent primary cancer for the vast majority of tumour entities.
5. The risk of radiation-induced second cancers is much greater in young and very young cancer patients.
6. A considerable fraction of radiation-induced second cancers occur in organs and tissues in or close to the high-dose volume, but some also appear in the low-dose (<2 Gy) volume.
7. There are pronounced differences in the types of radiation-induced second cancers between children, young adults and adult patients treated with radiotherapy. Moreover, the types of second cancers after radiotherapy are different from those induced by low-dose total-body irradiation, e.g. in the Japanese atomic bomb survivors.
8. There are different biological mechanisms leading to second cancers after radiotherapy, depending on dose distribution, gender and age of the irradiated patient. The dose-risk relationship, therefore, is unlikely to follow a simple mathematical function.
9. The risk of radiation-induced second cancers from radiotherapy should *never* be estimated using the effective dose method proposed by ICRP for radiation protection purposes.

## ■ BIBLIOGRAPHY

1. ANDANTE. Final Report Summary – ANDANTE (Multidisciplinary evaluation of the cancer risk from neutrons relative to photons using stem cells and the induction of second malignant neoplasms following paediatric radiation therapy). 2016; http://cordis.europa.eu/result/rcn/182088_en.html
2. Bekelman JE, Schultheiss T, Berrington De Gonzalez A. Subsequent malignancies after photon versus proton radiation therapy. *Int J Radiat Oncol Biol Phys* 2013;87: 10–12.
3. Berrington de Gonzalez A, Curtis RE, Kry SF et al. Proportion of second cancers attributable to radiotherapy treatment in adults: A cohort study in the US SEER cancer registries. *Lancet Oncol* 2011;12:353–360.
4. Berrington de Gonzalez A, Gilbert E, Curtis R et al. Second solid cancers after radiation therapy: A systematic review of the epidemiologic studies of the radiation dose-response relationship. *Int J Radiat Oncol Biol Phys* 2013;86:224–233.
5. Brenner DJ, Curtis RE, Hall EJ, Ron E. Second malignancies in prostate carcinoma patients after radiotherapy compared with surgery. *Cancer* 2000;88:398–406.
6. Chung CS, Yock TI, Nelson K, Xu Y, Keating NL, Tarbell NJ. Incidence of second malignancies among patients treated with proton versus photon radiation. *Int J Radiat Oncol Biol Phys* 2013;87:46–52.
7. Constine LS, Tarbell N, Hudson MM et al. Subsequent malignancies in children treated for Hodgkin's disease: Associations with gender and radiation dose. *Int J Radiat Oncol Biol Phys* 2008;72:24–33.
8. Darby SC, McGale P, Taylor CW, Peto R. Long-term mortality from heart disease and lung cancer after radiotherapy for early breast cancer: Prospective cohort study of about 300,000 women in US SEER cancer registries. *Lancet Oncol* 2005;6:557–565.
9. de Vathaire F, Hawkins M, Campbell S et al. Second malignant neoplasms after a first cancer in childhood: Temporal pattern of risk according to type of treatment. *Br J Cancer* 1999;79:1884–1893.
10. Diallo I, Haddy N, Adjadj E et al. Frequency distribution of second solid cancer locations in relation to the irradiated volume among 115 patients treated for childhood cancer. *Int J Radiat Oncol Biol Phys* 2009;74:876–883.
11. Doll R, Peto R. The causes of cancer: Quantitative estimates of avoidable risks of cancer in the United States today. *J Natl Cancer Inst* 1981;66:1191–1308.
12. Dores GM, Metayer C, Curtis RE et al. Second malignant neoplasms among long-term survivors of Hodgkin's disease: A population-based evaluation over 25 years. *J Clin Oncol* 2002;20:3484–3494.
13. Dörr W, Herrmann T. Cancer induction by radiotherapy: Dose dependence and spatial relationship to irradiated volume. *J Radiol Prot* 2002;22:A117–A121.
14. Dörr W, Herrmann T. Second primary tumors after radiotherapy for malignancies. Treatment-related parameters. *Strahlenther Onkol* 2002;178:357–362.
15. Grantzau T, Mellemkjaer L, Overgaard J. Second primary cancers after adjuvant radiotherapy in early breast cancer patients: A national population based study under the Danish Breast Cancer Cooperative Group (DBCG). *Radiother Oncol* 2013;106:42–49.
16. Grantzau T, Thomsen MS, Vaeth M, Overgaard J. Risk of second primary lung cancer in women after radiotherapy for breast cancer. *Radiother Oncol* 2014;111:366–373.

17. Hall EJ. Intensity-modulated radiation therapy, protons, and the risk of second cancers. *Int J Radiat Oncol Biol Phys* 2006;65:1–7.

18. International Commission on Radiological Protection (ICRP). 1990 Recommendations of the International Commission on Radiological Protection. ICRP publication 60. *Ann ICRP* 1991;21:1–201.

19. International Commission on Radiological Protection (ICRP). The 2007 Recommendations of the International Commission on Radiological Protection. ICRP publication 103. *Ann ICRP* 2007;37:1–332.

20. Kaplan HS, Rosenberg SA. The management of Hodgkin's disease. *Cancer* 1975;36:796–803.

21. Kleinerman RA, Boice JD, Storm HH et al. Second primary cancer after treatment for cervical cancer. An international cancer registries study. *Cancer* 1995;76:442–452.

22. Mertens AC, Liu Q, Neglia JP et al. Cause-specific late mortality among 5-year survivors of childhood cancer: The Childhood Cancer Survivor Study. *J Natl Cancer Inst* 2008;100:1368–1379.

23. Neglia JP, Friedman DL, Yasui Y et al. Second malignant neoplasms in five-year survivors of childhood cancer: Childhood cancer survivor study. *J Natl Cancer Inst* 2001;93:618–629.

24. Neglia JP, Robison LL, Stovall M et al. New primary neoplasms of the central nervous system in survivors of childhood cancer: A report from the Childhood Cancer Survivor Study. *J Natl Cancer Inst* 2006;98:1528–1537.

25. Olsen JH, Moller T, Anderson H et al. Lifelong cancer incidence in 47,697 patients treated for childhood cancer in the Nordic countries. *J Natl Cancer Inst* 2009;101:806–813.

26. Ottolenghi A, Baiocco G, Smyth V, Trott K, Consortium A. The ANDANTE project: A multidisciplinary approach to neutron RBE. *Radiat Prot Dosimetry* 2015;166:311–315.

27. Preston DL, Cullings H, Suyama A et al. Solid cancer incidence in atomic bomb survivors exposed in utero or as young children. *J Natl Cancer Inst* 2008;100:428–436.

28. Schellong G, Riepenhausen M, Ehlert K, Brämswig J, Dörffel W; German Working Group on the Long-Term Sequelae of Hodgkin's Disease, Schmutzler RK, Rhiem K, Bick U, German Consortium for Hereditary Breast and Ovarian Cancer. Breast cancer in young women after treatment for Hodgkin's disease during childhood or adolescence – An observational study with up to 33-year follow-up. *Dtsch Arztebl Int* 2014;111:3–9.

29. Schneider U, Sumila M, Robotka J. Site-specific dose-response relationships for cancer induction from the combined Japanese A-bomb and Hodgkin cohorts for doses relevant to radiotherapy. *Theor Biol Med Model* 2011;8:27.

30. Schneider U, Zwahlen D, Ross D, Kaser-Hotz B. Estimation of radiation-induced cancer from three-dimensional dose distributions: Concept of organ equivalent dose. *Int J Radiat Oncol Biol Phys* 2005;61:1510–1515.

31. Stovall M, Smith SA, Langholz BM et al. Women's Environmental Cancer and Radiation Epidemiology Study Collaborative Group. Dose to the contralateral breast from radiotherapy and risk of second primary breast cancer in the WECARE study. *Int J Radiat Oncol Biol Phys* 2008;72:1021–1030.

32. Swerdlow AJ, Barber JA, Hudson GV et al. Risk of second malignancy after Hodgkin's disease in a collaborative British cohort: The relation to age at treatment. *J Clin Oncol* 2000;18:498–509.

33. Swerdlow AJ, van Leeuwen FE. Late effects after treatment for Hodgkin's lymphoma. In: Dembo AJ, Linch DC and Lowenberg B, editors. *Textbook of Malignant Hematology.* Abingdon: Taylor & Francis Group; 2005. pp. 758–768.

34. Travis LB, Andersson M, Gospodarowicz M et al. Treatment-associated leukemia following testicular cancer. *J Natl Cancer Inst* 2000;92:1165–1171.

35. Travis LB, Curtis RE, Storm H et al. Risk of second malignant neoplasms among long-term survivors of testicular cancer. *J Natl Cancer Inst* 1997;89:1429–1439.

36. Travis LB, Ng AK, Allan JM et al. Second malignant neoplasms and cardiovascular disease following radiotherapy. *J Natl Cancer Inst* 2012;104:357–370.

37. Trott KR. Special radiobiological features of second cancer risk after particle radiotherapy. *Physica Medica: Eup J Med Phys* 2017;42:221–227.

38. Tukenova M, Guibout C, Hawkins M et al. Radiation therapy and late mortality from second sarcoma, carcinoma, and hematological malignancies after a solid cancer in childhood. *Int J Radiat Oncol Biol Phys* 2011;80:339–346.

39. UNSCEAR. Annex A: Epidemiological studies of radiation and cancer. In: *Effects of Ionizing Radiation.* Vol 1. New York, NY: United Nations; 2006.

40. van Leeuwen FE, Travis LB. Second cancers. In: DeVita VT, Hellman S and Rosenberg SA, editors. *Cancer: Principles and Practice of Oncology.* 7th ed. Philadelphia, PA: Lippincott Williams and Wilkins; 2005. pp. 2575–2602.

41. Wolden SL, Lamborn KR, Cleary SF, Tate DJ, Donaldson SS. Second cancers following pediatric Hodgkin's disease. *J Clin Oncol* 1998;16:536–544.

42. Parkin DM, Whelan SL, Ferlay J, Teppo L, Thomas DB, Eds. Cancer Incidence in Five Continents. Volume VIII. *IARC Sci Publ* 2002;155:1–781.

## ■ FURTHER READING

43. Henderson TO, Whitton J, Stovall M et al. Secondary sarcomas in childhood cancer survivors: A report from the Childhood Cancer Survivor Study. *J Natl Cancer Inst* 2007;99:300–308.

44. Mody R, Li S, Dover DC et al. Twenty five year follow-up among survivors of childhood acute lymphoblastic leukemia: A report from the Childhood Cancer Survivor Study. *Blood* 2008;111:5515–5523.

45. Mudie NY, Swerdlow AJ, Higgins CD et al. Risk of second malignancy after non-Hodgkin's lymphoma: A British Cohort Study. *J Clin Oncol* 2006;24:1568–1574.

# Glossary

$\alpha/\beta$ **ratio** The ratio of the two parameters $\alpha$ and $\beta$ in the linear-quadratic model used to describe cell-survival curves *in vitro*. More widely used as a single parameter *in vivo*, the $\alpha/\beta$ value, to quantify the fractionation sensitivity of tissues. A lower $\alpha/\beta$ value describes a higher sensitivity to changes in dose per fraction.

**Abortive cell division** The limited number of divisions of cells that are radiation damaged ('doomed' cells). The residual proliferative capacity of these cells contributes significantly to overall cell production during the early radiation response in normal tissues.

**Accelerated fractionation** Intensification of radiation therapy by increasing the average rate of dose delivery, by delivering multiple fractions per day, or by increasing the number of treatment days per week; a schedule in which the average rate of dose delivery exceeds the equivalent of 10 Gy per week in 2 Gy fractions.

**Accelerated proliferation** Increase in the stem cell (clonogen) proliferation rate after radiation or cytotoxic chemotherapy relative to its pre-treatment value.

**Acute hypoxia** Low oxygen concentrations associated with changes in blood flow through vessels (e.g. by transient closing of blood vessels). Also called *transient* or *perfusion limited* hypoxia.

**Analogue** A chemical compound structurally similar to another but differing by a single functional group.

**Angiogenesis** The process of formation of new blood vessels.

**Anoxia** The complete absence of oxygen.

**Apoptosis** A mode of rapid cell death after irradiation characterized by chromatin condensation, fragmentation and compartmentalization, often visualized by densely staining nuclear globules. Sometimes postulated to be 'programmed' and therefore a potentially controllable process.

**ARCON therapy** The use of Accelerated Radiotherapy with CarbOgen and Nicotinamide.

**Asymmetrical divisions** Divisions of stem cells into, on average, one new stem cell and one transit or differentiating cell. These divisions are called asymmetrical, as two 'different' cells are generated.

**Asymmetry loss** Switch of stem cell divisions from an asymmetrical to a symmetrical pattern during radiation-induced repopulation in normal tissues.

**Atrophy** Reduction in parenchymal cell numbers in a tissue, caused by radiation-induced impairment of microvascular function. It is a major pathogenic mechanism leading to late normal tissue responses after radiotherapy.

**Autophagy** A process in which cellular components are self-digested through the lysosome pathway. This process can extend cell survival during starvation conditions and remove damaged organelles, but can also lead to cell death.

**Autoradiography** Use of a photographic emulsion to detect the distribution of a radioactive label in a tissue specimen.

**Bath-and-shower effect** Decreasing the tolerance to partial organ irradiation by exposure of the surrounding tissue volume to a low dose that by itself does not induce detectable changes in that larger volume.

**BER** Base excision repair. DNA repair pathway for repairing damage to DNA bases.

**Biologically effective dose (BED)** In fractionated radiotherapy, the total dose that would be required in very small dose fractions to produce a particular effect, as indicated by the linear-quadratic equation. Otherwise known as *extrapolated total dose* (ETD). BED values calculated for different $\alpha/\beta$ values are not directly comparable. For time-dose calculations, EQD2 (equivalent dose in 2 Gy fractions) is preferred (Section 10.2).

**BNCT** Boron neutron capture therapy.

**Brachytherapy** Radiotherapy using sealed radioactive sources placed next to a body surface, or inserted into a body cavity or through needles implanted into tissues.

**Bragg peak** Region of maximum dose deposition near the end of the tracks of protons, $\alpha$-particles and heavier ions.

**Cancer stem cell** A cell within a tumour that possesses the capacity to self-renew and to generate the heterogeneous lineages of cancer cells that comprise the tumour. In the context of cancer therapy, this definition translates into a cell which can cause a tumour recurrence.

**CDK** Cyclin-dependent kinase. These proteins are responsible for movement through the cell cycle and are inactivated by various mechanisms during the DNA damage response, to cause cell-cycle checkpoints.

**Cell-cycle checkpoint** Cellular control mechanism to verify whether each phase of the cell cycle has been accurately completed before progression to the next phase. An important function is to continually assess DNA damage detected by *sensors*.

**Cell-cycle time** The time between one mitosis and the next.

**Cell death** In the context of radiobiology, cell death is generally equated with any process that leads to the permanent loss of clonogenic capacity (unlimited proliferation).

**Cell loss factor** The rate of cell loss from a tumour, as a proportion of the rate at which cells are being added to the tumour by mitosis. Sometimes designated by the symbol $\phi$. Cell loss factor = 1 – Tpot/Td, where Tpot is the potential doubling time and Td is the cell population doubling time.

**CGH** Comparative genomic hybridization. A large-scale method to detect amplifications and deletions in different regions of the genome by comparison with a reference cell or tissue using microarray technology (arrayCGH).

**CHART** Continuous hyperfractionated accelerated radiation therapy. A schedule delivering 54 Gy in 36 fractions, with three fractions per day on 12 consecutive days (i.e. including a weekend).

**Chromatin** The complex of DNA and proteins comprising the chromosomes.

**Chromosomal instability** An effect of irradiation in which new stable and unstable chromosomal aberrations continue to appear through many cell generations.

**Chronic hypoxia** Persistent low oxygen concentrations such as those existing in viable tumour cells close to regions of necrosis. Also called *diffusion-limited* hypoxia since it arises at distances $\sim$150 $\mu$m from blood vessels. A more correct term would be *consumption-limited* hypoxia as it is the result of increasingly lower oxygen concentrations at a distance from a blood vessel due to consumption of oxygen.

**Clonogenic cells** Cells that have the capacity to produce an expanding family of descendents (usually at least 50). Also called 'colony-forming cells' or 'clonogens'. This term is often used *in vivo* when actually tumour stem cells would be the more appropriate term as they are functionally not the same.

**Clonogenic survival** Defined as the fraction of cells that survive following exposure or treatment to an agent that causes cell death. Only cells that are able to form colonies (clonogenic cells) are considered to have survived the treatment (see *Cell death*).

**Colony** The family of usually more than 50 cells derived from a single clonogenic cell.

**Complementation** Identification of whether a (e.g. radiosensitive) phenotype in different mutants is due to the same gene. Studied by means of cell fusion.

**Consequential late effects** Late normal tissue complications which are influenced by the extent, i.e. severity and/or duration, of the *early* response in the same tissue or organ.

**DDR** The DNA damage response. A network of biological responses to DNA damage.

**Direct action** Ionization or excitation of atoms within DNA leading to free radicals, as distinct from the reaction with DNA of free radicals formed in nearby water molecules.

**$D_0$** A parameter in the multitarget equation: the radiation dose that reduces survival to $\exp(-1)$ (i.e. $\sim$0.37) of its previous value on the exponential portion of the cell survival curve.

**Dose modifying factor (DMF)** When a chemical or other agent acts as if to change the dose of radiation, DMF indicates the ratio: dose without/dose with the agent for the same level of a particular effect.

**Dose-rate effect** Increase in isoeffective radiation dose with decreasing radiation dose rate.

**Dose-reduction factor (DRF)** Term which has been used with different meanings, depending on context. For example, in low-dose rate studies, has been used to indicate the percentage or fraction reduction in dose to achieve the same effect, if the dose rate is raised (gives DRF values <1). Alternatively, has been used in studies of radioprotection as the ratio: dose with/dose without the protecting agent for the same level of effect (gives DRF values >1).

**DVH (dose volume histogram)** A histogram displaying the amount of a particular structure that receives a given dose. The cumulative form of the DVH, sometimes called the 'cDVH', is almost universally used in radiotherapy. It represents the volume of a structure that receives greater than or equal to a given dose, plotted as a function of dose. See Figure 7.2.

**Double trouble** A hot spot within a treated volume that receives not only a higher dose but also a higher dose per fraction, which means that the biological effectiveness per unit dose is also greater.

**Doubling time** Time for a cell population or tumour volume to double its size.

**Early endpoint** Clinical manifestation of an early normal tissue response to radiation therapy.

**Early normal tissue responses** Radiation-induced normal-tissue damage that is expressed in weeks to a few months after the onset of exposure (per definition within 90 days after onset of radiotherapy). $\alpha/\beta$ value tends to be large (>6 Gy).

**ED50** Radiation dose that is estimated to produce a specified (normal tissue) effect in 50% of subjects irradiated ('effective-dose-50%').

**Effective dose** The concept of effective dose has been introduced by the International Commission on Radiation Protection specifically to set dose limits for radiation workers and the general population. The effective dose is calculated by multiplying the dose equivalent (which is the mean organ dose multiplied by a radiation quality factor which accounts for the different effectiveness of different radiation qualities), by the respective organ/tissue weighting factor attributed to various critical organs by ICRP. This concept should not be used to describe normal tissue damage and cancer risk after radiotherapy or in medical radiology.

**Effectors** Proteins with the specific task of effecting (carrying out) the response to damage, e.g. apoptosis, cell cycle arrest or DNA repair.

**Elkind repair** Recovery of the 'shoulder' on a radiation dose cell-survival curve when irradiation follows several hours after a priming dose.

**EQD2** Equivalent total dose in 2 Gy fractions. Note that the EQD2$\alpha/\beta$ depends on the endpoint considered, related to the $\alpha/\beta$ value for this endpoint.

**EQD2$_T$** Equivalent dose in 2 Gy fractions but adjusted for a possible difference in overall treatment time by using a reference overall time, $T$.

**EUD** Equivalent uniform dose. Conversion of a non-uniform dose distribution within an organ to a uniform dose, which would result in the same biological effect. This is a model-dependent quantity which has been proposed for second cancer risk estimations.

**Exponential growth** Growth according to an exponential equation: $V = V_0 \exp(kt)$. The volume or population doubling time is constant and equal to $(\log_e 2)/k$.

**Extrapolated total dose (ETD)** Calculated isoeffective dose, at an infinitely low dose rate or fraction size (see *Biologically effective dose*).

**Extrapolation number** A parameter in the multitarget equation for cell survival versus dose: the point on the surviving fraction axis to which the straight part of the curve back-extrapolates.

**Field-size effect** The dependence of normal tissue damage on the size of the irradiated area (particularly in skin); in modern literature typically referred to as the 'volume effect'.

**FISH** Fluorescence *in situ* hybridization. Fluorescent dyes are attached to specific regions of the genome, thus aiding the identification of chromosomal damage.

**Flow cytometry** Analysis of cell suspensions in which a dilute stream of cells is passed through a laser beam. DNA content and other properties are measured by light scattering and fluorescence following staining with dyes or labelled antibodies.

**Fractionation sensitivity** The dependence of the isoeffective radiation dose for a particular biological endpoint on the dose per fraction. Usually quantified by the $\alpha/\beta$ value – a high fractionation sensitivity is characterized by a low $\alpha/\beta$ value (see $\alpha/\beta$ *ratio or value*).

**Free radical** A fragment of a molecule containing an unpaired electron, therefore very reactive.

**Functional imaging** Imaging methods aimed at detecting physiological changes, for example metabolism or blood flow, in a tissue (in contrast to structural, morphological or anatomical imaging). Examples are glucose metabolism (detected by [18]F-labelled FDG-PET) or oxygen consumption (blood oxygen level dependency [BOLD] MRI), or vascular function detected by dynamic contrast enhanced (DCE) CT. (See *Molecular imaging*).

**Functional sub-unit (FSU)** A concept of a (minimal) functional tissue structure (such as the alveolus in the lung). Their radiation-induced inactivation results in the reduced tissue function responses that can be seen after radiotherapy. Alternatively called tissue rescuing unit (TRU).

**Genomic or genetic instability** The failure to pass an accurate copy of the whole genome from a cell to its daughter cells, for example seen after irradiation.

**Genomics** Study of selected genes or the entire genome of the cell (DNA level).

**Gray (Gy)** 1 Gy is the SI unit equivalent to 1 joule of energy per 1 kg of mass. The gray is most commonly used to refer to absorbed radiation dose and has replaced the previous unit, the rad (1 Gy = 100 rad).

**Gray equivalents (GyE) or Cobalt gray equivalents (CGE)** GyE or CGE for densely ionizing radiation is equal to the measured physical dose in gray multiplied by the RBE factor. This is not an SI unit.

**Growth delay** Extra time required for an irradiated versus an unirradiated tumour to reach a given size.

**Growth fraction** The proportion of cells in a population that are actively cycling.

**Hierarchical tissues** Tissues comprising a lineage of stem cells, transit cells and postmitotic (differentiating or mature) cells.

**HR** Homologous recombination. DNA repair pathway for double-strand DNA breaks by using an undamaged homologous (identical) DNA sequence, usually from the sister chromatid.

**Hyperbaric oxygen (HBO)** The use of high oxygen pressures (2–3 atmospheres) to enhance oxygen availability in radiotherapy.

**Hyperfractionation** The use of dose fractions typically smaller than 1.8 Gy.

**Hyperthermia** The heating of tumours above normal physiological temperatures, to treat cancer.

**Hypofractionation** The use of dose fractions typically larger than 2.2 Gy.

**Hypoplasia** Reduction in cell numbers in a tissue, e.g. due to radiation-induced impairment of proliferation leading to early tissue responses.

**Hypoxia** Low oxygen tension; usually refers to the very low levels that are required to make cells maximally radioresistant.

**Hypoxic cell cytotoxins** Any agents, typically bioreductive drugs, that preferentially kill hypoxic cells.

**Hypoxic fraction** The fraction of hypoxic cells within a tumour. This term is used in different contexts. Historically, it refers to the fraction of viable radioresistant hypoxic cells in a tumour. More recently it has been used to represent the frequency of oxygen measurements below some arbitrary threshold of oxygen tension (e.g. 5 mm Hg).

**Image segmentation** The process of separating out mutually exclusive (i.e. non-overlapping) regions of interest in an image, for example outlining the lungs on a computed tomography scan.

**IMRT** Intensity-modulated radiation therapy. Irradiation technique using non-uniform radiation beam intensities for delivering radiation therapy. This allows high conformality treatment plans often with considerable sparing of critical organs at risk. Sometimes a distinction is made between IMXT (intensity modulated X-ray therapy) and IMPT (intensity modulated proton therapy).

**Incomplete repair** Incomplete recovery of radiation damage between fractions in fractionated radiotherapy, resulting in increased radiation effects.

**Indirect action** Damage to DNA by free radicals formed through the ionization of nearby water molecules.

**Initial slope** The steepness of the initial part of the cell survival curve, usually indicated by the value of $\alpha$ in the linear-quadratic model.

**Interphase death** The death of irradiated cells before they reach mitosis. Sometimes used as a synonym for apoptosis.

**Ionization** The process of removing electrons from (or adding electrons to) atoms or molecules, thereby creating ions.

**IRIF** Ionizing radiation induced foci. Used to describe the accumulation of DNA damage-response proteins that localize to sites of DNA damage after irradiation.

**Isoeffect plots** Graphs of the total dose for a given effect (e.g. ED50) plotted, for instance, against dose per fraction or dose rate.

**Labelling index** Proportion or percentage of cells positive for a certain signal, e.g. fraction of cells within the S-phase labelled by $^3$H-thymidine or other nucleotide analogues such as bromodeoxyuridine.

**Late endpoints** Clinical expression of late normal tissue responses.

**Late normal tissue responses** Radiation-induced normal tissue damage that in humans is expressed months to years after exposure (per definition later than 90 days after the onset of radiotherapy). $\alpha/\beta$ value tends to be small (<5 Gy).

**Latent time/period or latency interval** Time between (onset of) irradiation and clinical manifestation of a particular radiation effect/endpoint.

**LD50/30** Radiation dose to produce lethality in 50% of a population of individuals within 30 days; similarly LD50/7, etc.

**Linear energy transfer (LET)** The rate of energy loss along the track of an ionizing particle. Usually expressed in keV $\mu m^{-1}$.

**Linear-quadratic (LQ) model** Model in which the effect ($E$) is a linear-quadratic function of dose ($d$): $E = \alpha d + \beta d^2$. For cell survival: $S = \exp(-\alpha d - \beta d^2)$.

**Local tumour control** The complete regression of a tumour without later regrowth during follow-up; this requires that all cancer stem cells have been permanently inactivated.

**Log-phase culture** A cell culture growing exponentially.

**Mean inactivation dose ($D_{bar}$ or $\overline{D}$)** An estimate of the average radiation dose required to inactivate a cell. It is calculated as the area under the survival curve, plotted on linear coordinates.

**Microarray** An array of DNA spots of known sequence, usually on a glass slide, used to quantify amounts of genomic DNA or cDNA (made from mRNA) in cells or tissue. Can hold up to 50,000 spots, capable of monitoring expression of all known genes and their variants. Also referred to as gene expression microarrays or 'chips'.

**miRNA** Micro RNA. Small 19–22 nucleotide single-stranded non-coding RNAs expressed in cells which can regulate expression of genes by interacting with mRNAs.

**Mitigation** Interventions to reduce the severity or risk of radiation side effects, applied during or shortly after exposure and before clinically manifest symptoms occur (i.e. during the latent time).

**Mitotic catastrophe** Improper completion of cell division due to unrepaired or misrepaired DNA damage. Mitotic catastrophe occurs frequently after irradiation and is a major cause of cell death.

**Mitotic delay** Delay of entry into mitosis, resulting in an accumulation of cells in G2, as a result of treatment.

**Mitotic index** Proportion or percentage of cells in mitosis at any given time.

**MMR** Mismatch repair. DNA repair pathway for repairing mismatched bases in DNA, usually occurring through mis-incorporation by DNA polymerases.

**Molecular imaging** (Medical) imaging visualizing the spatial distribution of molecular targets, signalling pathways or cellular phenotypes. This is in contrast to traditional structural or anatomical imaging. Examples could be positron emission tomography or single photon emission computed tomography with an appropriately labelled tracer, magnetic resonance spectroscopy or optical imaging (see *Functional imaging*).

**Molecular targeted drugs** See *Targeted agents*.

**Multi-target equation** Model which assumes the presence of a number of critical targets in a cell, all of which require inactivation to kill the cell. Surviving fraction of a cell population is given by the formula $1 - [1 - \exp(D/D_0)]^n$.

**Necrosis** A form of cell injury which results in the premature death of cells in living tissue by autolysis. Necrosis is caused by factors external to the cell or tissue, such as irradiation, which result in the unregulated digestion of cellular components.

**NER** Nucleotide excision repair. DNA repair pathway for repairing bulky DNA lesions such as thymine dimers or cisplatin adducts.

**NHEJ** Non-homologous end joining. DNA repair pathway for repairing double-strand DNA breaks without using any homologous sequence as template.

**Non-stochastic effect** This term has been introduced by the International Commission on Radiation Protection specifically to protect workers from health effects for which a dose threshold could be identified. This term should not be used to describe normal tissue damage in radiotherapy.

**NTCP** Normal-tissue complication probability. Generally a term used in modelling normal tissue radiation response.

**Oxygen enhancement ratio (OER)** The ratio of dose given under anoxic conditions to the dose resulting in the same effect when given under some defined level of oxygen tension. If oxygen tensions >21% are used, the OER measured is usually termed the 'Full OER'. An OER of about half the full OER is usually obtained when the oxygen tension is between 0.5% and 1%.

**PET** Positron emission tomography.

**Plateau-phase cultures** Cell cultures grown to confluence so that proliferation is markedly reduced (also known as 'stationary phase').

**Plating efficiency (PE)** The proportion or percentage of *in vitro* plated cells that form colonies.

**Potential doubling time (Tpot)** The (theoretical) cell population doubling time in the assumed absence of cell loss. It is determined as the inverse of the cell production rate usually calculated from the labelling index and the duration of the S-phase of the cell cycle.

**Potentially lethal damage (PLD) repair** Operational term to describe an increase in cell survival that may occur during an interval between treatment and assay, caused by post-irradiation modification of cellular physiology or environment (e.g. sub-optimal growth conditions).

**Prodromal phase** Signs and symptoms in the first 48 hours following irradiation as a part of the response to partial or total-body irradiation ('radiation sickness').

**Programmed cell death** Cell death that occurs as the result of an active process carried out by molecules in the cell. Examples include apoptosis, autophagy, senescence and in some cases even necrosis.

**Proteomics** Study of the proteins expressed in cells, including structure and function.

**Quasi-threshold dose ($D_q$)** Point of extrapolation of the exponential portion of a multi-target survival curve to the level of zero clonogenic cell inactivation rate: $D_q = D_0 \ln(n)$.

**Radiation modifier** A substance (e.g. drug or gas) which in itself does not evoke an effect on cells or tissues, but which changes the effect of radiation.

**Radioresponsiveness** The clinical responsiveness to a course of radiation therapy, e.g. tumour shrinkage or improvement of signs and symptoms caused by the tumour such as pain. This depends on multiple factors, one of them hypothesized to be cellular radiosensitivity.

**Radiosensitivity, cellular** The sensitivity of cells to ionizing radiation *in vitro*. Usually indicated by the surviving fraction at 2 Gy (i.e. SF2) or by the parameters of the linear-quadratic or multi-target equations.

**Radiosensitizer** In general, any agent that increases the sensitivity of cells to radiation. Commonly applied to electron-affinic chemicals that mimic oxygen in fixing free-radical damage, although these should more correctly be referred to as *hypoxic cell sensitizers*.

**Reassortment or Redistribution** Return towards a more even cell-age distribution, following the selective killing of cells in certain phases of the cell cycle.

**Recovery** *At the cellular level*, an increase in cell survival as a function of time between dose fractions or during irradiation with low dose rates (see *Repair*). *At the tissue level*, an increase in isoeffective total dose with a decrease in dose per fraction or for irradiation at low dose rates.

**Regression rate** The rate at which the tumour volume shrinks during or after treatment.

**Relative biological effectiveness (RBE)** Ratio of dose of a reference radiation quality (usually $^{60}$Co γ-rays or 250 keV X-rays) and dose of a test radiation quality (e.g. protons or other particles) that produce an equal effect.

**Reoxygenation** The processes by which surviving hypoxic tumour stem cells become better oxygenated during the period after irradiation of a tumour.

**Repair** Restoration of the integrity of damaged macromolecules (see *Recovery*).

**Repair saturation** A proposed explanation of the shoulder on cell survival curves on the basis of the reduced effectiveness of repair after high radiation doses.

**Repopulation** Describes the increase of the number of surviving tumour stem cells during fractionated radiotherapy. Rapid repopulation of tumour stem cells during therapy is an important factor in treatment resistance. Also describes the regeneration response of early reactions (hypoplasia) of tissues to fractionated irradiation, which results in an increase in radiation tolerance with increasing overall treatment time.

**Reproductive integrity** Ability of cells to divide many times *in vitro* and thus be 'clonogenic'. *In vivo* it is the defining feature of stem cells.

**Senescence** A permanent arrest of cell division associated with differentiation, aging or cellular damage.

**Sensitizer enhancement ratio (SER)** The same as *Dose modifying factor* (DMF), but typically used to describe radiosensitizing agents so that SER >1.

**Sensors** Proteins with the specific task of sensing damage to DNA.

**SF2** Surviving fraction of cells following a dose of 2 Gy.

**Sievert (Sv)** The dose unit term *sievert* has been introduced by the International Commission on Radiation Protection specifically to calculate the effective dose which is used to protect workers from 'stochastic' health effects and to set dose limits for radiation workers and the general population. This term should not be used to describe normal tissue damage in radiotherapy.

**SNP** Single nucleotide polymorphism. Variations in DNA sequence between individuals at a single nucleotide that is the major source of genetic variation. Can affect protein function and expression, and thus response to damage.

**Spatial cooperation** The use of radiotherapy and chemotherapy to hit disease in different anatomical sites.

**Spheroid**  Clump of cells grown together in tissue-culture suspension.

**Split-dose recovery**  Decrease in radiation effect when a single radiation dose is split into fractions separated by times up to a few hours (also termed *Elkind recovery*, or recovery from sublethal damage).

**SSBR**  Single-strand break repair. DNA repair pathway for repairing a break occurring in only one of the two DNA strands.

**Stathmokinetic method**  Study of cell proliferation using agents that block cells in mitosis.

**Stem cells**  Cells with an unlimited proliferative capacity, capable of self-renewal and of differentiation to produce all the various types of cells in a lineage.

**Stochastic (non-deterministic) effect**  The term *stochastic effect* has been introduced by the International Commission on Radiation Protection specifically to protect workers from health effects for which no dose threshold could be identified, in particular radiation-induced cancer and genetic radiation effects to set dose limits for radiation workers and the general population. This term should not be used to describe normal tissue damage in radiotherapy.

**Sublethal damage (SLD)**  Non-lethal cellular injury that can be repaired. Interaction between SLD in a cell, can result in cytolethality. This process is described in the linear-quadratic model by the quadratic beta term.

**Supra-additivity or synergism**  A biological effect due to a combination that is greater than would be expected from the addition of the effects of the component agents.

**Symmetrical division**  Division of each stem cell into two stem cell daughters, occurring, e.g. during radiation-induced repopulation in normal tissues.

**Target cell**  A cell whose response to radiation is responsible for the clinical manifestation of a radiation response, e.g. in a normal tissue or tumour.

**Targeted agents**  Small molecules or antibodies that inhibit cellular pathways that are specific to cancer cells or substantially over-expressed in malignant cells compared with normal cells.

**Targeted radiotherapy**  Treatment of cancer by means of drugs that localise in tumours and carry therapeutic amounts of radioactivity.

**Target theory**  The idea that the shoulder on cell survival curves is due to the number of unrepaired lesions per cell.

**TBI**  Total-body irradiation.

**TCD50**  The radiation dose that gives a 50% tumour control probability.

**TCP**  Tumour control probability. Generally a term used in modelling tumour radiation response.

**Telangiectasia**  Pathologically dilated capillaries, observed in all irradiated tissues and organs in association with late radiation effects, e.g. atrophy.

**Theragnostics**  Use of molecular imaging to assist in prescribing the distribution of radiation dose in four dimensions, i.e. the three spatial dimensions plus time.

**Therapeutic index or ratio**  Denotes the relationship between the probability for tumour cure and the likelihood for normal tissue damage. An improved therapeutic ratio represents a more favourable ratio of efficacy to toxicity.

**Time-dose relationships**  The dependence of isoeffective radiation dose on the overall treatment time and number of fractions (or fraction size) in radiotherapy.

**Time factor**  Describes the change in isoeffective total dose for local tumour control or normal tissue complications that follows a change in the overall treatment duration.

**Tolerance dose**  The maximum radiation dose or intensity of fractionated radiotherapy that is associated with an acceptable probability of developing clinically relevant signs and symptoms of late normal tissue damage. (The actual frequency depends critically on the chosen severity, usually a rate of 1%–5% of patients with moderate to severe late normal tissue damage is being reported.) Values also depend on treatment protocol, irradiated volume, concomitant therapies, etc., but also on the clinical or health status of the organ/patient.

**Transcriptomics**  Study of genes which are expressed in cells at the RNA level.

**Transient hypoxia**  Low oxygen concentrations associated with the transient closing of blood vessels. Also called *acute* or *perfusion limited* hypoxia.

**Tumour bed effect (TBE)**  Slower rate of tumour re-growth after irradiation due to radiation injury to the vascular-connective tissue and reduced angiogenesis in the irradiated 'vascular bed'.

**Tumour cord**  Sleeve of viable tumour growing around a blood capillary.

**Vascular targeted therapies**  Treatments designed to specifically target tumour vasculature; includes angiogenesis inhibitors and vascular-disrupting agents.

**Vasculogenesis**  The process of blood vessel formation occurring by *de novo* production of endothelial cells from circulating cells. It is distinguished from angiogenesis in that the blood vessels are not formed by sprouting of endothelial cells from existing adjacent blood vessels, and is probably an important contributor to the reconstitution of tumour blood vessels after radiation therapy.

**Volume doubling time**  Time for a tumour to double in volume.

**Volume effect**  Dependence of radiation damage (a certain morbidity endpoint) on the volume of tissue irradiated and the anatomical distribution of radiation dose to an organ.

**Xenografts**  Transplants between species; usually applied to the transplantation of human tumours into immune-deficient mice and rats.

# Index